nal

Optum

HCPCS Level II

A resourceful compilation of HCPCS codes

Supports HIPAA compliance

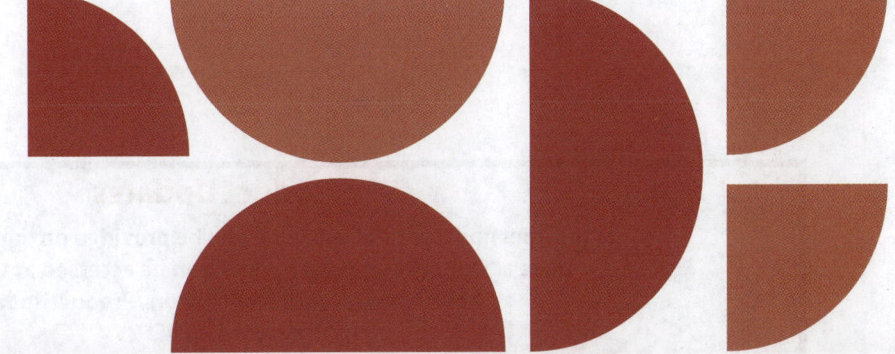

2025

optumcoding.com

Publisher's Notice

The Optum *2025 HCPCS Level II* is designed to be an accurate and authoritative source of information about this government coding system. Every effort has been made to verify the accuracy of the listings, and all information is believed reliable at the time of publication. Absolute accuracy cannot be guaranteed, however. This publication is made available with the understanding that the publisher is not engaged in rendering legal or other services that require a professional license.

Our Commitment to Accuracy

Optum is committed to producing accurate and reliable materials.

To report corrections, please email customerassistance@optum.com. You can also reach customer service by calling 1.800.464.3649, option 1.

To view Optum updates/correction notices, please visit http://www.optumcoding.com/ProductUpdates/

Copyright

Made in the USA

HB 978-1-62254-963-4

Acknowledgments

Marianne Randall, CPC, *Senior Product Manager*

Stacy Perry, *Manager, Desktop Publishing*

Elizabeth Leibold, RHIT, *Subject Matter Expert*

Tara Rose, CPC, CPC-I, CPMA, RHIA, CCS-P, *Subject Matter Expert*

Tracy Betzler, *Senior Desktop Publishing Specialist*

Hope M. Dunn, *Senior Desktop Publishing Specialist*

Katie Russell, *Desktop Publishing Specialist*

Lynn Speirs, *Editor*

Subject Matter Experts

Elizabeth Leibold, RHIT

Ms. Leibold has more than 30 years of experience in the health care profession. She has served in a variety of roles, ranging from patient registration to billing and collections, and has an extensive background in both physician and hospital outpatient coding and compliance. She has worked for large health care systems and health information management services companies, and has wide-ranging experience in facility and professional component coding, along with CPT expertise in interventional procedures, infusion services, emergency department, observation, and ambulatory surgery coding. Her areas of expertise include chart-to-claim coding audits and providing staff education to both tenured and new coding staff. She is an active member of the American Health Information Management Association (AHIMA) and Tennessee Health Information Management Association (THIMA).

Tara Rose, CPC, CPC-I, CPMA, RHIA, CCS-P

Ms. Rose has more than 15 years of experience in the health care profession. She has extensive experience in auditing, physician billing, and multi-specialty coding with assignment of CPT, HCPCS, and ICD-10-CM codes. She has served in roles as a coding consultant, trainer, clinical investigator, community college instructor, and coding lead. She has experience providing education to physicians and both new and experienced coders. Ms. Rose is a member of her local AAPC chapter and holds credentials from the American Health Information Management Association (AHIMA).

Product Updates

Significant updates to this manual will be provided on our product updates page at Optumcoding.com, which can be accessed at the following:
https://www.optumcoding.com/ProductUpdates/
Password: LEVEL25

Contents

Introduction

Note: All data current as of November 15, 2024.

HCPCS Level II codes, except for the dental code series, are developed and maintained by a joint editorial panel consisting of the Centers for Medicare and Medicaid Services (CMS), the Blue Cross Blue Shield Association, and the Health Insurance Association of America. HCPCS Level II codes may be used throughout the United States in all Medicare regions. They consist of one alpha character (A through V) followed by four digits. Optum does not change the code descriptions other than correcting typographical errors. There are some codes that appear to be duplicates. CMS has indicated that each of the codes is used to report a specific condition or service. At press time, CMS had not provided further clarification regarding these codes. Additional information may be found on the CMS website, https://www.cms.gov/medicare/coding-billing/healthcare-common-procedure-system.

Any supplier or manufacturer can submit a request for coding modification to the HCPCS Level II National codes. A document explaining the HCPCS modification process, as well as a detailed format for submitting a recommendation for a modification to HCPCS Level II codes, is available on the HCPCS website at https://www.cms.gov/medicare/coding-billing/healthcare-common-procedure-system. Besides the information requested in this format, a requestor should also submit any additional descriptive material, including the manufacturer's product literature and information that is believed would be helpful in furthering CMS's understanding of the medical features of the item for which a coding modification is being recommended. The HCPCS coding review process is an ongoing, continuous process.

The dental (D) codes are not included in the official 2025 HCPCS Level II code set. The American Dental Association (ADA) holds the copyright on those codes and instructed CMS to remove them. As a result, Optum has removed them from this product; however, Optum has additional resources available for customers requiring the dental codes. Please visit www.optumcoding.com or call 1.800.464.3649.

Significant updates to this manual will be provided on our product updates page at Optumcoding.com, which can be accessed at the following: https://www.optumcoding.com/ProductUpdates/. Password: LEVEL25

Getting Started with *HCPCS Level II Professional*

Coders should keep in mind that the insurance companies and government do not base payment solely on what was done for the patient. They need to know why the services were performed. In addition to using the HCPCS coding system for procedures and supplies, coders must also use the ICD-10-CM coding system to denote the diagnosis. This book will not discuss ICD-10-CM codes, which can be found in a current ICD-10-CM code book for diagnosis codes. To locate a HCPCS Level II code, follow these steps:

1. Identify the services or procedures that the patient received.

   Example:

   Patient administered PSA exam.

2. Look up the appropriate term in the index.

   Example:

   Screening

   prostate specific antigen test (PSA)

   Coding Tip: Coders who are unable to find the procedure or service in the index can look in the table of contents for the type of procedure or device to narrow the code choices. Also, coders should remember to check the unlisted procedure guidelines for additional choices.

3. Assign a tentative code.

   Example:

   Code G0103

   Coding Tip: To the right of the terminology, there may be a single code or multiple codes, a cross-reference, or an indication that the code has been deleted. Tentatively assign all codes listed.

4. Locate the code or codes in the appropriate section. When multiple codes are listed in the index, be sure to read the narrative of all codes listed to find the appropriate code based on the service performed.

   Example:

G0103	**Prostate cancer screening; prostate specific antigen test (PSA)**

5. Check for color bars, symbols, notes, and references.

G0103	**Prostate cancer screening; prostate specific antigen test (PSA)**	A

6. Review the appendixes for the reference definitions and other guidelines for coverage issues that apply.
7. Determine whether any modifiers should be appended.
8. Assign the code.

   Example:

   The code assigned is G0103.

Coding Standards

Levels of Use

Coders may find that the same procedure is coded at two or even three levels. Which code is correct? There are certain rules to follow if this should occur.

When both a CPT and a HCPCS Level II code have virtually identical narratives for a procedure or service, the CPT code should be used. If, however, the narratives are not identical (e.g., the CPT code narrative is generic, whereas the HCPCS Level II code is specific), the Level II code should be used.

Be sure to check for a national code when a CPT code description contains an instruction to include additional information, such as describing a specific medication or supply. There are many HCPCS Level II codes that specify supplies in more detail.

Special Reports

Submit a special report with the claim when a new, unusual, or variable procedure is provided or a modifier is used. Include the following information:

- A copy of the appropriate report (e.g., operative, x-ray), explaining the nature, extent, and need for the procedure
- Documentation of the medical necessity of the procedure
- Documentation of the time and effort necessary to perform the procedure

Organization of Optum *HCPCS Level II Professional*

The Optum 2025 *HCPCS Level II* contains mandated changes and new codes for use as of January 1, 2025. Deleted codes have also been indicated and cross-referenced to active codes when possible. New codes have been added to the appropriate sections, eliminating the time-consuming step of looking in two places for a code. However, keep in mind that the information in this book is a reproduction of the 2025 HCPCS; additional information on coverage issues may have been provided to Medicare contractors after publication. All contractors periodically update their systems and records throughout the year. If this book does not agree with your contractor, it is either because of a mid-year update or correction, or a specific local or regional coverage policy.

HCPCS Code Index

Because HCPCS is organized by code number rather than by service or supply name, the index enables the coder to locate any code without looking through individual ranges of codes. Just look up the medical or surgical supply, service, orthotic, or prosthetic in question to find the appropriate codes. This index also refers to many of the brand names by which these items are known.

Brand Name Drugs

Brand name drugs commonly reported with a code are listed underneath the code descriptor in blue font. This note will not appear if the brand name is part of the code descriptor.

Unlisted/Not Otherwise Classified (NOC)

CMS does not use consistent terminology when a code for a specific procedure is not listed. The code description may include any of the following terms: unlisted, not otherwise classified (NOC), unspecified, unclassified, other, and miscellaneous. If unsure there is no code for the service or supply provided or used, provide adequate documentation to the payer. Check with the payer for more information.

Icons

Codes in the Optum *HCPCS Level II Professional* follow the AMA CPT book conventions to indicate new, revised, and deleted codes.

● **New Codes**
Codes that have been added since the previous edition of the Optum HCPCS Level II book was printed.

▲ **Revised Codes**
Codes that have been revised since the previous edition of the Optum HCPCS Level II book was printed.

❍ **Recycled/Reinstated Codes**
Codes that have been recycled/reinstated since the previous edition of the Optum HCPCS Level II book was printed.

Strikethrough
Codes deleted from the current active codes appear with a strikethrough.

~~C9170 Injection, tarlatamab-dlle, 1 mg~~

Green Color Bar—Special Coverage Instructions
This color bar indicates special coverage instructions apply to these services and procedures. Medicare Internet-only Manuals (IOMs) reference numbers are typically provided to locate the specific instructions.

Pink Color Bar—Not Covered by or Invalid for Medicare
This color bar identifies services and procedures that are never covered benefits under Medicare. Medicare Internet-only Manuals (IOMs) reference numbers are typically provided to locate the specific instructions.

Yellow Color Bar—Carrier Discretion
This color bar indicates coverage for these services and procedures is left to "carrier discretion."

A **Age Edit**
This icon denotes codes intended for use with a specific age group, such as neonate, newborn, pediatric, and adult. This edit is based on age specifications in the HCPCS code descriptors, the product/service represented by the code may have age restrictions, and/or updates from the Integrated Outpatient Code Editor (I/OCE). Carefully review the code description to ensure the code you report most appropriately reflects the patient's age.

AHA: American Hospital Association *Coding Clinic® for HCPCS* citations assist users in finding expanded information about specific codes and their usage. This includes citations for the current year and the preceding five years.

CMS: The notation indicates that there is a specific CMS guideline pertaining to this code in the CMS Online Manual System which includes the Internet-only Manual (IOM). These CMS sources present the rules for submitting these services to the federal government or its contractors and a link to the IOMs is included in appendix 4 of this book.

♿ **DMEPOS**
Use this icon to identify when to consult the CMS durable medical equipment, prosthetics, orthotics, and supplies (DMEPOS) for payment of this durable medical item. For modifiers NU, RR, and UE: These modifiers are for use when DME equipment is either new, used, or rented. The RR modifiers must also be used in conjunction with rental modifiers KH, KI, or KJ.

♀ **Female Only**

♂ **Male Only**
Effective April 1, 2024, CMS has discontinued the logic for sex restricting editing. The Female Only and Male Only icons have been removed from the HCPCS Level II Expert book. For additional information, refer to the I/OCE Quarterly Data Files V251.R0 at https://www.cms.gov/medicare/coding-billing/outpatient-code-editor-oce/quarterly-release-files.

M **Maternity**
This icon identifies procedures that by definition should be used only for maternity patients generally between 9 and 64 years of age based on CMS I/OCE designations.

☑ **Quantity Alert**
Many codes in HCPCS report quantities that may not coincide with quantities available in the marketplace. For instance, a HCPCS code for an ostomy pouch with skin barrier reports each pouch, but the product is generally sold in a package of 10; "10" must be indicated in the quantity box on the CMS claim form to ensure proper reimbursement. This symbol indicates that care should be taken to verify quantities in this code. These quantity alerts do not represent Medicare Unlikely Edits (MUEs) and should not be used for MUEs.

⊘ **Skilled Nursing Facility (SNF)**
Use this icon to identify certain items and services excluded from SNF consolidated billing. These items may be billed directly to the Medicare contractor by the provider or supplier of the service or item.

A2–Z3 **ASC Payment Indicators**
This icon identifies the ASC status payment indicators. They indicate how the ASC payment rate was derived and/or how the procedure, item, or service is treated under the ASC payment system. For more information about these indicators and how they affect billing, consult Optum's *Revenue Cycle Pro*. **The ASC payment indicators contained in this publication were effective as of October 1, 2024.**

- A2 Surgical procedure on ASC list in CY 2007 or later; payment based on OPPS relative payment weight
- C5 Inpatient procedure
- F4 Corneal tissue acquisition, hepatitis B vaccine; paid at reasonable cost
- G2 Non-office-based surgical procedure added in CY 2008 or later; payment based on OPPS relative payment weight
- H2 Brachytherapy source paid separately when provided integral to a surgical procedure on ASC list; payment based on OPPS rate
- J7 OPPS pass-through device paid separately when provided integral to a surgical procedure on ASC list; payment based on OPPS rate
- J8 Device-intensive procedure paid at adjusted rate
- K2 Drugs and biologicals paid separately when provided integral to a surgical procedure on ASC list; payment based on OPPS rate
- K7 Unclassified drugs and biologicals; payment contractor-priced
- L1 Influenza vaccine; pneumococcal vaccine; packaged item/service; no separate payment made
- L6 New Technology Intraocular Lens (NTIOL); special payment
- N1 Packaged service/item; no separate payment made
- P2 Office-based surgical procedure added to ASC list in CY 2008 or later with MPFS nonfacility PE RVUs; payment based on OPPS relative payment weight
- P3 Office-based surgical procedure added to ASC list in CY 2008 or later with MPFS nonfacility PE RVUs; payment based on MPFS nonfacility PE RVUs
- R2 Office-based surgical procedure added to ASC list in CY 2008 or later without MPFS nonfacility PE RVUs; payment based on OPPS relative payment weight
- Z2 Radiology service paid separately when provided integral to a surgical procedure on ASC list; payment based on OPPS relative payment weight
- Z3 Radiology service paid separately when provided integral to a surgical procedure on ASC list; payment based on MPFS nonfacility PE RVUs

A-Y OPPS Status Indicators

Status indicators identify how individual HCPCS Level II codes are paid or not paid under the OPPS. The same status indicator is assigned to all the codes within an ambulatory payment classification (APC). Consult the payer or resource to learn which HCPCS codes fall within various APCs. **The OPSI contained in this publication were effective as of October 1, 2024.**

A Services furnished to a hospital outpatient that are paid under a fee schedule or payment system other than OPPS, for example:

- Ambulance Services
- Clinical Diagnostic Laboratory Services
- Non-Implantable Prosthetic and Orthotic Devices
- Physical, Occupational, and Speech Therapy
- Diagnostic Mammography
- Screening Mammography

B Codes that are not recognized by OPPS when submitted on an outpatient hospital Part B bill type (12x and 13x)

C Inpatient Procedures

E1 Items, Codes, and Services:

- Not covered by any Medicare outpatient benefit category
- Statutorily excluded by Medicare
- Not reasonable and necessary

F Corneal Tissue Acquisition; Certain CRNA Services

G Pass-Through Drugs and Biologicals

H Pass-Through Device Categories

J1 Hospital Part B services paid through a comprehensive APC

K Nonpass-Through Drugs and Nonimplantable Biologicals, Including Therapeutic Radiopharmaceuticals

L Influenza Vaccine; Pneumococcal Pneumonia Vaccine, Hepatitis B Vaccines, Covid-19 Vaccine, Monoclonal Antibody Therapy Product

M Items and Services Not Billable to the MAC

N Items and Services Packaged into APC Rates

P Partial Hospitalization or Intensive Outpatient Program

Q1 STV-Packaged Codes

Q2 T-Packaged Codes

Q3 Codes That May Be Paid Through a Composite APC

Q4 Conditionally Packaged Laboratory Tests

R Blood and Blood Products

S Significant Procedure, Not Discounted when Multiple

T Significant Procedure, Multiple Procedure Reduction Applies

U Brachytherapy Sources

V Clinic or Emergency Department Visit

Y Nonimplantable Durable Medical Equipment

Appendixes

Appendix 1: Table of Drugs and Biologicals

The brand names of drugs and biologicals listed are examples only and may not include all products available for that type. The table lists HCPCS codes from any available section including A codes, C codes, J codes, S codes, and Q codes under brand and generic names with amount, route of administration, and code numbers. While every effort is made to make the table comprehensive, it is not all-inclusive.

Appendix 2: Modifiers and Expanded Guidance

This appendix identifies current modifiers. A modifier is a two-position alpha or numeric code that is appended to a CPT or HCPCS code to clarify the services being reported. Modifiers provide a means by which a service can be altered without changing the procedure code. They add more information, such as anatomical site, to the code. In addition, they help eliminate the appearance of duplicate billing and unbundling. Modifiers are used to increase the accuracy in reimbursement and coding consistency, ease editing, and capture payment data.

Appendix 3: Abbreviations and Acronyms

This appendix contains a list of abbreviations and acronyms found throughout the HCPCS code set that may be helpful. It is not an all-inclusive list.

Appendix 4: Medicare Internet-only Manuals (IOMs)

Previously, this appendix contained a verbatim printout of the Medicare Internet-only Manual references pertaining to specific codes. This appendix now contains a link to the IOMs on the Centers for Medicare and Medicaid Services website. The IOM references to applicable to specific codes can still be found at the code level.

Appendix 5: New, Revised, and Deleted Codes

This appendix is a complete list of all new, revised, and deleted HCPCS codes for the current year. New and revised codes are listed along with their current code descriptors. Deleted codes are provided as a list of codes.

Appendix 6: Place of Service and Type of Service

This appendix contains lists of place-of-service codes that should be used on professional claims and type-of-service codes used by the Medicare Common Working File.

Anatomical Illustrations

Body Planes and Movements

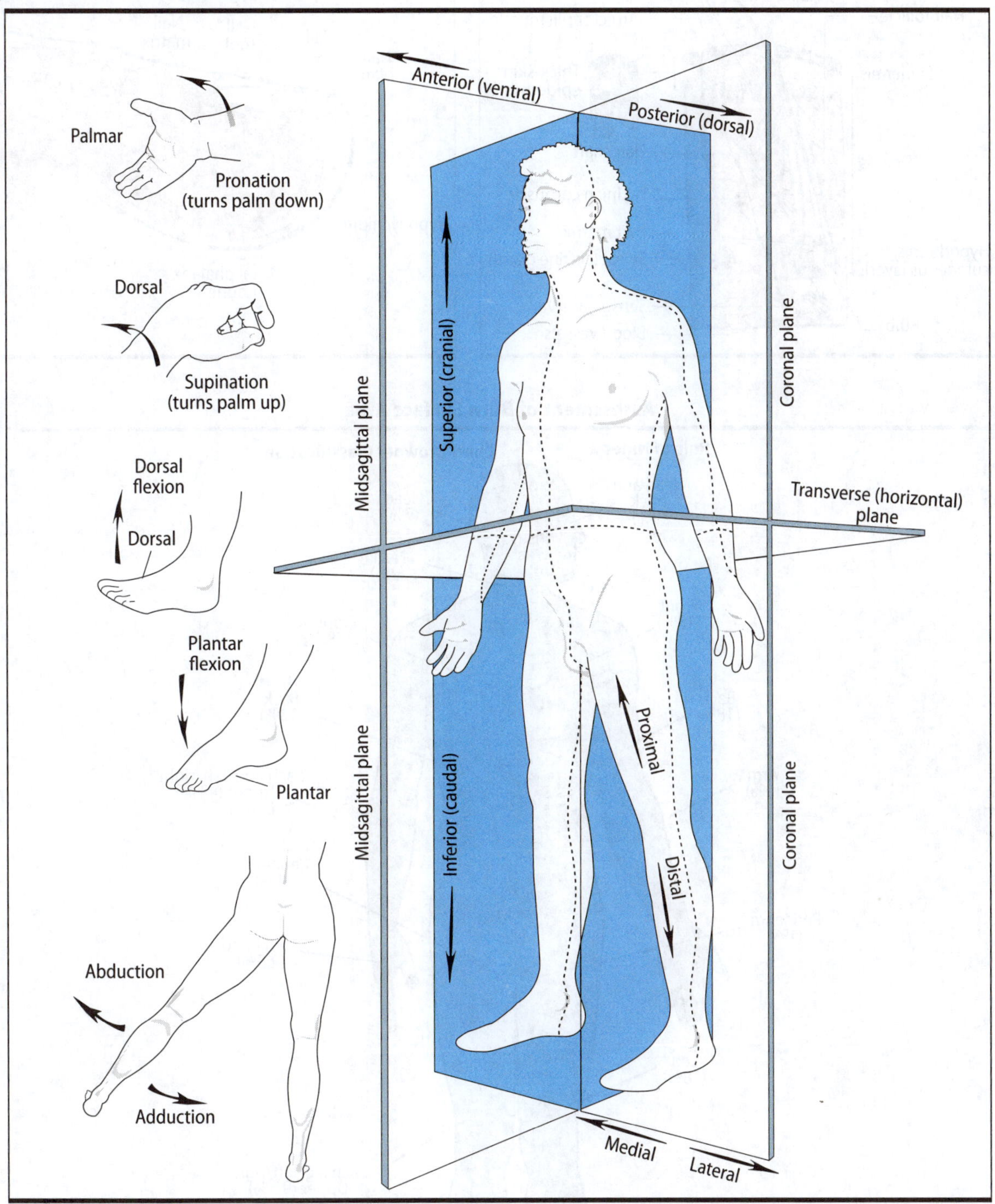

Integumentary System

Skin and Subcutaneous Tissue

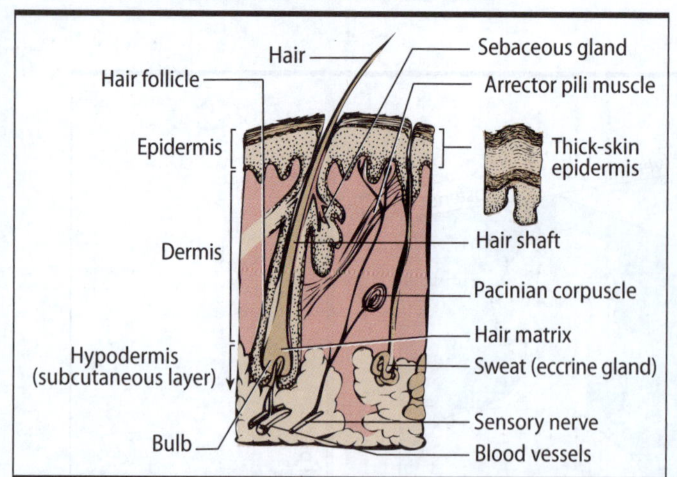

Hair
Hair follicle
Sebaceous gland
Arrector pili muscle
Epidermis
Thick-skin epidermis
Dermis
Hair shaft
Pacinian corpuscle
Hair matrix
Hypodermis (subcutaneous layer)
Sweat (eccrine gland)
Sensory nerve
Bulb
Blood vessels

Nail Anatomy

Nail plate
Nail bed
Nail root
Nail matrix
Hyponychium
Distal phalanx bone

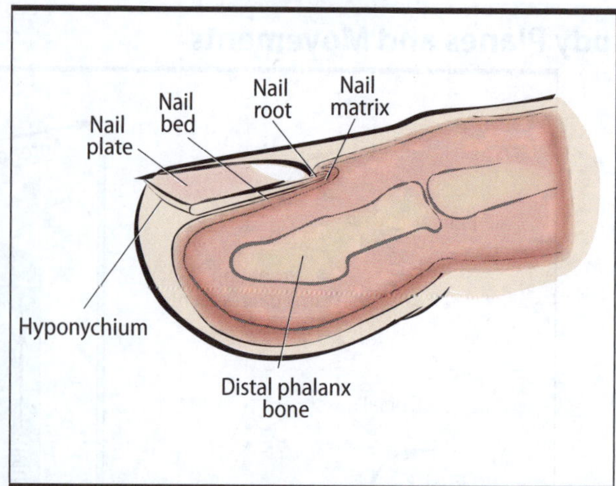

Assessment of Burn Surface Area

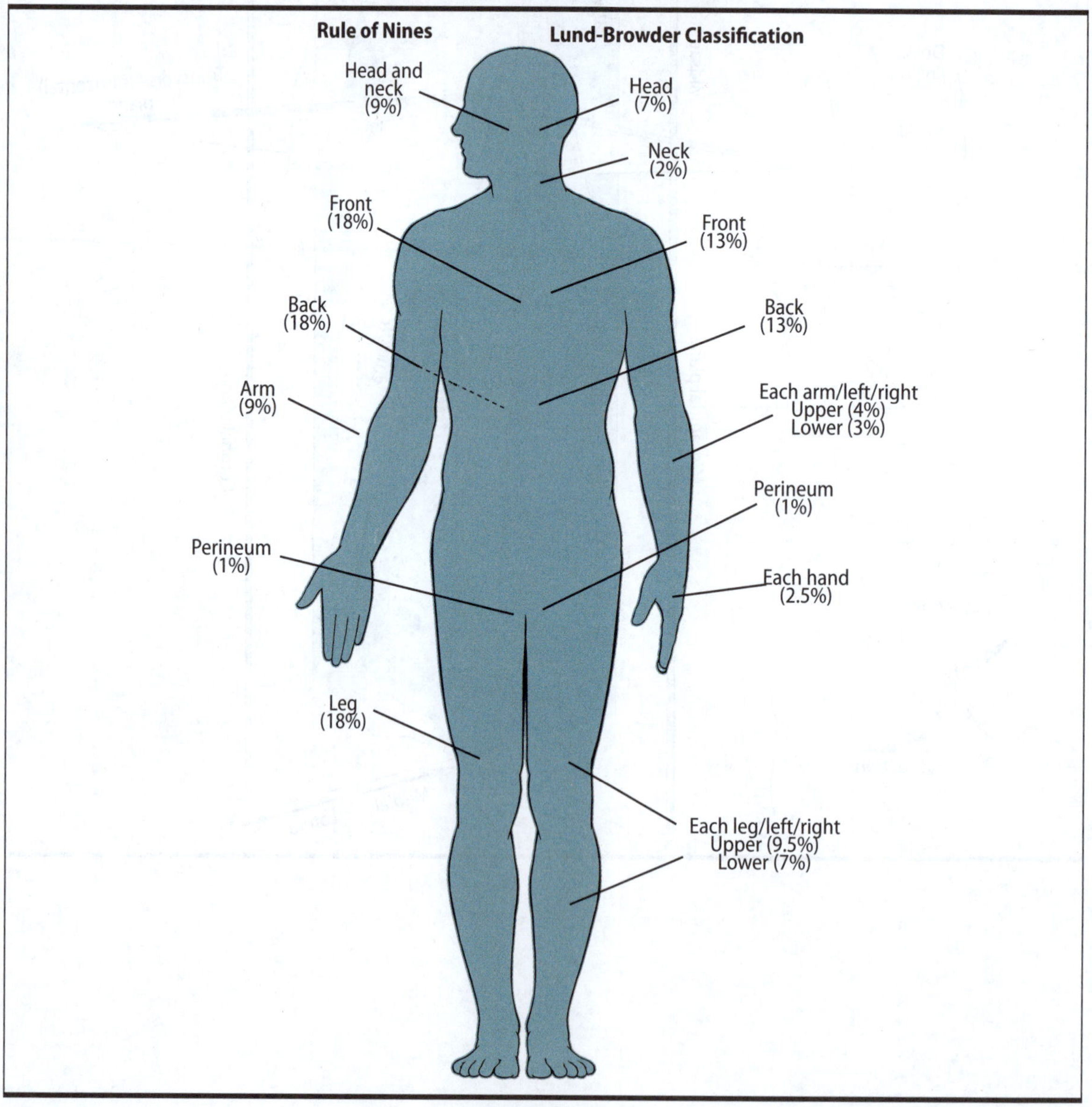

Rule of Nines
Lund-Browder Classification
Head and neck (9%)
Head (7%)
Neck (2%)
Front (18%)
Front (13%)
Back (18%)
Back (13%)
Arm (9%)
Each arm/left/right Upper (4%) Lower (3%)
Perineum (1%)
Perineum (1%)
Each hand (2.5%)
Leg (18%)
Each leg/left/right Upper (9.5%) Lower (7%)

Musculoskeletal System

Bones and Joints

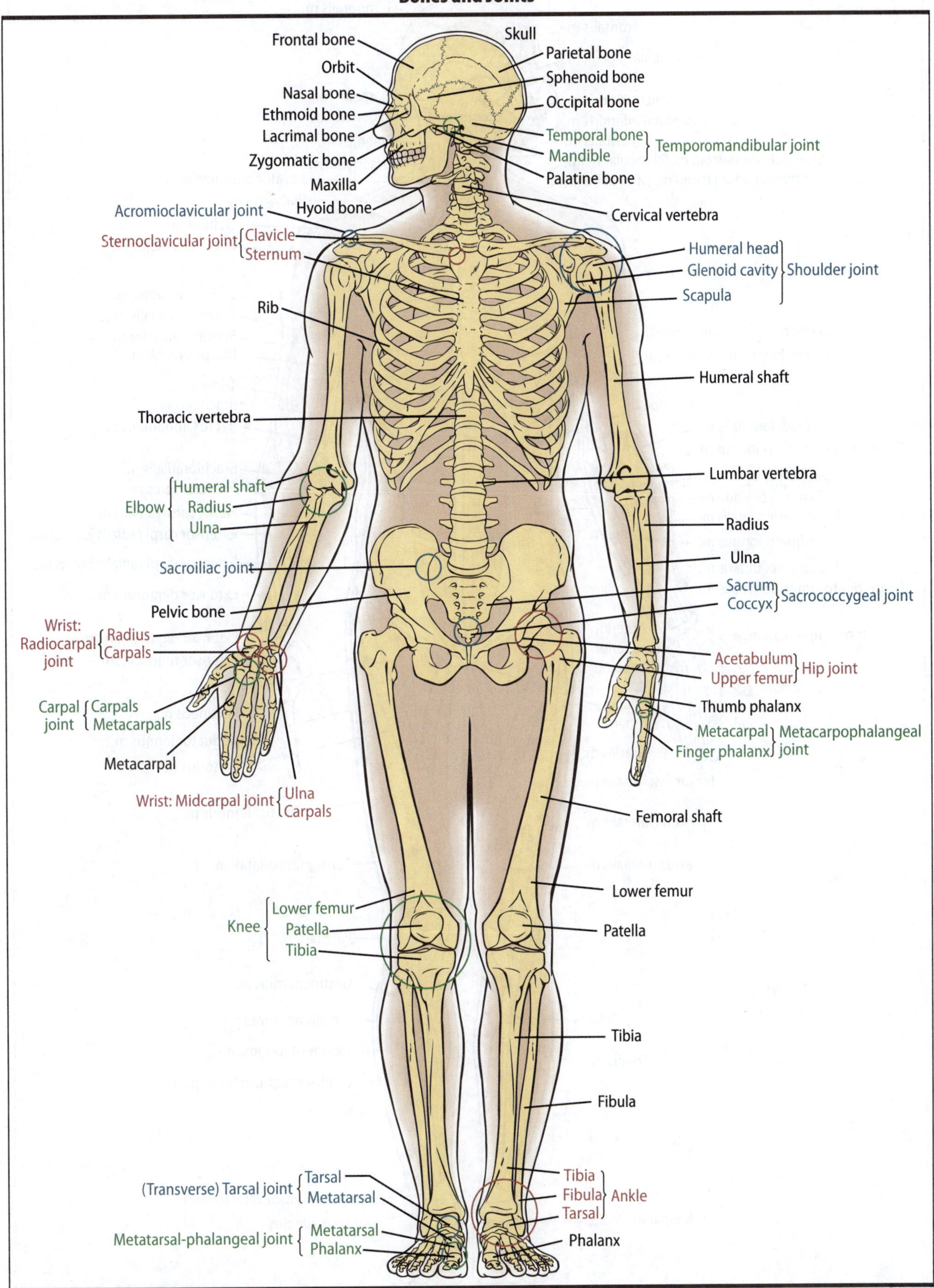

Muscles

Temporalis m.
Frontalis m.
Orbicularis oculi m.
Orbicularis oris m.
Depressor labii inferioris m.
Mentalis m.
Sternocleidomastoid m. (clavicular head)
Sternocleidomastoid m. (sternal head)
Masseter m.
Zygomaticus major m.
Splenius m.
Omohyoid m.
Levator scapulae m.
Platysma m.
Deltoid m.
Pectoralis major m.
Latissimus dorsi m.
Coracobrachialis m.
Serratus anterior m.
Biceps brachii m.
Biceps brachii m. (short head)
Biceps brachii m. (long head)
Triceps m.
Brachialis m.
Rectus abdominis m.
Linea alba
Brachioradialis m.
Extensor carpi radialis longus m.
Bicipital aponeurosis
External oblique m.
Flexor carpi radialis m.
Palmaris longus m.
Flexor carpi ulnaris m.
Flexor digitorum superficialis m.
Brachioradialis m.
Pronator teres m.
Flexor carpi radialis m.
Extensor carpi radialis longus m.
Extensor carpi radialis brevis m.
Extensor digitorum m.
Extensor digiti minimi m.
Extensor retinaculum
Extensor retinaculum
Anterior superior iliac spine
Pubic tubercle
Iliopsoas m.
Pectineus m.
Adductor longus m.
Sartorius m.
Gracilis m.
Tensor fascia latae m.
Vastus lateralis m.
Rectus femoris m.
Vastus medialis m.
Tensor fascia latae m.
Patella
Gastrocnemius m.
Tibia
Tibialis anterior m.
Peroneus longus m.
Soleus m.
Extensor digitorum longus m.
Superior extensor retinaculum
Medial malleolus
Lateral malleolus

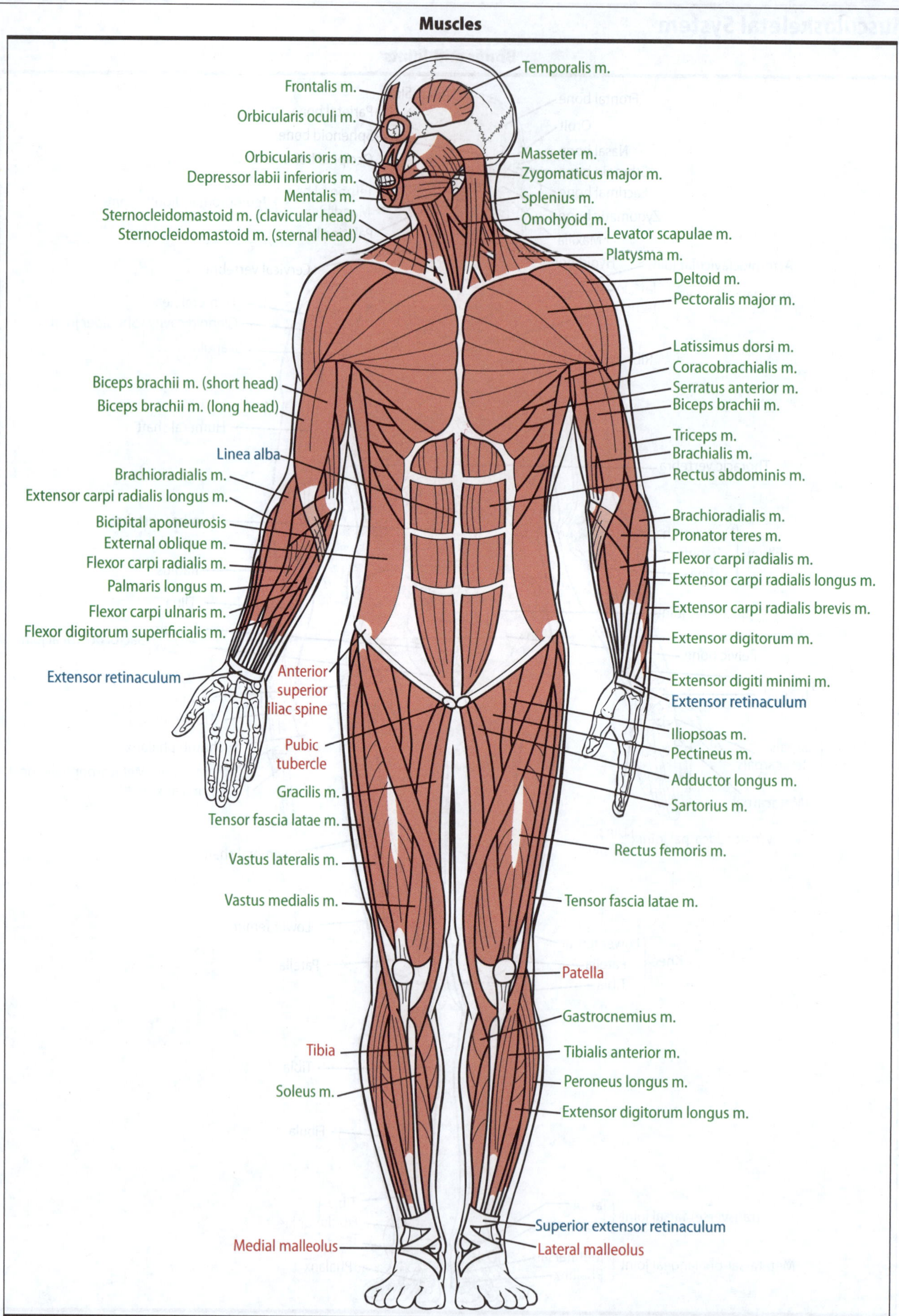

Head and Facial Bones

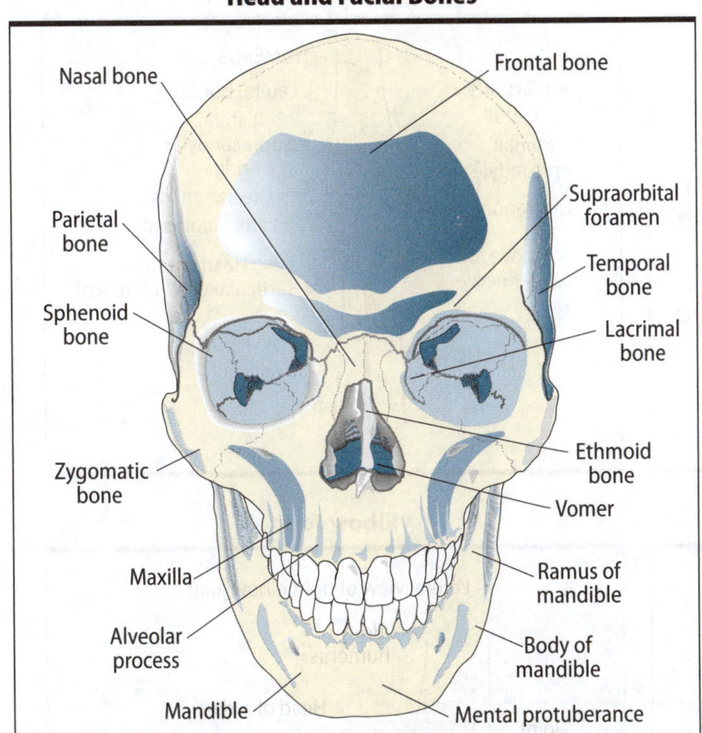

Nose

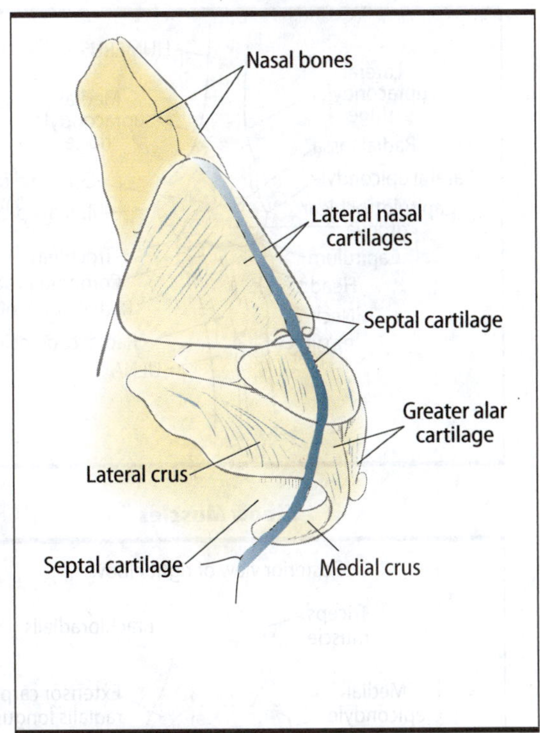

Shoulder (Anterior View)

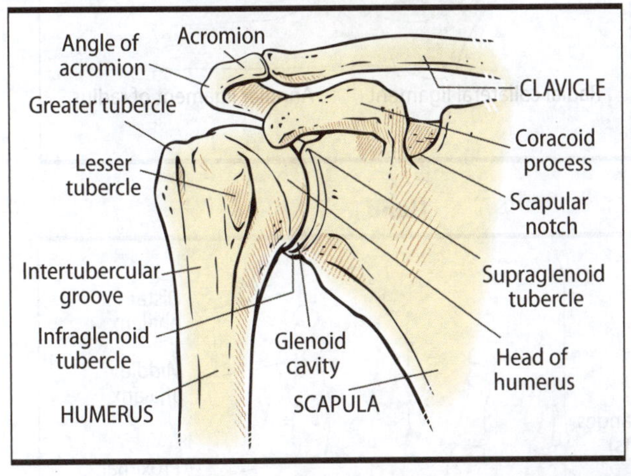

Shoulder (Posterior View)

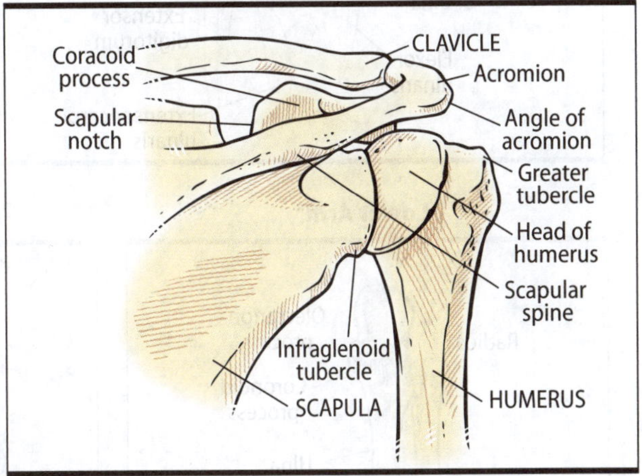

Shoulder Muscles

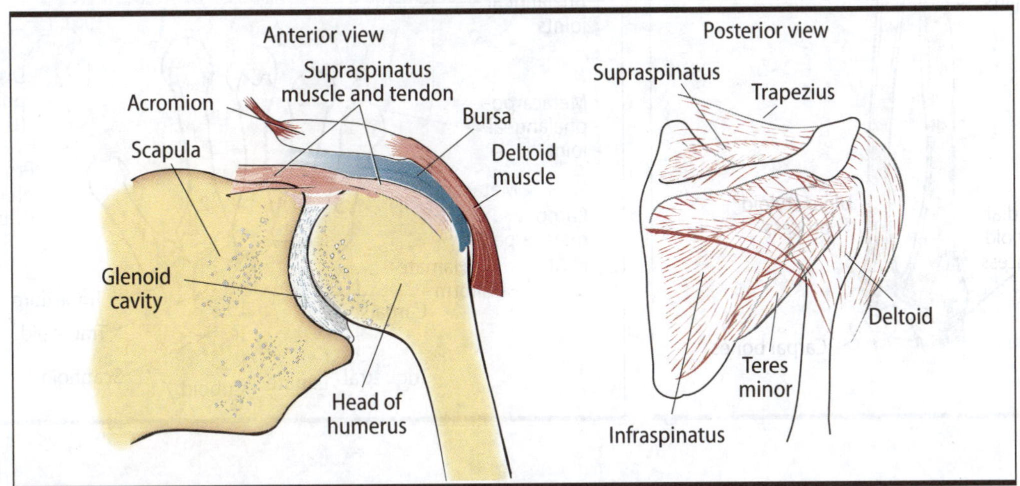

Elbow (Anterior View)

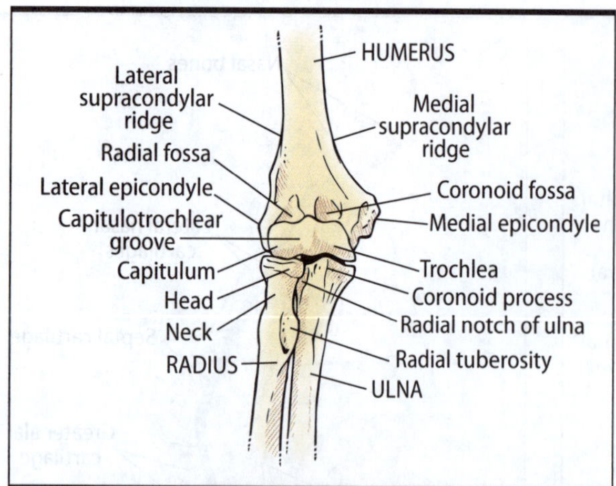

Elbow (Posterior View)

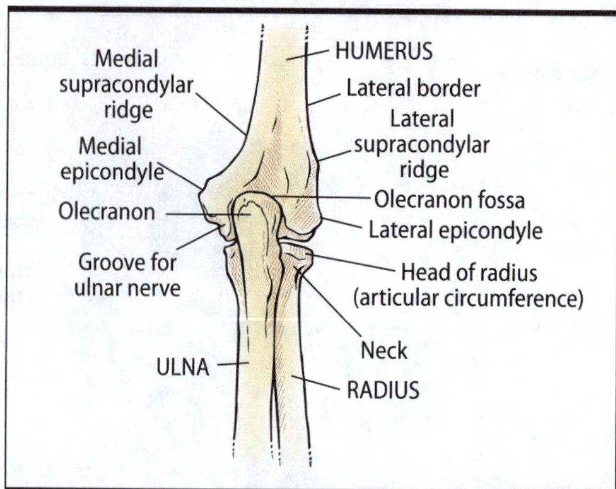

Elbow Muscles

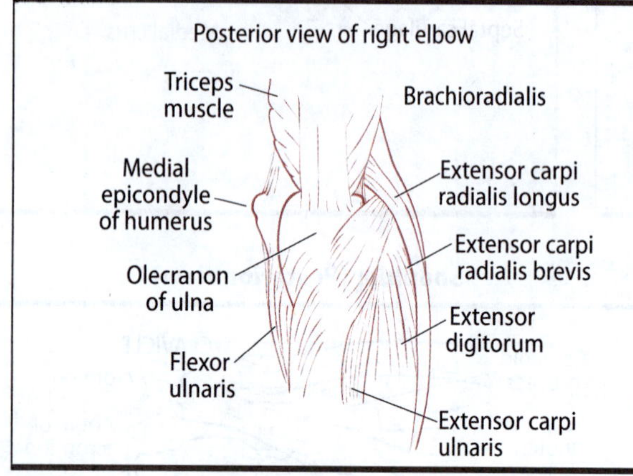

Elbow Joint

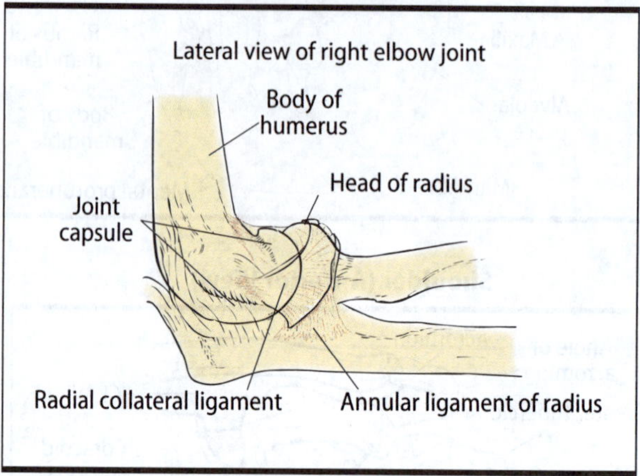

Lower Arm

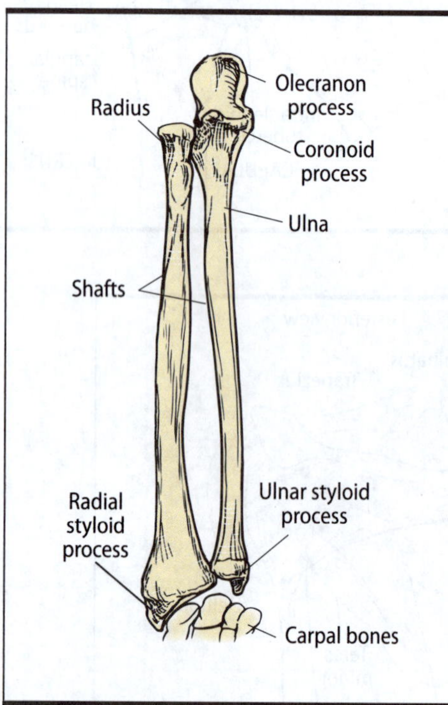

Hand

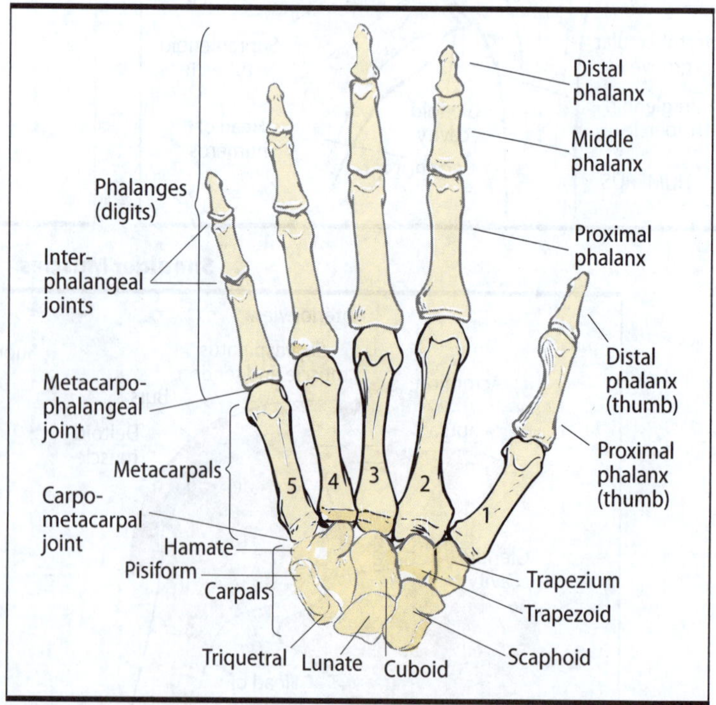

Hip (Anterior View)

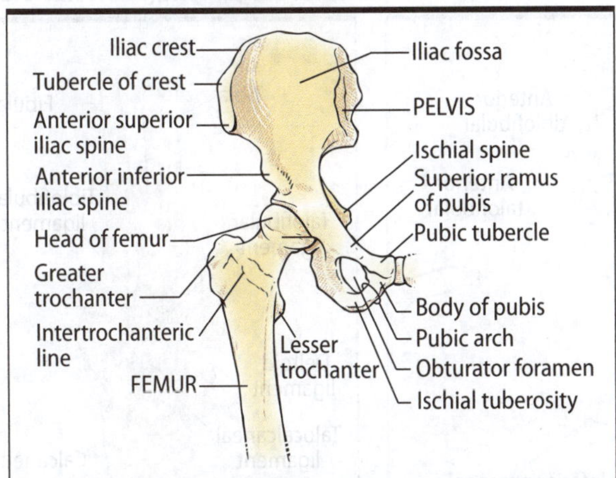

Hip (Posterior View)

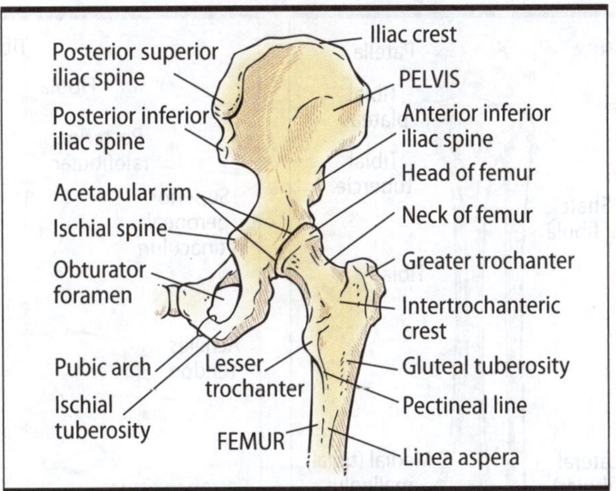

Knee (Anterior View)

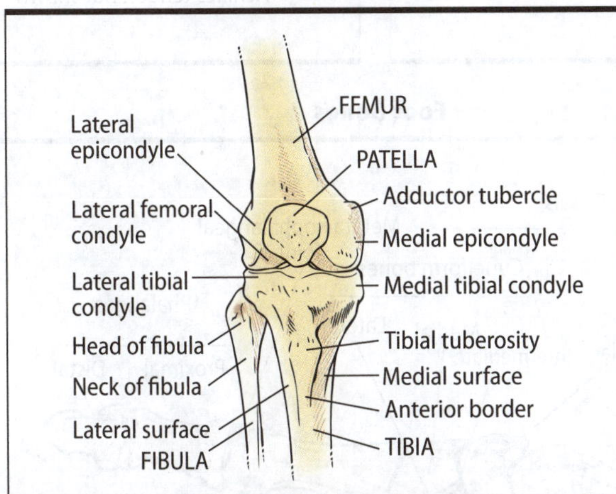

Knee (Posterior View)

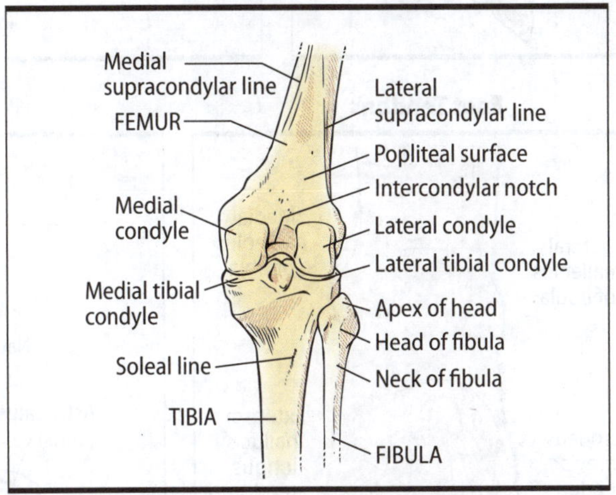

Knee Joint (Anterior View)

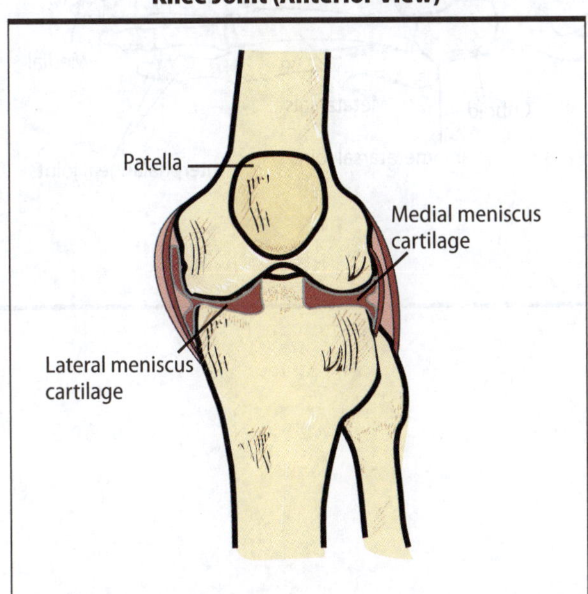

Knee Joint (Lateral View)

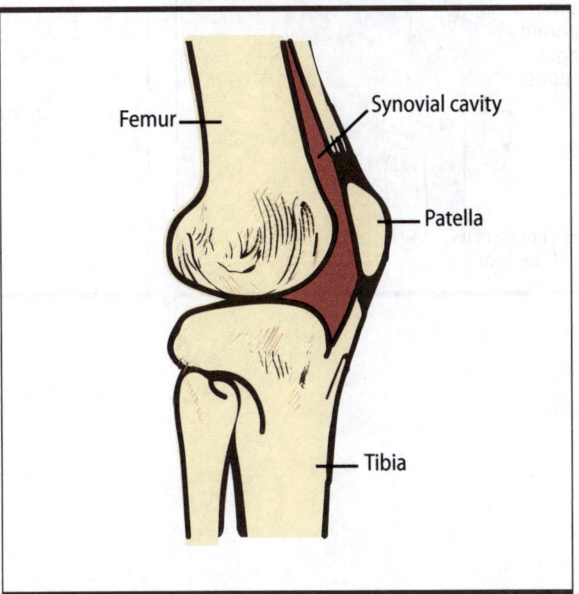

Lower Leg

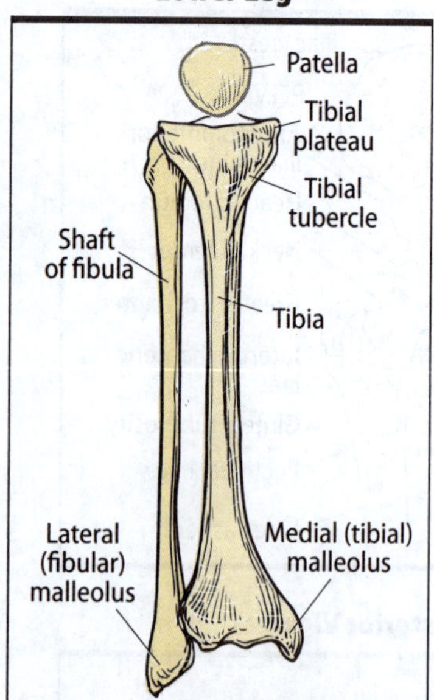

Ankle Ligament (Lateral View)

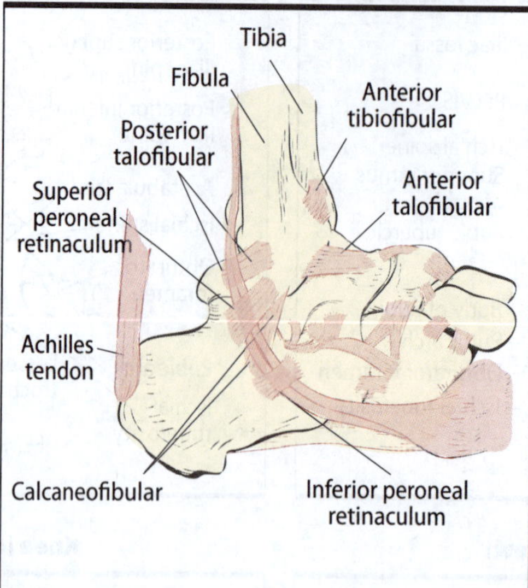

Ankle Ligament (Posterior View)

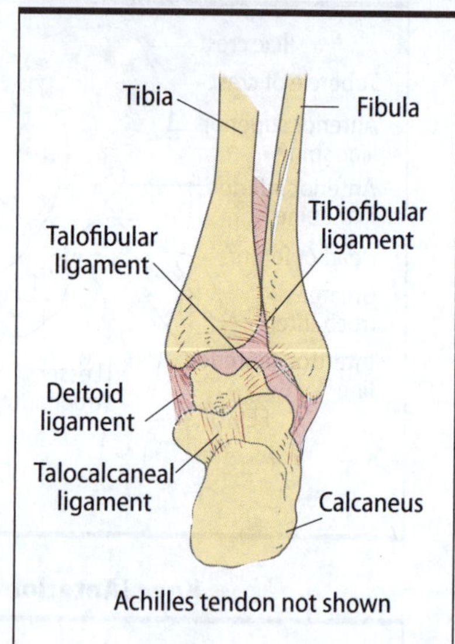

Achilles tendon not shown

Foot Tendons

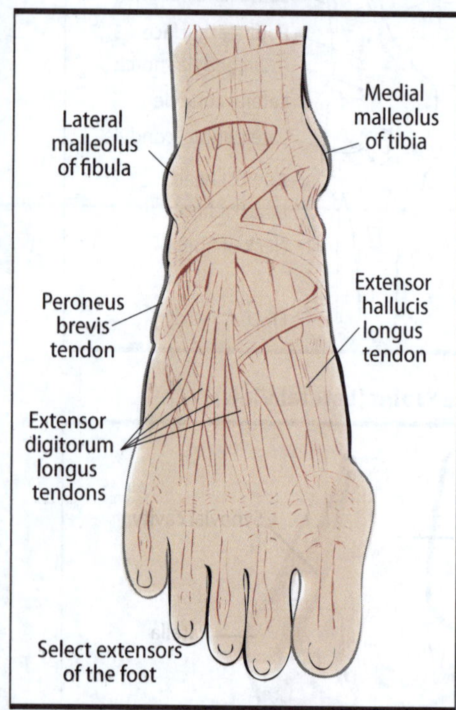

Select extensors of the foot

Foot Bones

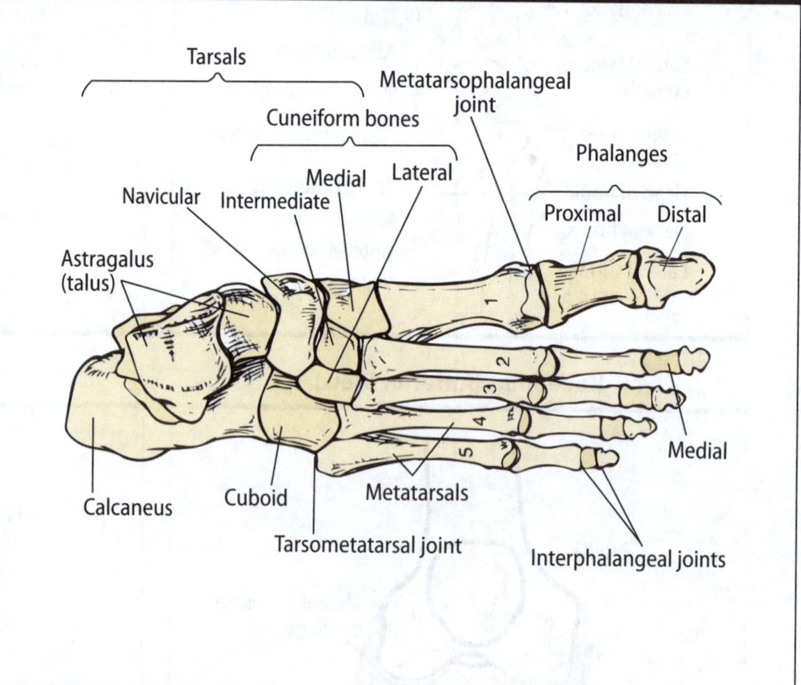

Respiratory System

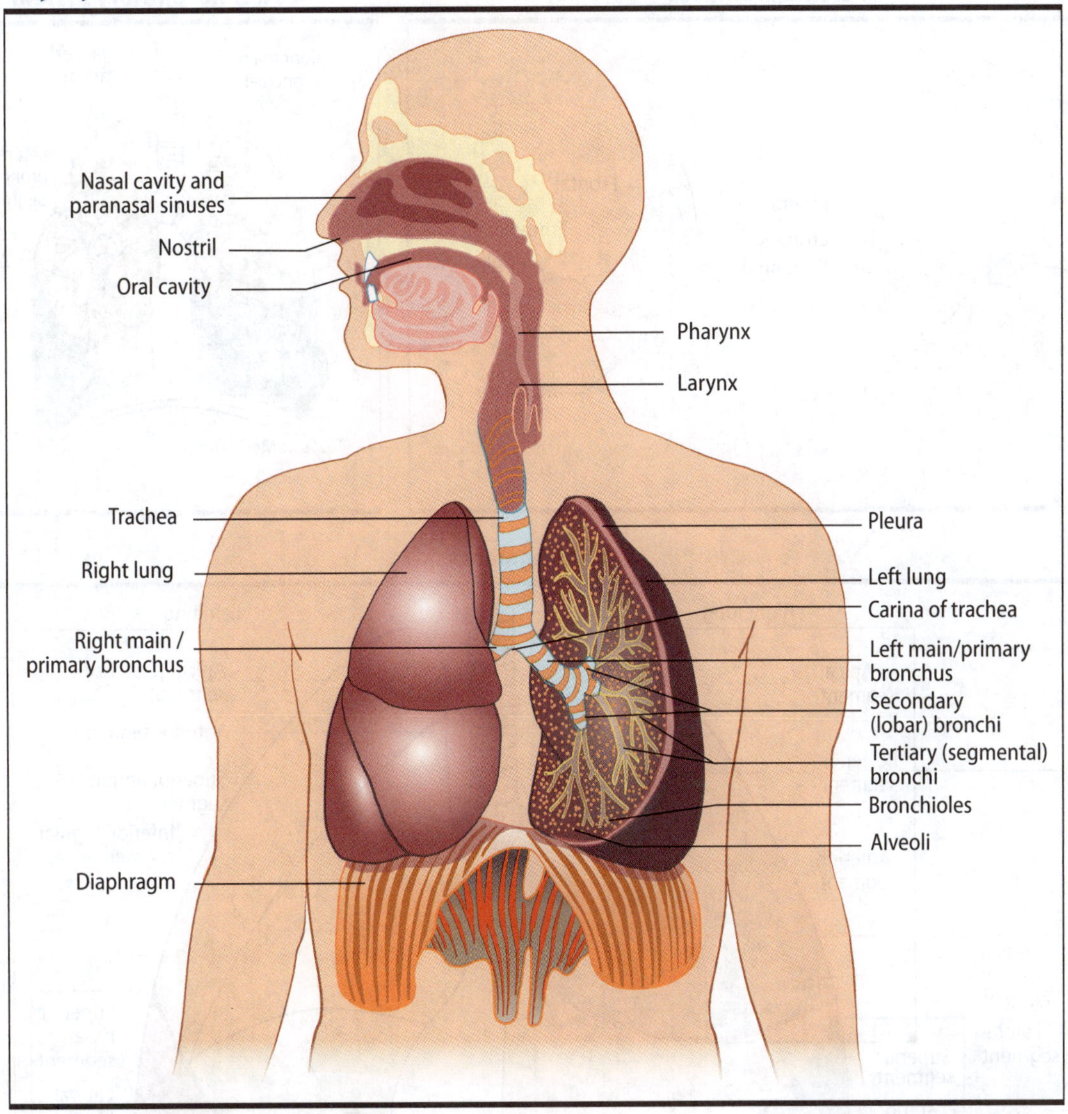

Nasal cavity and paranasal sinuses
Nostril
Oral cavity
Pharynx
Larynx
Trachea
Right lung
Right main / primary bronchus
Pleura
Left lung
Carina of trachea
Left main/primary bronchus
Secondary (lobar) bronchi
Tertiary (segmental) bronchi
Bronchioles
Alveoli
Diaphragm

Upper Respiratory System

Paranasal sinuses drain into nose via ducts under nasal conchae
Frontal sinus
Olfactory bulb and nerves
Sphenoid sinus
Window in nasal septum reveals lateral nasal wall
Orifice of auditory tube
Naris
Soft palate
Nasal cavity from front
Epiglottis
Nasal conchae
Larynx
Vocal cords
Meati
Cricoid cartilage
Trachea
Septum

Nasal Turbinates

Mid frontal cutaway view
Ethmoid air cells (sinus)
Eye orbit
Superior turbinate
Middle turbinate
Inferior turbinate
Maxillary sinus

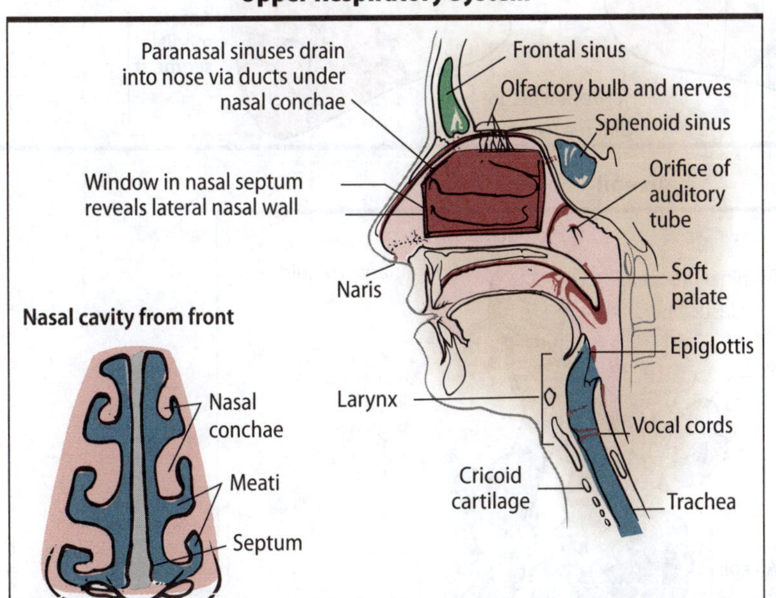

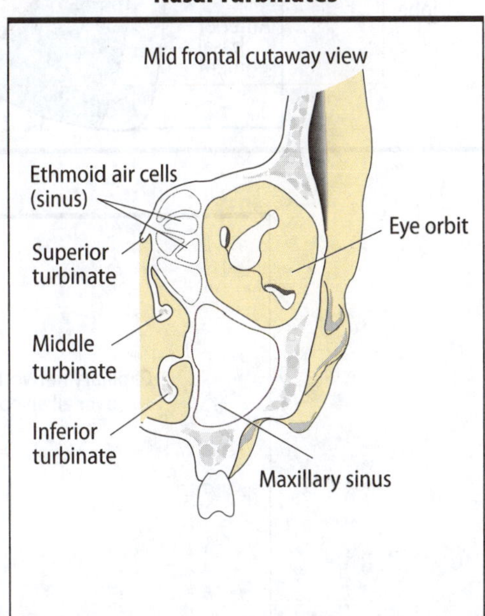

Anatomical Illustrations

Paranasal Sinuses

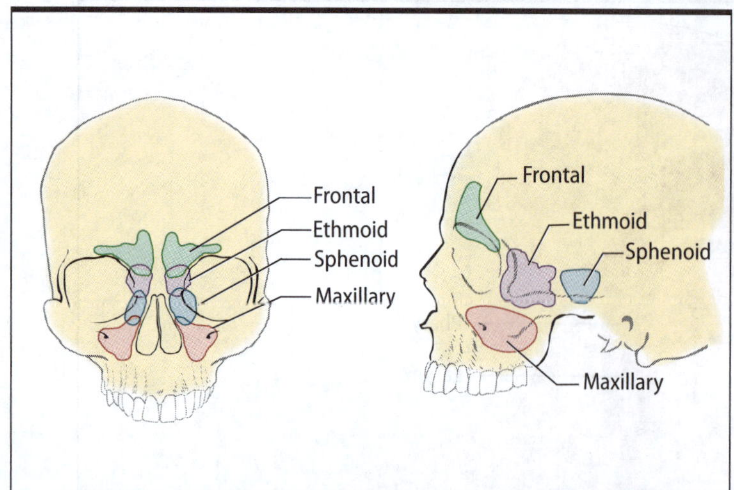

Lower Respiratory System

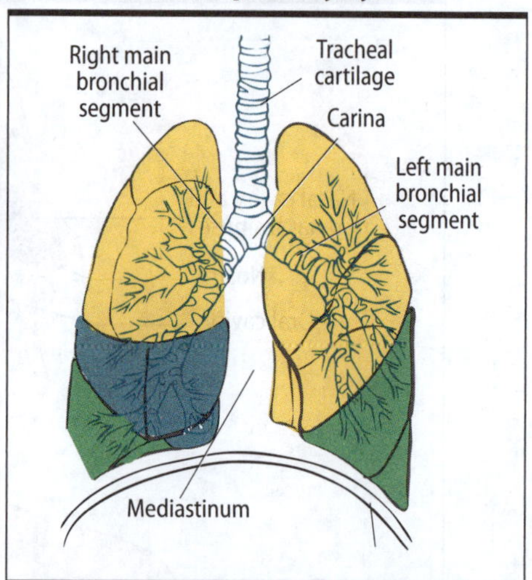

Lung Segments

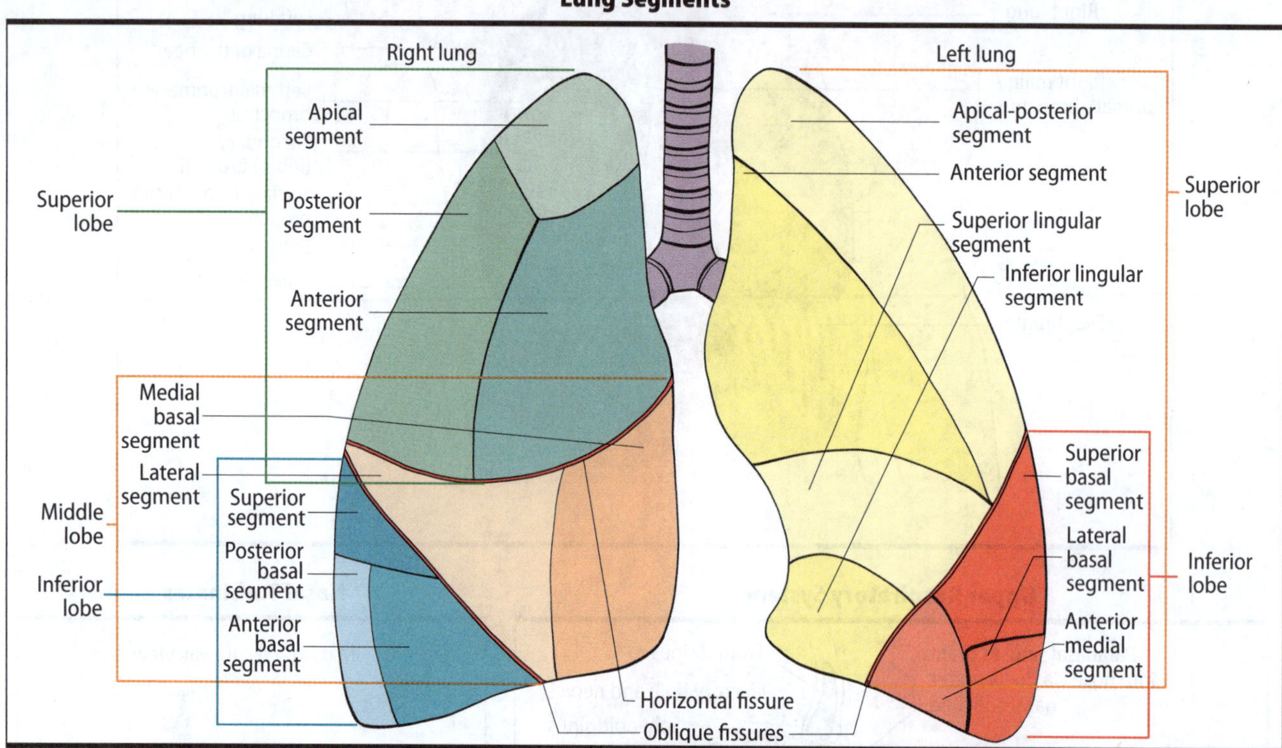

Alveoli

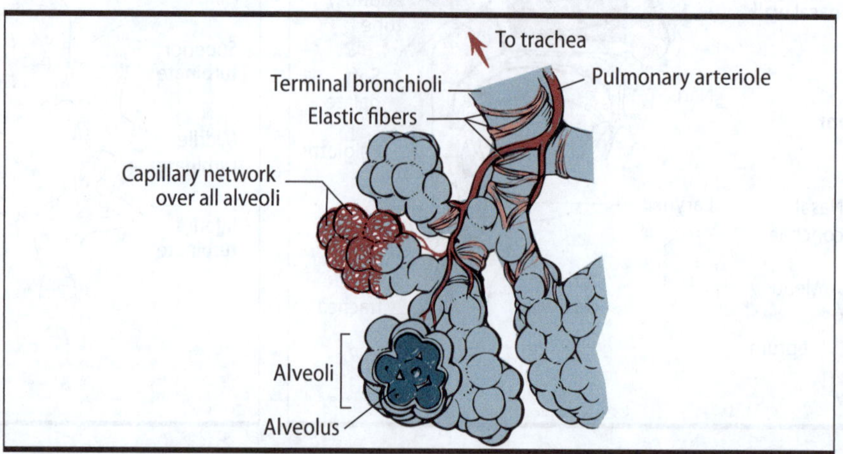

Arterial System

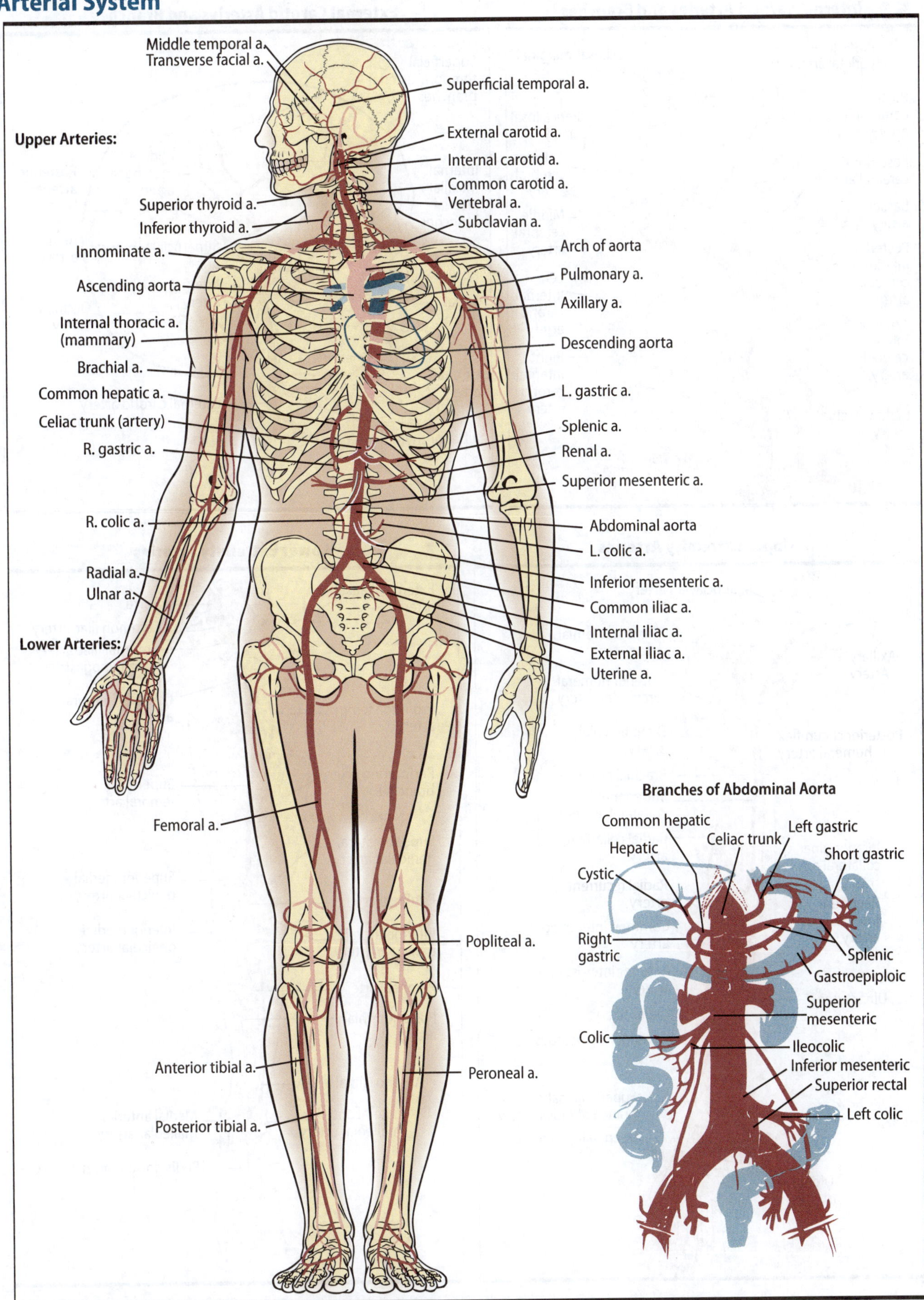

Internal Carotid Arteries and Branches

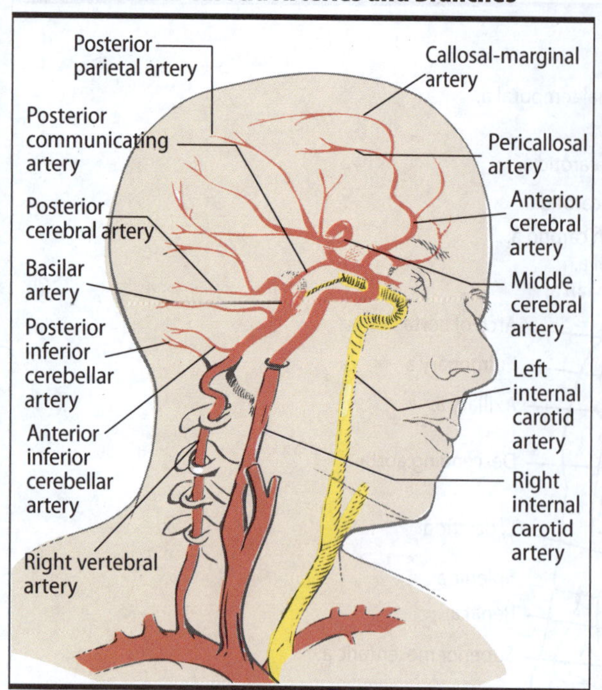

External Carotid Arteries and Branches

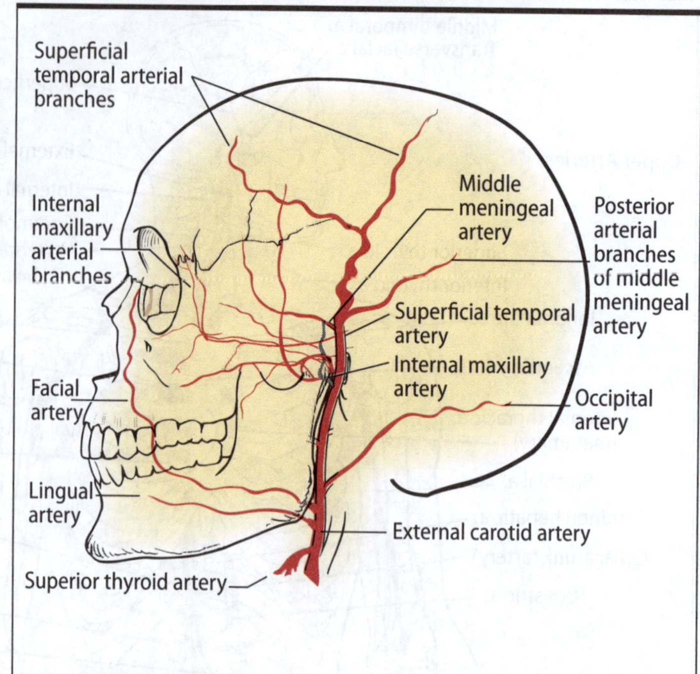

Upper Extremity Arteries

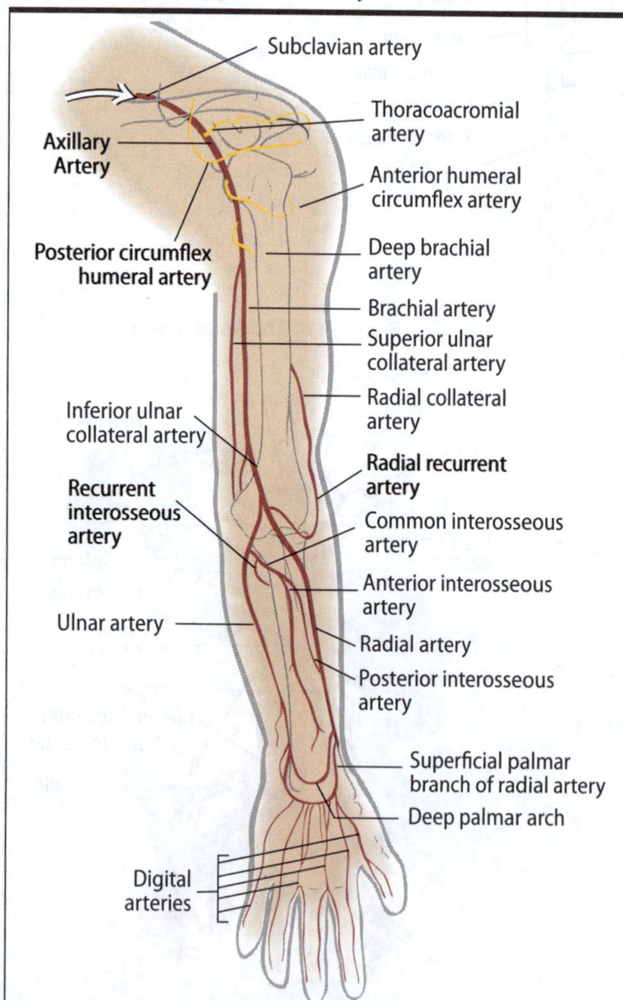

Lower Extremity Arteries

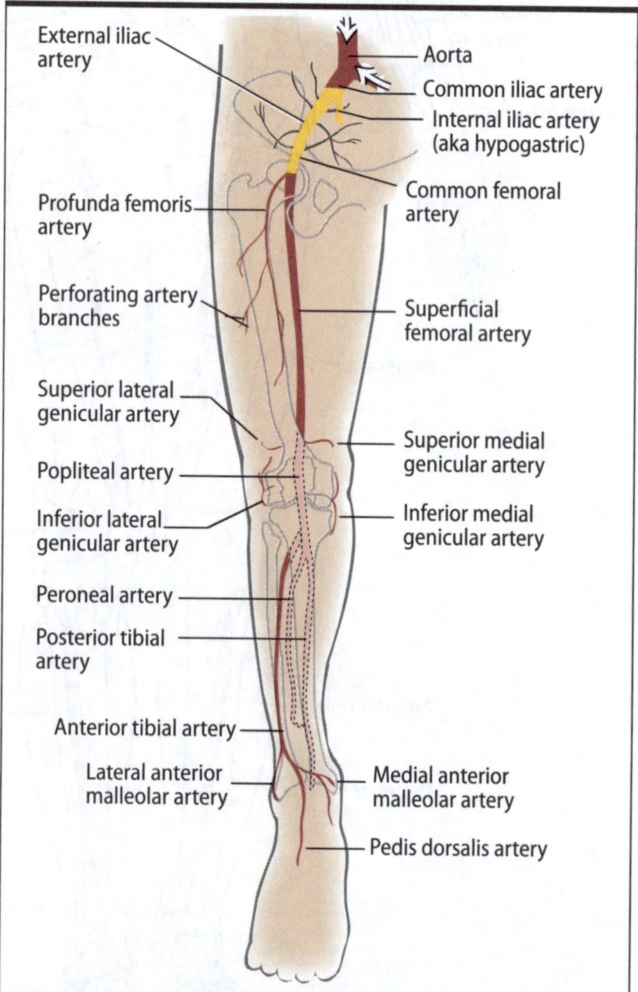

Venous System

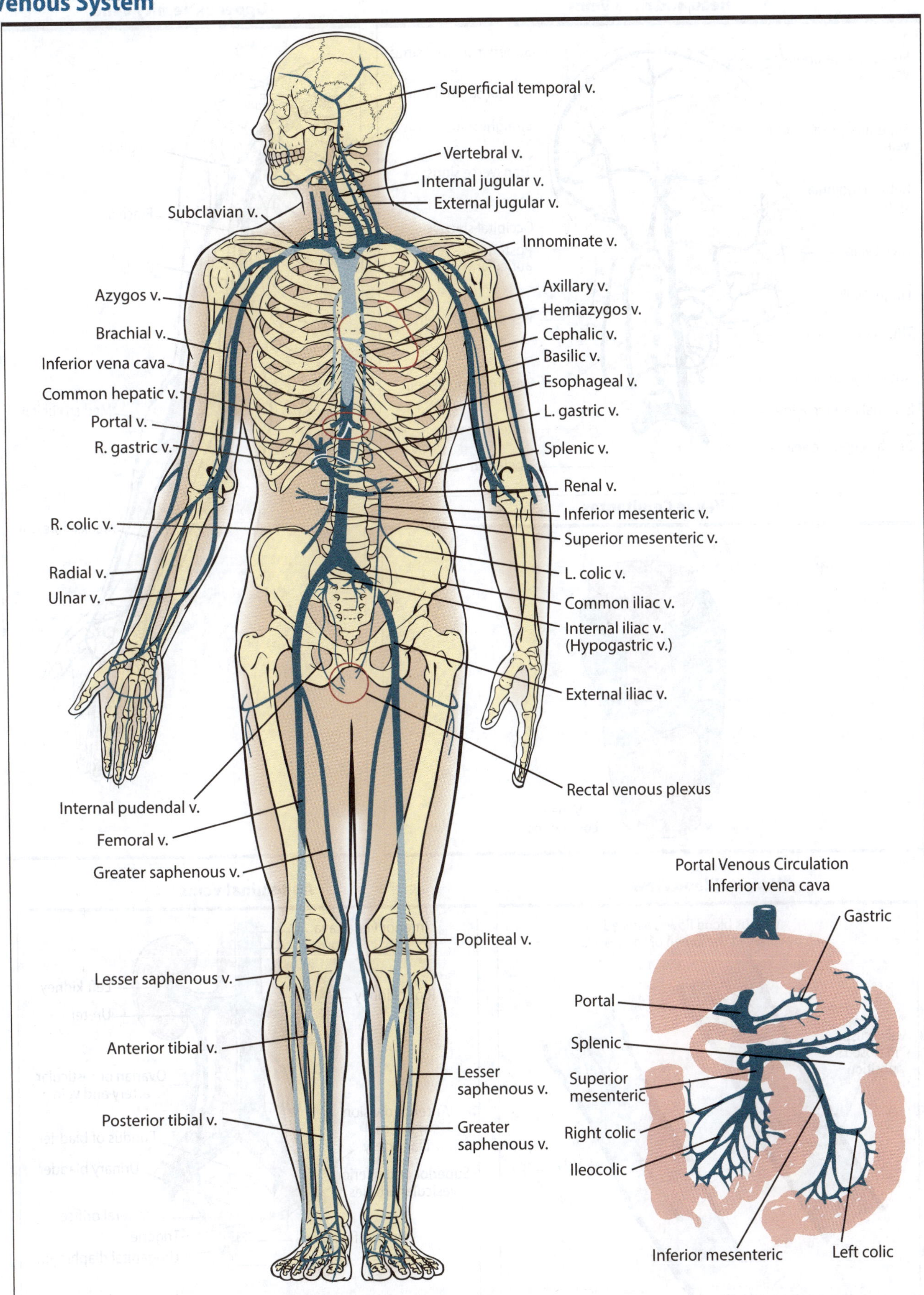

Head and Neck Veins

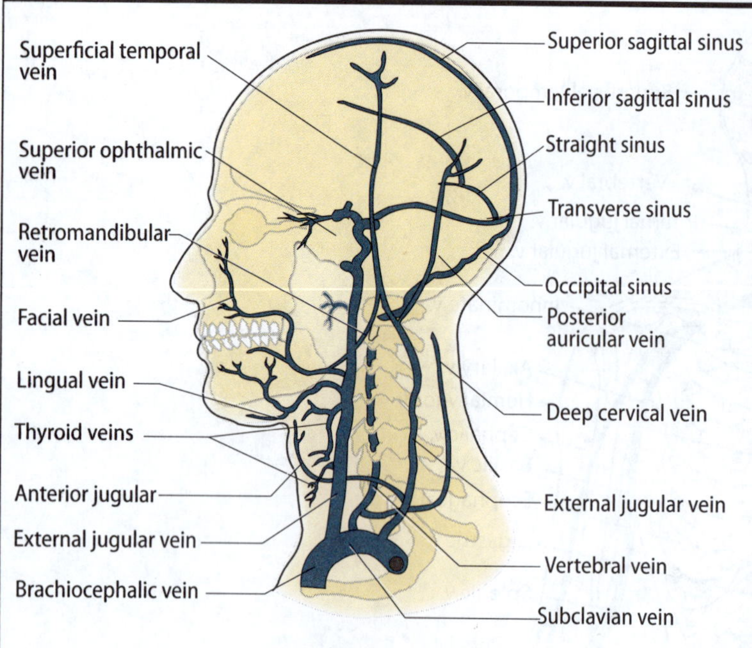

Upper Extremity Veins

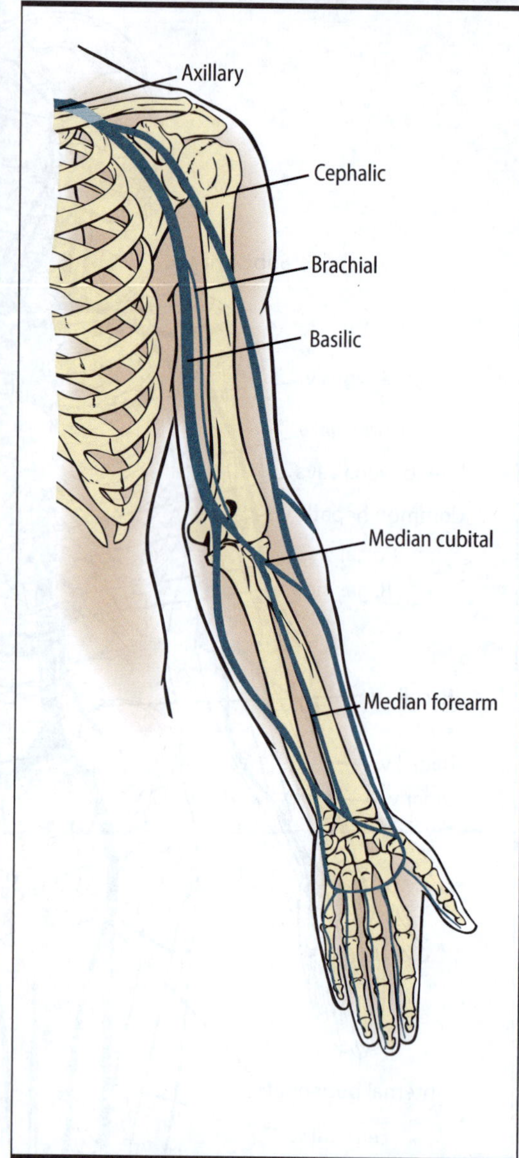

Venae Comitantes

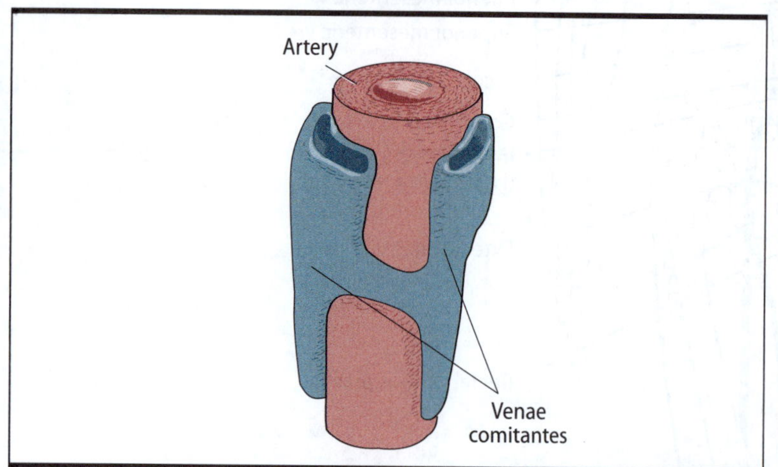

Venous Blood Flow

Venous blood flow is assisted by valves in the lumen of the vessels
Valve cusps in closed position
Valve cusps in open position

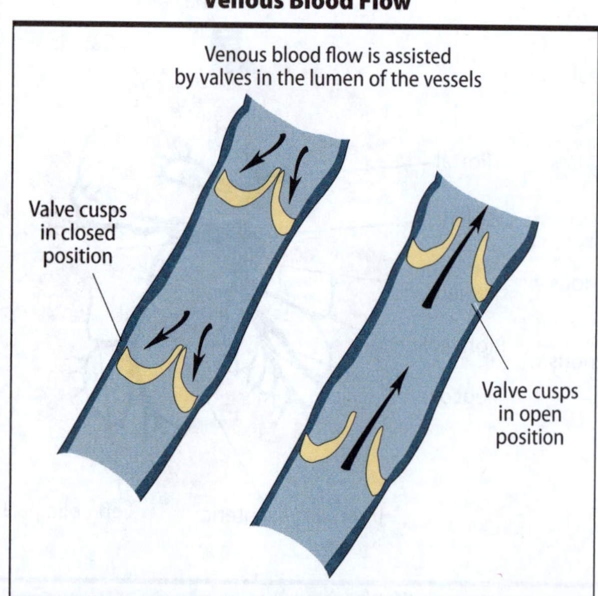

Abdominal Veins

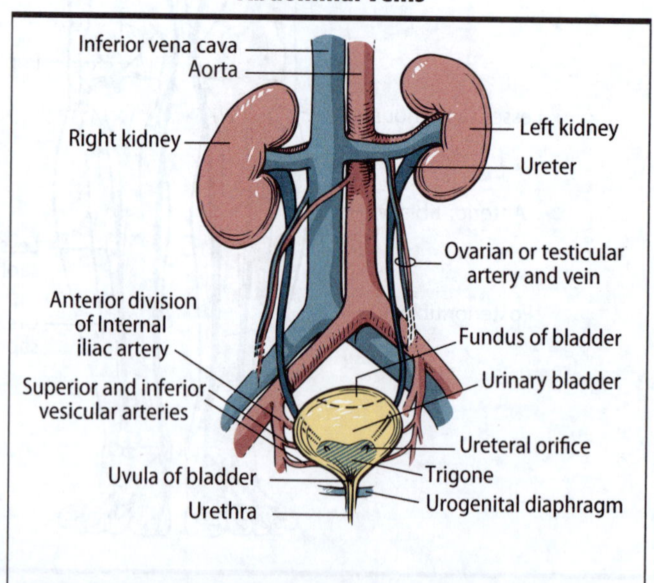

Cardiovascular System

Coronary Veins

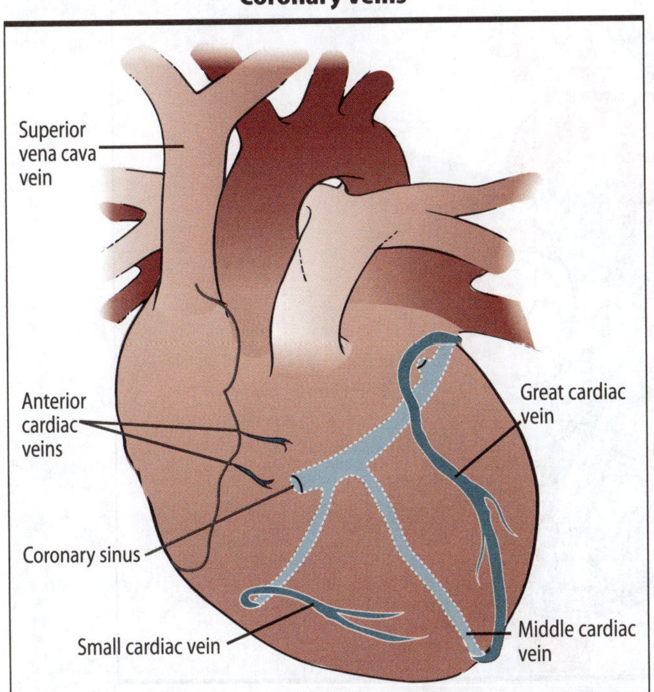

Anatomy of the Heart

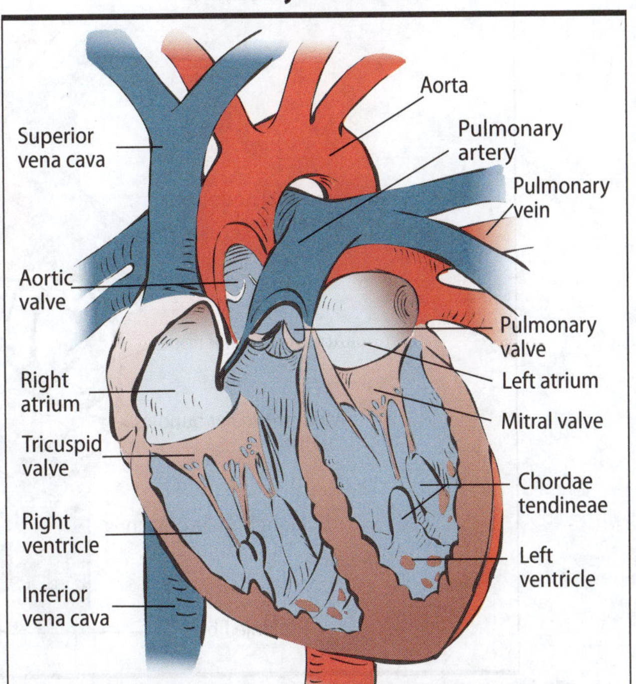

Heart Cross Section

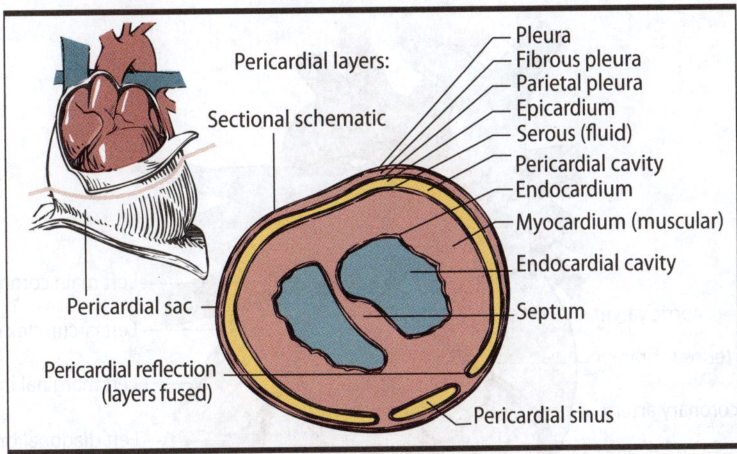

Heart Valves

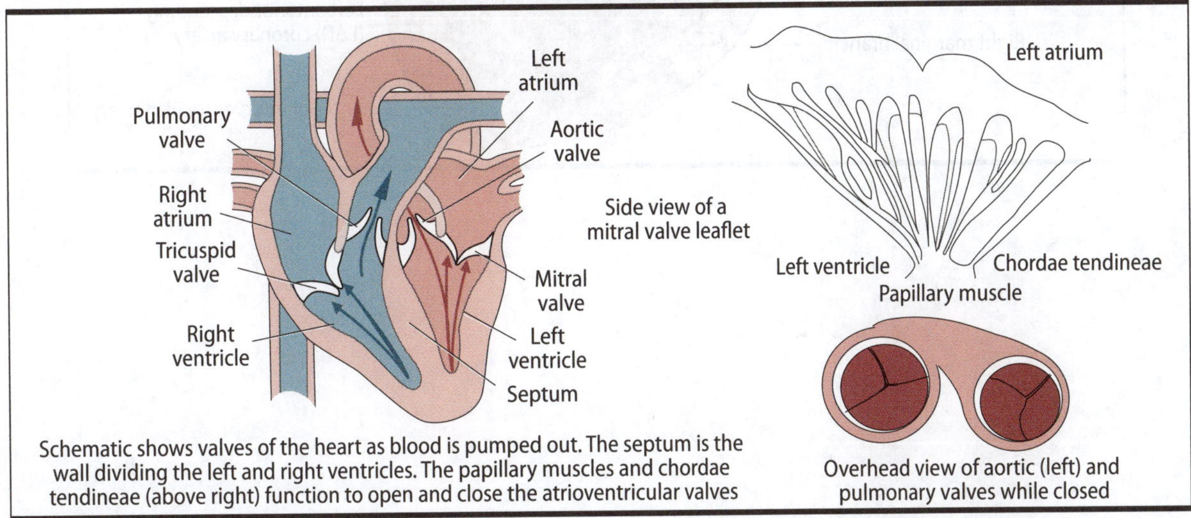

Schematic shows valves of the heart as blood is pumped out. The septum is the wall dividing the left and right ventricles. The papillary muscles and chordae tendineae (above right) function to open and close the atrioventricular valves

Overhead view of aortic (left) and pulmonary valves while closed

Heart Conduction System

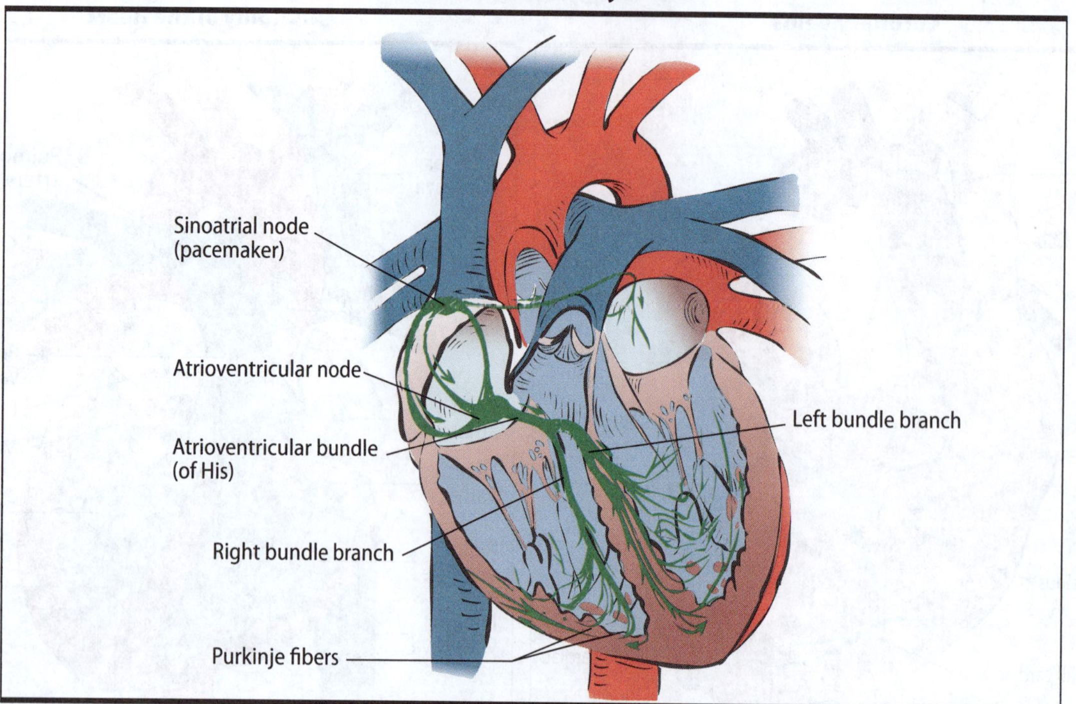

Coronary Arteries

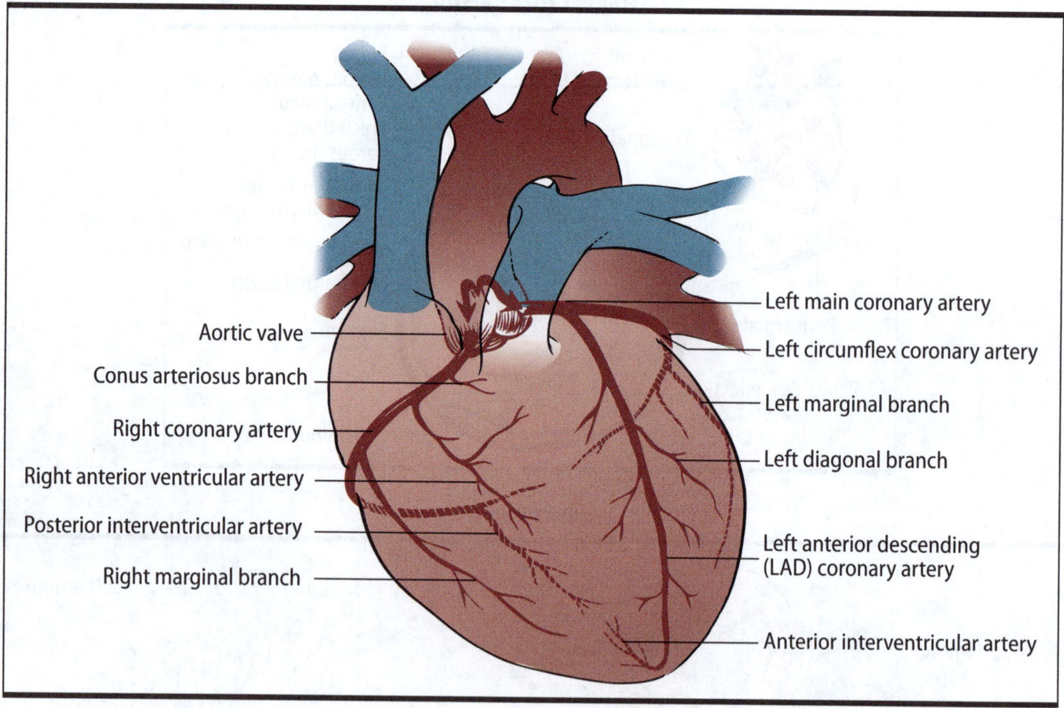

Lymphatic System

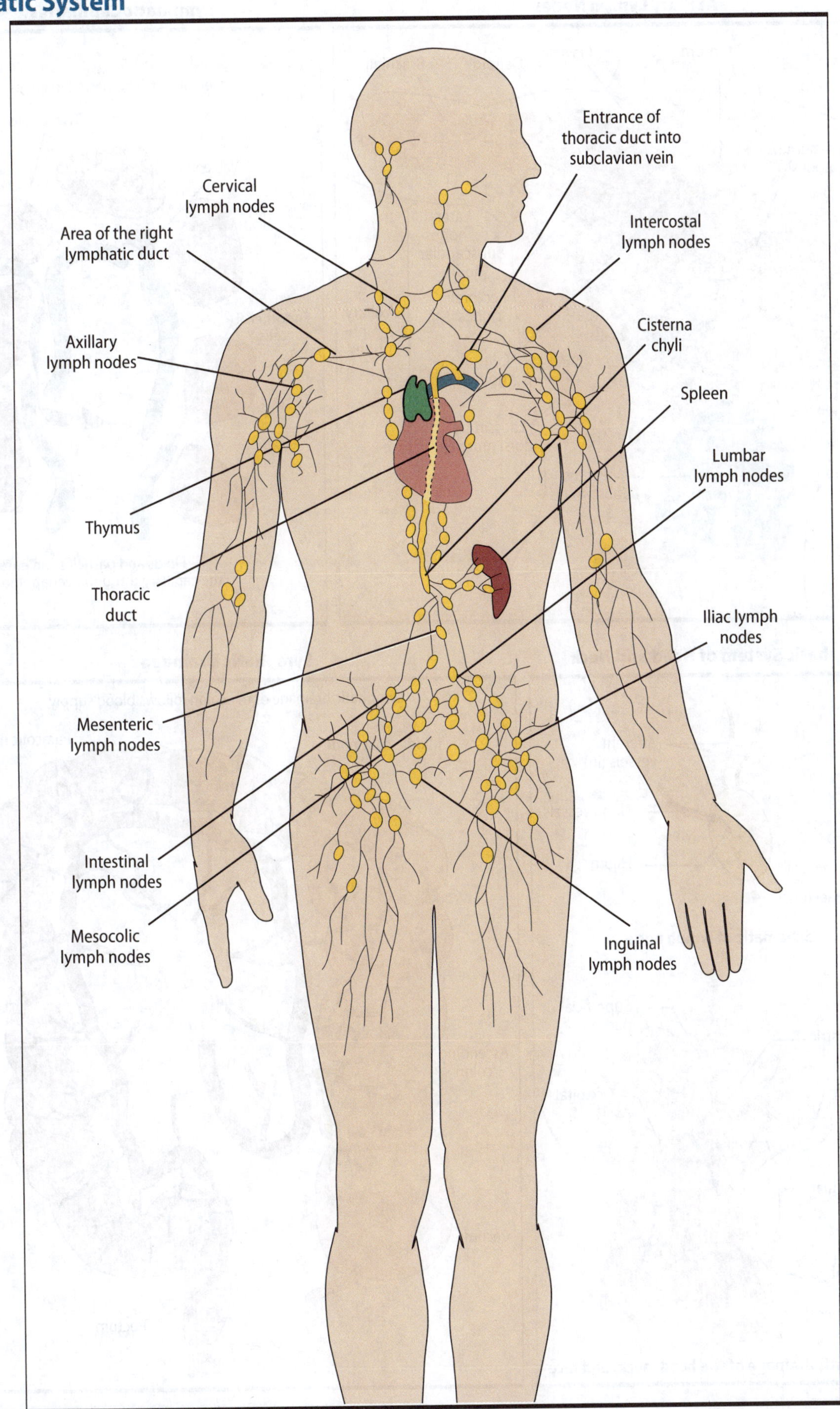

Anatomical Illustrations

Axillary Lymph Nodes

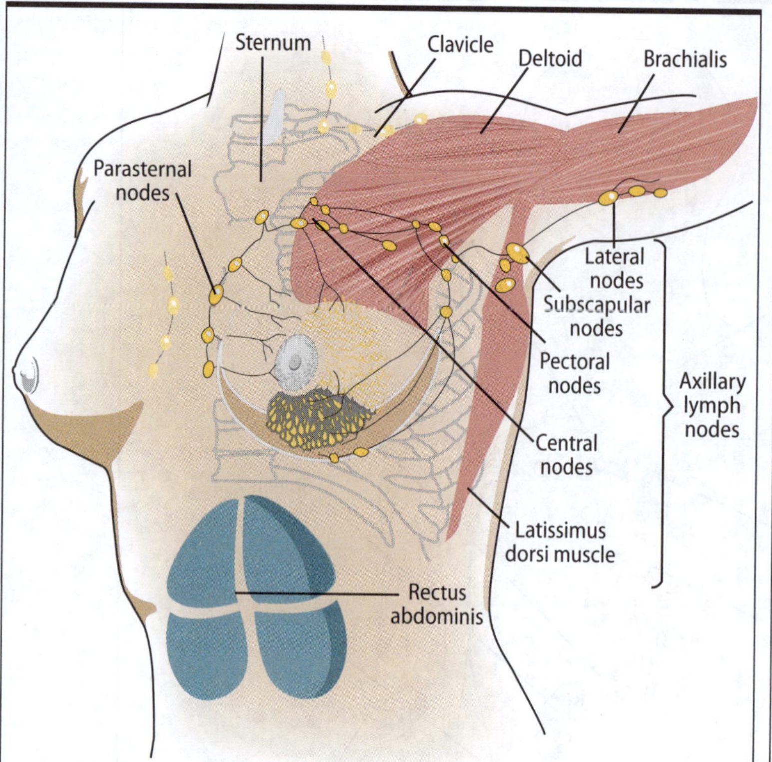

Lymphatic Capillaries

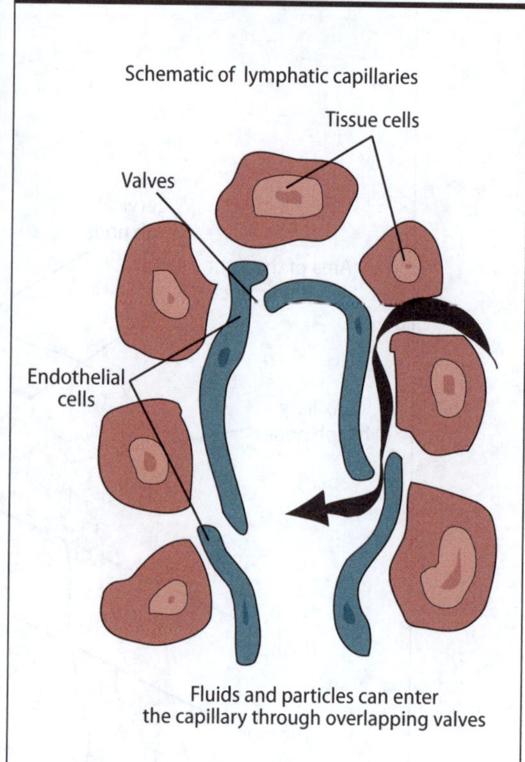

Lymphatic System of Head and Neck

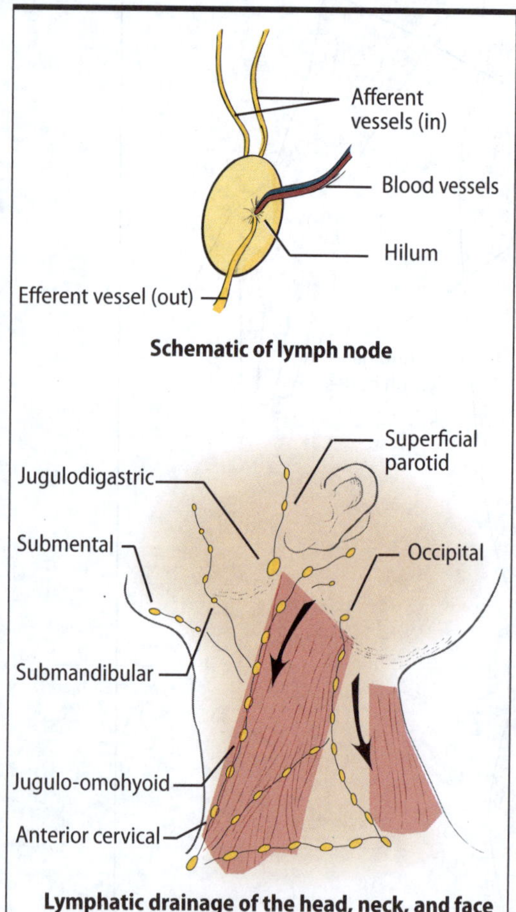

Lymphatic Drainage

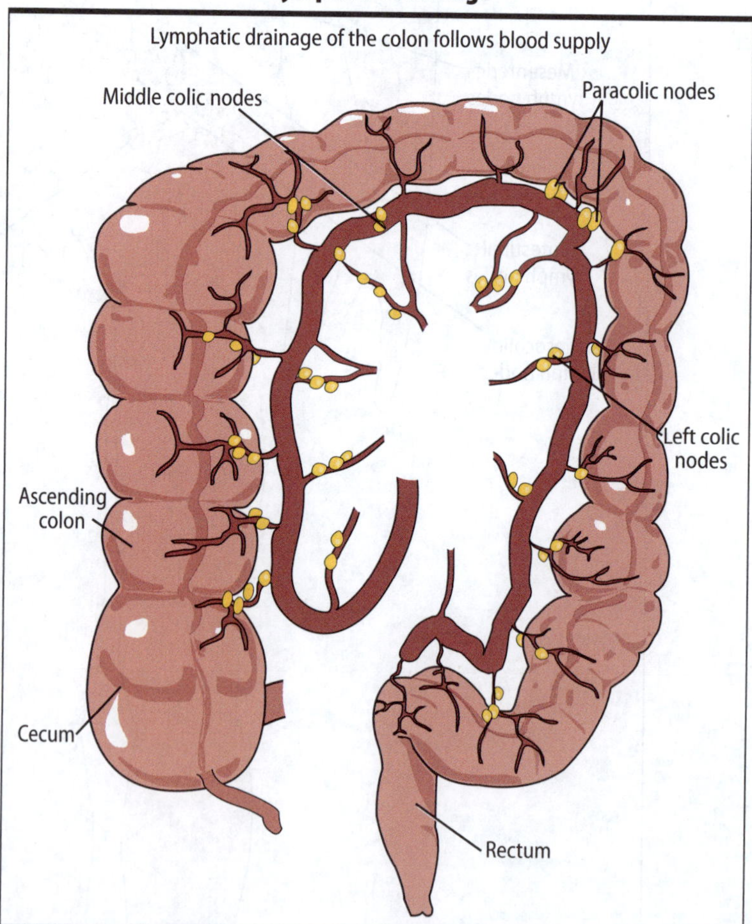

Spleen Internal Structures

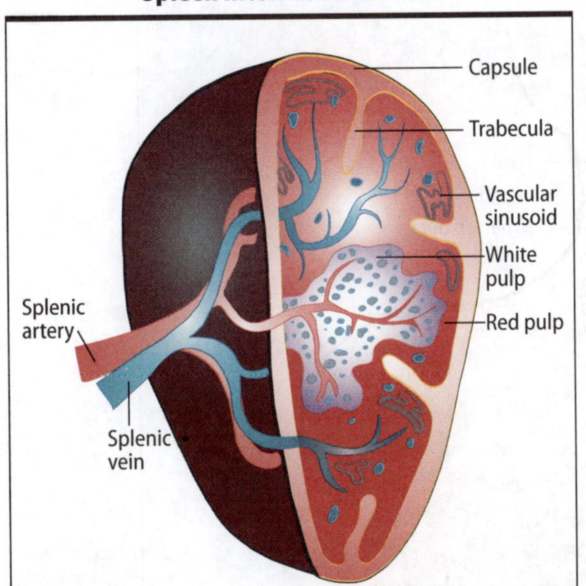

Spleen External Structures

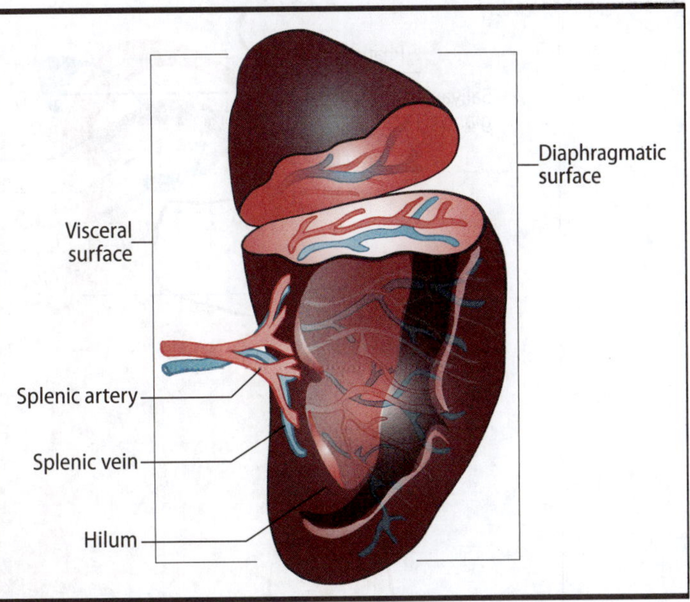

Digestive System

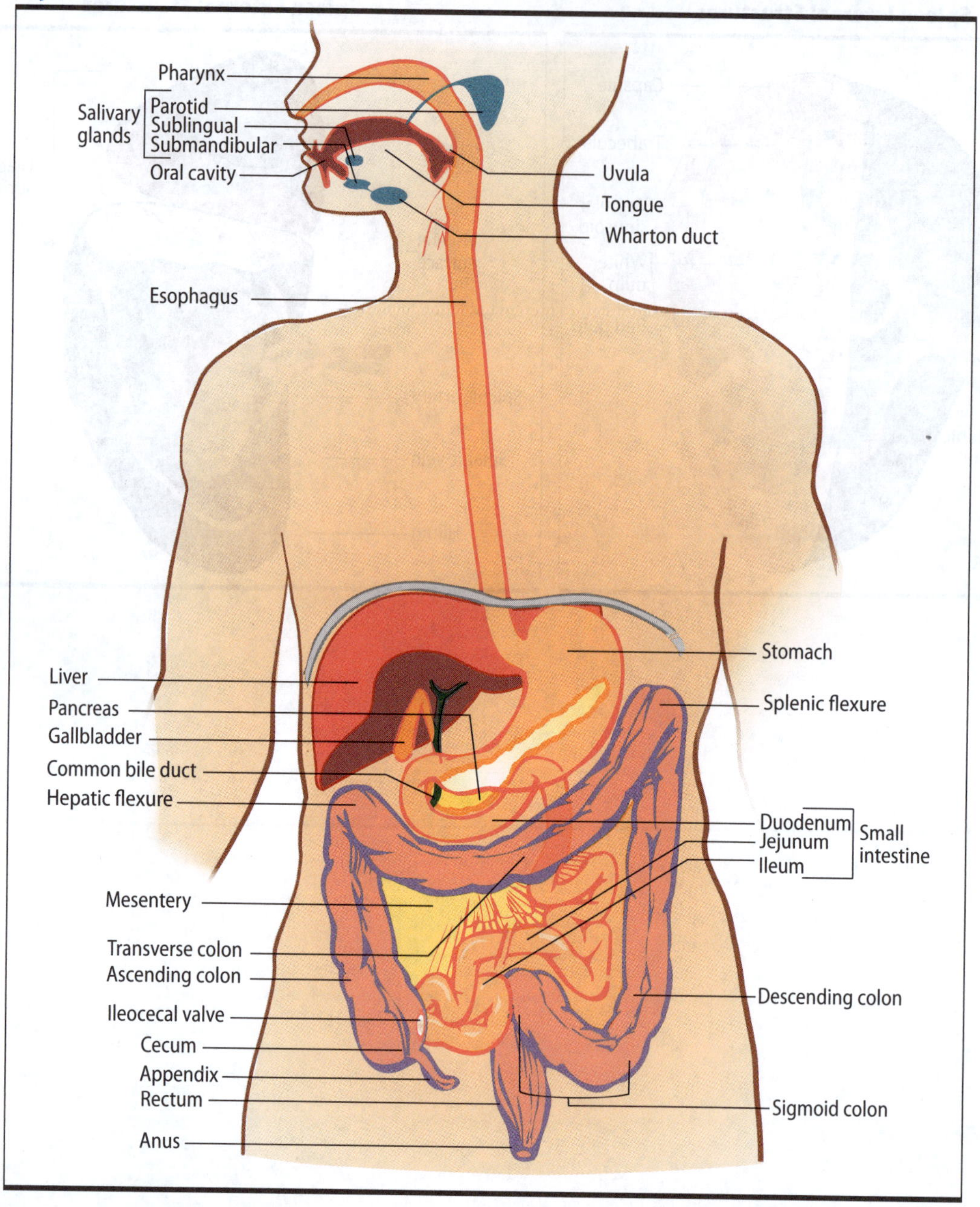

Gallbladder

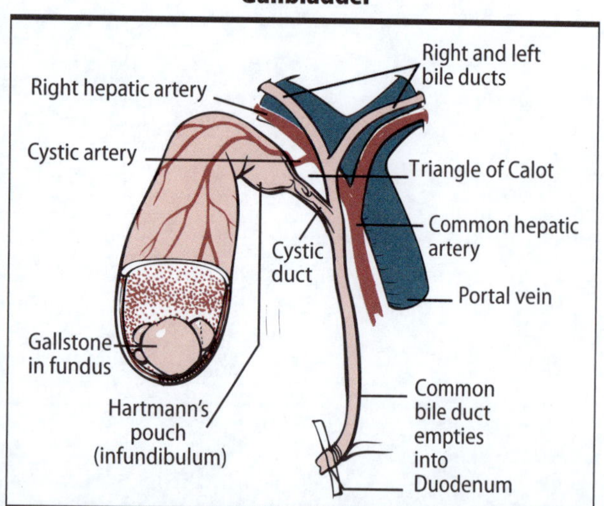

Stomach

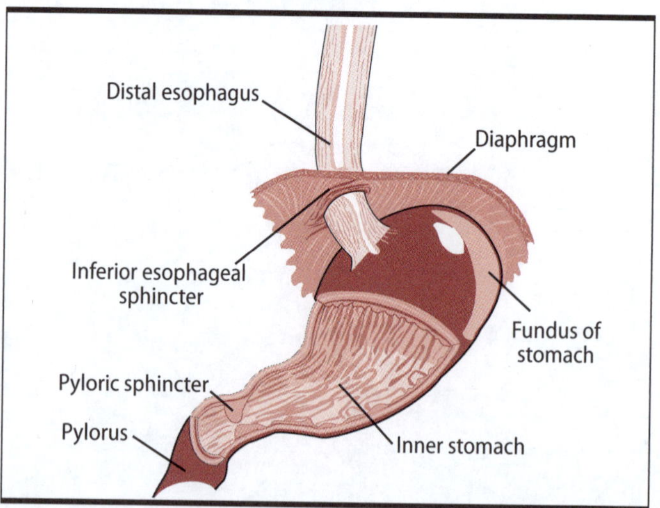

Mouth (Upper)

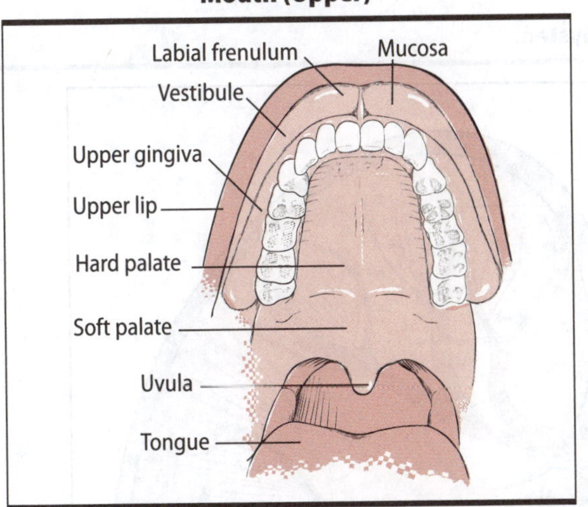

Mouth (Lower)

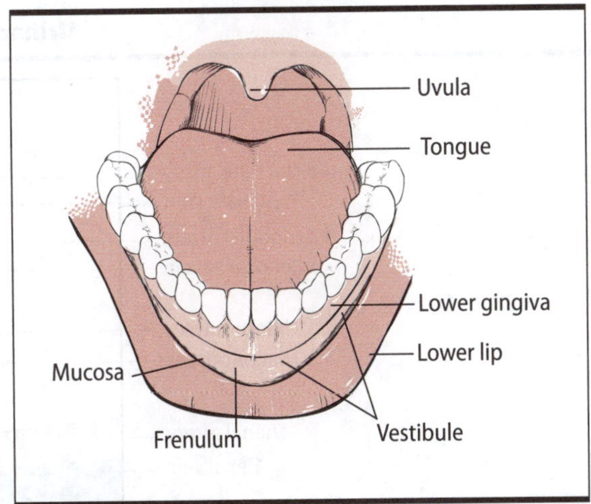

Pancreas

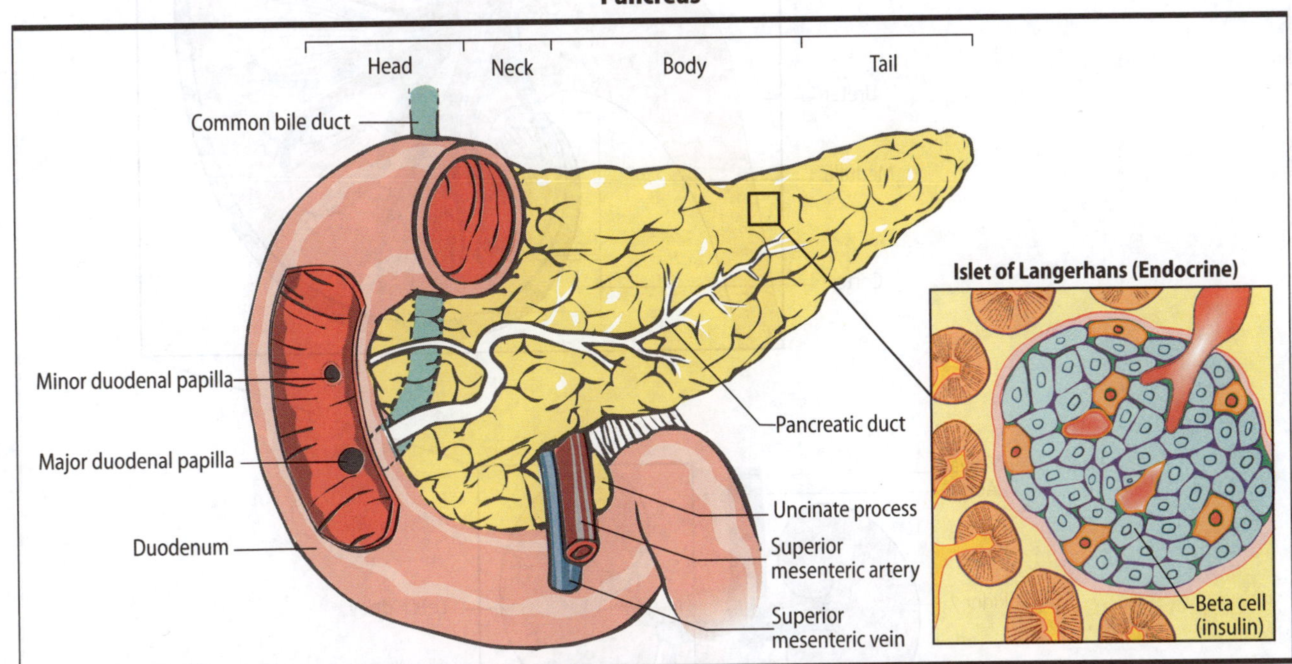

Liver

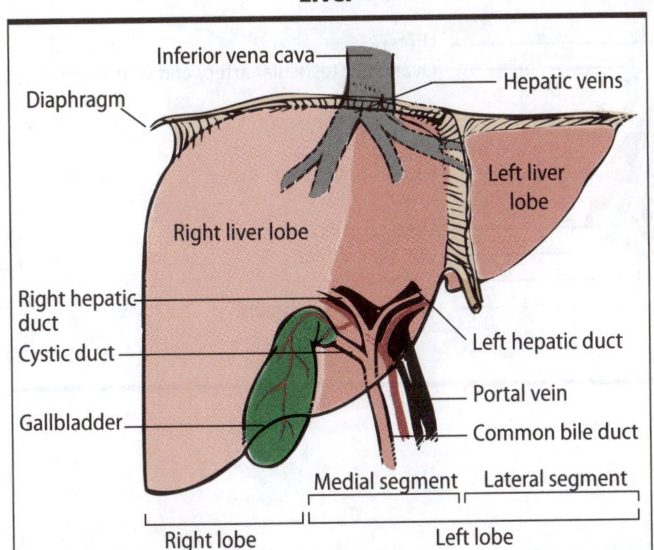

Anus

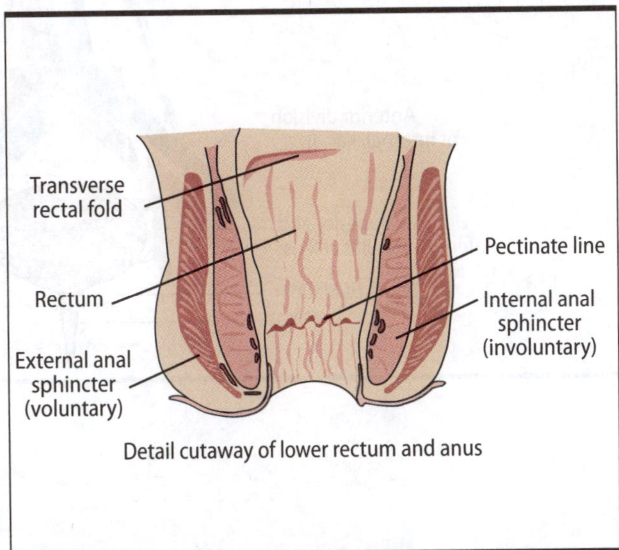

Detail cutaway of lower rectum and anus

Anatomical Illustrations

Genitourinary System

Urinary System

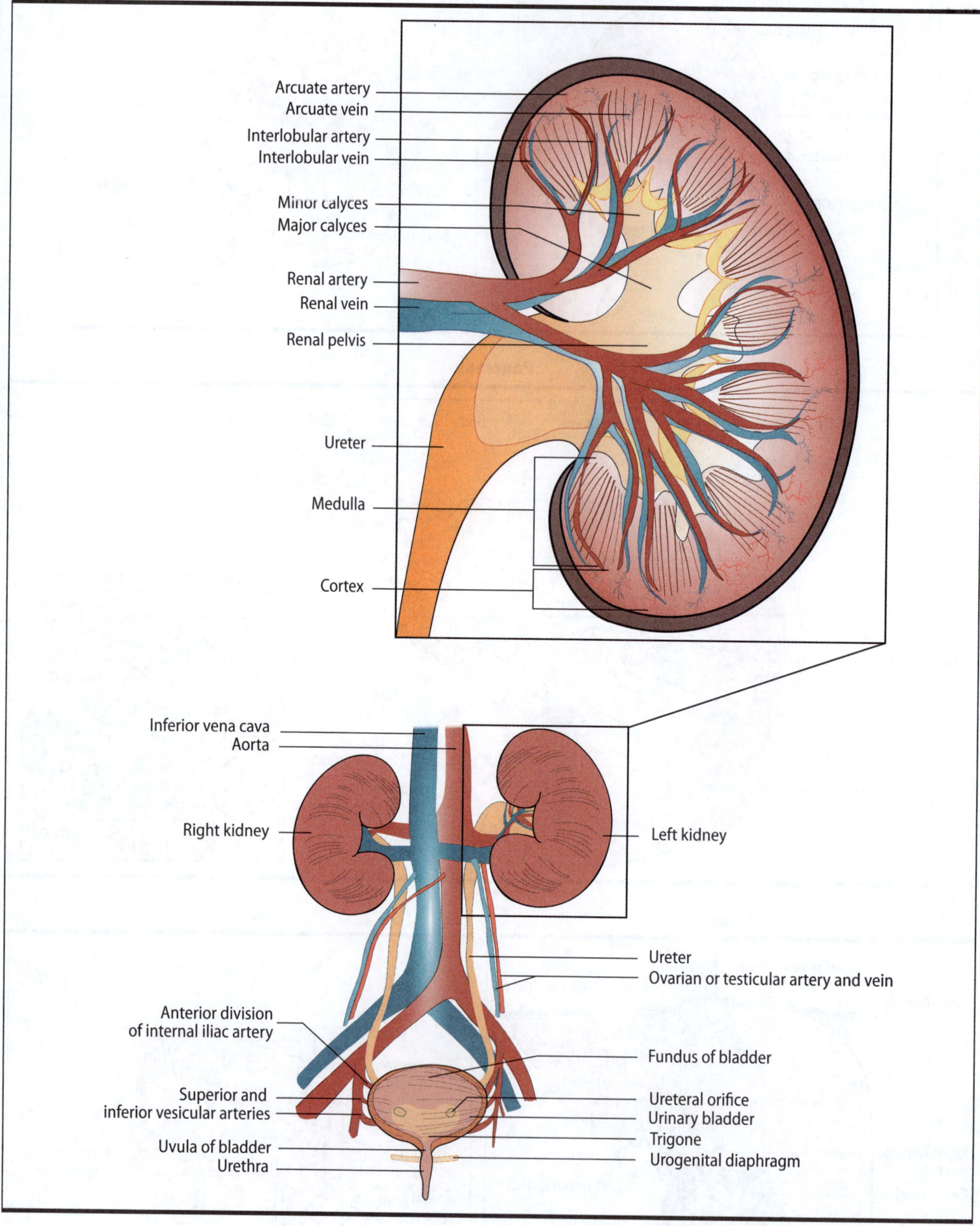

Nephron

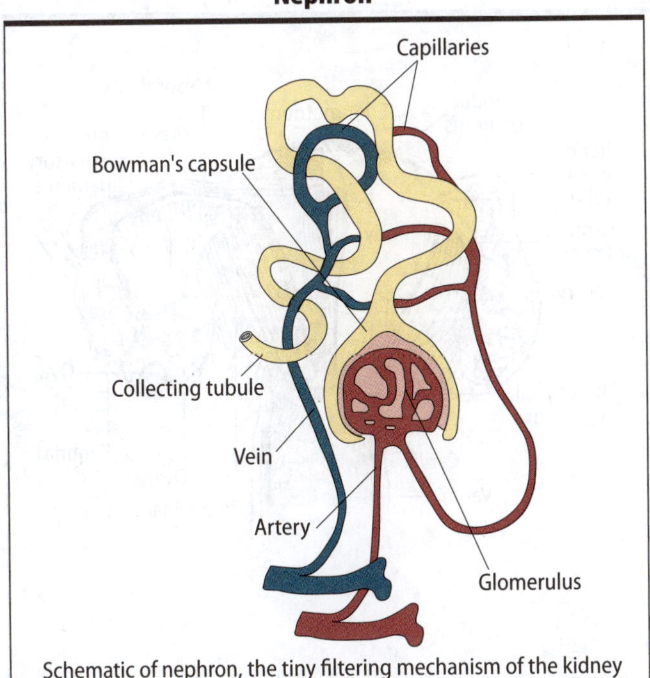

Schematic of nephron, the tiny filtering mechanism of the kidney

Male Genitourinary

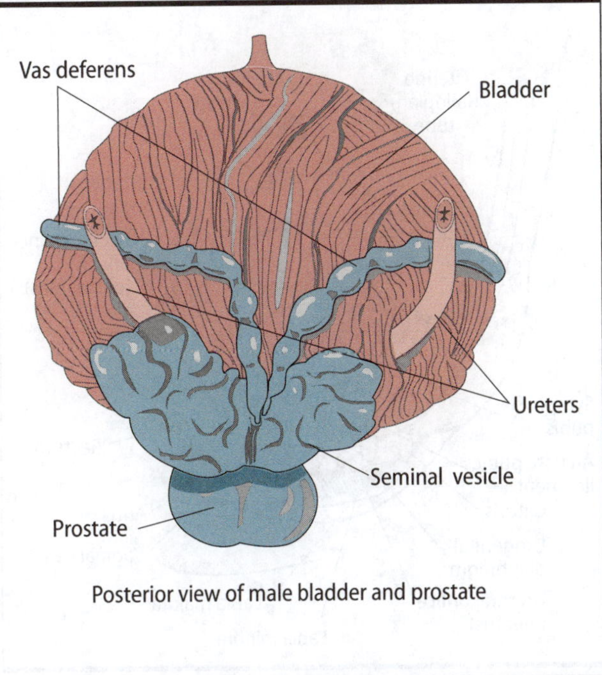

Posterior view of male bladder and prostate

Testis and Associated Structures

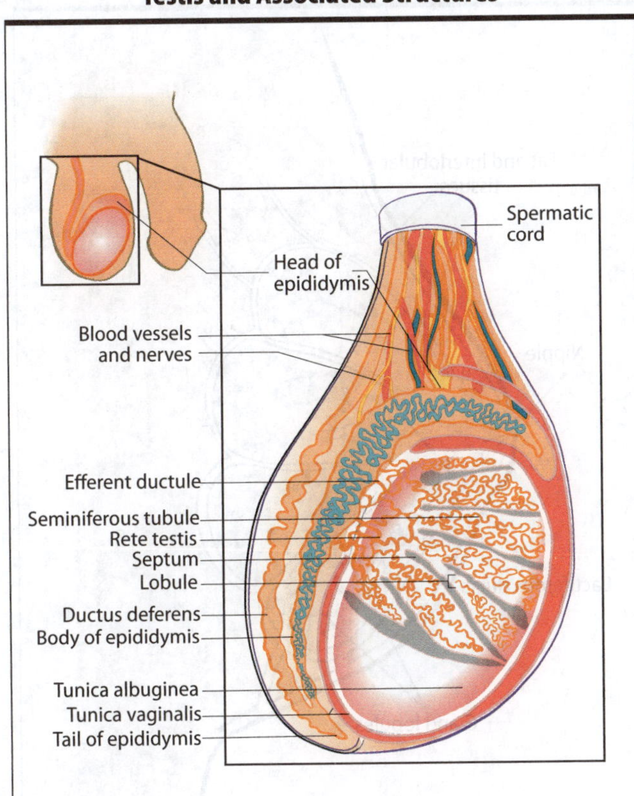

Male Genitourinary System

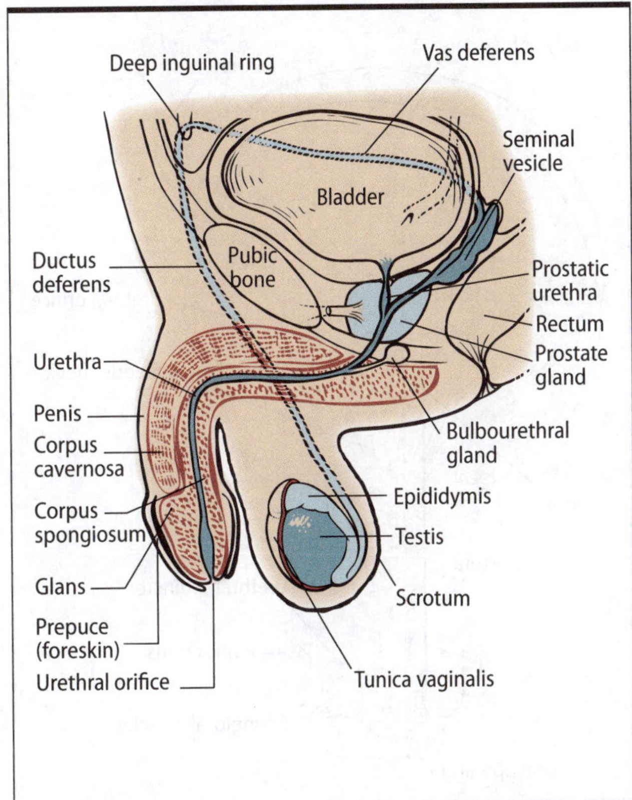

Female Genitourinary

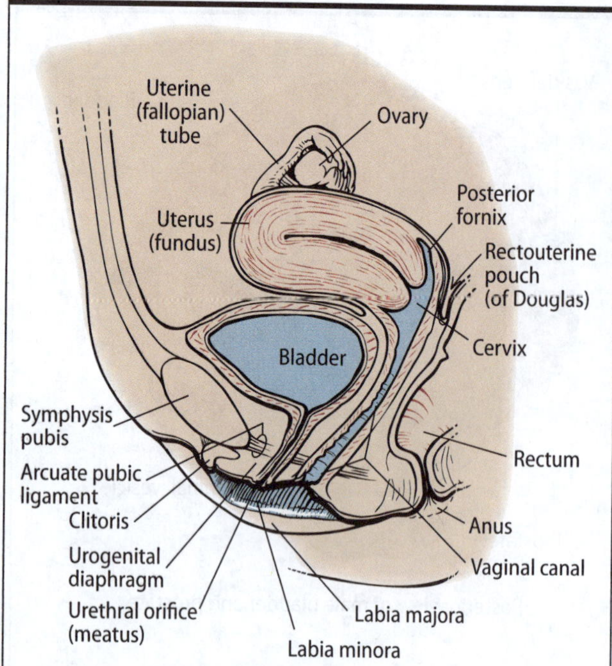

Female Reproductive System

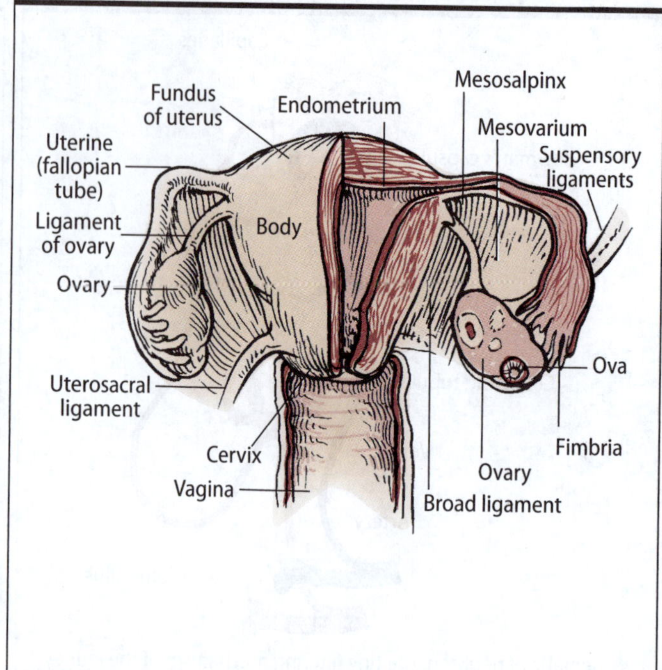

Female Bladder

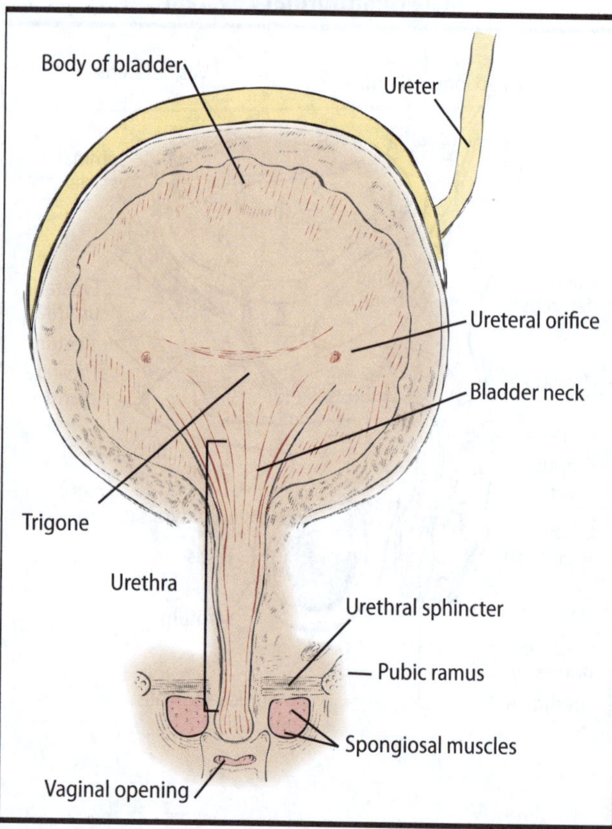

Female Breast

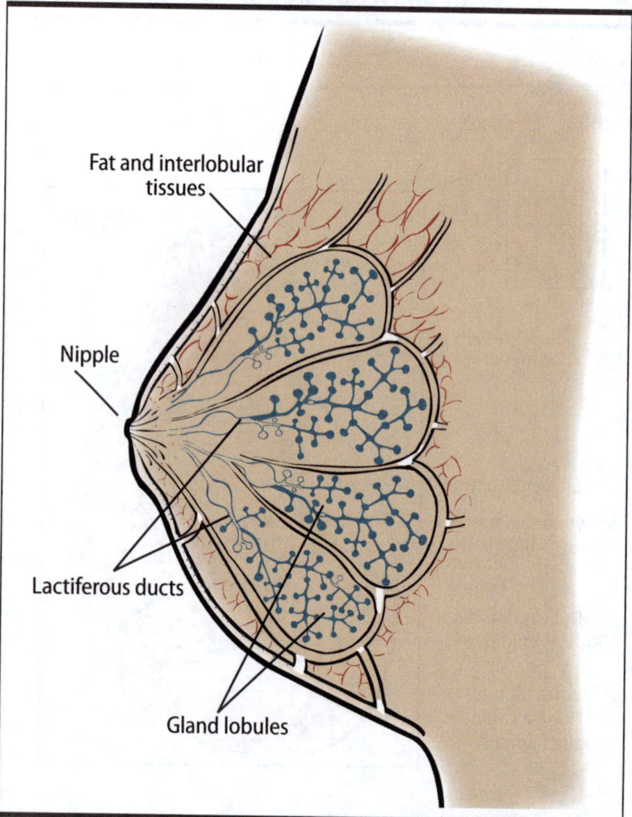

Endocrine System

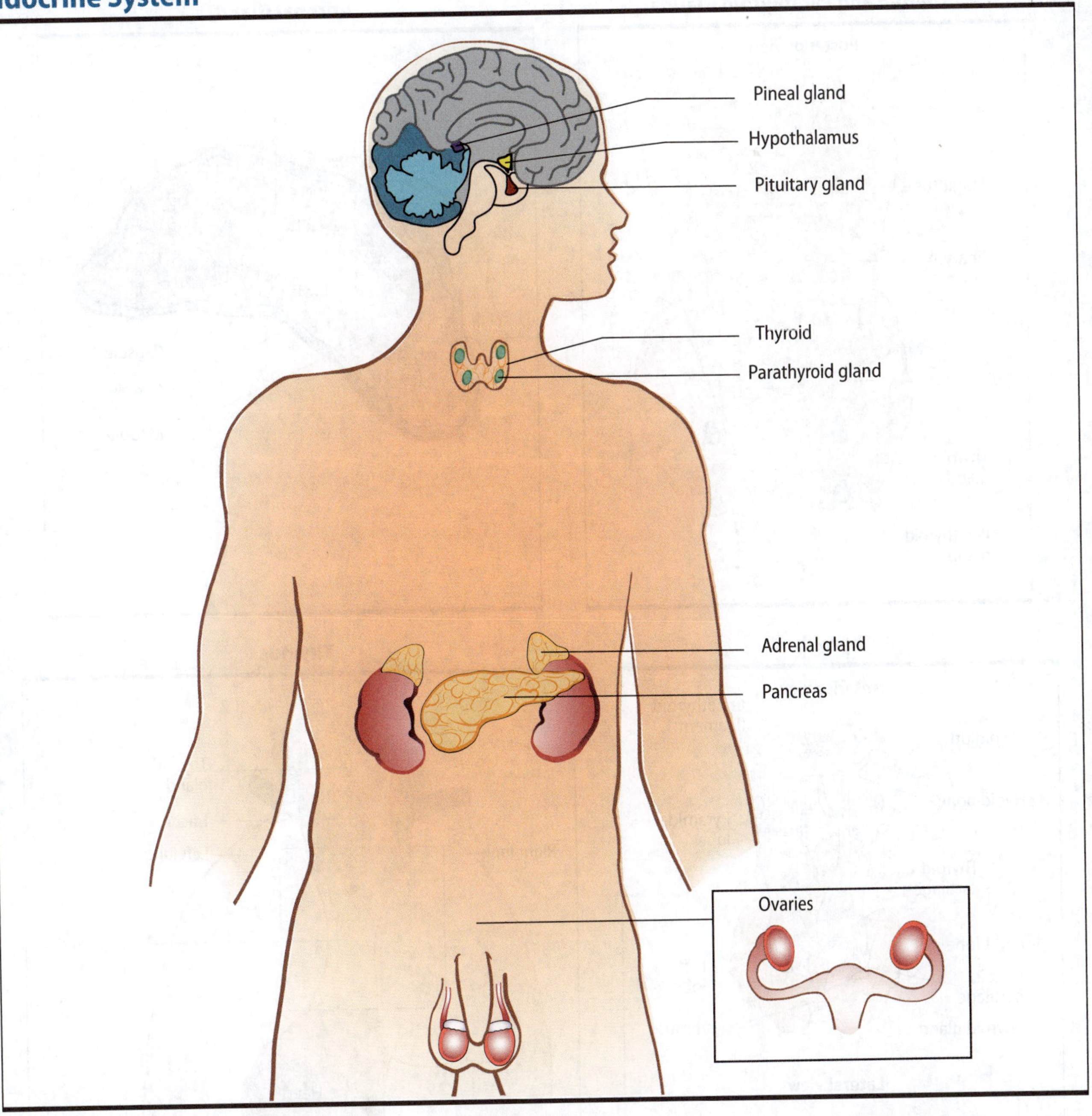

Pineal gland

Hypothalamus

Pituitary gland

Thyroid

Parathyroid gland

Adrenal gland

Pancreas

Ovaries

Structure of an Ovary

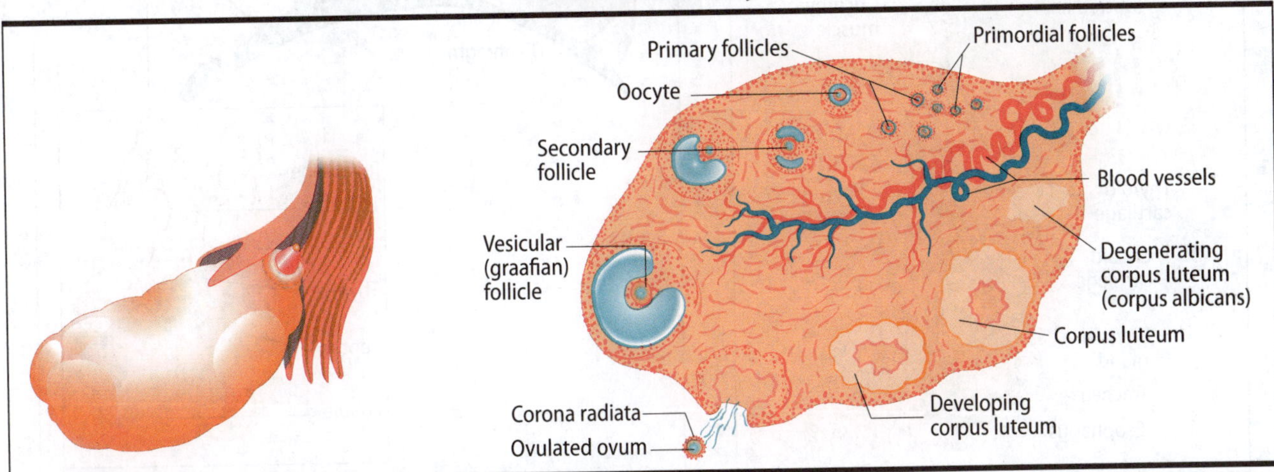

Thyroid and Parathyroid Glands

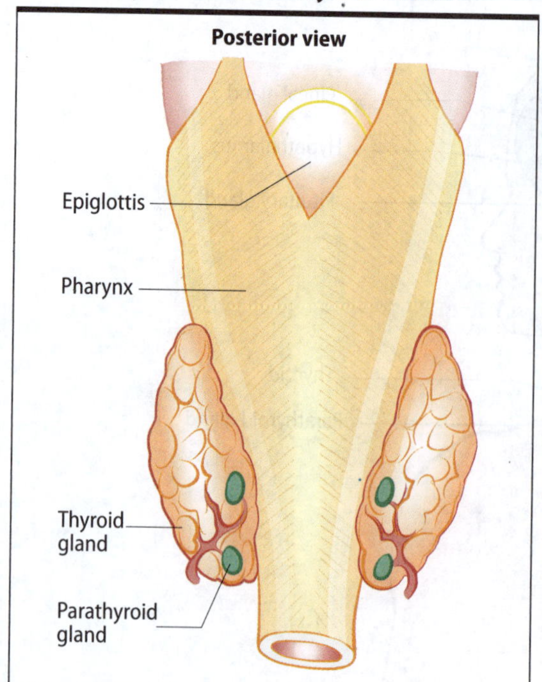

Adrenal Gland

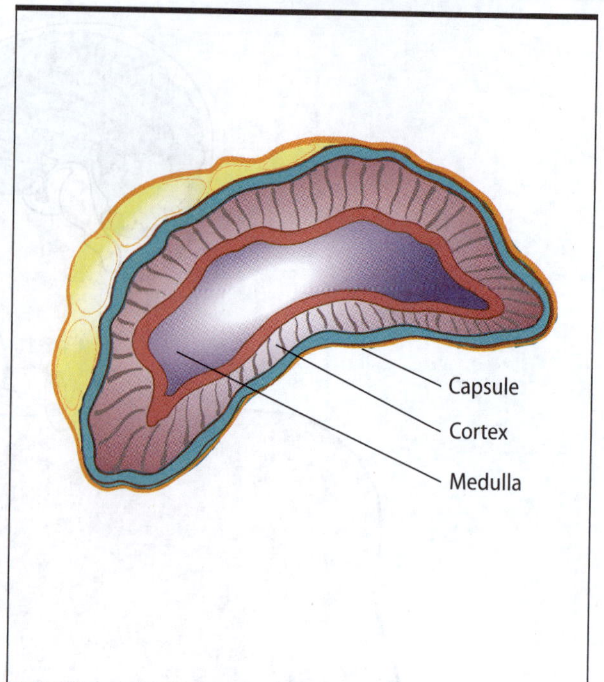

Thyroid

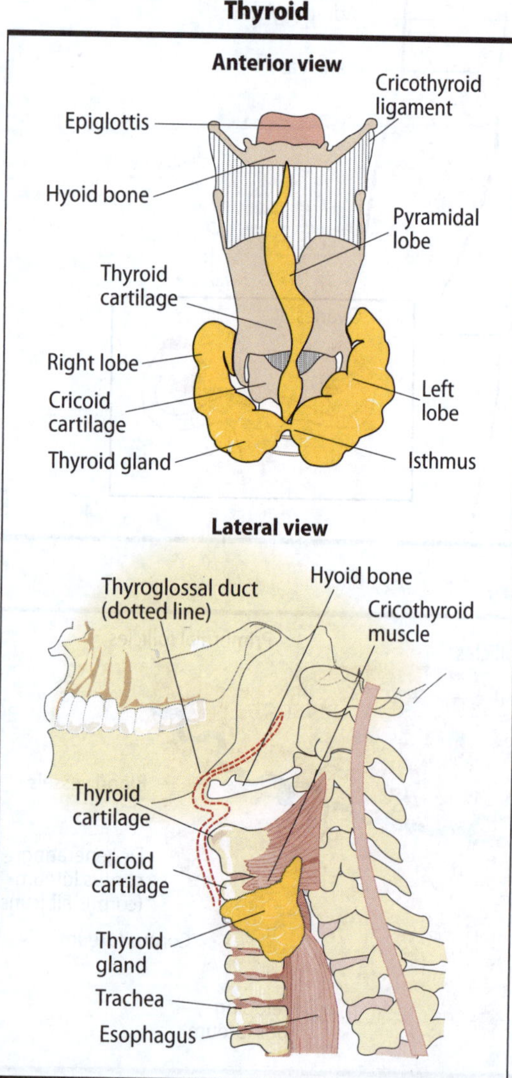

Thymus

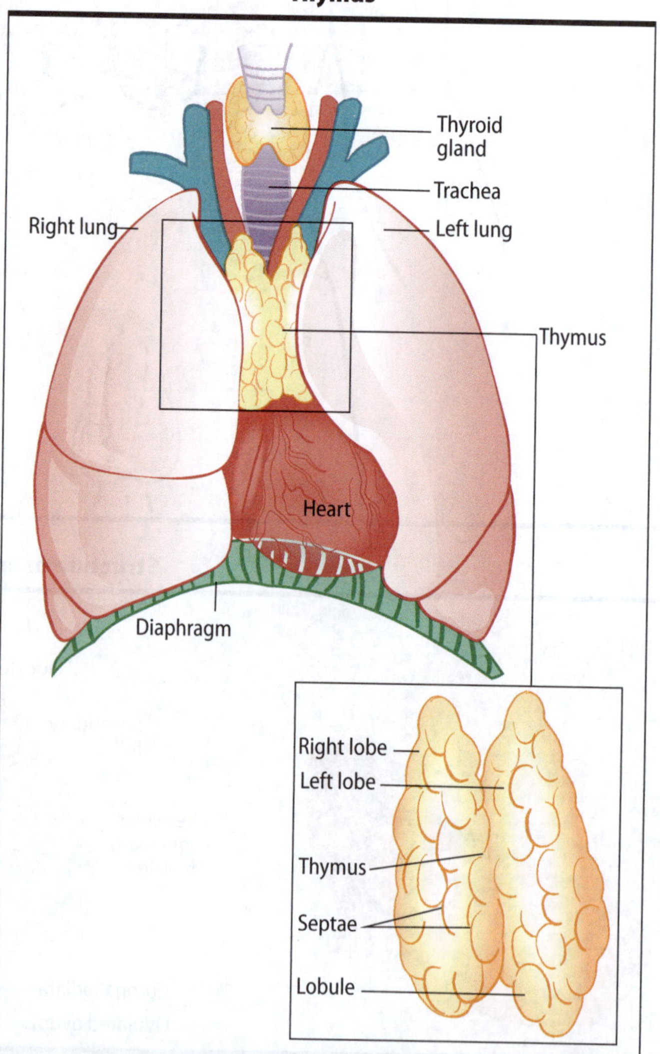

Nervous System

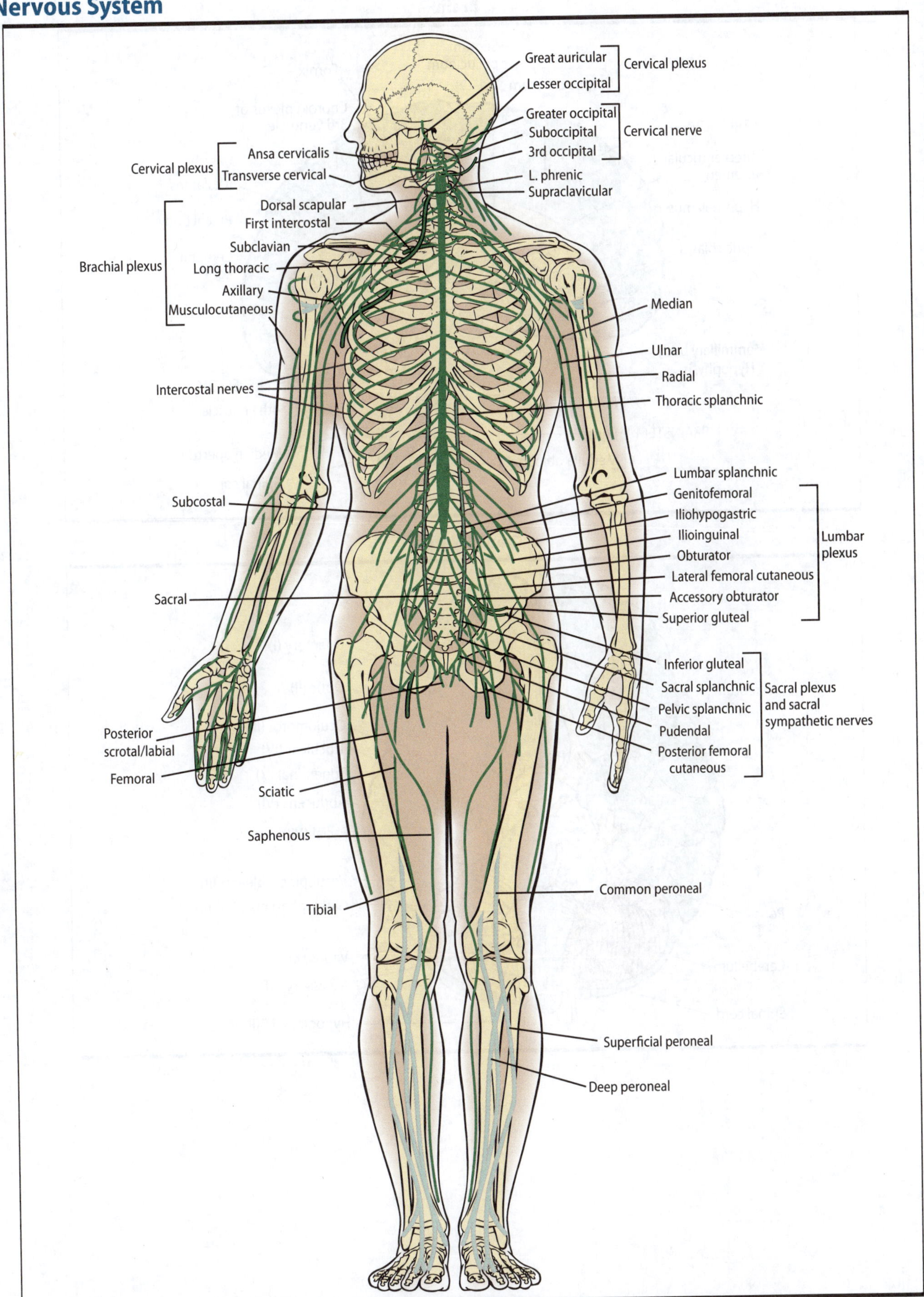

Brain

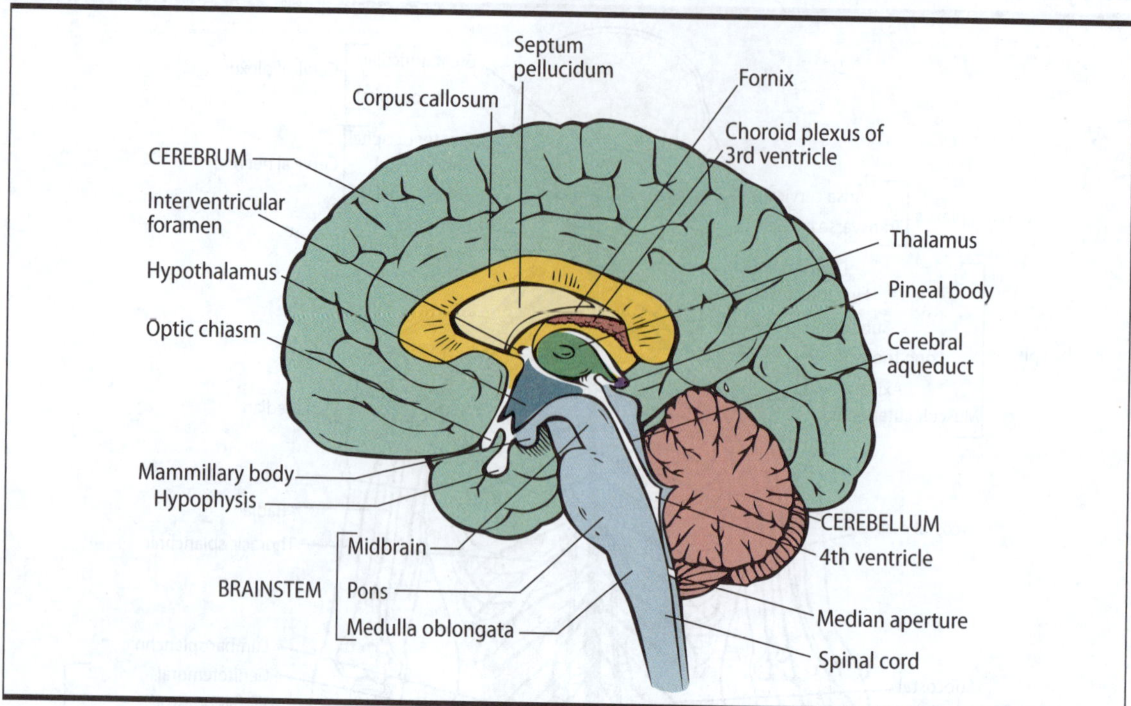

Cranial Nerves

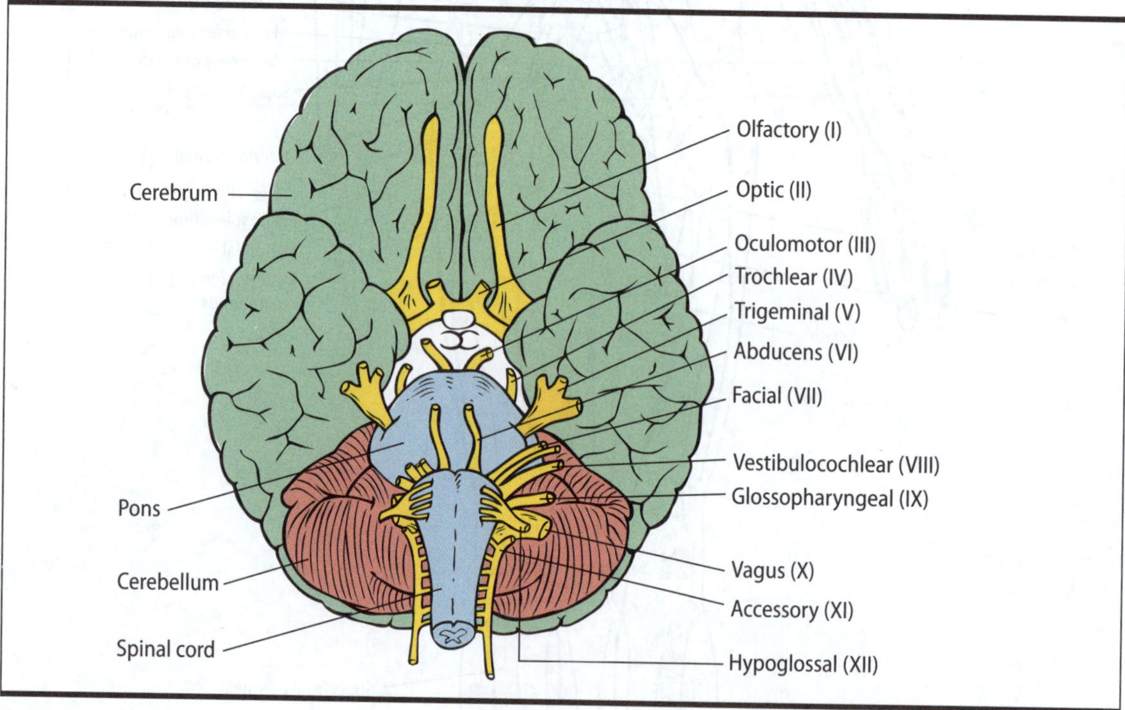

Spinal Cord and Spinal Nerves

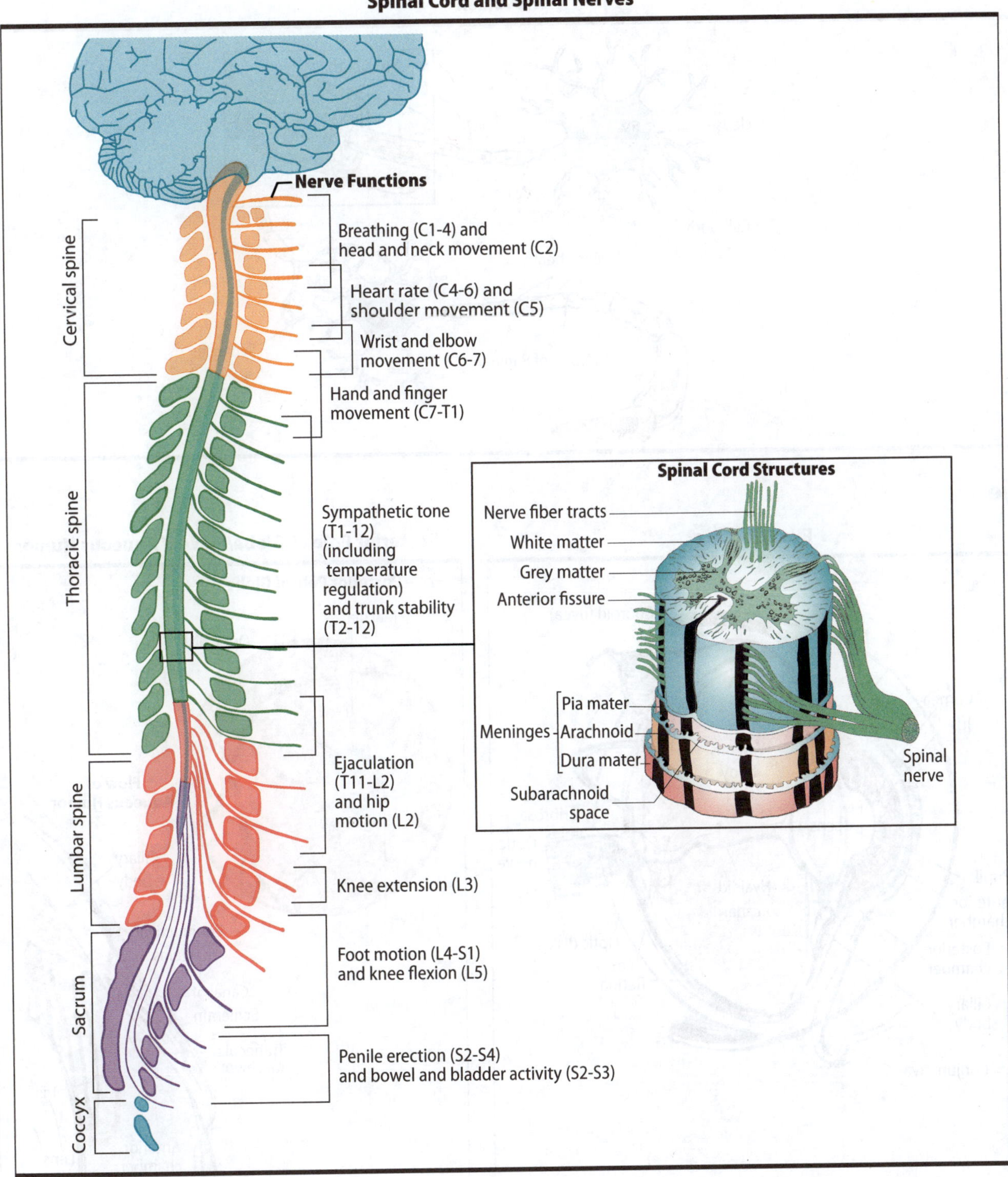

Nerve Cell

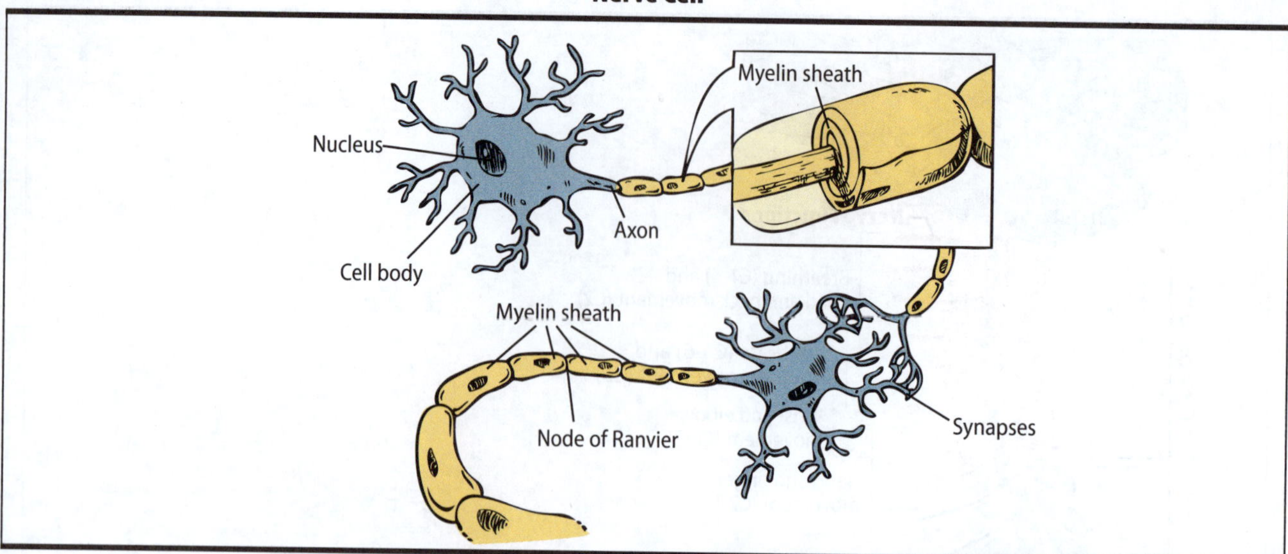

Eye

Eye Structure

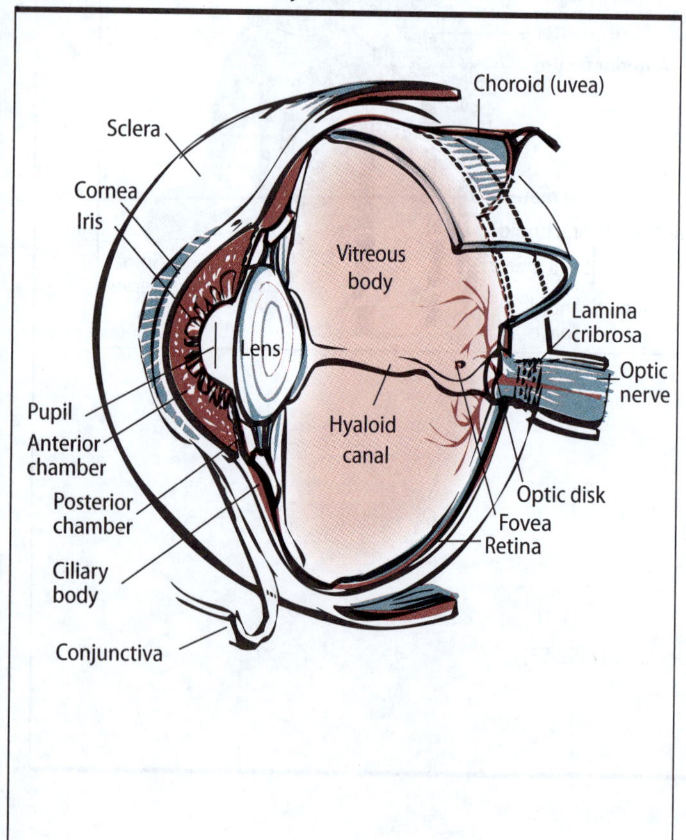

Posterior Pole of Globe/Flow of Aqueous Humor

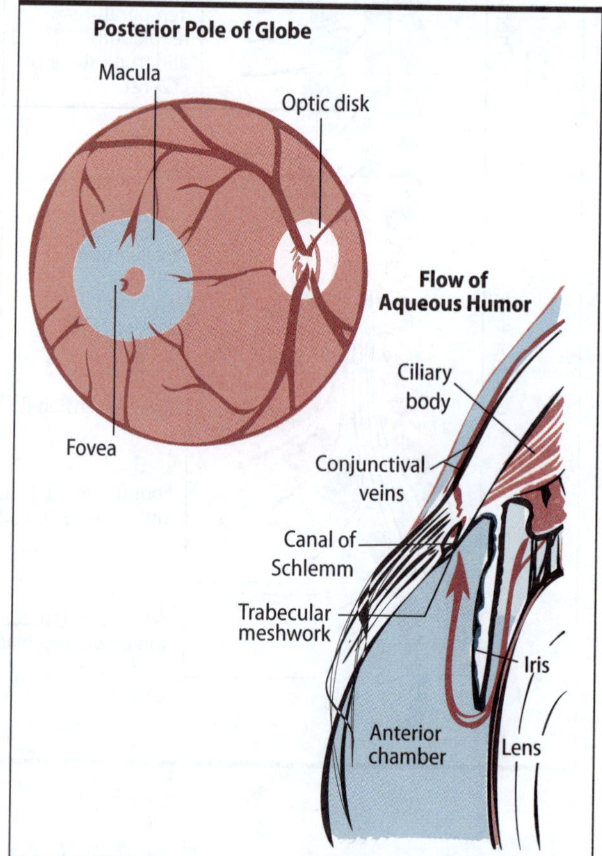

Eye Musculature

Superior rectus
Superior oblique
Lateral rectus
Medial rectus
Inferior rectus
Inferior oblique

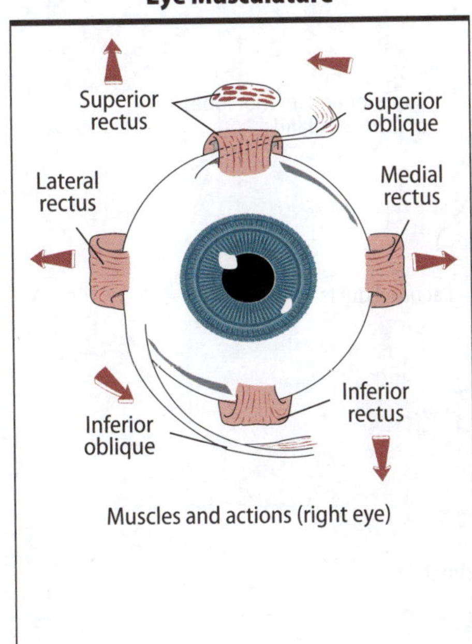

Muscles and actions (right eye)

Eyelid Structures

Superior fornix of conjunctiva
Opening of tarsal gland
Cornea
Lens
Iris
Inferior fornix of conjunctiva
Orbital part of superior eyelid
Sulcus of eyelid
Tarsal part of superior eyelid
Lacrimal puncta
Pupil
Iris
Lower eyelid

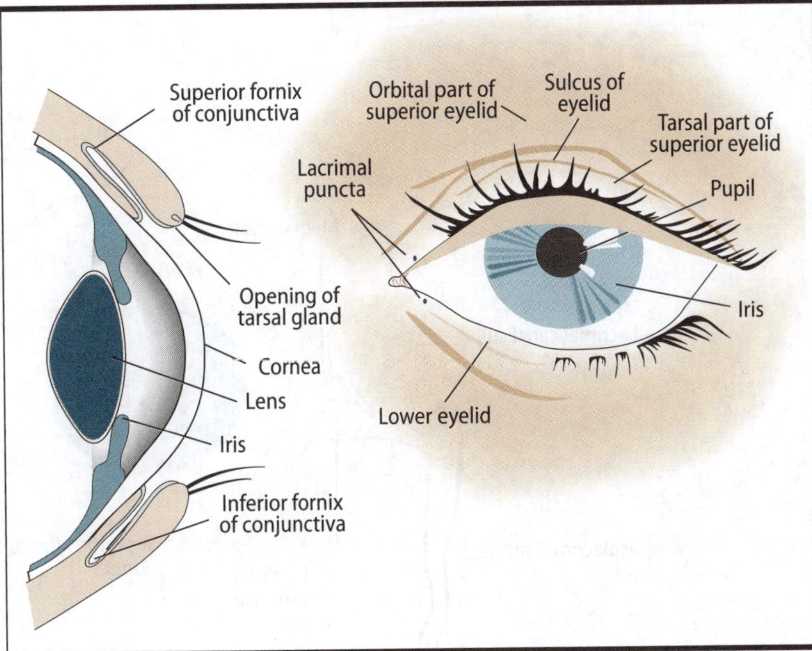

Ear and Lacrimal System

Ear Anatomy

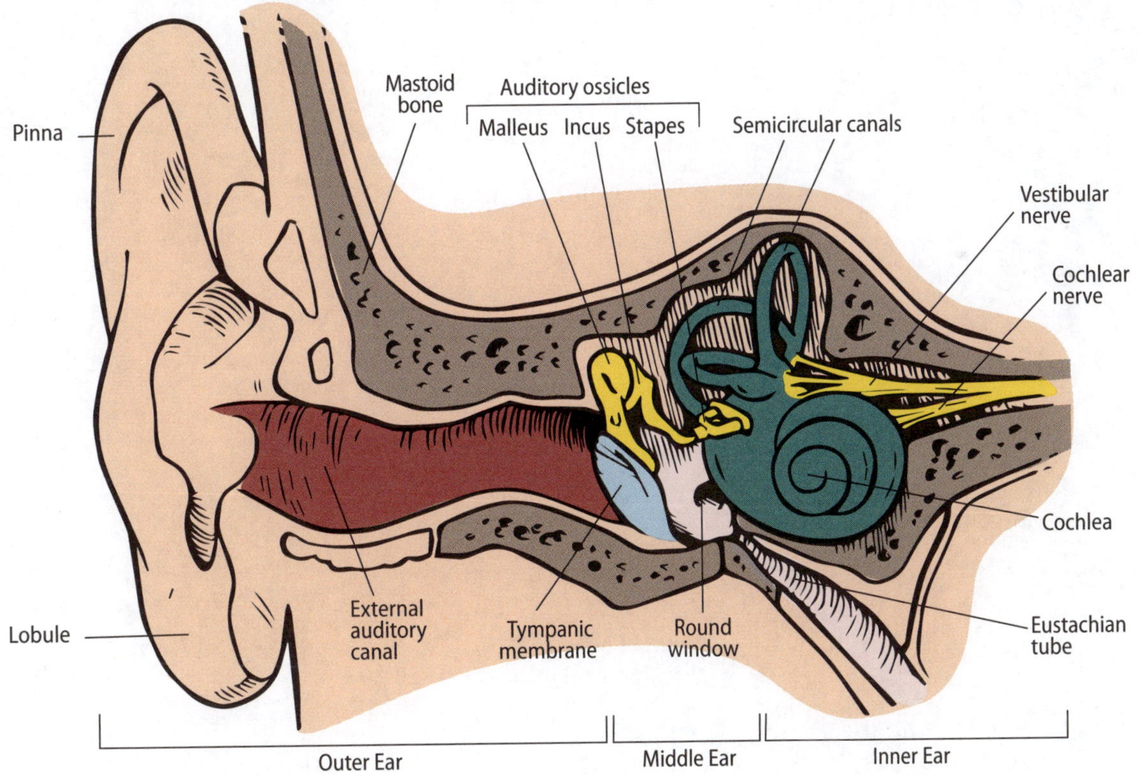

Pinna
Mastoid bone
Auditory ossicles
Malleus
Incus
Stapes
Semicircular canals
Vestibular nerve
Cochlear nerve
Cochlea
Eustachian tube
Round window
Tympanic membrane
External auditory canal
Lobule
Outer Ear
Middle Ear
Inner Ear

Lacrimal System

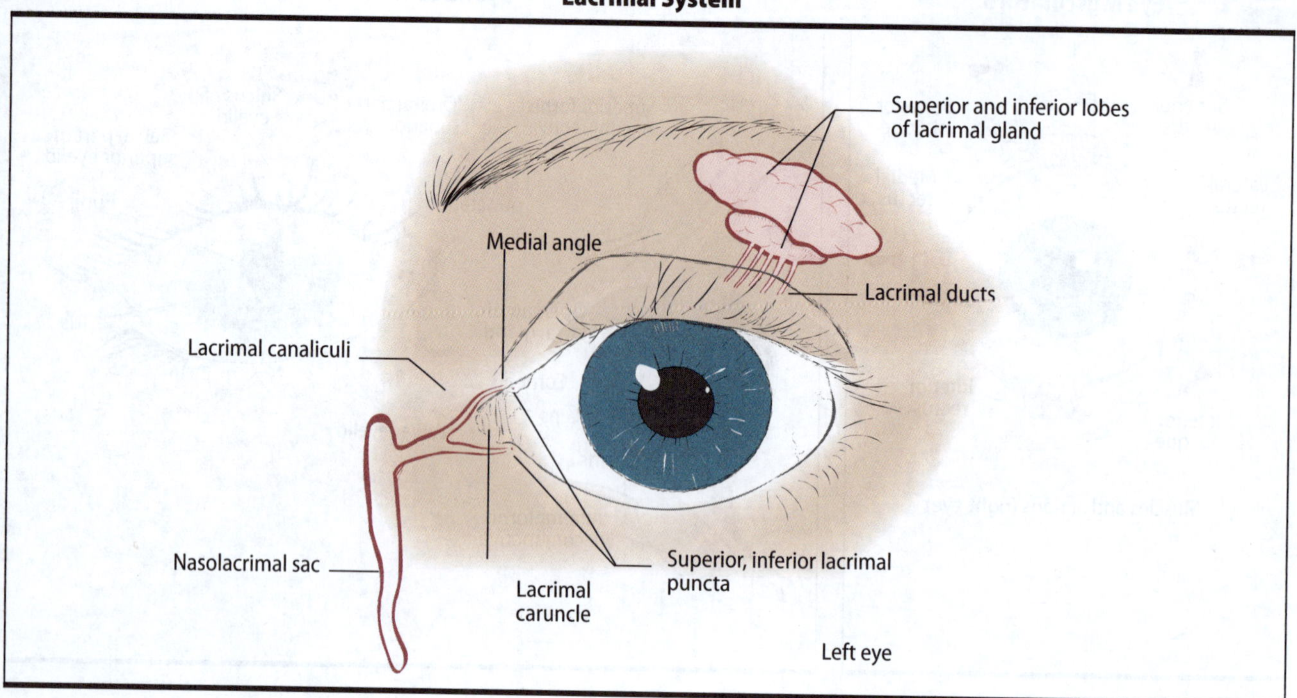

A

E

I

N

O

P

BLS - basic life support
ALS - advance life support

Transportation Services Including Ambulance A0021-A0999

This code range includes ground and air ambulance, nonemergency transportation (taxi, bus, automobile, wheelchair van), and ancillary transportation-related fees.

HCPCS Level II codes for ambulance services must be reported with modifiers that indicate pick-up origins and destinations. The modifier describing the arrangement (QM, QN) is listed first. The modifiers describing the origin and destination are listed second. Origin and destination modifiers are created by combining two alpha characters from the following list. Each alpha character, with the exception of X, represents either an origin or a destination. Each pair of alpha characters creates one modifier. The first position represents the origin and the second the destination. The modifiers most commonly used are:

D	Diagnostic or therapeutic site other than "P" or "H" when these are used as origin codes
E	Residential, domiciliary, custodial facility (other than 1819 facility)
G	Hospital-based ESRD facility
H	Hospital
I	Site of transfer (e.g., airport or helicopter pad) between modes of ambulance transport
J	Free standing ESRD facility
N	Skilled nursing facility (SNF)
P	Physician's office
R	Residence
S	Scene of accident or acute event
X	Intermediate stop at physician's office on way to hospital (destination code only)

Note: Modifier X can only be used as a destination code in the second position of a modifier. See S0215. For Medicaid, see T codes and T modifiers.

Ambulance Transport and Supplies

A0021 **Ambulance service, outside state per mile, transport (Medicaid only)** E1
CMS: 100-04,15,20.4

A0080 **Nonemergency transportation, per mile - vehicle provided by volunteer (individual or organization), with no vested interest** E1
CMS: 100-04,15,20.4

A0090 **Nonemergency transportation, per mile - vehicle provided by individual (family member, self, neighbor) with vested interest** E1
CMS: 100-04,15,20.4

A0100 **Nonemergency transportation; taxi** E1
CMS: 100-04,15,20.4

A0110 **Nonemergency transportation and bus, intra- or interstate carrier** E1
CMS: 100-04,15,20.4

A0120 **Nonemergency transportation: mini-bus, mountain area transports, or other transportation systems** E1
CMS: 100-04,15,20.4

A0130 **Nonemergency transportation: wheelchair van** E1
CMS: 100-04,15,20.4

A0140 **Nonemergency transportation and air travel (private or commercial) intra- or interstate** E1
CMS: 100-04,15,20.4

A0160 **Nonemergency transportation: per mile - caseworker or social worker** E1
CMS: 100-04,15,20.4

A0170 **Transportation ancillary: parking fees, tolls, other** E1
CMS: 100-04,15,20.4

A0180 **Nonemergency transportation: ancillary: lodging-recipient** E1
CMS: 100-04,15,20.4

A0190 **Nonemergency transportation: ancillary: meals, recipient** E1
CMS: 100-04,15,20.4

A0200 **Nonemergency transportation: ancillary: lodging, escort** E1
CMS: 100-04,15,20.4

A0210 **Nonemergency transportation: ancillary: meals, escort** E1
CMS: 100-04,15,20.4

A0225 **Ambulance service, neonatal transport, base rate, emergency transport, one way** E1
CMS: 100-02,10,10.1.2; 100-02,10,10.2.1; 100-02,10,30.1; 100-02,10,30.1.1; 100-04,15,20.4

A0380 **BLS mileage (per mile)** E1 ☑
See code(s): A0425
CMS: 100-02,10,10.1.2; 100-02,10,10.2.1; 100-02,10,10.3.3; 100-02,10,30.1; 100-02,10,30.1.1; 100-04,15,20.4; 100-04,15,30.2

A0382 **BLS routine disposable supplies** E1
CMS: 100-02,10,10.1.2; 100-02,10,10.2.1; 100-02,10,30.1; 100-02,10,30.1.1; 100-04,15,20.4

A0384 **BLS specialized service disposable supplies; defibrillation (used by ALS ambulances and BLS ambulances in jurisdictions where defibrillation is permitted in BLS ambulances)** E1
CMS: 100-02,10,10.1.2; 100-02,10,10.2.1; 100-02,10,30.1; 100-02,10,30.1.1; 100-04,15,20.4

A0390 **ALS mileage (per mile)** E1 ☑
See code(s): A0425
CMS: 100-02,10,10.1.2; 100-02,10,10.2.1; 100-02,10,10.3.3; 100-02,10,30.1; 100-02,10,30.1.1; 100-04,15,20.4; 100-04,15,30.2

A0392 **ALS specialized service disposable supplies; defibrillation (to be used only in jurisdictions where defibrillation cannot be performed in BLS ambulances)** E1
CMS: 100-02,10,10.1.2; 100-02,10,10.2.1; 100-02,10,30.1; 100-02,10,30.1.1; 100-04,15,20.4

A0394 **ALS specialized service disposable supplies; IV drug therapy** E1
CMS: 100-02,10,10.1.2; 100-02,10,10.2.1; 100-02,10,30.1; 100-02,10,30.1.1; 100-04,15,20.4

A0396 **ALS specialized service disposable supplies; esophageal intubation** E1
CMS: 100-02,10,10.1.2; 100-02,10,10.2.1; 100-02,10,30.1; 100-02,10,30.1.1; 100-04,15,20.4

A0398 **ALS routine disposable supplies** E1
CMS: 100-02,10,10.1.2; 100-02,10,10.2.1; 100-02,10,30.1; 100-02,10,30.1.1; 100-04,15,20.4

Waiting Time

Units	Time
1	1/2 to 1 hr.
2	1 to 1-1/2 hrs.
3	1-1/2 to 2 hrs.
4	2 to 2-1/2 hrs.
5	2-1/2 to 3 hrs.
6	3 to 3-1/2 hrs.
7	3-1/2 to 4 hrs.
8	4 to 4-1/2 hrs.
9	4-1/2 to 5 hrs.
10	5 to 5-1/2 hrs.

A0420 **Ambulance waiting time (ALS or BLS), one-half (1/2) hour increments** E1
CMS: 100-02,10,10.1.2; 100-02,10,10.2.1; 100-02,10,30.1; 100-02,10,30.1.1; 100-04,15,20.4

Other Ambulance Services

A0422 **Ambulance (ALS or BLS) oxygen and oxygen supplies, life sustaining situation** E1
CMS: 100-02,10,10.1.2; 100-02,10,10.2.1; 100-02,10,30.1; 100-02,10,30.1.1; 100-04,15,20.4

A0424 **Extra ambulance attendant, ground (ALS or BLS) or air (fixed or rotary winged); (requires medical review)** E1
Pertinent documentation to evaluate medical appropriateness should be included when this code is reported.
CMS: 100-02,10,10.1.2; 100-02,10,10.2.1; 100-02,10,30.1; 100-02,10,30.1.1; 100-04,15,20.4; 100-04,15,30.2.1

A0425 **Ground mileage, per statute mile** A ☑
CMS: 100-02,10,10.1.2; 100 02,10,10.2.1; 100-02,10,10.2.2; 100-02,10,10.3.3; 100-02,10,20; 100-02,10,30.1; 100-02,10,30.1.1; 100-02,10.20; 100-04,15,10.3; 100-04,15,20.1.4; 100-04,15,20.4; 100-04,15,20.6; 100-04,15,30; 100-04,15,30.1.2; 100-04,15,30.2.1; 100-04,15,40

A0426 **Ambulance service, advanced life support, nonemergency transport, level 1 (ALS 1)** A
CMS: 100-02,10,10.1.2; 100-02,10,10.2.1; 100-02,10,10.2.2; 100-02,10,10.3.3; 100-02,10,20; 100-02,10,30.1; 100-02,10,30.1.1; 100-02,10.20; 100-04,15,10.3; 100-04,15,20.1.4; 100-04,15,20.4; 100-04,15,30; 100-04,15,30.1.2; 100-04,15,30.2; 100-04,15,30.2.1; 100-04,15,40

A0427 **Ambulance service, advanced life support, emergency transport, level 1 (ALS 1 - emergency)** A
CMS: 100-02,10,10.1.2; 100-02,10,10.2.1; 100-02,10,10.2.2; 100-02,10,10.3.3; 100-02,10,20; 100-02,10,30.1; 100-02,10,30.1.1; 100-02,10.20; 100-04,15,10.3; 100-04,15,20.1.4; 100-04,15,20.4; 100-04,15,30; 100-04,15,30.1.2; 100-04,15,30.2; 100-04,15,30.2.1; 100-04,15,40

A0428 **Ambulance service, basic life support, nonemergency transport, (BLS)** A
CMS: 100-02,10,10.1.2; 100-02,10,10.2.1; 100-02,10,10.2.2; 100-02,10,10.3.3; 100-02,10,20; 100-02,10,30.1; 100-02,10,30.1.1; 100-02,10.20; 100-04,15,10.3; 100-04,15,20.1.4; 100-04,15,20.4; 100-04,15,20.6; 100-04,15,30; 100-04,15,30.1.2; 100-04,15,30.2; 100-04,15,30.2.1; 100-04,15,40

A0429 **Ambulance service, basic life support, emergency transport (BLS, emergency)** A
CMS: 100-02,10,10.1.2; 100-02,10,10.2.1; 100-02,10,10.2.2; 100-02,10,10.3.3; 100-02,10,20; 100-02,10,30.1; 100-02,10,30.1.1; 100-02,10.20; 100-04,15,10.3; 100-04,15,20.1.4; 100-04,15,20.4; 100-04,15,30; 100-04,15,30.1.2; 100-04,15,30.2; 100-04,15,30.2.1; 100-04,15,40

A0430 **Ambulance service, conventional air services, transport, one way (fixed wing)** A
CMS: 100-02,10,10.1.2; 100-02,10,10.2.1; 100-02,10,10.2.2; 100-02,10,10.3.3; 100-02,10,20; 100-02,10,30.1; 100-02,10,30.1.1; 100-02,10.20; 100-04,15,10.3; 100-04,15,20.1.4; 100-04,15,20.3; 100-04,15,20.4; 100-04,15,30; 100-04,15,30.1.2; 100-04,15,30.2; 100-04,15,30.2.1; 100-04,15,40

A0431 **Ambulance service, conventional air services, transport, one way (rotary wing)** A
CMS: 100-02,10,10.1.2; 100-02,10,10.2.1; 100-02,10,10.2.2; 100-02,10,10.3.3; 100-02,10,20; 100-02,10,30.1; 100-02,10,30.1.1; 100-02,10.20; 100-04,15,10.3; 100-04,15,20.1.4; 100-04,15,20.3; 100-04,15,20.4; 100-04,15,30; 100-04,15,30.1.2; 100-04,15,30.2; 100-04,15,30.2.1; 100-04,15,40

A0432 **Paramedic intercept (PI), rural area, transport furnished by a volunteer ambulance company which is prohibited by state law from billing third-party payers** A
CMS: 100-02,10,10.1.2; 100-02,10,10.2.1; 100-02,10,10.2.2; 100-02,10,10.3.3; 100-02,10,20; 100-02,10,30.1; 100-02,10,30.1.1; 100-02,10.20; 100-04,15,10.3; 100-04,15,20.1.4; 100-04,15,20.4; 100-04,15,30; 100-04,15,30.1.2; 100-04,15,30.2; 100-04,15,30.2.1; 100-04,15,40

A0433 **Advanced life support, level 2 (ALS 2)** A
CMS: 100-02,10,10.1.2; 100-02,10,10.2.1; 100-02,10,10.2.2; 100-02,10,10.3.3; 100-02,10,20; 100-02,10,30.1; 100-02,10,30.1.1; 100-02,10.20; 100-04,15,10.3; 100-04,15,20.1.4; 100-04,15,20.4; 100-04,15,30; 100-04,15,30.1.2; 100-04,15,30.2; 100-04,15,30.2.1; 100-04,15,40

A0434 **Specialty care transport (SCT)** A
CMS: 100-02,10,10.1.2; 100-02,10,10.2.1; 100-02,10,10.2.2; 100-02,10,10.3.3; 100-02,10,20; 100-02,10,30.1; 100-02,10,30.1.1; 100-02,10.20; 100-04,15,10.3; 100-04,15,20.1.4; 100-04,15,20.4; 100-04,15,30; 100-04,15,30.1.2; 100-04,15,30.2; 100-04,15,30.2.1; 100-04,15,40

A0435 **Fixed wing air mileage, per statute mile** A
CMS: 100-02,10,10.1.2; 100-02,10,10.2.1; 100-02,10,10.2.2; 100-02,10,10.3.3; 100-02,10,20; 100-02,10,30.1; 100-02,10,30.1.1; 100-02,10.20; 100-04,15,10.3; 100-04,15,20.1.4; 100-04,15,20.3; 100-04,15,20.4; 100-04,15,30; 100-04,15,30.1.2; 100-04,15,30.2; 100-04,15,30.2.1; 100-04,15,40

A0436 **Rotary wing air mileage, per statute mile** A
CMS: 100-02,10,10.1.2; 100-02,10,10.2.1; 100-02,10,10.2.2; 100-02,10,10.3.3; 100-02,10,20; 100-02,10,30.1; 100-02,10,30.1.1; 100-02,10.20; 100-04,15,10.3; 100-04,15,20.1.4; 100-04,15,20.3; 100-04,15,20.4; 100-04,15,30; 100-04,15,30.1.2; 100-04,15,30.2; 100-04,15,30.2.1; 100-04,15,40

A0888 **Noncovered ambulance mileage, per mile (e.g., for miles traveled beyond closest appropriate facility)** E1
CMS: 100-02,10,10.1.2; 100-02,10,10.2.1; 100-02,10,20; 100-02,10,30.1; 100-02,10,30.1.1; 100-04,15,20.4; 100-04,15,30.1.2; 100-04,15,30.2.4

A0998 **Ambulance response and treatment, no transport** E1
CMS: 100-02,10,10.1.2; 100-02,10,10.2.1; 100-02,10,30.1; 100-02,10,30.1.1; 100-04,15,20.4

A0999 **Unlisted ambulance service** A
CMS: 100-02,10,10.1; 100-02,10,10.1.2; 100-02,10,10.2.1; 100-02,10,20; 100-02,10,30.1; 100-02,10,30.1.1; 100-04,15,20.4

Medical and Surgical Supplies A2001-A9999

This section covers a wide variety of medical, surgical, and some durable medical equipment (DME) related supplies and accessories. DME-related supplies, accessories, maintenance, and repair required to ensure the proper functioning of this equipment is generally covered by Medicare under the prosthetic devices provision.

Skin Substitutes

A2001 **InnovaMatrix AC, per sq cm** N N1
AHA: 1Q,22

A2002 **Mirragen Advanced Wound Matrix, per sq cm** N N1
AHA: 1Q,22

A2004 **XCelliStem, 1 mg** N N1
AHA: 1Q,22

A2005 **Microlyte Matrix, per sq cm** N N1
AHA: 1Q,22

A2006 **NovoSorb SynPath dermal matrix, per sq cm** N N1
AHA: 1Q,22

A2007 **Restrata, per sq cm** N N1
AHA: 1Q,22

A2008 **TheraGenesis, per sq cm** N N1
AHA: 1Q,22

A2009 **Symphony, per sq cm** N N1
AHA: 1Q,22

A2010 **Apis, per sq cm** N N1
AHA: 1Q,22

A2011 **Supra SDRM, per sq cm** N N1
AHA: 2Q,22

A2012 SUPRATHEL, per sq cm N N1
AHA: 2Q,22

A2013 InnovaMatrix FS, per sq cm N N1
AHA: 2Q,22

A2014 Omeza Collagen Matrix, per 100 mg N N1
AHA: 4Q,22

A2015 Phoenix Wound Matrix, per sq cm N N1
AHA: 4Q,22

A2016 PermeaDerm B, per sq cm N N1
AHA: 4Q,22

A2017 PermeaDerm Glove, each N N1
AHA: 4Q,22

A2018 PermeaDerm C, per sq cm N N1
AHA: 4Q,22

A2019 Kerecis Omega3 MariGen Shield, per sq cm N N1
AHA: 2Q,23

A2020 AC5 Advanced Wound System (AC5) N N1
AHA: 2Q,23

A2021 NeoMatriX, per sq cm N N1
AHA: 2Q,23

A2022 InnovaBurn or InnovaMatrix XL, per sq cm N N1
AHA: 4Q,23

A2023 InnovaMatrix PD, 1 mg N N1
AHA: 4Q,23

▲ **A2024** Resolve Matrix or XenoPatch, per sq cm N N1
AHA: 4Q,23

A2025 Miro3D, per cu cm N N1
AHA: 4Q,23

● **A2026** Restrata MiniMatrix, 5 mg N
AHA: 2Q,24

● **A2027** MatriDerm, per sq cm

● **A2028** MicroMatrix Flex, per mg

● **A2029** MiroTract Wound Matrix sheet, per cc

A4100 Skin substitute, FDA-cleared as a device, not otherwise specified N N1
AHA: 2Q,22

Injection Supplies

A4206 Syringe with needle, sterile, 1 cc or less, each N ☑

A4207 Syringe with needle, sterile 2 cc, each N ☑

A4208 Syringe with needle, sterile 3 cc, each N ☑

A4209 Syringe with needle, sterile 5 cc or greater, each N ☑

A4210 Needle-free injection device, each E1 ☑
Sometimes covered by commercial payers with preauthorization and physician letter stating need (e.g., for insulin injection in young children).

A4211 Supplies for self-administered injections N
When a drug that is usually injected by the patient (e.g., insulin or calcitonin) is injected by the physician, it is excluded from Medicare coverage unless administered in an emergency situation (e.g., diabetic coma).

A4212 Noncoring needle or stylet with or without catheter N

A4213 Syringe, sterile, 20 cc or greater, each N ☑

A4215 Needle, sterile, any size, each N

A4216 Sterile water, saline and/or dextrose, diluent/flush, 10 ml N ☑ ♿

A4217 Sterile water/saline, 500 ml N ☑ ♿ (AU)
CMS: 100-04,20,30.9

A4218 Sterile saline or water, metered dose dispenser, 10 ml N ☑

A4220 Refill kit for implantable infusion pump N

A4221 Supplies for maintenance of noninsulin drug infusion catheter, per week (list drugs separately) N ♿

A4222 Infusion supplies for external drug infusion pump, per cassette or bag (list drugs separately) N ♿

A4223 Infusion supplies not used with external infusion pump, per cassette or bag (list drugs separately) N ☑

A4224 Supplies for maintenance of insulin infusion catheter, per week N ♿

A4225 Supplies for external insulin infusion pump, syringe type cartridge, sterile, each N ♿

A4226 Supplies for maintenance of insulin infusion pump with dosage rate adjustment using therapeutic continuous glucose sensing, per week E1

A4230 Infusion set for external insulin pump, nonneedle cannula type N ☑
Covered by some commercial payers as ongoing supply to preauthorized pump.

A4231 Infusion set for external insulin pump, needle type N ☑
Covered by some commercial payers as ongoing supply to preauthorized pump.

A4232 Syringe with needle for external insulin pump, sterile, 3 cc E1 ☑
Covered by some commercial payers as ongoing supply to preauthorized pump.

Batteries

A4233 Replacement battery, alkaline (other than J cell), for use with medically necessary home blood glucose monitor owned by patient, each E1 ☑ ♿ (NU)
CMS: 100-04,23,60.1

A4234 Replacement battery, alkaline, J cell, for use with medically necessary home blood glucose monitor owned by patient, each E1 ☑ ♿ (NU)
CMS: 100-04,23,60.1

A4235 Replacement battery, lithium, for use with medically necessary home blood glucose monitor owned by patient, each E1 ☑ ♿ (NU)
CMS: 100-04,23,60.1

A4236 Replacement battery, silver oxide, for use with medically necessary home blood glucose monitor owned by patient, each E1 ☑ ♿ (NU)
CMS: 100-04,23,60.1

Other Supplies

A4238 Supply allowance for adjunctive, nonimplanted continuous glucose monitor (CGM), includes all supplies and accessories, 1 month supply = 1 unit of service Y (KF)

A4239 Supply allowance for nonadjunctive, nonimplanted continuous glucose monitor (CGM), includes all supplies and accessories, 1 month supply = 1 unit of service Y (KF)

A4244 Alcohol or peroxide, per pint N ☑

A4245 Alcohol wipes, per box N ☑

A4246 Betadine or pHisoHex solution, per pint N ☑

A4247 Betadine or iodine swabs/wipes, per box N ☑

A4248 Chlorhexidine containing antiseptic, 1 ml N ☑

A4250 **Urine test or reagent strips or tablets (100 tablets or strips)** E1 ☑
CMS: 100-02,15,110

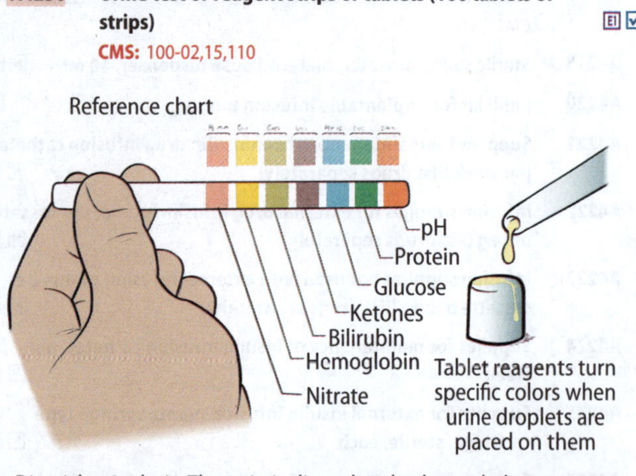

Dipstick urinalysis: The strip is dipped and color-coded squares are read at timed intervals (e.g., pH immediately; ketones at 15 seconds, etc.). Results are compared against a reference chart

A4252 **Blood ketone test or reagent strip, each** E1 ☑

A4253 **Blood glucose test or reagent strips for home blood glucose monitor, per 50 strips** N ☑ & (NU)
Medicare covers glucose strips for diabetic patients using home glucose monitoring devices prescribed by their physicians.
CMS: 100-04,23,60.1

A4255 **Platforms for home blood glucose monitor, 50 per box** N ☑ &
Some Medicare contractors cover monitor platforms for diabetic patients using home glucose monitoring devices prescribed by their physicians. Some commercial payers also provide this coverage to noninsulin dependent diabetics.

A4256 **Normal, low, and high calibrator solution/chips** N &
Some Medicare contractors cover calibration solutions or chips for diabetic patients using home glucose monitoring devices prescribed by their physicians. Some commercial payers also provide this coverage to noninsulin dependent diabetics.
CMS: 100-04,23,60.1

A4257 **Replacement lens shield cartridge for use with laser skin piercing device, each** E1 ☑ &

A4258 **Spring-powered device for lancet, each** N ☑ &
Some Medicare contractors cover lancing devices for diabetic patients using home glucose monitoring devices prescribed by their physicians. Medicare jurisdiction: DME regional contractor. Some commercial payers also provide this coverage to noninsulin dependent diabetics.
CMS: 100-04,23,60.1

A4259 **Lancets, per box of 100** N ☑ &
Medicare covers lancets for diabetic patients using home glucose monitoring devices prescribed by their physicians. Medicare jurisdiction: DME regional contractor. Some commercial payers also provide this coverage to noninsulin dependent diabetics.
CMS: 100-04,23,60.1

A4261 **Cervical cap for contraceptive use** M E1

A4262 **Temporary, absorbable lacrimal duct implant, each** N ☑
Always report concurrent to the implant procedure.

A4263 **Permanent, long-term, nondissolvable lacrimal duct implant, each** N ☑
Always report concurrent to the implant procedure.

A4264 **Permanent implantable contraceptive intratubal occlusion device(s) and delivery system** M E1 ☑

A4265 **Paraffin, per pound** N ☑ &

A4266 **Diaphragm for contraceptive use** M E1

A4267 **Contraceptive supply, condom, male, each** E1 ☑

A4268 **Contraceptive supply, condom, female, each** M E1 ☑

A4269 **Contraceptive supply, spermicide (e.g., foam, gel), each** M E1 ☑

A4270 **Disposable endoscope sheath, each** N ☑

▲ **A4271** **Integrated lancing and blood sample testing cartridges for home blood glucose monitor, per 50 tests** A
AHA: 2Q,24

A4280 **Adhesive skin support attachment for use with external breast prosthesis, each** N ☑ &

Two part prosthesis

Adhesive skin support (A4280)

Any of several breast prostheses fits over skin support

A4281 **Tubing for breast pump, replacement** M E1

A4282 **Adapter for breast pump, replacement** M E1

A4283 **Cap for breast pump bottle, replacement** M E1

A4284 **Breast shield and splash protector for use with breast pump, replacement** M E1

A4285 **Polycarbonate bottle for use with breast pump, replacement** M E1

A4286 **Locking ring for breast pump, replacement** M E1

A4287 **Disposable collection and storage bag for breast milk, any size, any type, each** Y

A4290 **Sacral nerve stimulation test lead, each** N ☑
CMS: 100-04,32,40.1; 100-04,32,40.2.1; 100-04,32,40.4

Vascular Catheters and Drug Delivery Systems

A4300 Implantable access catheter, (e.g., venous, arterial, epidural subarachnoid, or peritoneal, etc.) external access N

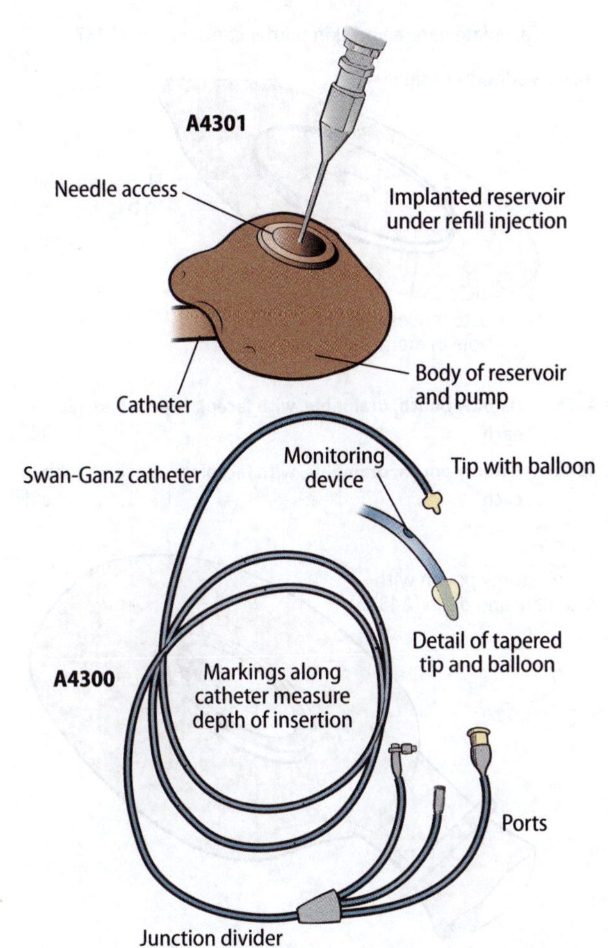

A4301 Implantable access total catheter, port/reservoir (e.g., venous, arterial, epidural, subarachnoid, peritoneal, etc.) N

A4305 Disposable drug delivery system, flow rate of 50 ml or greater per hour N ☑

A4306 Disposable drug delivery system, flow rate of less than 50 ml per hour N ☑

Incontinence Appliances and Care Supplies

Covered by Medicare when the medical record indicates incontinence is permanent, or of long and indefinite duration.

A4310 Insertion tray without drainage bag and without catheter (accessories only) N ♿

A4311 Insertion tray without drainage bag with indwelling catheter, Foley type, two-way latex with coating (Teflon, silicone, silicone elastomer or hydrophilic, etc.) N ♿

A4312 Insertion tray without drainage bag with indwelling catheter, Foley type, two-way, all silicone N ♿

A4313 Insertion tray without drainage bag with indwelling catheter, Foley type, three-way, for continuous irrigation N ♿

A4314 Insertion tray with drainage bag with indwelling catheter, Foley type, two-way latex with coating (Teflon, silicone, silicone elastomer or hydrophilic, etc.) N ♿

A4315 Insertion tray with drainage bag with indwelling catheter, Foley type, two-way, all silicone N ♿

A4316 Insertion tray with drainage bag with indwelling catheter, Foley type, three-way, for continuous irrigation N ♿

A4320 Irrigation tray with bulb or piston syringe, any purpose N ♿

A4321 Therapeutic agent for urinary catheter irrigation N ♿

A4322 Irrigation syringe, bulb or piston, each N ☑ ♿

A4326 Male external catheter with integral collection chamber, any type, each N ☑ ♿

A4327 Female external urinary collection device; meatal cup, each N ☑ ♿

A4328 Female external urinary collection device; pouch, each A N ☑ ♿

A4330 Perianal fecal collection pouch with adhesive, each N ☑ ♿

A4331 Extension drainage tubing, any type, any length, with connector/adaptor, for use with urinary leg bag or urostomy pouch, each N ☑ ♿

A4332 Lubricant, individual sterile packet, each N ☑ ♿

A4333 Urinary catheter anchoring device, adhesive skin attachment, each N ☑ ♿

A4334 Urinary catheter anchoring device, leg strap, each N ☑ ♿

A4335 Incontinence supply; miscellaneous N

A4336 Incontinence supply, urethral insert, any type, each N ☑ ♿

A4337 Incontinence supply, rectal insert, any type, each N

A4338 Indwelling catheter; Foley type, two-way latex with coating (Teflon, silicone, silicone elastomer, or hydrophilic, etc.), each N ☑ ♿

A4340 Indwelling catheter; specialty type, (e.g., Coude, mushroom, wing, etc.), each N ☑ ♿

A4341 Indwelling intraurethral drainage device with valve, patient inserted, replacement only, each N
AHA: 2Q,23

A4342 Accessories for patient inserted indwelling intraurethral drainage device with valve, replacement only, each N
AHA: 2Q,23

A4344 Indwelling catheter, foley type, two-way, all silicone or polyurethane, each N N1 ☑ ♿
AHA: 4Q,23

A4346 Indwelling catheter; Foley type, three-way for continuous irrigation, each N ☑ ♿

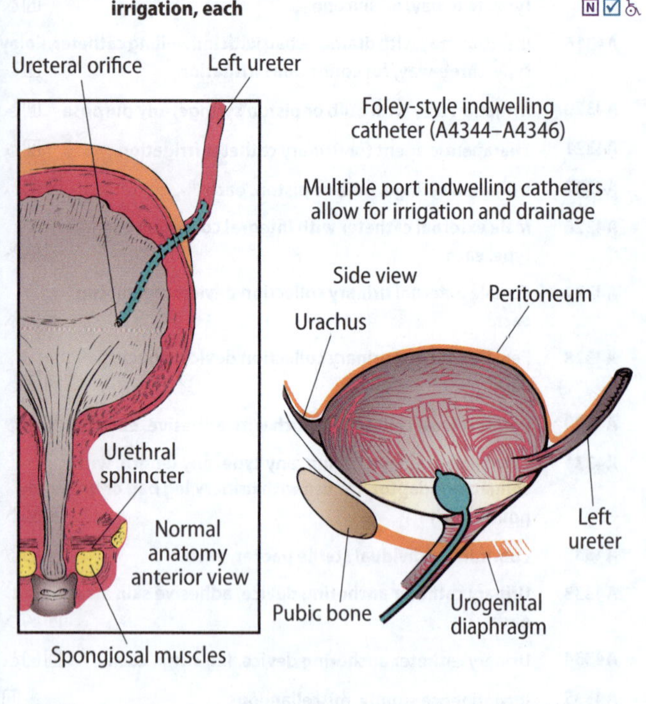

A4349 Male external catheter, with or without adhesive, disposable, each N ☑ ♿

A4351 Intermittent urinary catheter; straight tip, with or without coating (Teflon, silicone, silicone elastomer, or hydrophilic, etc.), each N ☑ ♿

A4352 Intermittent urinary catheter; Coude (curved) tip, with or without coating (Teflon, silicone, silicone elastomeric, or hydrophilic, etc.), each N ☑ ♿

A4353 Intermittent urinary catheter, with insertion supplies N ♿

A4354 Insertion tray with drainage bag but without catheter N ♿

A4355 Irrigation tubing set for continuous bladder irrigation through a three-way indwelling Foley catheter, each N ☑ ♿

A4356 External urethral clamp or compression device (not to be used for catheter clamp), each N ☑ ♿

A4357 Bedside drainage bag, day or night, with or without antireflux device, with or without tube, each N ☑ ♿

A4358 Urinary drainage bag, leg or abdomen, vinyl, with or without tube, with straps, each N ☑ ♿

A4360 Disposable external urethral clamp or compression device, with pad and/or pouch, each N ☑ ♿

Ostomy Supplies

A4361 Ostomy faceplate, each N ☑ ♿

A4362 Skin barrier; solid, 4 x 4 or equivalent; each N ☑ ♿

A4363 Ostomy clamp, any type, replacement only, each E1 ♿

A4364 Adhesive, liquid or equal, any type, per oz N ☑ ♿

A4366 Ostomy vent, any type, each N ☑ ♿

A4367 Ostomy belt, each N ☑ ♿

A4368 Ostomy filter, any type, each N ☑ ♿

A4369 Ostomy skin barrier, liquid (spray, brush, etc.), per oz N ☑ ♿

A4371 Ostomy skin barrier, powder, per oz N ☑ ♿

A4372 Ostomy skin barrier, solid 4 x 4 or equivalent, standard wear, with built-in convexity, each N ☑ ♿

A4373 Ostomy skin barrier, with flange (solid, flexible or accordion), with built-in convexity, any size, each N ☑ ♿

Faceplate flange and skin barrier combination (A4373)

Barrier adheres to skin
Flange attaches to bag
Waste moves through hole in membrane

A4375 Ostomy pouch, drainable, with faceplate attached, plastic, each N ☑ ♿

A4376 Ostomy pouch, drainable, with faceplate attached, rubber, each N ☑ ♿

Colostomy pouch with faceplate and drain (A4376)

A4377 Ostomy pouch, drainable, for use on faceplate, plastic, each N ☑ ♿

A4378 Ostomy pouch, drainable, for use on faceplate, rubber, each N ☑ ♿

A4379 Ostomy pouch, urinary, with faceplate attached, plastic, each N ☑ ♿

A4380 Ostomy pouch, urinary, with faceplate attached, rubber, each N ☑ ♿

A4381 Ostomy pouch, urinary, for use on faceplate, plastic, each N ☑ ♿

A4382 Ostomy pouch, urinary, for use on faceplate, heavy plastic, each N ☑ ♿

A4383 Ostomy pouch, urinary, for use on faceplate, rubber, each N ☑ ♿

A4384 Ostomy faceplate equivalent, silicone ring, each N ☑ ♿

A4385 Ostomy skin barrier, solid 4 x 4 or equivalent, extended wear, without built-in convexity, each N ☑ ♿

A4387 Ostomy pouch, closed, with barrier attached, with built-in convexity (one piece), each N ☑ ♿

A4388 Ostomy pouch, drainable, with extended wear barrier attached, (one piece), each N ☑ ♿

A4389 Ostomy pouch, drainable, with barrier attached, with built-in convexity (one piece), each

A4390 Ostomy pouch, drainable, with extended wear barrier attached, with built-in convexity (one piece), each

A4391 Ostomy pouch, urinary, with extended wear barrier attached (one piece), each

A4392 Ostomy pouch, urinary, with standard wear barrier attached, with built-in convexity (one piece), each

A4393 Ostomy pouch, urinary, with extended wear barrier attached, with built-in convexity (one piece), each

A4394 Ostomy deodorant, with or without lubricant, for use in ostomy pouch, per fl oz

A4395 Ostomy deodorant for use in ostomy pouch, solid, per tablet

A4396 Ostomy belt with peristomal hernia support

A4398 Ostomy irrigation supply; bag, each

A4399 Ostomy irrigation supply; cone/catheter, with or without brush

A4400 Ostomy irrigation set

A4402 Lubricant, per oz

A4404 Ostomy ring, each

A4405 Ostomy skin barrier, nonpectin-based, paste, per oz

A4406 Ostomy skin barrier, pectin-based, paste, per oz

A4407 Ostomy skin barrier, with flange (solid, flexible, or accordion), extended wear, with built-in convexity, 4 x 4 in or smaller, each

A4408 Ostomy skin barrier, with flange (solid, flexible or accordion), extended wear, with built-in convexity, larger than 4 x 4 in, each

A4409 Ostomy skin barrier, with flange (solid, flexible or accordion), extended wear, without built-in convexity, 4 x 4 in or smaller, each

A4410 Ostomy skin barrier, with flange (solid, flexible or accordion), extended wear, without built-in convexity, larger than 4 x 4 in, each

A4411 Ostomy skin barrier, solid 4 x 4 or equivalent, extended wear, with built-in convexity, each

A4412 Ostomy pouch, drainable, high output, for use on a barrier with flange (two-piece system), without filter, each

A4413 Ostomy pouch, drainable, high output, for use on a barrier with flange (two-piece system), with filter, each

A4414 Ostomy skin barrier, with flange (solid, flexible or accordion), without built-in convexity, 4 x 4 in or smaller, each

A4415 Ostomy skin barrier, with flange (solid, flexible or accordion), without built-in convexity, larger than 4 x 4 in, each

A4416 Ostomy pouch, closed, with barrier attached, with filter (one piece), each

A4417 Ostomy pouch, closed, with barrier attached, with built-in convexity, with filter (one piece), each

A4418 Ostomy pouch, closed; without barrier attached, with filter (one piece), each

A4419 Ostomy pouch, closed; for use on barrier with nonlocking flange, with filter (two piece), each

A4420 Ostomy pouch, closed; for use on barrier with locking flange (two piece), each

A4421 Ostomy supply; miscellaneous

Determine if an alternative HCPCS Level II or a CPT code better describes the service being reported. This code should be used only if a more specific code is unavailable.

A4422 Ostomy absorbent material (sheet/pad/crystal packet) for use in ostomy pouch to thicken liquid stomal output, each

A4423 Ostomy pouch, closed; for use on barrier with locking flange, with filter (two piece), each

A4424 Ostomy pouch, drainable, with barrier attached, with filter (one piece), each

A4425 Ostomy pouch, drainable; for use on barrier with nonlocking flange, with filter (two-piece system), each

A4426 Ostomy pouch, drainable; for use on barrier with locking flange (two-piece system), each

A4427 Ostomy pouch, drainable; for use on barrier with locking flange, with filter (two-piece system), each

A4428 Ostomy pouch, urinary, with extended wear barrier attached, with faucet-type tap with valve (one piece), each

A4429 Ostomy pouch, urinary, with barrier attached, with built-in convexity, with faucet-type tap with valve (one piece), each

A4430 Ostomy pouch, urinary, with extended wear barrier attached, with built-in convexity, with faucet-type tap with valve (one piece), each

A4431 Ostomy pouch, urinary; with barrier attached, with faucet-type tap with valve (one piece), each

A4432 Ostomy pouch, urinary; for use on barrier with nonlocking flange, with faucet-type tap with valve (two piece), each

A4433 Ostomy pouch, urinary; for use on barrier with locking flange (two piece), each

A4434 Ostomy pouch, urinary; for use on barrier with locking flange, with faucet-type tap with valve (two piece), each

A4435 Ostomy pouch, drainable, high output, with extended wear barrier (one-piece system), with or without filter, each

A4436 Irrigation supply; sleeve, reusable, per month

A4437 Irrigation supply; sleeve, disposable, per month

Miscellaneous Supplies

● **A4438** Adhesive clip applied to the skin to secure external electrical nerve stimulator controller, each

AHA: 2Q,24

A4450 Tape, nonwaterproof, per 18 sq in (AU, AV, AW)

See also code A4452.

CMS: 100-04,20,30.9

A4452 Tape, waterproof, per 18 sq in (AU, AV, AW)

See also code A4450.

CMS: 100-04,20,30.9

A4453 Rectal catheter for use with the manual pump-operated enema system, replacement only

A4455 Adhesive remover or solvent (for tape, cement or other adhesive), per oz

A4456 Adhesive remover, wipes, any type, each

A4457 Enema tube, with or without adapter, any type, replacement only, each

A4458 Enema bag with tubing, reusable

A4459 Manual pump-operated enema system, includes balloon, catheter and all accessories, reusable, any type N

A4461 Surgical dressing holder, nonreusable, each N ☑ ♿

A4463 Surgical dressing holder, reusable, each N ☑ ♿

A4465 Nonelastic binder for extremity N

A4467 Belt, strap, sleeve, garment, or covering, any type E

A4468 Exsufflation belt, includes all supplies and accessories E

A4470 Gravlee jet washer N

A4480 VABRA aspirator N
CMS: 100-03,230.6; 100-03,240.4

A4481 Tracheostoma filter, any type, any size, each N ☑ ♿

A4483 Moisture exchanger, disposable, for use with invasive mechanical ventilation N ♿

A4490 Surgical stockings above knee length, each E ☑
CMS: 100-02,15,110

A4495 Surgical stockings thigh length, each E ☑
CMS: 100-02,15,110

A4500 Surgical stockings below knee length, each E ☑
CMS: 100-02,15,110

A4510 Surgical stockings full-length, each E ☑
CMS: 100-02,15,110

A4520 Incontinence garment, any type, (e.g., brief, diaper), each E ☑

A4540 Distal transcutaneous electrical nerve stimulator, stimulates peripheral nerves of the upper arm E
AHA: 1Q,24

A4541 Monthly supplies for use of device coded at E0733 Y

A4542 Supplies and accessories for external upper limb tremor stimulator of the peripheral nerves of the wrist Y

● **A4543** Supplies for transcutaneous electrical nerve stimulator, for nerves in the auricular region, per month

● **A4544** Electrode for external lower extremity nerve stimulator for restless legs syndrome

● **A4545** Supplies and accessories for external tibial nerve stimulator (e.g., socks, gel pads, electrodes, etc.), needed for one month

A4550 Surgical trays B
CMS: 100-04,12,40.1

A4553 Nondisposable underpads, all sizes E

A4554 Disposable underpads, all sizes E ☑

A4555 Electrode/transducer for use with electrical stimulation device used for cancer treatment, replacement only E

A4556 Electrodes (e.g., apnea monitor), per pair N ☑ ♿
If service is not separately payable, or incident to a physician's service, bill through the local carrier. If other, bill the DME MAC.
Some payers only cover apnea monitors for newborn or pediatric use. Review specific carrier policy for apnea monitors and supplies.

A4557 Lead wires (e.g., apnea monitor), per pair N ☑ ♿
If service is not separately payable, or incident to a physician's service, bill through the local carrier. If other, bill the DME MAC.
Some payers only cover apnea monitors for newborn or pediatric use. Review specific carrier policy for apnea monitors and supplies.

A4558 Conductive gel or paste, for use with electrical device (e.g., TENS, NMES), per oz N ☑ ♿

A4559 Coupling gel or paste, for use with ultrasound device, per oz N ☑ ♿

A4560 Neuromuscular electrical stimulator (NMES), disposable, replacement only E
AHA: 2Q,23

▲ **A4561** Pessary, reusable, rubber, any type N ♿
AHA: 2Q,24

▲ **A4562** Pessary, reusable, non rubber, any type N ♿
Medicare jurisdiction: DME regional contractor.
AHA: 2Q,24

A4563 Rectal control system for vaginal insertion, for long term use, includes pump and all supplies and accessories, any type each A

● **A4564** Pessary, disposable, any type A
AHA: 2Q,24

A4565 Slings N ♿

A4566 Shoulder sling or vest design, abduction restrainer, with or without swathe control, prefabricated, includes fitting and adjustment E

A4570 Splint E
Dressings applied by a physician are included as part of the professional service.

A4575 Topical hyperbaric oxygen chamber, disposable A

A4580 Cast supplies (e.g., plaster) E
See Q4001-Q4048.

A4590 Special casting material (e.g., fiberglass) E
See Q4001-Q4048.

● **A4593** Neuromodulation stimulator system, adjunct to rehabilitation therapy regime, controller E
AHA: 2Q,24

● **A4594** Neuromodulation stimulator system, adjunct to rehabilitation therapy regime, mouthpiece, each E
AHA: 2Q,24

A4595 Electrical stimulator supplies, 2 lead, per month, (e.g., TENS, NMES) N ♿
CMS: 100-03,10.2

A4596 Cranial electrotherapy stimulation (CES) system supplies and accessories, per month N
AHA: 4Q,22

A4600 Sleeve for intermittent limb compression device, replacement only, each E ☑

A4601 Lithium-ion battery, rechargeable, for nonprosthetic use, replacement E

A4602 Replacement battery for external infusion pump owned by patient, lithium, 1.5 volt, each N ♿ (NU)

A4604 Tubing with integrated heating element for use with positive airway pressure device N ♿ (NU)
CMS: 100-04,36,50.14

A4605 Tracheal suction catheter, closed system, each N ☑ ♿ (NU)

A4606 Oxygen probe for use with oximeter device, replacement N

A4608 Transtracheal oxygen catheter, each N ☑ ♿

Supplies for Oxygen and Related Respiratory Equipment

A4611 Battery, heavy-duty; replacement for patient-owned ventilator E

A4612 Battery cables; replacement for patient-owned ventilator E

A4613 Battery charger; replacement for patient-owned ventilator E ☑

A4614 Peak expiratory flow rate meter, hand held N ♿

A4615 Cannula, nasal
CMS: 100-04,20,100.2

A4616 Tubing (oxygen), per foot
CMS: 100-04,20,100.2

A4617 Mouthpiece
CMS: 100-04,20,100.2

A4618 Breathing circuits (NU, RR, UE)
CMS: 100-04,20,100.2

A4619 Face tent (NU)
CMS: 100-04,20,100.2

A4620 Variable concentration mask
CMS: 100-04,20,100.2

A4623 Tracheostomy, inner cannula

A4624 Tracheal suction catheter, any type other than closed system, each (NU)

A4625 Tracheostomy care kit for new tracheostomy

A4626 Tracheostomy cleaning brush, each

A4627 Spacer, bag or reservoir, with or without mask, for use with metered dose inhaler
CMS: 100-02,15,110

A4628 Oral and/or oropharyngeal suction catheter, each (NU)
AHA: 2Q,23

A4629 Tracheostomy care kit for established tracheostomy

Replacement Supplies for DME

A4630 Replacement batteries, medically necessary, transcutaneous electrical stimulator, owned by patient (NU)

A4633 Replacement bulb/lamp for ultraviolet light therapy system, each (NU)

A4634 Replacement bulb for therapeutic light box, tabletop model

A4635 Underarm pad, crutch, replacement, each (NU, RR, UE)

A4636 Replacement, handgrip, cane, crutch, or walker, each (NU, RR, UE)
CMS: 100-04,36,50.15

A4637 Replacement, tip, cane, crutch, walker, each (NU, RR, UE)
CMS: 100-04,36,50.15

A4638 Replacement battery for patient-owned ear pulse generator, each (NU, RR, UE)

A4639 Replacement pad for infrared heating pad system, each (RR)

A4640 Replacement pad for use with medically necessary alternating pressure pad owned by patient (NU, RR, UE)

Radiopharmaceuticals

A4641 Radiopharmaceutical, diagnostic, not otherwise classified
CMS: 100-04,13,60.3; 100-04,13,60.3.2

A4642 Indium In-111 satumomab pendetide, diagnostic, per study dose, up to 6 mCi
Use this code for Oncoscint.

Miscellaneous Supplies

A4648 Tissue marker, implantable, any type, each
AHA: 3Q,24; 2Q,18

A4649 Surgical supply; miscellaneous
Determine if an alternative HCPCS Level II or a CPT code better describes the service being reported. This code should be used only if a more specific code is unavailable.
AHA: 3Q,23

A4650 Implantable radiation dosimeter, each

A4651 Calibrated microcapillary tube, each

A4652 Microcapillary tube sealant

Dialysis Supplies

A4653 Peritoneal dialysis catheter anchoring device, belt, each

A4657 Syringe, with or without needle, each
CMS: 100-04,8,60.2.1; 100-04,8,60.4.4; 100-04,8,60.4.6.3

A4660 Sphygmomanometer/blood pressure apparatus with cuff and stethoscope

A4663 Blood pressure cuff only

A4670 Automatic blood pressure monitor

A4671 Disposable cycler set used with cycler dialysis machine, each

A4672 Drainage extension line, sterile, for dialysis, each

A4673 Extension line with easy lock connectors, used with dialysis

A4674 Chemicals/antiseptics solution used to clean/sterilize dialysis equipment, per 8 oz

A4680 Activated carbon filter for hemodialysis, each

A4690 Dialyzer (artificial kidneys), all types, all sizes, for hemodialysis, each

A4706 Bicarbonate concentrate, solution, for hemodialysis, per gallon

A4707 Bicarbonate concentrate, powder, for hemodialysis, per packet

A4708 Acetate concentrate solution, for hemodialysis, per gallon

A4709 Acid concentrate, solution, for hemodialysis, per gallon

A4714 Treated water (deionized, distilled, or reverse osmosis) for peritoneal dialysis, per gallon

A4719 "Y set" tubing for peritoneal dialysis

A4720 Dialysate solution, any concentration of dextrose, fluid volume greater than 249 cc, but less than or equal to 999 cc, for peritoneal dialysis

A4721 Dialysate solution, any concentration of dextrose, fluid volume greater than 999 cc but less than or equal to 1999 cc, for peritoneal dialysis

A4722 Dialysate solution, any concentration of dextrose, fluid volume greater than 1999 cc but less than or equal to 2999 cc, for peritoneal dialysis

A4723 Dialysate solution, any concentration of dextrose, fluid volume greater than 2999 cc but less than or equal to 3999 cc, for peritoneal dialysis

A4724 Dialysate solution, any concentration of dextrose, fluid volume greater than 3999 cc but less than or equal to 4999 cc, for peritoneal dialysis

A4725 Dialysate solution, any concentration of dextrose, fluid volume greater than 4999 cc but less than or equal to 5999 cc, for peritoneal dialysis

A4726 Dialysate solution, any concentration of dextrose, fluid volume greater than 5999 cc, for peritoneal dialysis

A4728 Dialysate solution, nondextrose containing, 500 ml

A4730 Fistula cannulation set for hemodialysis, each

A4736 Topical anesthetic, for dialysis, per g

A4737 Injectable anesthetic, for dialysis, per 10 ml

A4740 Shunt accessory, for hemodialysis, any type, each

A4750 Blood tubing, arterial or venous, for hemodialysis, each

A4755 Blood tubing, arterial and venous combined, for hemodialysis, each

A4760 Dialysate solution test kit, for peritoneal dialysis, any type, each

A4765 Dialysate concentrate, powder, additive for peritoneal dialysis, per packet

A4766 Dialysate concentrate, solution, additive for peritoneal dialysis, per 10 ml

A4770 Blood collection tube, vacuum, for dialysis, per 50

A4771 Serum clotting time tube, for dialysis, per 50

A4772 Blood glucose test strips, for dialysis, per 50

A4773 Occult blood test strips, for dialysis, per 50

A4774 Ammonia test strips, for dialysis, per 50

A4802 Protamine sulfate, for hemodialysis, per 50 mg

A4860 Disposable catheter tips for peritoneal dialysis, per 10

A4870 Plumbing and/or electrical work for home hemodialysis equipment

A4890 Contracts, repair and maintenance, for hemodialysis equipment

A4911 Drain bag/bottle, for dialysis, each

A4913 Miscellaneous dialysis supplies, not otherwise specified

Pertinent documentation to evaluate medical appropriateness should be included when this code is reported. Determine if an alternative HCPCS Level II or a CPT code better describes the service being reported. This code should be used only if a more specific code is unavailable.

CMS: 100-04,8,20; 100-04,8,60.2.1

A4918 Venous pressure clamp, for hemodialysis, each

A4927 Gloves, nonsterile, per 100

A4928 Surgical mask, per 20

A4929 Tourniquet for dialysis, each

A4930 Gloves, sterile, per pair

A4931 Oral thermometer, reusable, any type, each

A4932 Rectal thermometer, reusable, any type, each

Ostomy Pouches and Supplies

A5051 Ostomy pouch, closed; with barrier attached (one piece), each

A5052 Ostomy pouch, closed; without barrier attached (one piece), each

A5053 Ostomy pouch, closed; for use on faceplate, each

A5054 Ostomy pouch, closed; for use on barrier with flange (two piece), each

A5055 Stoma cap

A5056 Ostomy pouch, drainable, with extended wear barrier attached, with filter, (one piece), each

A5057 Ostomy pouch, drainable, with extended wear barrier attached, with built in convexity, with filter, (one piece), each

A5061 Ostomy pouch, drainable; with barrier attached, (one piece), each

A5062 Ostomy pouch, drainable; without barrier attached (one piece), each

A5063 Ostomy pouch, drainable; for use on barrier with flange (two-piece system), each

A5071 Ostomy pouch, urinary; with barrier attached (one piece), each

A5072 Ostomy pouch, urinary; without barrier attached (one piece), each

A5073 Ostomy pouch, urinary; for use on barrier with flange (two piece), each

A5081 Stoma plug or seal, any type

A5082 Continent device; catheter for continent stoma

A5083 Continent device, stoma absorptive cover for continent stoma

A5093 Ostomy accessory; convex insert

Incontinence Supplies

A5102 Bedside drainage bottle with or without tubing, rigid or expandable, each

A5105 Urinary suspensory with leg bag, with or without tube, each

A5112 Urinary drainage bag, leg or abdomen, latex, with or without tube, with straps, each

A5113 Leg strap; latex, replacement only, per set

A5114 Leg strap; foam or fabric, replacement only, per set

A5120 Skin barrier, wipes or swabs, each (AU, AV)

A5121 Skin barrier; solid, 6 x 6 or equivalent, each

A5122 Skin barrier; solid, 8 x 8 or equivalent, each

A5126 Adhesive or nonadhesive; disk or foam pad

A5131 Appliance cleaner, incontinence and ostomy appliances, per 16 oz

A5200 Percutaneous catheter/tube anchoring device, adhesive skin attachment

Diabetic Shoes, Fitting, and Modifications

According to Medicare, documentation from the prescribing physician must certify the diabetic patient has one of the following conditions: peripheral neuropathy with evidence of callus formation; history of preulcerative calluses; history of ulceration; foot deformity; previous amputation; or poor circulation. The footwear must be fitted and furnished by a podiatrist, pedorthist, orthotist, or prosthetist.

A5500 For diabetics only, fitting (including follow-up), custom preparation and supply of off-the-shelf depth-inlay shoe manufactured to accommodate multidensity insert(s), per shoe

CMS: 100-02,15,140

A5501 For diabetics only, fitting (including follow-up), custom preparation and supply of shoe molded from cast(s) of patient's foot (custom molded shoe), per shoe

CMS: 100-02,15,140

A5503 For diabetics only, modification (including fitting) of off-the-shelf depth-inlay shoe or custom molded shoe with roller or rigid rocker bottom, per shoe
CMS: 100-02,15,140

A5504 For diabetics only, modification (including fitting) of off-the-shelf depth-inlay shoe or custom molded shoe with wedge(s), per shoe
CMS: 100-02,15,140

A5505 For diabetics only, modification (including fitting) of off-the-shelf depth-inlay shoe or custom molded shoe with metatarsal bar, per shoe
CMS: 100-02,15,140

A5506 For diabetics only, modification (including fitting) of off-the-shelf depth-inlay shoe or custom molded shoe with off-set heel(s), per shoe
CMS: 100-02,15,140

A5507 For diabetics only, not otherwise specified modification (including fitting) of off-the-shelf depth-inlay shoe or custom molded shoe, per shoe
CMS: 100-02,15,140

A5508 For diabetics only, deluxe feature of off-the-shelf depth-inlay shoe or custom molded shoe, per shoe
CMS: 100-02,15,140

A5510 For diabetics only, direct formed, compression molded to patient's foot without external heat source, multiple-density insert(s) prefabricated, per shoe
CMS: 100-02,15,140

A5512 For diabetics only, multiple density insert, direct formed, molded to foot after external heat source of 230 degrees Fahrenheit or higher, total contact with patient's foot, including arch, base layer minimum of 1/4 inch material of Shore A 35 durometer or 3/16 inch material of Shore A 40 durometer (or higher), prefabricated, each

A5513 For diabetics only, multiple density insert, custom molded from model of patient's foot, total contact with patient's foot, including arch, base layer minimum of 3/16 inch material of Shore A 35 durometer (or higher), includes arch filler and other shaping material, custom fabricated, each

A5514 For diabetics only, multiple density insert, made by direct carving with CAM technology from a rectified CAD model created from a digitized scan of the patient, total contact with patient's foot, including arch, base layer minimum of 3/16 inch material of Shore A 35 durometer (or higher), includes arch filler and other shaping material, custom fabricated, each

Dressings

A6000 Noncontact wound-warming wound cover for use with the noncontact wound-warming device and warming card

A6010 Collagen based wound filler, dry form, sterile, per g of collagen

A6011 Collagen based wound filler, gel/paste, per g of collagen

A6021 Collagen dressing, sterile, size 16 sq in or less, each

A6022 Collagen dressing, sterile, size more than 16 sq in but less than or equal to 48 sq in, each

A6023 Collagen dressing, sterile, size more than 48 sq in, each

A6024 Collagen dressing wound filler, sterile, per 6 in

A6025 Gel sheet for dermal or epidermal application, (e.g., silicone, hydrogel, other), each

A6154 Wound pouch, each

A6196 Alginate or other fiber gelling dressing, wound cover, sterile, pad size 16 sq in or less, each dressing

A6197 Alginate or other fiber gelling dressing, wound cover, sterile, pad size more than 16 sq in but less than or equal to 48 sq in, each dressing

A6198 Alginate or other fiber gelling dressing, wound cover, sterile, pad size more than 48 sq in, each dressing

A6199 Alginate or other fiber gelling dressing, wound filler, sterile, per 6 in

A6203 Composite dressing, sterile, pad size 16 sq in or less, with any size adhesive border, each dressing

A6204 Composite dressing, sterile, pad size more than 16 sq in, but less than or equal to 48 sq in, with any size adhesive border, each dressing

A6205 Composite dressing, sterile, pad size more than 48 sq in, with any size adhesive border, each dressing

A6206 Contact layer, sterile, 16 sq in or less, each dressing

A6207 Contact layer, sterile, more than 16 sq in but less than or equal to 48 sq in, each dressing

A6208 Contact layer, sterile, more than 48 sq in, each dressing

A6209 Foam dressing, wound cover, sterile, pad size 16 sq in or less, without adhesive border, each dressing

A6210 Foam dressing, wound cover, sterile, pad size more than 16 sq in but less than or equal to 48 sq in, without adhesive border, each dressing

A6211 Foam dressing, wound cover, sterile, pad size more than 48 sq in, without adhesive border, each dressing

A6212 Foam dressing, wound cover, sterile, pad size 16 sq in or less, with any size adhesive border, each dressing

A6213 Foam dressing, wound cover, sterile, pad size more than 16 sq in but less than or equal to 48 sq in, with any size adhesive border, each dressing

A6214 Foam dressing, wound cover, sterile, pad size more than 48 sq in, with any size adhesive border, each dressing

A6215 Foam dressing, wound filler, sterile, per g

A6216 Gauze, nonimpregnated, nonsterile, pad size 16 sq in or less, without adhesive border, each dressing

A6217 Gauze, nonimpregnated, nonsterile, pad size more than 16 sq in but less than or equal to 48 sq in, without adhesive border, each dressing

A6218 Gauze, nonimpregnated, nonsterile, pad size more than 48 sq in, without adhesive border, each dressing

A6219 Gauze, nonimpregnated, sterile, pad size 16 sq in or less, with any size adhesive border, each dressing

A6220 Gauze, nonimpregnated, sterile, pad size more than 16 sq in but less than or equal to 48 sq in, with any size adhesive border, each dressing

A6221 Gauze, nonimpregnated, sterile, pad size more than 48 sq in, with any size adhesive border, each dressing

A6222 Gauze, impregnated with other than water, normal saline, or hydrogel, sterile, pad size 16 sq in or less, without adhesive border, each dressing

A6223 Gauze, impregnated with other than water, normal saline, or hydrogel, sterile, pad size more than 16 sq in but less than or equal to 48 sq in, without adhesive border, each dressing

A6224 Gauze, impregnated with other than water, normal saline, or hydrogel, sterile, pad size more than 48 sq in, without adhesive border, each dressing N ☑ ♿

A6228 Gauze, impregnated, water or normal saline, sterile, pad size 16 sq in or less, without adhesive border, each dressing N ☑

A6229 Gauze, impregnated, water or normal saline, sterile, pad size more than 16 sq in but less than or equal to 48 sq in, without adhesive border, each dressing N ☑ ♿

A6230 Gauze, impregnated, water or normal saline, sterile, pad size more than 48 sq in, without adhesive border, each dressing N ☑

A6231 Gauze, impregnated, hydrogel, for direct wound contact, sterile, pad size 16 sq in or less, each dressing N ☑ ♿

A6232 Gauze, impregnated, hydrogel, for direct wound contact, sterile, pad size greater than 16 sq in but less than or equal to 48 sq in, each dressing N ☑ ♿

A6233 Gauze, impregnated, hydrogel, for direct wound contact, sterile, pad size more than 48 sq in, each dressing N ☑ ♿

A6234 Hydrocolloid dressing, wound cover, sterile, pad size 16 sq in or less, without adhesive border, each dressing N ☑ ♿

A6235 Hydrocolloid dressing, wound cover, sterile, pad size more than 16 sq in but less than or equal to 48 sq in, without adhesive border, each dressing N ☑ ♿

A6236 Hydrocolloid dressing, wound cover, sterile, pad size more than 48 sq in, without adhesive border, each dressing N ☑ ♿

A6237 Hydrocolloid dressing, wound cover, sterile, pad size 16 sq in or less, with any size adhesive border, each dressing N ☑ ♿

A6238 Hydrocolloid dressing, wound cover, sterile, pad size more than 16 sq in but less than or equal to 48 sq in, with any size adhesive border, each dressing N ☑ ♿

A6239 Hydrocolloid dressing, wound cover, sterile, pad size more than 48 sq in, with any size adhesive border, each dressing N ☑

A6240 Hydrocolloid dressing, wound filler, paste, sterile, per oz N ☑ ♿

A6241 Hydrocolloid dressing, wound filler, dry form, sterile, per g N ☑ ♿

A6242 Hydrogel dressing, wound cover, sterile, pad size 16 sq in or less, without adhesive border, each dressing N ☑ ♿

A6243 Hydrogel dressing, wound cover, sterile, pad size more than 16 sq in but less than or equal to 48 sq in, without adhesive border, each dressing N ☑ ♿

A6244 Hydrogel dressing, wound cover, sterile, pad size more than 48 sq in, without adhesive border, each dressing N ☑ ♿

A6245 Hydrogel dressing, wound cover, sterile, pad size 16 sq in or less, with any size adhesive border, each dressing N ☑ ♿

A6246 Hydrogel dressing, wound cover, sterile, pad size more than 16 sq in but less than or equal to 48 sq in, with any size adhesive border, each dressing N ☑ ♿

A6247 Hydrogel dressing, wound cover, sterile, pad size more than 48 sq in, with any size adhesive border, each dressing N ☑ ♿

A6248 Hydrogel dressing, wound filler, gel, per fl oz N ☑ ♿

A6250 Skin sealants, protectants, moisturizers, ointments, any type, any size N

Surgical dressings applied by a physician are included as part of the professional service. Surgical dressings obtained by the patient to perform homecare as prescribed by the physician are covered.

A6251 Specialty absorptive dressing, wound cover, sterile, pad size 16 sq in or less, without adhesive border, each dressing N ☑ ♿

A6252 Specialty absorptive dressing, wound cover, sterile, pad size more than 16 sq in but less than or equal to 48 sq in, without adhesive border, each dressing N ☑ ♿

A6253 Specialty absorptive dressing, wound cover, sterile, pad size more than 48 sq in, without adhesive border, each dressing N ☑ ♿

A6254 Specialty absorptive dressing, wound cover, sterile, pad size 16 sq in or less, with any size adhesive border, each dressing N ☑ ♿

A6255 Specialty absorptive dressing, wound cover, sterile, pad size more than 16 sq in but less than or equal to 48 sq in, with any size adhesive border, each dressing N ☑ ♿

A6256 Specialty absorptive dressing, wound cover, sterile, pad size more than 48 sq in, with any size adhesive border, each dressing N ☑

A6257 Transparent film, sterile, 16 sq in or less, each dressing N ☑ ♿

Surgical dressings applied by a physician are included as part of the professional service. Surgical dressings obtained by the patient to perform homecare as prescribed by the physician are covered. Use this code for Polyskin, Tegaderm, and Tegaderm HP.

A6258 Transparent film, sterile, more than 16 sq in but less than or equal to 48 sq in, each dressing N ☑ ♿

Surgical dressings applied by a physician are included as part of the professional service. Surgical dressings obtained by the patient to perform homecare as prescribed by the physician are covered.

A6259 Transparent film, sterile, more than 48 sq in, each dressing N ☑ ♿

Surgical dressings applied by a physician are included as part of the professional service. Surgical dressings obtained by the patient to perform homecare as prescribed by the physician are covered.

A6260 Wound cleansers, any type, any size N

Surgical dressings applied by a physician are included as part of the professional service. Surgical dressings obtained by the patient to perform homecare as prescribed by the physician are covered.

A6261 Wound filler, gel/paste, per fl oz, not otherwise specified N ☑

Surgical dressings applied by a physician are included as part of the professional service. Surgical dressings obtained by the patient to perform homecare as prescribed by the physician are covered.

A6262 Wound filler, dry form, per g, not otherwise specified N ☑

A6266 Gauze, impregnated, other than water, normal saline, or zinc paste, sterile, any width, per linear yd N ☑ ♿

Surgical dressings applied by a physician are included as part of the professional service. Surgical dressings obtained by the patient to perform homecare as prescribed by the physician are covered.

A6402 Gauze, nonimpregnated, sterile, pad size 16 sq in or less, without adhesive border, each dressing N ☑ ♿

Surgical dressings applied by a physician are included as part of the professional service. Surgical dressings obtained by the patient to perform homecare as prescribed by the physician are covered.

A6403 Gauze, nonimpregnated, sterile, pad size more than 16 sq in but less than or equal to 48 sq in, without adhesive border, each dressing N ☑ ♿

Surgical dressings applied by a physician are included as part of the professional service. Surgical dressings obtained by the patient to perform homecare as prescribed by the physician are covered.

A6404 Gauze, nonimpregnated, sterile, pad size more than 48 sq in, without adhesive border, each dressing N ☑

A6407 Packing strips, nonimpregnated, sterile, up to 2 in in width, per linear yd N ☑ ♿

A6410 Eye pad, sterile, each N ☑ ♿

A6411 Eye pad, nonsterile, each N ☑ ♿

A6412 Eye patch, occlusive, each N ☑

A6413 Adhesive bandage, first aid type, any size, each E ☑

A6441 Padding bandage, nonelastic, nonwoven/nonknitted, width greater than or equal to 3 in and less than 5 in, per yd N ☑ ♿

A6442 Conforming bandage, nonelastic, knitted/woven, nonsterile, width less than 3 in, per yd N ☑ ♿

A6443 Conforming bandage, nonelastic, knitted/woven, nonsterile, width greater than or equal to 3 in and less than 5 in, per yd N ☑ ♿

A6444 Conforming bandage, nonelastic, knitted/woven, nonsterile, width greater than or equal to 5 in, per yd N ☑ ♿

A6445 Conforming bandage, nonelastic, knitted/woven, sterile, width less than 3 in, per yd N ☑ ♿

A6446 Conforming bandage, nonelastic, knitted/woven, sterile, width greater than or equal to 3 in and less than 5 in, per yd N ☑ ♿

A6447 Conforming bandage, nonelastic, knitted/woven, sterile, width greater than or equal to 5 in, per yd N ☑ ♿

A6448 Light compression bandage, elastic, knitted/woven, width less than 3 in, per yd N ☑ ♿

A6449 Light compression bandage, elastic, knitted/woven, width greater than or equal to 3 in and less than 5 in, per yd N ☑ ♿

A6450 Light compression bandage, elastic, knitted/woven, width greater than or equal to 5 in, per yd N ☑ ♿

A6451 Moderate compression bandage, elastic, knitted/woven, load resistance of 1.25 to 1.34 ft lbs at 50% maximum stretch, width greater than or equal to 3 in and less than 5 in, per yd N ☑ ♿

A6452 High compression bandage, elastic, knitted/woven, load resistance greater than or equal to 1.35 ft lbs at 50% maximum stretch, width greater than or equal to 3 in and less than 5 in, per yd N ☑ ♿

A6453 Self-adherent bandage, elastic, nonknitted/nonwoven, width less than 3 in, per yd N ☑ ♿

A6454 Self-adherent bandage, elastic, nonknitted/nonwoven, width greater than or equal to 3 in and less than 5 in, per yd N ☑ ♿

A6455 Self-adherent bandage, elastic, nonknitted/nonwoven, width greater than or equal to 5 in, per yd N ☑ ♿

A6456 Zinc paste impregnated bandage, nonelastic, knitted/woven, width greater than or equal to 3 in and less than 5 in, per yd N ☑ ♿

A6457 Tubular dressing with or without elastic, any width, per linear yd N ♿

A6460 Synthetic resorbable wound dressing, sterile, pad size 16 sq in or less, without adhesive border, each dressing N

A6461 Synthetic resorbable wound dressing, sterile, pad size more than 16 sq in but less than or equal to 48 sq in, without adhesive border, each dressing N

Compression Garments

A6501 Compression burn garment, bodysuit (head to foot), custom fabricated N ♿

A6502 Compression burn garment, chin strap, custom fabricated N ♿

A6503 Compression burn garment, facial hood, custom fabricated N ♿

A6504 Compression burn garment, glove to wrist, custom fabricated N ♿

A6505 Compression burn garment, glove to elbow, custom fabricated N ♿

A6506 Compression burn garment, glove to axilla, custom fabricated N ♿

A6507 Compression burn garment, foot to knee length, custom fabricated N ♿

A6508 Compression burn garment, foot to thigh length, custom fabricated N ♿

A6509 Compression burn garment, upper trunk to waist including arm openings (vest), custom fabricated N ♿

A6510 Compression burn garment, trunk, including arms down to leg openings (leotard), custom fabricated N ♿

A6511 Compression burn garment, lower trunk including leg openings (panty), custom fabricated N ♿

A6512 Compression burn garment, not otherwise classified N

A6513 Compression burn mask, face and/or neck, plastic or equal, custom fabricated B ♿

A6520 Gradient compression garment, glove, padded, for nighttime use, each A

A6521 Gradient compression garment, glove, padded, for nighttime use, custom, each A

A6522 Gradient compression garment, arm, padded, for nighttime use, each A

A6523 Gradient compression garment, arm, padded, for nighttime use, custom, each A

A6524 Gradient compression garment, lower leg and foot, padded, for nighttime use, each A

A6525 Gradient compression garment, lower leg and foot, padded, for nighttime use, custom, each A

A6526 Gradient compression garment, full leg and foot, padded, for nighttime use, each A

A6527 Gradient compression garment, full leg and foot, padded, for nighttime use, custom, each A

A6528 Gradient compression garment, bra, for nighttime use, each A

A6529 Gradient compression garment, bra, for nighttime use, custom, each A

A6530 Gradient compression stocking, below knee, 18-30 mm Hg, each A ☑

A6531 Gradient compression stocking, below knee, 30-40 mm Hg, used as a surgical dressing, each A ☑ ♿ (AW)

A6532 Gradient compression stocking, below knee, 40-50 mm Hg, used as a surgical dressing, each A ☑ ♿ (AW)

A6533 Gradient compression stocking, thigh length, 18-30 mm Hg, each A ☑

A6534 Gradient compression stocking, thigh length, 30-40 mm Hg, each A ☑

A6535 Gradient compression stocking, thigh length, 40 mm Hg or greater, each A ☑

A6536 Gradient compression stocking, full-length/chap style, 18-30 mm Hg, each A ☑

A6537 Gradient compression stocking, full-length/chap style, 30-40 mm Hg, each A ☑

A6538 Gradient compression stocking, full length/chap style, 40 mm Hg or greater, each A ☑

A6539 Gradient compression stocking, waist length, 18-30 mm Hg, each

A6540 Gradient compression stocking, waist length, 30-40 mm Hg, each

A6541 Gradient compression stocking, waist length, 40 mm Hg or greater, each

A6544 Gradient compression stocking, garter belt

A6545 Gradient compression wrap, nonelastic, below knee, 30-50 mm Hg, used as a surgical dressing, each (AW)

A6549 Gradient compression garment, not otherwise specified

A6550 Wound care set, for negative pressure wound therapy electrical pump, includes all supplies and accessories
CMS: 100-02,7,40.1.2.8

A6552 Gradient compression stocking, below knee, 30-40 mm Hg, each

A6553 Gradient compression stocking, below knee, 30-40 mm Hg, custom, each

A6554 Gradient compression stocking, below knee, 40 mm Hg or greater, each

A6555 Gradient compression stocking, below knee, 40 mm Hg or greater, custom, each

A6556 Gradient compression stocking, thigh length, 18-30 mm Hg, custom, each

A6557 Gradient compression stocking, thigh length, 30-40 mm Hg, custom, each

A6558 Gradient compression stocking, thigh length, 40 mm Hg or greater, custom, each

A6559 Gradient compression stocking, full length/chap style, 18-30 mm Hg, custom, each

A6560 Gradient compression stocking, full length/chap style, 30-40 mm Hg, custom, each

A6561 Gradient compression stocking, full length/chap style, 40 mm Hg or greater, custom, each

A6562 Gradient compression stocking, waist length, 18-30 mm Hg, custom, each

A6563 Gradient compression stocking, waist length, 30-40 mm Hg, custom, each

A6564 Gradient compression stocking, waist length, 40 mm Hg or greater, custom, each

A6565 Gradient compression gauntlet, custom, each

A6566 Gradient compression garment, neck/head, each

A6567 Gradient compression garment, neck/head, custom, each

A6568 Gradient compression garment, torso and shoulder, each

A6569 Gradient compression garment, torso/shoulder, custom, each

A6570 Gradient compression garment, genital region, each

A6571 Gradient compression garment, genital region, custom, each

A6572 Gradient compression garment, toe caps, each

A6573 Gradient compression garment, toe caps, custom, each

A6574 Gradient compression arm sleeve and glove combination, custom, each

A6575 Gradient compression arm sleeve and glove combination, each

A6576 Gradient compression arm sleeve, custom, medium weight, each

A6577 Gradient compression arm sleeve, custom, heavy weight, each

A6578 Gradient compression arm sleeve, each

A6579 Gradient compression glove, custom, medium weight, each

A6580 Gradient compression glove, custom, heavy weight, each

A6581 Gradient compression glove, each

A6582 Gradient compression gauntlet, each

A6583 Gradient compression wrap with adjustable straps, below knee, 30-50 mm Hg, each

A6584 Gradient compression wrap with adjustable straps, not otherwise specified

A6585 Gradient pressure wrap with adjustable straps, above knee, each

A6586 Gradient pressure wrap with adjustable straps, full leg, each

A6587 Gradient pressure wrap with adjustable straps, foot, each

A6588 Gradient pressure wrap with adjustable straps, arm, each

A6589 Gradient pressure wrap with adjustable straps, bra, each

External Urinary Catheters

A6590 External urinary catheters; disposable, with wicking material, for use with suction pump, per month
AHA: 2Q,23

A6591 External urinary catheter; non-disposable, for use with suction pump, per month
AHA: 2Q,23

Gradient Compression Accessories/Supplies

A6593 Accessory for gradient compression garment or wrap with adjustable straps, not otherwise specified

A6594 Gradient compression bandaging supply, bandage liner, lower extremity, any size or length, each

A6595 Gradient compression bandaging supply, bandage liner, upper extremity, any size or length, each

A6596 Gradient compression bandaging supply, conforming gauze, per linear yd, any width, each

A6597 Gradient compression bandage roll, elastic long stretch, linear yd, any width, each

A6598 Gradient compression bandage roll, elastic medium stretch, per linear yd, any width, each

A6599 Gradient compression bandage roll, inelastic short stretch, per linear yd, any width, each

A6600 Gradient compression bandaging supply, high density foam sheet, per 250 sq cm, each

A6601 Gradient compression bandaging supply, high density foam pad, any size or shape, each

A6602 Gradient compression bandaging supply, high density foam roll for bandage, per linear yd, any width, each

A6603 Gradient compression bandaging supply, low density channel foam sheet, per 250 sq cm, each

A6604 Gradient compression bandaging supply, low density flat foam sheet, per 250 sq cm, each

A6605 Gradient compression bandaging supply, padded foam, per linear yd, any width, each

A6606 Gradient compression bandaging supply, padded textile, per linear yd, any width, each [A]

A6607 Gradient compression bandaging supply, tubular protective absorption layer, per linear yd, any width, each [A]

A6608 Gradient compression bandaging supply, tubular protective absorption padded layer, per linear yd, any width, each [A]

A6609 Gradient compression bandaging supply, not otherwise specified [A]

A6610 Gradient compression stocking, below knee, 18-30 mm Hg, custom, each [A]

Respiratory Supplies

A7000 Canister, disposable, used with suction pump, each [Y] ☑ ♿ (NU)

A7001 Canister, nondisposable, used with suction pump, each [Y] ☑ ♿ (NU)

A7002 Tubing, used with suction pump, each [Y] ☑ ♿ (NU)

A7003 Administration set, with small volume nonfiltered pneumatic nebulizer, disposable [Y] ♿ (NU)

A7004 Small volume nonfiltered pneumatic nebulizer, disposable [Y] ♿ (NU)

A7005 Administration set, with small volume nonfiltered pneumatic nebulizer, nondisposable [Y] ♿ (NU)

A7006 Administration set, with small volume filtered pneumatic nebulizer [Y] ♿ (NU)

A7007 Large volume nebulizer, disposable, unfilled, used with aerosol compressor [Y] ♿ (NU)

A7008 Large volume nebulizer, disposable, prefilled, used with aerosol compressor [Y] ♿ (NU)

A7009 Reservoir bottle, nondisposable, used with large volume ultrasonic nebulizer [Y] ♿ (NU)

A7010 Corrugated tubing, disposable, used with large volume nebulizer, 100 ft [Y] ☑ ♿ (NU)

A7012 Water collection device, used with large volume nebulizer [Y] ♿ (NU)

A7013 Filter, disposable, used with aerosol compressor or ultrasonic generator [Y] ♿ (NU)

A7014 Filter, nondisposable, used with aerosol compressor or ultrasonic generator [Y] ♿ (NU)

A7015 Aerosol mask, used with DME nebulizer [Y] ♿ (NU)

A7016 Dome and mouthpiece, used with small volume ultrasonic nebulizer [Y] ♿ (NU)

A7017 Nebulizer, durable, glass or autoclavable plastic, bottle type, not used with oxygen [Y] ♿ (NU, RR, UE)

A7018 Water, distilled, used with large volume nebulizer, 1000 ml [Y] ☑ ♿

A7020 Interface for cough stimulating device, includes all components, replacement only [Y] ♿ (NU)

● **A7021** Supplies and accessories for lung expansion airway clearance, continuous high frequency oscillation, and nebulization device (e.g., handset, nebulizer kit, biofilter) (NU)

A7023 Mechanical allergen particle barrier/inhalation filter, cream, nasal, topical [E]

A7025 High frequency chest wall oscillation system vest, replacement for use with patient-owned equipment, each [N] ☑ ♿ (RR)

A7026 High frequency chest wall oscillation system hose, replacement for use with patient-owned equipment, each [Y] ☑ ♿ (NU)

A7027 Combination oral/nasal mask, used with continuous positive airway pressure device, each [Y] ☑ ♿ (NU)

A7028 Oral cushion for combination oral/nasal mask, replacement only, each [Y] ☑ ♿ (NU)

A7029 Nasal pillows for combination oral/nasal mask, replacement only, pair [Y] ☑ ♿ (NU)

A7030 Full face mask used with positive airway pressure device, each [Y] ☑ ♿ (NU)
CMS: 100-04,36,50.14

A7031 Face mask interface, replacement for full face mask, each [Y] ☑ ♿ (NU)
CMS: 100-04,36,50.14

A7032 Cushion for use on nasal mask interface, replacement only, each [Y] ☑ ♿ (NU)
CMS: 100-03,240.4; 100-04,36,50.14

A7033 Pillow for use on nasal cannula type interface, replacement only, pair [Y] ☑ ♿ (NU)
CMS: 100-03,240.4; 100-04,36,50.14

A7034 Nasal interface (mask or cannula type) used with positive airway pressure device, with or without head strap [Y] ♿ (NU)
CMS: 100-03,240.4; 100-04,36,50.14

A7035 Headgear used with positive airway pressure device [Y] ♿ (NU)
CMS: 100-03,240.4; 100-04,36,50.14

A7036 Chinstrap used with positive airway pressure device [Y] ♿ (NU)
CMS: 100-03,240.4; 100-04,36,50.14

A7037 Tubing used with positive airway pressure device [Y] ♿ (NU)
CMS: 100-03,240.4; 100-04,36,50.14

A7038 Filter, disposable, used with positive airway pressure device [Y] ♿ (NU)
CMS: 100-04,36,50.14

A7039 Filter, nondisposable, used with positive airway pressure device [Y] ♿ (NU)
CMS: 100-04,36,50.14

A7040 One way chest drain valve [N] ♿

A7041 Water seal drainage container and tubing for use with implanted chest tube [N] ♿

A7044 Oral interface used with positive airway pressure device, each [Y] ☑ ♿ (NU)
CMS: 100-03,240.4; 100-04,36,50.14

A7045 Exhalation port with or without swivel used with accessories for positive airway devices, replacement only [Y] ♿ (NU, RR, UE)
CMS: 100-03,240.4; 100-04,36,50.14

A7046 Water chamber for humidifier, used with positive airway pressure device, replacement, each [Y] ☑ ♿ (NU)
CMS: 100-04,36,50.14

A7047 Oral interface used with respiratory suction pump, each [N] ☑ ♿ (NU)

A7048 Vacuum drainage collection unit and tubing kit, including all supplies needed for collection unit change, for use with implanted catheter, each [N] ♿

A7049 Expiratory positive airway pressure intranasal resistance valve [E]
AHA: 2Q,23

Tracheostomy Supplies

A7501 Tracheostoma valve, including diaphragm, each [N] ☑ ♿

A7502 Replacement diaphragm/faceplate for tracheostoma valve, each [N] ☑ ♿

A7503 Filter holder or filter cap, reusable, for use in a tracheostoma heat and moisture exchange system, each N ☑ ♿

A7504 Filter for use in a tracheostoma heat and moisture exchange system, each N ☑ ♿

A7505 Housing, reusable without adhesive, for use in a heat and moisture exchange system and/or with a tracheostoma valve, each N ☑ ♿

A7506 Adhesive disc for use in a heat and moisture exchange system and/or with tracheostoma valve, any type each N ☑ ♿

A7507 Filter holder and integrated filter without adhesive, for use in a tracheostoma heat and moisture exchange system, each N ☑ ♿

A7508 Housing and integrated adhesive, for use in a tracheostoma heat and moisture exchange system and/or with a tracheostoma valve, each N ☑ ♿

A7509 Filter holder and integrated filter housing, and adhesive, for use as a tracheostoma heat and moisture exchange system, each N ☑ ♿

A7520 Tracheostomy/laryngectomy tube, noncuffed, polyvinyl chloride (PVC), silicone or equal, each N ☑ ♿

A7521 Tracheostomy/laryngectomy tube, cuffed, polyvinyl chloride (PVC), silicone or equal, each N ☑ ♿

A7522 Tracheostomy/laryngectomy tube, stainless steel or equal (sterilizable and reusable), each N ☑ ♿

A7523 Tracheostomy shower protector, each N ☑

A7524 Tracheostoma stent/stud/button, each N ☑ ♿

A7525 Tracheostomy mask, each N ☑ ♿

A7526 Tracheostomy tube collar/holder, each N ☑ ♿

A7527 Tracheostomy/laryngectomy tube plug/stop, each N ☑ ♿

Protective Helmet

A8000 Helmet, protective, soft, prefabricated, includes all components and accessories Y ♿ (NU, RR, UE)

A8001 Helmet, protective, hard, prefabricated, includes all components and accessories Y ♿ (NU, RR, UE)

A8002 Helmet, protective, soft, custom fabricated, includes all components and accessories Y ♿ (NU, RR, UE)

A8003 Helmet, protective, hard, custom fabricated, includes all components and accessories Y ♿ (NU, RR, UE)

A8004 Soft interface for helmet, replacement only Y ♿ (NU, RR, UE)

Other Supplies and Devices

A9150 Nonprescription drugs B

A9152 Single vitamin/mineral/trace element, oral, per dose, not otherwise specified E1 ☑

A9153 Multiple vitamins, with or without minerals and trace elements, oral, per dose, not otherwise specified E1 ☑

A9155 Artificial saliva, 30 ml B ☑

A9156 Oral mucoadhesive, any type (liquid, gel, paste, etc.), per 1 ml N N1

Use this code for MuGard.

AHA: 4Q,23

A9180 Pediculosis (lice infestation) treatment, topical, for administration by patient/caretaker E1

A9268 Programmer for transient, orally ingested capsule E1

AHA: 4Q,23

A9269 Programmable, transient, orally ingested capsule, for use with external programmer, per month E1

AHA: 4Q,23

A9270 Noncovered item or service E1

CMS: 100-04,11,100.1; 100-04,20,30.9; 100-04,23,20.9.1.1

A9272 Wound suction, disposable, includes dressing, all accessories and components, any type, each A ☑

CMS: 100-04,10,40.2

A9273 Cold or hot fluid bottle, ice cap or collar, heat and/or cold wrap, any type E1

A9274 External ambulatory insulin delivery system, disposable, each, includes all supplies and accessories E1 ☑

A9275 Home glucose disposable monitor, includes test strips E1

A9276 Sensor; invasive (e.g., subcutaneous), disposable, for use with nondurable medical equipment interstitial continuous glucose monitoring system (CGM), one unit = 1 day supply E1 ☑

A9277 Transmitter; external, for use with nondurable medical equipment interstitial continuous glucose monitoring system (CGM) E1

A9278 Receiver (monitor); external, for use with nondurable medical equipment interstitial continuous glucose monitoring system (CGM) E1

A9279 Monitoring feature/device, stand-alone or integrated, any type, includes all accessories, components and electronics, not otherwise classified E1

A9280 Alert or alarm device, not otherwise classified E1

A9281 Reaching/grabbing device, any type, any length, each E1 ☑

A9282 Wig, any type, each E1 ☑

A9283 Foot pressure off loading/supportive device, any type, each E1 ☑

A9284 Spirometer, nonelectronic, includes all accessories N

A9285 Inversion/eversion correction device A

A9286 Hygienic item or device, disposable or nondisposable, any type, each E1

A9291 Prescription digital cognitive and/or behavioral therapy, FDA-cleared, per course of treatment E1

AHA: 4Q,22

A9292 Prescription digital visual therapy, software-only, FDA cleared, per course of treatment E1

AHA: 4Q,23

● **A9293** Fertility cycle (contraception & conception) tracking software application, FDA cleared, per month, includes accessories (e.g., thermometer) E1

AHA: 2Q,24

A9300 Exercise equipment E1

Radiopharmaceuticals

A9500 Technetium Tc-99m sestamibi, diagnostic, per study dose N N1 ☑ ⊘

Use this code for Cardiolite.

A9501 Technetium Tc-99m teboroxime, diagnostic, per study dose N N1 ☑ ⊘

A9502 Technetium Tc-99m tetrofosmin, diagnostic, per study dose N N1 ☑ ⊘

Use this code for Myoview.

A9503 Technetium Tc-99m medronate, diagnostic, per study dose, up to 30 mCi
Use this code for CIS-MDP, Draximage MDP-10, Draximage MDP-25, MDP-Bracco, Technetium Tc-99m MPI-MDP.

A9504 Technetium Tc-99m apcitide, diagnostic, per study dose, up to 20 mCi
Use this code for Acutect.

A9505 Thallium Tl-201 thallous chloride, diagnostic, per mCi
Use this code for MIBG, Thallous Chloride USP.

● **A9506** Graphite crucible for preparation of technetium Tc 99m-labeled carbon aerosol, one crucible
Use this code for Technegas.
AHA: 3Q,24

A9507 Indium In-111 capromab pendetide, diagnostic, per study dose, up to 10 millicuries
Use this code for Prostascint.

A9508 Iodine I-131 iobenguane sulfate, diagnostic, per 0.5 mCi
Use this code for MIBG.

A9509 Iodine I-123 sodium iodide, diagnostic, per mCi

A9510 Technetium Tc-99m disofenin, diagnostic, per study dose, up to 15 mCi
Use this code for Hepatolite.

A9512 Technetium Tc-99m pertechnetate, diagnostic, per mCi
Use this code for Technelite, Ultra-Technekow.

A9513 Lutetium Lu 177, dotatate, therapeutic, 1 mCi
Use this code for Lutathera.
AHA: 1Q,19

A9515 Choline C-11, diagnostic, per study dose up to 20 mCi

A9516 Iodine I-123 sodium iodide, diagnostic, per 100 mcCi, up to 999 mcCi

A9517 Iodine I-131 sodium iodide capsule(s), therapeutic, per mCi

A9520 Technetium Tc-99m, tilmanocept, diagnostic, up to 0.5 mCi

A9521 Technetium Tc-99m exametazime, diagnostic, per study dose, up to 25 mCi
Use this code for Ceretec.

A9524 Iodine I-131 iodinated serum albumin, diagnostic, per 5 mcCi

A9526 Nitrogen N-13 ammonia, diagnostic, per study dose, up to 40 mCi
CMS: 100-04,13,60.3; 100-04,13,60.3.2
AHA: 1Q,22

A9527 Iodine I-125, sodium iodide solution, therapeutic, per mCi

A9528 Iodine I-131 sodium iodide capsule(s), diagnostic, per mCi

A9529 Iodine I-131 sodium iodide solution, diagnostic, per mCi

A9530 Iodine I-131 sodium iodide solution, therapeutic, per mCi

A9531 Iodine I-131 sodium iodide, diagnostic, per mCi (up to 100 mcCi)

A9532 Iodine I-125 serum albumin, diagnostic, per 5 mcCi

A9536 Technetium Tc-99m depreotide, diagnostic, per study dose, up to 35 mCi

A9537 Technetium Tc-99m mebrofenin, diagnostic, per study dose, up to 15 mCi

A9538 Technetium Tc-99m pyrophosphate, diagnostic, per study dose, up to 25 mCi
Use this code for CIS-PYRO, Phosphotec, Technescan Pyp Kit.

A9539 Technetium Tc-99m pentetate, diagnostic, per study dose, up to 25 mCi
Use this code for AN-DTPA, DTPA, MPI-DTPA Kit-Chelate, MPI Indium DTPA IN-111, Pentetate Calcium Trisodium, Pentate Zinc Trisodium.

A9540 Technetium Tc-99m macroaggregated albumin, diagnostic, per study dose, up to 10 mCi

A9541 Technetium Tc-99m sulfur colloid, diagnostic, per study dose, up to 20 mCi

A9542 Indium In-111 ibritumomab tiuxetan, diagnostic, per study dose, up to 5 mCi
Use this code for Zevalin.

A9543 Yttrium Y-90 ibritumomab tiuxetan, therapeutic, per treatment dose, up to 40 mCi

A9546 Cobalt Co-57/58, cyanocobalamin, diagnostic, per study dose, up to 1 mcCi

A9547 Indium In-111 oxyquinoline, diagnostic, per 0.5 mCi

A9548 Indium In-111 pentetate, diagnostic, per 0.5 mCi

A9550 Technetium Tc-99m sodium gluceptate, diagnostic, per study dose, up to 25 mCi

A9551 Technetium Tc-99m succimer, diagnostic, per study dose, up to 10 mCi
Use this code for MPI-DMSA Kidney Reagent.

A9552 Fluorodeoxyglucose F-18 FDG, diagnostic, per study dose, up to 45 mCi
CMS: 100-03,220.6.13; 100-03,220.6.17; 100-04,13,60.15; 100-04,13,60.16; 100-04,13,60.3.2
AHA: 1Q,22

A9553 Chromium Cr-51 sodium chromate, diagnostic, per study dose, up to 250 mcCi
Use this code for Chromitope Sodium.

A9554 Iodine I-125 sodium iothalamate, diagnostic, per study dose, up to 10 mcCi
Use this code for Glofil-125.

A9555 Rubidium Rb-82, diagnostic, per study dose, up to 60 mCi
Use this code for Cardiogen 82.
CMS: 100-03,220.6.1; 100-04,13,60.3.2
AHA: 1Q,22

A9556 Gallium Ga-67 citrate, diagnostic, per mCi

A9557 Technetium Tc-99m bicisate, diagnostic, per study dose, up to 25 mCi
Use this code for Neurolite.

A9558 Xenon Xe-133 gas, diagnostic, per 10 mCi

A9559 Cobalt Co-57 cyanocobalamin, oral, diagnostic, per study dose, up to 1 mcCi

A9560 Technetium Tc-99m labeled red blood cells, diagnostic, per study dose, up to 30 mCi

A9561 Technetium Tc-99m oxidronate, diagnostic, per study dose, up to 30 mCi
Use this code for TechneScan.

A9562 Technetium Tc-99m mertiatide, diagnostic, per study dose, up to 15 mCi
Use this code for TechneScan MAG-3.

A9563 Sodium phosphate P-32, therapeutic, per mCi

A9564 Chromic phosphate P-32 suspension, therapeutic, per mCi
Use this code for Phosphocol (P32).

A9566 Technetium Tc-99m fanolesomab, diagnostic, per study dose, up to 25 mCi

A9567 Technetium Tc-99m pentetate, diagnostic, aerosol, per study dose, up to 75 mCi
Use this code for AN-DTPA, DTPA, MPI-DTPA Kit-Chelate, MPI Indium DTPA IN-111, Pentate Calcium Trisodium, Pentate Zinc Trisodium.

A9568 Technetium Tc-99m arcitumomab, diagnostic, per study dose, up to 45 mCi
Use this code for CEA Scan.

A9569 Technetium Tc-99m exametazime labeled autologous white blood cells, diagnostic, per study dose

A9570 Indium In-111 labeled autologous white blood cells, diagnostic, per study dose

A9571 Indium In-111 labeled autologous platelets, diagnostic, per study dose

A9572 Indium In-111 pentetreotide, diagnostic, per study dose, up to 6 mCi
Use this code for Octreoscan.

A9573 Injection, gadopiclenol, 1 ml
Use this code for Vueway.
AHA: 4Q,23

A9575 Injection, gadoterate meglumine, 0.1 ml
Use this code for Dotarem.

A9576 Injection, gadoteridol, (ProHance multipack), per ml

A9577 Injection, gadobenate dimeglumine (MultiHance), per ml

A9578 Injection, gadobenate dimeglumine (MultiHance multipack), per ml

A9579 Injection, gadolinium-based magnetic resonance contrast agent, not otherwise specified (NOS), per ml
Use this code for Omniscan, Magnevist.
CMS: 100-03,1,220.2

A9580 Sodium fluoride F-18, diagnostic, per study dose, up to 30 mCi
CMS: 100-03,220.6.19; 100-04,13,60.18; 100-04,13,60.3.2

A9581 Injection, gadoxetate disodium, 1 ml
Use this code for Eovist.

A9582 Iodine I-123 iobenguane, diagnostic, per study dose, up to 15 mCi

A9583 Injection, gadofosveset trisodium, 1 ml
Use this code for Ablavar, Vasovist.

A9584 Iodine I-123 ioflupane, diagnostic, per study dose, up to 5 mCi
Use this code for DaTscan.

A9585 Injection, gadobutrol, 0.1 ml
Use this code for Gadavist.

A9586 Florbetapir F18, diagnostic, per study dose, up to 10 mCi
Use this code for Amyvid.
CMS: 100-04,13,60.12; 100-04,17, 80.12; 100-04,32,60.12

A9587 Gallium Ga-68, dotatate, diagnostic, 0.1 mCi
Use this code for Netspot.
CMS: 100-04,13,60.3.2

A9588 Fluciclovine F-18, diagnostic, 1 mCi
Use this code for Axumin.
CMS: 100-04,13,60.3.2

A9589 Instillation, hexaminolevulinate HCl, 100 mg
Use this code for Cysview.
CMS: 100-04,13,60.3.2
AHA: 1Q,19

A9590 Iodine I-131, iobenguane, 1 mCi
Use this code for Azedra.
CMS: 100-04,13,60.3.2

A9591 Fluoroestradiol F-18, diagnostic, 1 mCi
Use this code for Cerianna.
CMS: 100-04,13,60.3.2
AHA: 1Q,21

A9592 Copper Cu-64, dotatate, diagnostic, 1 mCi
Use this code for Detectnet.
CMS: 100-04,13,60.3.2
AHA: 1Q,21

A9593 Gallium Ga-68 PSMA-11, diagnostic, (UCSF), 1 mCi
CMS: 100-04,13,60.3.2
AHA: 3Q,21

A9594 Gallium Ga-68 PSMA-11, diagnostic, (UCLA), 1 mCi
CMS: 100-04,13,60.3.2
AHA: 3Q,21

A9595 Piflufolastat F-18, diagnostic, 1 mCi
Use this code for Pylarify.
CMS: 100-04,13,60.3.2
AHA: 1Q,22

A9596 Gallium Ga-68 gozetotide, diagnostic, (Illuccix), 1 mCi
CMS: 100-04,13,60.3.2
AHA: 3Q,22

A9597 Positron emission tomography radiopharmaceutical, diagnostic, for tumor identification, not otherwise classified
CMS: 100-04,13,60.3.2

A9598 Positron emission tomography radiopharmaceutical, diagnostic, for nontumor identification, not otherwise classified
CMS: 100-04,13,60.3.2

A9600 Strontium Sr-89 chloride, therapeutic, per mCi
Use this code for Metastron.

A9601 Flortaucipir F 18 injection, diagnostic, 1 mCi
Use this code for Tauvid.
AHA: 3Q,22

A9602 Fluorodopa F-18, diagnostic, per mCi
AHA: 4Q,22

A9603 Injection, pafolacianine, 0.1 mg
Use this code for Cytalux.
AHA: 4Q,23

A9604 Samarium Sm-153 lexidronam, therapeutic, per treatment dose, up to 150 mCi
Use this code for Quadramet.

A9606 Radium RA-223 dichloride, therapeutic, per UCI
Use this code for Xofigo.

A9607 Lutetium Lu 177 vipivotide tetraxetan, therapeutic, 1 mCi
Use this code for Pluvicto.
AHA: 4Q,22

A9608 **Flotufolastat F18, diagnostic, 1 mCi** G K2
Use this code for Posluma.
AHA: 1Q,24

A9609 **Fludeoxyglucose F18, up to 15 mCi** N N1
AHA: 1Q,24

● **A9610** **Xenon Xe-129 hyperpolarized gas, diagnostic, per study dose**
Use this code for Xenoview.

● **A9615** **Injection, pegulicianine, 1 mg**
Use this code for Lumisight.

A9697 **Injection, carboxydextran-coated superparamagnetic iron oxide, per study dose** N N1
Use this code for Magtrace.
AHA: 4Q,23

A9698 **Nonradioactive contrast imaging material, not otherwise classified, per study** N N1 ☑ ⊘

A9699 **Radiopharmaceutical, therapeutic, not otherwise classified** N ☑ ⊘

A9700 **Supply of injectable contrast material for use in echocardiography, per study** N N1

A9800 **Gallium Ga-68 gozetotide, diagnostic, (Locametz), 1 mCi** G K2
AHA: 4Q,22

Miscellaneous

A9900 **Miscellaneous DME supply, accessory, and/or service component of another HCPCS code** Y

A9901 **DME delivery, set up, and/or dispensing service component of another HCPCS code** A

A9999 **Miscellaneous DME supply or accessory, not otherwise specified** Y

Medical and Surgical Supplies

A9608 — A9999

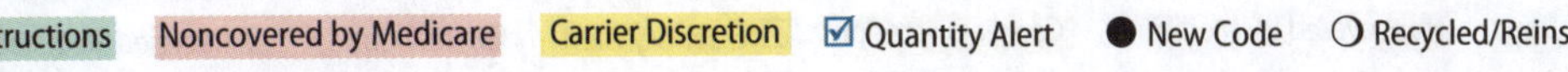
Special Coverage Instructions | Noncovered by Medicare | Carrier Discretion | ☑ Quantity Alert | ● New Code | ○ Recycled/Reinstated | ▲ Revised Code

Enteral and Parenteral Therapy B4034-B9999

This section includes codes for supplies, formulae, nutritional solutions, and infusion pumps.

Enteral Formulae and Enteral Medical Supplies

B4034 **Enteral feeding supply kit; syringe fed, per day, includes but not limited to feeding/flushing syringe, administration set tubing, dressings, tape** Y ☑
CMS: 100-03,180.2; 100-04,20,160.2

B4035 **Enteral feeding supply kit; pump fed, per day, includes but not limited to feeding/flushing syringe, administration set tubing, dressings, tape** Y ☑
CMS: 100-03,180.2; 100-04,20,160.2

B4036 **Enteral feeding supply kit; gravity fed, per day, includes but not limited to feeding/flushing syringe, administration set tubing, dressings, tape** Y ☑
CMS: 100-03,180.2; 100-04,20,160.2

B4081 **Nasogastric tubing with stylet** Y
CMS: 100-03,180.2; 100-04,20,160.2

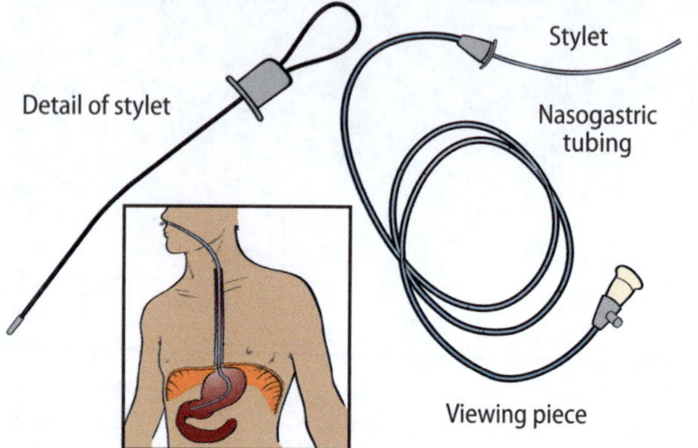

B4082 **Nasogastric tubing without stylet** Y
CMS: 100-03,180.2; 100-04,20,160.2

B4083 **Stomach tube - Levine type** Y
CMS: 100-03,180.2; 100-04,20,160.2

B4087 **Gastrostomy/jejunostomy tube, standard, any material, any type, each** Y ☑
CMS: 100-03,180.2

B4088 **Gastrostomy/jejunostomy tube, low-profile, any material, any type, each** Y ☑
CMS: 100-03,180.2

B4100 **Food thickener, administered orally, per oz** EI ☑
CMS: 100-03,180.2

B4102 **Enteral formula, for adults, used to replace fluids and electrolytes (e.g., clear liquids), 500 ml = 1 unit** Y ☑
CMS: 100-03,180.2

B4103 **Enteral formula, for pediatrics, used to replace fluids and electrolytes (e.g., clear liquids), 500 ml = 1 unit** Y ☑
CMS: 100-03,180.2

B4104 **Additive for enteral formula (e.g., fiber)** EI
CMS: 100-03,180.2

B4105 **In-line cartridge containing digestive enzyme(s) for enteral feeding, each** Y
CMS: 100-03,180.2

B4148 **Enteral feeding supply kit; elastomeric control fed, per day, includes but not limited to feeding/flushing syringe, administration set tubing, dressings, tape** Y
CMS: 100-03,180.2
AHA: 4Q,23

B4149 **Enteral formula, manufactured blenderized natural foods with intact nutrients, includes proteins, fats, carbohydrates, vitamins and minerals, may include fiber, administered through an enteral feeding tube, 100 calories = 1 unit** Y ☑
CMS: 100-03,180.2

B4150 **Enteral formula, nutritionally complete with intact nutrients, includes proteins, fats, carbohydrates, vitamins and minerals, may include fiber, administered through an enteral feeding tube, 100 calories = 1 unit** Y ☑
Use this code for Enrich, Ensure, Ensure HN, Ensure Powder, Isocal, Lonalac Powder, Meritene, Meritene Powder, Osmolite, Osmolite HN, Portagen Powder, Sustacal, Renu, Sustagen Powder, Travasorb.
CMS: 100-03,180.2; 100-04,20,160.2

B4152 **Enteral formula, nutritionally complete, calorically dense (equal to or greater than 1.5 kcal/ml) with intact nutrients, includes proteins, fats, carbohydrates, vitamins and minerals, may include fiber, administered through an enteral feeding tube, 100 calories = 1 unit** Y ☑
Use this code for Magnacal, Isocal HCN, Sustacal HC, Ensure Plus, Ensure Plus HN.
CMS: 100-03,180.2; 100-04,20,160.2

B4153 **Enteral formula, nutritionally complete, hydrolyzed proteins (amino acids and peptide chain), includes fats, carbohydrates, vitamins and minerals, may include fiber, administered through an enteral feeding tube, 100 calories = 1 unit** Y ☑
Use this code for Criticare HN, Vivonex t.e.n. (Total Enteral Nutrition), Vivonex HN, Vital (Vital HN), Travasorb HN, Isotein HN, Precision HN, Precision Isotonic.
CMS: 100-03,180.2; 100-04,20,160.2

B4154 **Enteral formula, nutritionally complete, for special metabolic needs, excludes inherited disease of metabolism, includes altered composition of proteins, fats, carbohydrates, vitamins and/or minerals, may include fiber, administered through an enteral feeding tube, 100 calories = 1 unit** Y ☑
Use this code for Hepatic-aid, Travasorb Hepatic, Travasorb MCT, Travasorb Renal, Traum-aid, Tramacal, Aminaid.
CMS: 100-03,180.2; 100-04,20,160.2

B4155 **Enteral formula, nutritionally incomplete/modular nutrients, includes specific nutrients, carbohydrates (e.g., glucose polymers), proteins/amino acids (e.g., glutamine, arginine), fat (e.g., medium chain triglycerides) or combination, administered through an enteral feeding tube, 100 calories = 1 unit** Y ☑
Use this code for Propac, Gevral Protein, Promix, Casec, Moducal, Controlyte, Polycose Liquid or Powder, Sumacal, Microlipids, MCT Oil, Nutri-source.
CMS: 100-03,180.2; 100-04,20,160.2

B4157 **Enteral formula, nutritionally complete, for special metabolic needs for inherited disease of metabolism, includes proteins, fats, carbohydrates, vitamins and minerals, may include fiber, administered through an enteral feeding tube, 100 calories = 1 unit** Y ☑
CMS: 100-03,180.2

B4158 **Enteral formula, for pediatrics, nutritionally complete with intact nutrients, includes proteins, fats, carbohydrates, vitamins and minerals, may include fiber and/or iron, administered through an enteral feeding tube, 100 calories = 1 unit** Y ☑
CMS: 100-03,180.2

B4159 Enteral formula, for pediatrics, nutritionally complete soy based with intact nutrients, includes proteins, fats, carbohydrates, vitamins and minerals, may include fiber and/or iron, administered through an enteral feeding tube, 100 calories = 1 unit Y ☑
CMS: 100-03,180.2

B4160 Enteral formula, for pediatrics, nutritionally complete calorically dense (equal to or greater than 0.7 kcal/ml) with intact nutrients, includes proteins, fats, carbohydrates, vitamins and minerals, may include fiber, administered through an enteral feeding tube, 100 calories = 1 unit Y ☑
CMS: 100-03,180.2

B4161 Enteral formula, for pediatrics, hydrolyzed/amino acids and peptide chain proteins, includes fats, carbohydrates, vitamins and minerals, may include fiber, administered through an enteral feeding tube, 100 calories = 1 unit Y ☑
CMS: 100-03,180.2

B4162 Enteral formula, for pediatrics, special metabolic needs for inherited disease of metabolism, includes proteins, fats, carbohydrates, vitamins and minerals, may include fiber, administered through an enteral feeding tube, 100 calories = 1 unit Y ☑
CMS: 100-03,180.2

Parenteral Nutrition Solutions and Supplies

B4164 Parenteral nutrition solution: carbohydrates (dextrose), 50% or less (500 ml = 1 unit), home mix Y ☑
CMS: 100-03,180.2; 100-04,20,160.2

B4168 Parenteral nutrition solution; amino acid, 3.5%, (500 ml = 1 unit) - home mix Y ☑
CMS: 100-03,180.2; 100-04,20,160.2

B4172 Parenteral nutrition solution; amino acid, 5.5% through 7%, (500 ml = 1 unit) - home mix Y ☑
CMS: 100-03,180.2; 100-04,20,160.2

B4176 Parenteral nutrition solution; amino acid, 7% through 8.5%, (500 ml = 1 unit) - home mix Y ☑
CMS: 100-03,180.2; 100-04,20,160.2

B4178 Parenteral nutrition solution: amino acid, greater than 8.5% (500 ml = 1 unit) - home mix Y ☑
CMS: 100-03,180.2; 100-04,20,160.2

B4180 Parenteral nutrition solution: carbohydrates (dextrose), greater than 50% (500 ml = 1 unit), home mix Y ☑
CMS: 100-03,180.2; 100-04,20,160.2

B4185 Parenteral nutrition solution, not otherwise specified, 10 g lipids B ☑
CMS: 100-03,180.2

B4187 Omegaven, 10 g lipids B
CMS: 100-03,180.2

B4189 Parenteral nutrition solution: compounded amino acid and carbohydrates with electrolytes, trace elements, and vitamins, including preparation, any strength, 10 to 51 g of protein, premix Y ☑
CMS: 100-03,180.2; 100-04,20,160.2

B4193 Parenteral nutrition solution: compounded amino acid and carbohydrates with electrolytes, trace elements, and vitamins, including preparation, any strength, 52 to 73 g of protein, premix Y ☑
CMS: 100-03,180.2; 100-04,20,160.2

B4197 Parenteral nutrition solution; compounded amino acid and carbohydrates with electrolytes, trace elements and vitamins, including preparation, any strength, 74 to 100 g of protein - premix Y ☑
CMS: 100-03,180.2; 100-04,20,160.2

B4199 Parenteral nutrition solution; compounded amino acid and carbohydrates with electrolytes, trace elements and vitamins, including preparation, any strength, over 100 g of protein - premix Y ☑
CMS: 100-03,180.2; 100-04,20,160.2

B4216 Parenteral nutrition; additives (vitamins, trace elements, Heparin, electrolytes), home mix, per day Y
CMS: 100-03,180.2; 100-04,20,160.2

B4220 Parenteral nutrition supply kit; premix, per day Y
CMS: 100-03,180.2; 100-04,20,160.2

B4222 Parenteral nutrition supply kit; home mix, per day Y
CMS: 100-03,180.2; 100-04,20,160.2

B4224 Parenteral nutrition administration kit, per day Y
CMS: 100-03,180.2; 100-04,20,160.2

B5000 Parenteral nutrition solution: compounded amino acid and carbohydrates with electrolytes, trace elements, and vitamins, including preparation, any strength, renal - Amirosyn RF, NephrAmine, RenAmine - premix Y
Use this code for Amirosyn-RF, NephrAmine, RenAmin.
CMS: 100-03,180.2; 100-04,20,160.2

B5100 Parenteral nutrition solution compounded amino acid and carbohydrates with electrolytes, trace elements, and vitamins, including preparation, any strength, hepatic-HepatAmine-premix Y
Use this code for FreAmine HBC, HepatAmine.
CMS: 100-03,180.2; 100-04,20,160.2

B5200 Parenteral nutrition solution compounded amino acid and carbohydrates with electrolytes, trace elements, and vitamins, including preparation, any strength, stress-branch chain amino acids-FreAmine-HBC-premix Y
CMS: 100-03,180.2; 100-04,20,160.2

Enteral and Parenteral Pumps

B9002 Enteral nutrition infusion pump, any type Y
CMS: 100-03,180.2; 100-04,20,160.2

B9004 Parenteral nutrition infusion pump, portable Y
CMS: 100-03,180.2; 100-04,20,160.2

B9006 Parenteral nutrition infusion pump, stationary Y
CMS: 100-03,180.2; 100-04,20,160.2

B9998 NOC for enteral supplies Y
CMS: 100-03,180.2

B9999 NOC for parenteral supplies Y
Determine if an alternative HCPCS Level II or a CPT code better describes the service being reported. This code should be used only if a more specific code is unavailable.
CMS: 100-03,180.2

B4159 Enteral formula, for pediatrics, nutritionally complete soy based with intact nutrients, includes proteins, fats, carbohydrates, vitamins and minerals, may include fiber, administered through an enteral feeding tube, 100 calories = 1 unit
CMS: 100-03,180.2

B4160 Enteral formula, for pediatrics, nutritionally complete calorically dense (equal to or greater than 0.7 kcal/ml) with intact nutrients, includes proteins, fats, carbohydrates, vitamins and minerals, may include fiber, administered through an enteral feeding tube, 100 calories = 1 unit
CMS: [illegible]

B4161 Enteral formula, for pediatrics, hydrolyzed/amino acids and peptide chain proteins, includes fats, carbohydrates, vitamins and minerals, may include fiber, administered through an enteral feeding tube, 100 calories = 1 unit
CMS: [illegible]

B4162 Enteral formula, for pediatrics, special metabolic needs for inherited disease of metabolism, includes proteins, fats, carbohydrates, vitamins and minerals, may include fiber, administered through an enteral feeding tube, 100 calories = 1 unit
CMS: [illegible]

Parenteral Nutrition Solutions and Supplies

B4164 Parenteral nutrition solution: carbohydrates (dextrose), 50% or less (500 ml = 1 unit), home mix
CMS: [illegible]

B4168 Parenteral nutrition solution; amino acid, 3.5%, (500 ml = 1 unit) - home mix
CMS: [illegible]

B4172 Parenteral nutrition solution; amino acid, 5.5% through 7% (500 ml = 1 unit) - home mix
CMS: [illegible]

B4176 Parenteral nutrition solution; amino acid, 7% through 8.5% (500 ml = 1 unit) - home mix
CMS: [illegible]

B4178 Parenteral nutrition solution: amino acid, greater than 8.5% (500 ml = 1 unit) - home mix
CMS: [illegible]

B4180 Parenteral nutrition solution: carbohydrates (dextrose), greater than 50% (500 ml = 1 unit), home mix
CMS: [illegible]

B4185 Parenteral nutrition solution, not otherwise specified, 10 g lipids
CMS: [illegible]

B4187 Omegaven, 10 g lipids
CMS: [illegible]

B4189 Parenteral nutrition solution: compounded amino acid and carbohydrates with electrolytes, trace elements, and vitamins, including preparation, any strength, 10 to 51 g of protein, premix
CMS: [illegible]

B4193 Parenteral nutrition solution: compounded amino acid and carbohydrates with electrolytes, trace elements, and vitamins, including preparation, any strength, 52 to 73 g of protein, premix
CMS: [illegible]

B4197 Parenteral nutrition solution; compounded amino acid and carbohydrates with electrolytes, trace elements and vitamins, including preparation, any strength, 74 to 100 g of protein - premix
CMS: [illegible]

B4199 Parenteral nutrition solution; compounded amino acid and carbohydrates with electrolytes, trace elements and vitamins, including preparation, any strength, over 100 g of protein - premix
CMS: [illegible]

B4216 Parenteral nutrition; additives (vitamins, trace elements, Heparin, electrolytes), home mix, per day
CMS: [illegible]

B4220 Parenteral nutrition supply kit; premix, per day
CMS: [illegible]

B4222 Parenteral nutrition supply kit; home mix, per day
CMS: [illegible]

B4224 Parenteral nutrition administration kit, per day
CMS: [illegible]

B5000 Parenteral nutrition solution: compounded amino acid and carbohydrates with electrolytes, trace elements, and vitamins, including preparation, any strength, renal - Aminosyn-RF, NephrAmine, RenAmine - premix
CMS: [illegible]

B5100 Parenteral nutrition solution: compounded amino acid and carbohydrates with electrolytes, trace elements, and vitamins, including preparation, any strength, hepatic - HepatAmine - premix
CMS: [illegible]

B5200 Parenteral nutrition solution: compounded amino acid and carbohydrates with electrolytes, trace elements, and vitamins, including preparation, any strength, stress - branch chain amino acids - FreAmine-HBC - premix
CMS: [illegible]

Enteral and Parenteral Pumps

B9002 Enteral nutrition infusion pump, any type
CMS: [illegible]

B9004 Parenteral nutrition infusion pump, portable
CMS: [illegible]

B9006 Parenteral nutrition infusion pump, stationary
CMS: [illegible]

B9998 NOC for enteral supplies
CMS: [illegible]

B9999 NOC for parenteral supplies
[illegible]
CMS: [illegible]

Outpatient PPS C1052-C9901

This section reports drug, biological, and device codes that must be used by OPPS hospitals. Non-OPPS hospitals, Critical Access Hospitals (CAHs), Indian Health Service Hospitals (HIS), hospitals located in American Samoa, Guam, Saipan, or the Virgin Islands, and Maryland waiver hospitals may report these codes at their discretion. The codes can only be reported for facility (technical) services.

The C series of HCPCS may include device categories, new technology procedures, and drugs, biologicals and radiopharmaceuticals that do not have other HCPCS codes assigned. Some of these items and services are eligible for transitional pass-through payments for OPPS hospitals, have separate APC payments, or are items that are packaged. Hospitals are encouraged to report all appropriate C codes regardless of payment status.

C1052 **Hemostatic agent, gastrointestinal, topical** N N1
CMS: 100-04,4,60.4.2

C1062 **Intravertebral body fracture augmentation with implant (e.g., metal, polymer)** N N1
CMS: 100-04,4,60.4.2

C1600 **Catheter, transluminal intravascular lesion preparation device, bladed, sheathed (insertable)** H J7
AHA: 1Q,24

C1601 **Endoscope, single-use (i.e., disposable), pulmonary, imaging/illumination device (insertable)** H J7
AHA: 1Q,24

C1602 **Orthopedic/device/drug matrix/absorbable bone void filler, antimicrobial-eluting (implantable)** H J7
AHA: 1Q,24

C1603 **Retrieval device, insertable, laser (used to retrieve intravascular inferior vena cava filter)** H J7
AHA: 1Q,24

C1604 **Graft, transmural transvenous arterial bypass (implantable), with all delivery system components** H N1
AHA: 1Q,24

● **C1605** **Pacemaker, leadless, dual chamber (right atrial and right ventricular implantable components), rate-responsive, including all necessary components for implantation** N1
AHA: 3Q,24

● **C1606** **Adapter, single-use (i.e., disposable), for attaching ultrasound system to upper gastrointestinal endoscope** J7
AHA: 3Q,24

C1713 **Anchor/screw for opposing bone-to-bone or soft tissue-to-bone (implantable)** N N1
CMS: 100-04,4,60.4.2; 100-04,4,60.4.3
AHA: 4Q,22; 3Q,22; 2Q,21; 1Q,21; 4Q,20; 2Q,18; 1Q,18

C1714 **Catheter, transluminal atherectomy, directional** N N1
CMS: 100-04,4,60.4.2

C1715 **Brachytherapy needle** N N1 ⃠
CMS: 100-04,4,60.4.2

C1716 **Brachytherapy source, nonstranded, gold-198, per source** U H2 ☑ ⃠
CMS: 100-04,4,60.4.2

C1717 **Brachytherapy source, nonstranded, high dose rate iridium-192, per source** U H2 ☑ ⃠
CMS: 100-04,4,60.4.2

C1719 **Brachytherapy source, nonstranded, nonhigh dose rate iridium-192, per source** U H2 ☑ ⃠
CMS: 100-04,4,60.4.2

C1721 **Cardioverter-defibrillator, dual chamber (implantable)** N N1
CMS: 100-04,14,40.8; 100-04,4,60.4.2

C1722 **Cardioverter-defibrillator, single chamber (implantable)** N N1
CMS: 100-04,14,40.8; 100-04,4,60.4.2

C1724 **Catheter, transluminal atherectomy, rotational** N N1
CMS: 100-04,4,60.4.1; 100-04,4,60.4.2

C1725 **Catheter, transluminal angioplasty, nonlaser (may include guidance, infusion/perfusion capability)** N N1
To appropriately report drug-coated transluminal angioplasty catheters, use HCPCS code C2623.
CMS: 100-04,4,60.4.2; 100-04,4,60.4.3

C1726 **Catheter, balloon dilatation, nonvascular** N N1
CMS: 100-04,4,60.4.2; 100-04,4,60.4.3

C1727 **Catheter, balloon tissue dissector, nonvascular (insertable)** N N1
CMS: 100-04,4,60.4.2; 100-04,4,60.4.3

C1728 **Catheter, brachytherapy seed administration** N N1 ⃠
CMS: 100-04,4,60.4.2

C1729 **Catheter, drainage** N N1
CMS: 100-04,4,60.4.2; 100-04,4,60.4.3

C1730 **Catheter, electrophysiology, diagnostic, other than 3D mapping (19 or fewer electrodes)** N N1
CMS: 100-04,4,60.4.2; 100-04,4,60.4.3

C1731 **Catheter, electrophysiology, diagnostic, other than 3D mapping (20 or more electrodes)** N N1
CMS: 100-04,4,60.4.2; 100-04,4,60.4.3

C1732 **Catheter, electrophysiology, diagnostic/ablation, 3D or vector mapping** N N1
CMS: 100-04,4,60.4.2; 100-04,4,60.4.3

C1733 **Catheter, electrophysiology, diagnostic/ablation, other than 3D or vector mapping, other than cool-tip** N N1
CMS: 100-04,4,60.4.2; 100-04,4,60.4.3

C1734 **Orthopedic/device/drug matrix for opposing bone-to-bone or soft tissue-to bone (implantable)** N N1
CMS: 100-04,4,60.4.2
AHA: 1Q,20

● **C1735** **Catheter(s), intravascular for renal denervation, radiofrequency, including all single-use system components**

● **C1736** **Catheter(s), intravascular for renal denervation, ultrasound, including all single-use system components**

● **C1737** **Joint fusion and fixation device(s), sacroiliac and pelvis, including all system components (implantable)**

● **C1738** **Powered, single-use (i.e., disposable) endoscopic ultrasound-guided biopsy device**

● **C1739** **Tissue marker, imaging and nonimaging device (implantable)**

C1747 **Endoscope, single-use (i.e., disposable), urinary tract, imaging/illumination device (insertable)** H J7
AHA: 3Q,23; 1Q,23

C1748 **Endoscope, single-use (i.e. disposable), upper GI, imaging/illumination device (insertable)** N N1
CMS: 100-04,4,60.4.2
AHA: 3Q,23; 2Q,20

C1749 **Endoscope, retrograde imaging/illumination colonoscope device (implantable)** N N1
CMS: 100-04,4,60.4.2

C1750 **Catheter, hemodialysis/peritoneal, long-term** N N1
CMS: 100-04,4,60.4.2

C1751 **Catheter, infusion, inserted peripherally, centrally or midline (other than hemodialysis)** N N1
CMS: 100-04,4,60.4.1; 100-04,4,60.4.2
AHA: 2Q,19

C1752 **Catheter, hemodialysis/peritoneal, short-term** N N1
CMS: 100-04,4,60.4.2

C1753 Catheter, intravascular ultrasound N N1
CMS: 100-04,4,60.4.2

C1754 Catheter, intradiscal N N1
CMS: 100-04,4,60.4.2

C1755 Catheter, intraspinal N N1
CMS: 100-04,4,60.4.2

C1756 Catheter, pacing, transesophageal N N1
CMS: 100-04,4,60.4.2

C1757 Catheter, thrombectomy/embolectomy N N1
CMS: 100-04,4,60.4.2

C1758 Catheter, ureteral N N1

C1759 Catheter, intracardiac echocardiography N N1
CMS: 100-04,4,60.4.2

C1760 Closure device, vascular (implantable/insertable) N N1
CMS: 100-04,4,60.4.2; 100-04,4,60.4.3

C1761 Catheter, transluminal intravascular lithotripsy, coronary H N1
CMS: 100-04,4,60.4.2
AHA: 2Q,23; 4Q,21; 3Q,21

C1762 Connective tissue, human (includes fascia lata) N N1
CMS: 100-04,4,60.4.2; 100-04,4,60.4.3

C1763 Connective tissue, nonhuman (includes synthetic) N N1
CMS: 100-04,4,60.4.2; 100-04,4,60.4.3
AHA: 4Q,22

C1764 Event recorder, cardiac (implantable) N N1
CMS: 100-04,14,40.8; 100-04,4,60.4.2

C1765 Adhesion barrier N N1
CMS: 100-04,4,60.4.2; 100-04,4,60.4.3

C1766 Introducer/sheath, guiding, intracardiac electrophysiological, steerable, other than peel-away N N1
CMS: 100-04,4,60.4.2

C1767 Generator, neurostimulator (implantable), nonrechargeable N N1
CMS: 100-04,14,40.8; 100-04,32,40.1; 100-04,32,40.2.1; 100-04,32,40.2.4; 100-04,32,40.4; 100-04,4,60.4.2
AHA: 1Q,21

C1768 Graft, vascular N N1
CMS: 100-04,4,60.4.2

C1769 Guide wire N N1
CMS: 100-04,4,60.4.2
AHA: 1Q,22; 3Q,19; 2Q,19

C1770 Imaging coil, magnetic resonance (insertable) N N1
CMS: 100-04,4,60.4.2

C1771 Repair device, urinary, incontinence, with sling graft N N1
CMS: 100-04,14,40.8; 100-04,4,60.4.2; 100-04,4,60.4.3

C1772 Infusion pump, programmable (implantable) N N1
CMS: 100-04,14,40.8; 100-04,4,60.4.2

C1773 Retrieval device, insertable (used to retrieve fractured medical devices) N N1
CMS: 100-04,4,60.4.2; 100-04,4,60.4.3

C1776 Joint device (implantable) N N1
CMS: 100-04,14,40.8; 100-04,4,60.4.2; 100-04,4,60.4.3
AHA: 3Q,21; 1Q,20; 3Q,18

C1777 Lead, cardioverter-defibrillator, endocardial single coil (implantable) N N1
CMS: 100-04,4,60.4.2

C1778 Lead, neurostimulator (implantable) N N1
CMS: 100-04,14,40.8; 100-04,32,40.1; 100-04,32,40.2.1; 100-04,32,40.2.4; 100-04,32,40.4; 100-04,4,60.4.2
AHA: 4Q,22; 1Q,21; 3Q,19; 1Q,19

C1779 Lead, pacemaker, transvenous VDD single pass N N1
CMS: 100-04,14,40.8; 100-04,4,60.4.2; 100-04,4,60.4.3

C1780 Lens, intraocular (new technology) N N1
CMS: 100-04,4,60.4.2; 100-04,4,60.4.3

C1781 Mesh (implantable) N N1
Use this code for OrthADAPT Bioimplant.
CMS: 100-04,4,60.4.2; 100-04,4,60.4.3
AHA: 4Q,22; 1Q,19

C1782 Morcellator N N1
CMS: 100-04,4,60.4.2; 100-04,4,60.4.3

C1783 Ocular implant, aqueous drainage assist device N N1
CMS: 100-04,4,60.4.2

C1784 Ocular device, intraoperative, detached retina N N1
CMS: 100-04,4,60.4.2; 100-04,4,60.4.3

C1785 Pacemaker, dual chamber, rate-responsive (implantable) N N1
CMS: 100-04,14,40.8; 100-04,21,320.4.7; 100-04,32,320.4.1; 100-04,32,320.4.2; 100-04,32,320.4.4; 100-04,32,320.4.6; 100-04,32,320.4.7; 100-04,4,60.4.2

C1786 Pacemaker, single chamber, rate-responsive (implantable) N N1
CMS: 100-04,14,40.8; 100-04,21,320.4.7; 100-04,32,320.4.1; 100-04,32,320.4.2; 100-04,32,320.4.4; 100-04,32,320.4.6; 100-04,32,320.4.7; 100-04,4,60.4.2

C1787 Patient programmer, neurostimulator N N1
CMS: 100-04,4,60.4.2; 100-04,4,60.4.3

C1788 Port, indwelling (implantable) N N1
CMS: 100-04,4,60.4.2
AHA: 2Q,19

C1789 Prosthesis, breast (implantable) N N1
CMS: 100-04,4,60.4.2

C1813 Prosthesis, penile, inflatable N N1
CMS: 100-04,14,40.8; 100-04,4,60.4.2

C1814 Retinal tamponade device, silicone oil N N1
CMS: 100-04,4,60.4.2; 100-04,4,60.4.3

C1815 Prosthesis, urinary sphincter (implantable) N N1
CMS: 100-04,14,40.8; 100-04,4,60.4.2

C1816 Receiver and/or transmitter, neurostimulator (implantable) N N1
CMS: 100-04,4,60.4.2
AHA: 4Q,22

C1817 Septal defect implant system, intracardiac N N1
CMS: 100-04,4,60.4.2; 100-04,4,60.4.3

C1818 Integrated keratoprosthesis N N1
CMS: 100-04,4,60.4.2; 100-04,4,60.4.3

C1819 Surgical tissue localization and excision device (implantable) N N1
CMS: 100-04,4,60.4.2

C1820 Generator, neurostimulator (implantable), with rechargeable battery and charging system N N1
Use to report neurostimulator generators that are not high frequency.
CMS: 100-04,14,40.8; 100-04,32,40.2.1; 100-04,32,40.2.4; 100-04,32,40.4; 100-04,4,10.12; 100-04,4,60.4.2

C1821 Interspinous process distraction device (implantable) N N1
CMS: 100-04,4,60.4.2

C1822 **Generator, neurostimulator (implantable), high frequency, with rechargeable battery and charging system** N N1
Use to report neurostimulator generators that are high frequency.
CMS: 100-04,4,60.4.2

C1823 **Generator, neurostimulator (implantable), nonrechargeable, with transvenous sensing and stimulation leads** N N1
CMS: 100-04,4,260.1; 100-04,4,260.1.1; 100-04,4,60.4.2
AHA: 1Q,23; 1Q,19

C1824 **Generator, cardiac contractility modulation (implantable)** N N1
CMS: 100-04,4,60.4.2
AHA: 1Q,20

C1825 **Generator, neurostimulator (implantable), nonrechargeable with carotid sinus baroreceptor stimulation lead(s)** N N1
CMS: 100-04,4,60.4.2

C1826 **Generator, neurostimulator (implantable), includes closed feedback loop leads and all implantable components, with rechargeable battery and charging system** H J7
AHA: 1Q,23

C1827 **Generator, neurostimulator (implantable), nonrechargeable, with implantable stimulation lead and external paired stimulation controller** H J7
AHA: 1Q,23

C1830 **Powered bone marrow biopsy needle** N N1
CMS: 100-04,4,60.4.2

C1831 **Interbody cage, anterior, lateral or posterior, personalized (implantable)** H N1
CMS: 100-04,4,60.4.2
AHA: 1Q,23; 1Q,22; 4Q,21

C1832 **Autograft suspension, including cell processing and application, and all system components** H J7
CMS: 100-04,4,60.4.2
AHA: 1Q,22

C1833 **Monitor, cardiac, including intracardiac lead and all system components (implantable)** H J7
CMS: 100-04,4,60.4.2
AHA: 1Q,22

C1839 **Iris prosthesis** N N1
CMS: 100-04,4,60.4.2
AHA: 1Q,20

C1840 **Lens, intraocular (telescopic)** N N1
CMS: 100-04,4,60.4.2

C1874 **Stent, coated/covered, with delivery system** N N1
CMS: 100-04,4,60.4.2; 100-04,4,60.4.3
AHA: 2Q,23

C1875 **Stent, coated/covered, without delivery system** N N1
CMS: 100-04,4,60.4.2; 100-04,4,60.4.3
AHA: 2Q,23; 2Q,20

C1876 **Stent, noncoated/noncovered, with delivery system** N N1
CMS: 100-04,4,60.4.2; 100-04,4,60.4.3

C1877 **Stent, noncoated/noncovered, without delivery system** N N1
CMS: 100-04,4,60.4.2

C1878 **Material for vocal cord medialization, synthetic (implantable)** N N1
CMS: 100-04,4,60.4.2; 100-04,4,60.4.3

C1880 **Vena cava filter** N N1
CMS: 100-04,4,60.4.2

C1881 **Dialysis access system (implantable)** N N1
CMS: 100-04,14,40.8; 100-04,4,60.4.2

C1882 **Cardioverter-defibrillator, other than single or dual chamber (implantable)** N N1
CMS: 100-04,14,40.8; 100-04,4,60.4.2; 100-04,4,60.4.3

C1883 **Adapter/extension, pacing lead or neurostimulator lead (implantable)** N N1
CMS: 100-04,32,40.1; 100-04,32,40.2.1; 100-04,32,40.2.4; 100-04,32,40.4; 100-04,4,60.4.2; 100-04,4,60.4.3

C1884 **Embolization protective system** N N1
CMS: 100-04,4,60.4.2; 100-04,4,60.4.3

C1885 **Catheter, transluminal angioplasty, laser** N N1
CMS: 100-04,4,60.4.2; 100-04,4,60.4.3

C1886 **Catheter, extravascular tissue ablation, any modality (insertable)** N N1
CMS: 100-04,4,60.4.2

C1887 **Catheter, guiding (may include infusion/perfusion capability)** N N1
CMS: 100-04,4,60.4.2; 100-04,4,60.4.3

C1888 **Catheter, ablation, noncardiac, endovascular (implantable)** N N1
CMS: 100-04,4,60.4.2; 100-04,4,60.4.3

C1889 **Implantable/insertable device, not otherwise classified** N N1

C1890 **No implantable/insertable device used with device-intensive procedures** E1 J7
CMS: 100-04,4,260.1; 100-04,4,260.1.1
AHA: 1Q,19

C1891 **Infusion pump, nonprogrammable, permanent (implantable)** N N1
CMS: 100-04,14,40.8; 100-04,4,60.4.2

C1892 **Introducer/sheath, guiding, intracardiac electrophysiological, fixed-curve, peel-away** N N1
CMS: 100-04,4,60.4.2; 100-04,4,60.4.3

C1893 **Introducer/sheath, guiding, intracardiac electrophysiological, fixed-curve, other than peel-away** N N1
CMS: 100-04,4,60.4.2

C1894 **Introducer/sheath, other than guiding, other than intracardiac electrophysiological, nonlaser** N N1
CMS: 100-04,4,60.4.1; 100-04,4,60.4.2
AHA: 2Q,19

C1895 **Lead, cardioverter-defibrillator, endocardial dual coil (implantable)** N N1
CMS: 100-04,4,60.4.2

C1896 **Lead, cardioverter-defibrillator, other than endocardial single or dual coil (implantable)** N N1
CMS: 100-04,4,60.4.2

C1897 **Lead, neurostimulator test kit (implantable)** N N1
CMS: 100-04,14,40.8; 100-04,32,40.1; 100-04,32,40.2.1; 100-04,32,40.2.4; 100-04,32,40.4; 100-04,4,60.4.2

C1898 **Lead, pacemaker, other than transvenous VDD single pass** N N1
CMS: 100-04,14,40.8; 100-04,4,60.4.2

C1899 **Lead, pacemaker/cardioverter-defibrillator combination (implantable)** N N1
CMS: 100-04,4,60.4.2

C1900 **Lead, left ventricular coronary venous system** N N1
CMS: 100-04,14,40.8; 100-04,4,60.4.2; 100-04,4,60.4.3

C1982 **Catheter, pressure generating, one-way valve, intermittently occlusive** N N1
CMS: 100-04,4,60.4.2
AHA: 1Q,20

C2596 Probe, image guided, robotic, waterjet ablation N N1
CMS: 100-04,4,60.4.2
AHA: 1Q,20

C2613 Lung biopsy plug with delivery system N N1
CMS: 100-04,4,60.4.2

C2614 Probe, percutaneous lumbar discectomy N N1
CMS: 100-04,4,60.4.2

C2615 Sealant, pulmonary, liquid N N1
CMS: 100-04,4,60.4.2; 100-04,4,60.4.3

C2616 Brachytherapy source, nonstranded, yttrium-90, per source U H2
CMS: 100-04,4,60.4.2

C2617 Stent, noncoronary, temporary, without delivery system N N1
CMS: 100-04,4,60.4.2; 100-04,4,60.4.3

C2618 Probe/needle, cryoablation N N1
CMS: 100-04,4,60.4.2

C2619 Pacemaker, dual chamber, nonrate-responsive (implantable) N N1
CMS: 100-04,14,40.8; 100-04,21,320.4.7; 100-04,32,320.4.1; 100-04,32,320.4.2; 100-04,32,320.4.4; 100-04,32,320.4.6; 100-04,32,320.4.7; 100-04,4,60.4.2

C2620 Pacemaker, single chamber, nonrate-responsive (implantable) N N1
CMS: 100-04,14,40.8; 100-04,21,320.4.7; 100-04,32,320.4.1; 100-04,32,320.4.2; 100-04,32,320.4.4; 100-04,32,320.4.6; 100-04,32,320.4.7; 100-04,4,60.4.2

C2621 Pacemaker, other than single or dual chamber (implantable) N N1
CMS: 100-04,14,40.8; 100-04,4,60.4.2; 100-04,4,60.4.3

C2622 Prosthesis, penile, noninflatable N N1
CMS: 100-04,14,40.8; 100-04,4,60.4.2

C2623 Catheter, transluminal angioplasty, drug-coated, nonlaser N N1
CMS: 100-04,4,60.4.2

C2624 Implantable wireless pulmonary artery pressure sensor with delivery catheter, including all system components N N1
CMS: 100-04,4,60.4.2

C2625 Stent, noncoronary, temporary, with delivery system N N1
CMS: 100-04,4,60.4.2; 100-04,4,60.4.3

C2626 Infusion pump, nonprogrammable, temporary (implantable) N N1
CMS: 100-04,14,40.8; 100-04,4,60.4.2; 100-04,4,60.4.3

C2627 Catheter, suprapubic/cystoscopic N N1
CMS: 100-04,4,60.4.2

C2628 Catheter, occlusion N N1
CMS: 100-04,4,60.4.2

C2629 Introducer/sheath, other than guiding, other than intracardiac electrophysiological, laser N N1
CMS: 100-04,4,60.4.2

C2630 Catheter, electrophysiology, diagnostic/ablation, other than 3D or vector mapping, cool-tip N N1
CMS: 100-04,4,60.4.2; 100-04,4,60.4.3

C2631 Repair device, urinary, incontinence, without sling graft N N1
CMS: 100-04,14,40.8; 100-04,4,60.4.2; 100-04,4,60.4.3

C2634 Brachytherapy source, nonstranded, high activity, iodine-125, greater than 1.01 mCi (NIST), per source U H2

C2635 Brachytherapy source, nonstranded, high activity, palladium-103, greater than 2.2 mCi (NIST), per source U H2

C2636 Brachytherapy linear source, nonstranded, palladium-103, per 1 mm U H2

C2637 Brachytherapy source, nonstranded, ytterbium-169, per source B

C2638 Brachytherapy source, stranded, iodine-125, per source U H2

C2639 Brachytherapy source, nonstranded, iodine-125, per source U H2

C2640 Brachytherapy source, stranded, palladium-103, per source U H2

C2641 Brachytherapy source, nonstranded, palladium-103, per source U H2

C2642 Brachytherapy source, stranded, cesium-131, per source U H2

C2643 Brachytherapy source, nonstranded, cesium-131, per source U H2

C2644 Brachytherapy source, cesium-131 chloride solution, per mCi E

C2645 Brachytherapy planar source, palladium-103, per sq mm U H2

C2698 Brachytherapy source, stranded, not otherwise specified, per source U H2

C2699 Brachytherapy source, nonstranded, not otherwise specified, per source U H2

C5271 Application of low cost skin substitute graft to trunk, arms, legs, total wound surface area up to 100 sq cm; first 25 sq cm or less wound surface area T G2

C5272 Application of low cost skin substitute graft to trunk, arms, legs, total wound surface area up to 100 sq cm; each additional 25 sq cm wound surface area, or part thereof (list separately in addition to code for primary procedure) N N1

C5273 Application of low cost skin substitute graft to trunk, arms, legs, total wound surface area greater than or equal to 100 sq cm; first 100 sq cm wound surface area, or 1% of body area of infants and children T G2

C5274 Application of low cost skin substitute graft to trunk, arms, legs, total wound surface area greater than or equal to 100 sq cm; each additional 100 sq cm wound surface area, or part thereof, or each additional 1% of body area of infants and children, or part thereof (list separately in addition to code for primary procedure) N N1

C5275 Application of low cost skin substitute graft to face, scalp, eyelids, mouth, neck, ears, orbits, genitalia, hands, feet, and/or multiple digits, total wound surface area up to 100 sq cm; first 25 sq cm or less wound surface area T G2

C5276 Application of low cost skin substitute graft to face, scalp, eyelids, mouth, neck, ears, orbits, genitalia, hands, feet, and/or multiple digits, total wound surface area up to 100 sq cm; each additional 25 sq cm wound surface area, or part thereof (list separately in addition to code for primary procedure) N N1

C5277 Application of low cost skin substitute graft to face, scalp, eyelids, mouth, neck, ears, orbits, genitalia, hands, feet, and/or multiple digits, total wound surface area greater than or equal to 100 sq cm; first 100 sq cm wound surface area, or 1% of body area of infants and children T G2

C5278 Application of low cost skin substitute graft to face, scalp, eyelids, mouth, neck, ears, orbits, genitalia, hands, feet, and/or multiple digits, total wound surface area greater than or equal to 100 sq cm; each additional 100 sq cm wound surface area, or part thereof, or each additional 1% of body area of infants and children, or part thereof (list separately in addition to code for primary procedure) N N1 ☑

C7500 Debridement, bone including epidermis, dermis, subcutaneous tissue, muscle and/or fascia, if performed, first 20 sq cm or less with manual preparation and insertion of deep (e.g., subfascial) drug-delivery device(s) E1 G2

AHA: 1Q,23

C7501 Percutaneous breast biopsies using stereotactic guidance, with placement of breast localization device(s) (e.g., clip, metallic pellet), when performed, and imaging of the biopsy specimen, when performed, all lesions unilateral and bilateral (for single lesion biopsy, use appropriate code) E1 G2

AHA: 1Q,23

C7502 Percutaneous breast biopsies using magnetic resonance guidance, with placement of breast localization device(s) (e.g., clip, metallic pellet), when performed, and imaging of the biopsy specimen, when performed, all lesions unilateral or bilateral (for single lesion biopsy, use appropriate code) E1 G2

AHA: 1Q,23

C7503 Open biopsy or excision of deep cervical node(s) with intraoperative identification (e.g., mapping) of sentinel lymph node(s) including injection of nonradioactive dye when performed E1 G2

AHA: 1Q,23

C7504 Percutaneous vertebroplasties (bone biopsies included when performed), first cervicothoracic and any additional cervicothoracic or lumbosacral vertebral bodies, unilateral or bilateral injection, inclusive of all imaging guidance E1 G2

AHA: 1Q,23

C7505 Percutaneous vertebroplasties (bone biopsies included when performed), first lumbosacral and any additional cervicothoracic or lumbosacral vertebral bodies, unilateral or bilateral injection, inclusive of all imaging guidance E1 G2

AHA: 1Q,23

C7506 Arthrodesis, interphalangeal joints, with or without internal fixation E1 G2

AHA: 1Q,23

C7507 Percutaneous vertebral augmentations, first thoracic and any additional thoracic or lumbar vertebral bodies, including cavity creations (fracture reductions and bone biopsies included when performed) using mechanical device (e.g., kyphoplasty), unilateral or bilateral cannulations, inclusive of all imaging guidance E1 G2

AHA: 1Q,23

C7508 Percutaneous vertebral augmentations, first lumbar and any additional thoracic or lumbar vertebral bodies, including cavity creations (fracture reductions and bone biopsies included when performed) using mechanical device (e.g., kyphoplasty), unilateral or bilateral cannulations, inclusive of all imaging guidance E1 G2

AHA: 1Q,23

C7509 Bronchoscopy, rigid or flexible, diagnostic with cell washing(s) when performed, with computer-assisted image-guided navigation, including fluoroscopic guidance when performed E1 G2

AHA: 1Q,23

C7510 Bronchoscopy, rigid or flexible, with bronchial alveolar lavage(s), with computer-assisted image-guided navigation, including fluoroscopic guidance when performed E1 G2

AHA: 1Q,23

C7511 Bronchoscopy, rigid or flexible, with single or multiple bronchial or endobronchial biopsy(ies), single or multiple sites, with computer-assisted image-guided navigation, including fluoroscopic guidance when performed E1 G2

AHA: 1Q,23

C7512 Bronchoscopy, rigid or flexible, with single or multiple bronchial or endobronchial biopsy(ies), single or multiple sites, with transendoscopic endobronchial ultrasound (EBUS) during bronchoscopic diagnostic or therapeutic intervention(s) for peripheral lesion(s), including fluoroscopic guidance when performed E1 G2

AHA: 1Q,23

C7513 Dialysis circuit, introduction of needle(s) and/or catheter(s), with diagnostic angiography of the dialysis circuit, including all direct puncture(s) and catheter placement(s), injection(s) of contrast, all necessary imaging from the arterial anastomosis and adjacent artery through entire venous outflow including the inferior or superior vena cava, fluoroscopic guidance, with transluminal balloon angioplasty of central dialysis segment, performed through dialysis circuit, including all required imaging, radiological supervision and interpretation, image documentation and report E1 G2

AHA: 2Q,24; 1Q,23

C7514 Dialysis circuit, introduction of needle(s) and/or catheter(s), with diagnostic angiography of the dialysis circuit, including all direct puncture(s) and catheter placement(s), injection(s) of contrast, all necessary imaging from the arterial anastomosis and adjacent artery through entire venous outflow including the inferior or superior vena cava, fluoroscopic guidance, with all angioplasty in the central dialysis segment, and transcatheter placement of intravascular stent(s), central dialysis segment, performed through dialysis circuit, including all required imaging, radiological supervision and interpretation, image documentation and report E1 G2

AHA: 1Q,23

C7515 Dialysis circuit, introduction of needle(s) and/or catheter(s), with diagnostic angiography of the dialysis circuit, including all direct puncture(s) and catheter placement(s), injection(s) of contrast, all necessary imaging from the arterial anastomosis and adjacent artery through entire venous outflow including the inferior or superior vena cava, fluoroscopic guidance, with dialysis circuit permanent endovascular embolization or occlusion of main circuit or any accessory veins, including all required imaging, radiological supervision and interpretation, image documentation and report E1 G2

AHA: 1Q,23

C7516 Catheter placement in coronary artery(s) for coronary angiography, including intraprocedural injection(s) for coronary angiography, with endoluminal imaging of initial coronary vessel or graft using intravascular ultrasound (IVUS) or optical coherence tomography (OCT) during diagnostic evaluation and/or therapeutic intervention including imaging supervision, interpretation and report E1 G2

AHA: 1Q,23

C7517 Catheter placement in coronary artery(s) for coronary angiography, including intraprocedural injection(s) for coronary angiography, with iliac and/or femoral artery angiography, nonselective, bilateral or ipsilateral to catheter insertion, performed at the same time as cardiac catheterization and/or coronary angiography, includes positioning or placement of the catheter in the distal aorta or ipsilateral femoral or iliac artery, injection of dye, production of permanent images, and radiologic supervision and interpretation E1 G2
AHA: 1Q,23

C7518 Catheter placement in coronary artery(ies) for coronary angiography, including intraprocedural injection(s) for coronary angiography, imaging supervision and interpretation, with catheter placement(s) in bypass graft(s) (internal mammary, free arterial, venous grafts) including intraprocedural injection(s) for bypass graft angiography with endoluminal imaging of initial coronary vessel or graft using intravascular ultrasound (IVUS) or optical coherence tomography (OCT) during diagnostic evaluation and/or therapeutic intervention including imaging, supervision, interpretation and report E1
AHA: 1Q,23

C7519 Catheter placement in coronary artery(ies) for coronary angiography, including intraprocedural injection(s) for coronary angiography, imaging supervision and interpretation, with catheter placement(s) in bypass graft(s) (internal mammary, free arterial, venous grafts) including intraprocedural injection(s) for bypass graft angiography with intravascular doppler velocity and/or pressure derived coronary flow reserve measurement (initial coronary vessel or graft) during coronary angiography including pharmacologically induced stress E1
AHA: 1Q,23

C7520 Catheter placement in coronary artery(ies) for coronary angiography, including intraprocedural injection(s) for coronary angiography, imaging supervision and interpretation, with catheter placement(s) in bypass graft(s) (internal mammary, free arterial, venous grafts) includes intraprocedural injection(s) for bypass graft angiography with iliac and/or femoral artery angiography, nonselective, bilateral or ipsilateral to catheter insertion, performed at the same time as cardiac catheterization and/or coronary angiography, includes positioning or placement of the catheter in the distal aorta or ipsilateral femoral or iliac artery, injection of dye, production of permanent images, and radiologic supervision and interpretation E1 G2
AHA: 1Q,23

C7521 Catheter placement in coronary artery(ies) for coronary angiography, including intraprocedural injection(s) for coronary angiography with right heart catheterization with endoluminal imaging of initial coronary vessel or graft using intravascular ultrasound (IVUS) or optical coherence tomography (OCT) during diagnostic evaluation and/or therapeutic intervention including imaging supervision, interpretation and report E1 G2
AHA: 1Q,23

C7522 Catheter placement in coronary artery(ies) for coronary angiography, including intraprocedural injection(s) for coronary angiography, imaging supervision and interpretation with right heart catheterization, with intravascular doppler velocity and/or pressure derived coronary flow reserve measurement (initial coronary vessel or graft) during coronary angiography including pharmacologically induced stress E1 G2
AHA: 1Q,23

C7523 Catheter placement in coronary artery(ies) for coronary angiography, including intraprocedural injection(s) for coronary angiography, imaging supervision and interpretation, with left heart catheterization including intraprocedural injection(s) for left ventriculography, when performed, with endoluminal imaging of initial coronary vessel or graft using intravascular ultrasound (IVUS) or optical coherence tomography (OCT) during diagnostic evaluation and/or therapeutic intervention including imaging supervision, interpretation and report E1 G2
AHA: 1Q,23

C7524 Catheter placement in coronary artery(ies) for coronary angiography, including intraprocedural injection(s) for coronary angiography, imaging supervision and interpretation, with left heart catheterization including intraprocedural injection(s) for left ventriculography, when performed, with intravascular doppler velocity and/or pressure derived coronary flow reserve measurement (initial coronary vessel or graft) during coronary angiography including pharmacologically induced stress E1 G2
AHA: 1Q,23

C7525 Catheter placement in coronary artery(ies) for coronary angiography, including intraprocedural injection(s) for coronary angiography, imaging supervision and interpretation, with left heart catheterization including intraprocedural injection(s) for left ventriculography, when performed, catheter placement(s) in bypass graft(s) (internal mammary, free arterial, venous grafts) with bypass graft angiography with endoluminal imaging of initial coronary vessel or graft using intravascular ultrasound (IVUS) or optical coherence tomography (OCT) during diagnostic evaluation and/or therapeutic intervention including imaging supervision, interpretation and report E1 G2
AHA: 1Q,23

C7526 Catheter placement in coronary artery(ies) for coronary angiography, including intraprocedural injection(s) for coronary angiography, imaging supervision and interpretation, with left heart catheterization including intraprocedural injection(s) for left ventriculography, when performed, catheter placement(s) in bypass graft(s) (internal mammary, free arterial, venous grafts) with bypass graft angiography with intravascular doppler velocity and/or pressure derived coronary flow reserve measurement (initial coronary vessel or graft) during coronary angiography including pharmacologically induced stress E1 G2
AHA: 1Q,23

C7527 Catheter placement in coronary artery(ies) for coronary angiography, including intraprocedural injection(s) for coronary angiography, imaging supervision and interpretation, with right and left heart catheterization including intraprocedural injection(s) for left ventriculography, when performed, with endoluminal imaging of initial coronary vessel or graft using intravascular ultrasound (IVUS) or optical coherence tomography (OCT) during diagnostic evaluation and/or therapeutic intervention including imaging supervision, interpretation and report E1 G2
AHA: 1Q,23

C7528 Catheter placement in coronary artery(ies) for coronary angiography, including intraprocedural injection(s) for coronary angiography, imaging supervision and interpretation, with right and left heart catheterization including intraprocedural injection(s) for left ventriculography, when performed, with intravascular doppler velocity and/or pressure derived coronary flow reserve measurement (initial coronary vessel or graft) during coronary angiography including pharmacologically induced stress E1 G2
AHA: 1Q,23

C7529 Catheter placement in coronary artery(ies) for coronary angiography, including intraprocedural injection(s) for coronary angiography, imaging supervision and interpretation, with right and left heart catheterization including intraprocedural injection(s) for left ventriculography, when performed, catheter placement(s) in bypass graft(s) (internal mammary, free arterial, venous grafts) with bypass graft angiography with intravascular doppler velocity and/or pressure derived coronary flow reserve measurement (initial coronary vessel or graft) during coronary angiography including pharmacologically induced stress E1 G2
AHA: 1Q,23

C7530 Dialysis circuit, introduction of needle(s) and/or catheter(s), with diagnostic angiography of the dialysis circuit, including all direct puncture(s) and catheter placement(s), injection(s) of contrast, all necessary imaging from the arterial anastomosis and adjacent artery through entire venous outflow including the inferior or superior vena cava, fluoroscopic guidance, with transluminal balloon angioplasty, peripheral dialysis segment, including all imaging and radiological supervision and interpretation necessary to perform the angioplasty and all angioplasty in the central dialysis segment, with transcatheter placement of intravascular stent(s), central dialysis segment, performed through dialysis circuit, including all imaging, radiological supervision and interpretation, documentation and report E1 G2
AHA: 1Q,23

C7531 Revascularization, endovascular, open or percutaneous, femoral, popliteal artery(ies), unilateral, with transluminal angioplasty with intravascular ultrasound (initial noncoronary vessel) during diagnostic evaluation and/or therapeutic intervention, including radiological supervision and interpretation E1 J8
AHA: 1Q,23

C7532 Transluminal balloon angioplasty (except lower extremity artery(ies) for occlusive disease, intracranial, coronary, pulmonary, or dialysis circuit), initial artery, open or percutaneous, including all imaging and radiological supervision and interpretation necessary to perform the angioplasty within the same artery, with intravascular ultrasound (initial noncoronary vessel) during diagnostic evaluation and/or therapeutic intervention, including radiological supervision and interpretation E1 J8
AHA: 1Q,23

C7533 Percutaneous transluminal coronary angioplasty, single major coronary artery or branch with transcatheter placement of radiation delivery device for subsequent coronary intravascular brachytherapy E1 J8
AHA: 1Q,23

C7534 Revascularization, endovascular, open or percutaneous, femoral, popliteal artery(ies), unilateral, with atherectomy, includes angioplasty within the same vessel, when performed with intravascular ultrasound (initial noncoronary vessel) during diagnostic evaluation and/or therapeutic intervention, including radiological supervision and interpretation E1
AHA: 1Q,23

C7535 Revascularization, endovascular, open or percutaneous, femoral, popliteal artery(ies), unilateral, with transluminal stent placement(s), includes angioplasty within the same vessel, when performed, with intravascular ultrasound (initial noncoronary vessel) during diagnostic evaluation and/or therapeutic intervention, including radiological supervision and interpretation E1 J8
AHA: 1Q,23

C7537 Insertion of new or replacement of permanent pacemaker with atrial transvenous electrode(s), with insertion of pacing electrode, cardiac venous system, for left ventricular pacing, at time of insertion of implantable defibrillator or pacemaker pulse generator (e.g., for upgrade to dual chamber system) E1 J8
AHA: 1Q,23

C7538 Insertion of new or replacement of permanent pacemaker with ventricular transvenous electrode(s), with insertion of pacing electrode, cardiac venous system, for left ventricular pacing, at time of insertion of implantable defibrillator or pacemaker pulse generator (e.g., for upgrade to dual chamber system) E1 J8
AHA: 1Q,23

C7539 Insertion of new or replacement of permanent pacemaker with atrial and ventricular transvenous electrode(s), with insertion of pacing electrode, cardiac venous system, for left ventricular pacing, at time of insertion of implantable defibrillator or pacemaker pulse generator (e.g., for upgrade to dual chamber system) E1 J8
AHA: 1Q,23

C7540 Removal of permanent pacemaker pulse generator with replacement of pacemaker pulse generator, dual lead system, with insertion of pacing electrode, cardiac venous system, for left ventricular pacing, at time of insertion of implantable defibrillator or pacemaker pulse generator (e.g., for upgrade to dual chamber system) E1 J8
AHA: 1Q,23

C7541 Diagnostic endoscopic retrograde cholangiopancreatography (ERCP), including collection of specimen(s) by brushing or washing, when performed, with endoscopic cannulation of papilla with direct visualization of pancreatic/common bile ducts(s) E1
AHA: 1Q,23

C7542 Endoscopic retrograde cholangiopancreatography (ERCP) with biopsy, single or multiple, with endoscopic cannulation of papilla with direct visualization of pancreatic/common bile ducts(s) E1
AHA: 1Q,23

C7543 Endoscopic retrograde cholangiopancreatography (ERCP) with sphincterotomy/papillotomy, with endoscopic cannulation of papilla with direct visualization of pancreatic/common bile ducts(s) E1
AHA: 1Q,23

C7544 Endoscopic retrograde cholangiopancreatography (ERCP) with removal of calculi/debris from biliary/pancreatic duct(s), with endoscopic cannulation of papilla with direct visualization of pancreatic/common bile ducts(s) E1
AHA: 1Q,23

C7545 Percutaneous exchange of biliary drainage catheter (e.g., external, internal-external, or conversion of internal-external to external only), with removal of calculi/debris from biliary duct(s) and/or gallbladder, including destruction of calculi by any method (e.g., mechanical, electrohydraulic, lithotripsy) when performed, including diagnostic cholangiography(ies) when performed, imaging guidance (e.g., fluoroscopy), and all associated radiological supervision and interpretation E1 G2
AHA: 1Q,23

C7546 Removal and replacement of externally accessible nephroureteral catheter (e.g., external/internal stent) requiring fluoroscopic guidance, with ureteral stricture balloon dilation, including imaging guidance and all associated radiological supervision and interpretation E1
AHA: 1Q,23

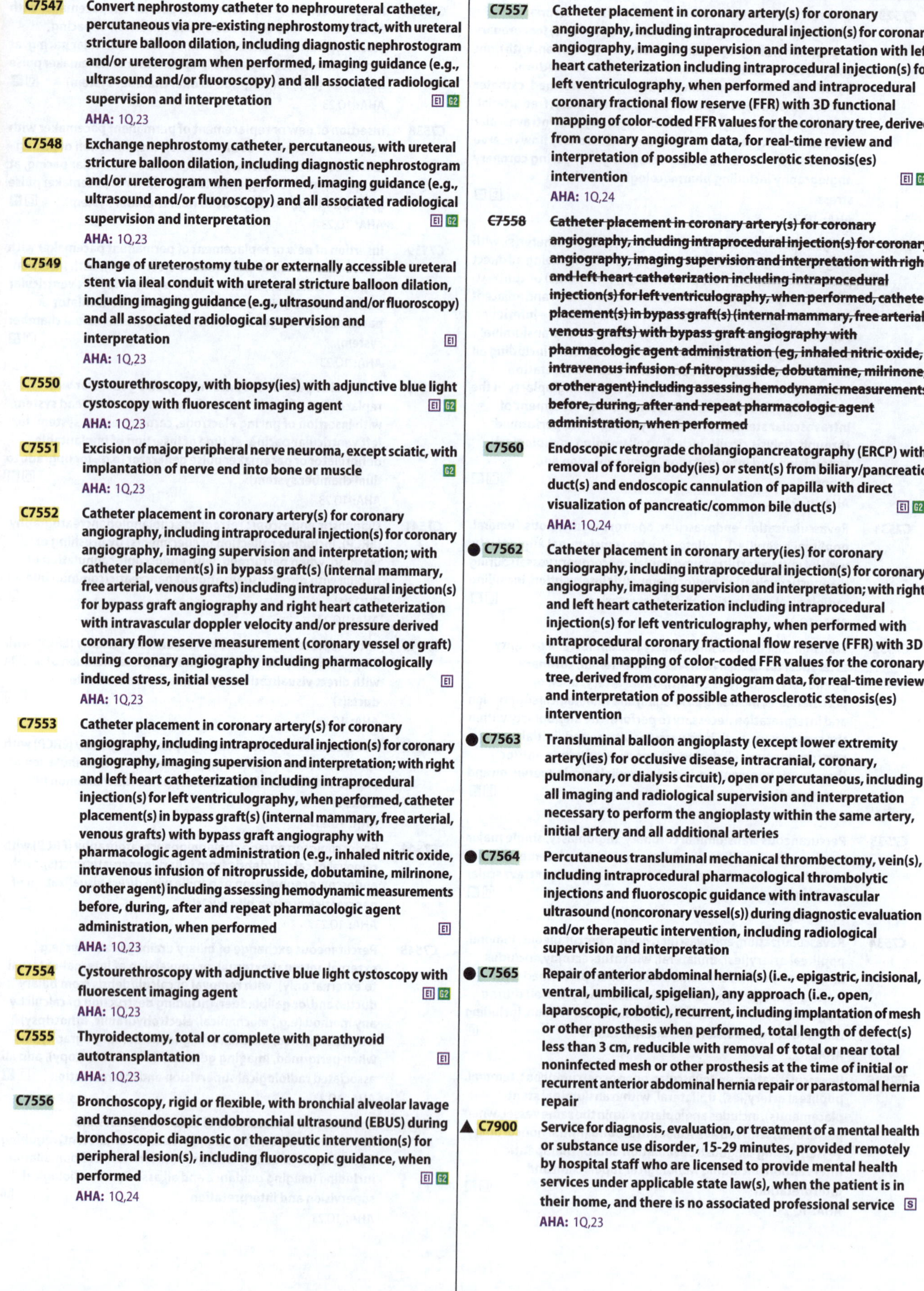

C7547 Convert nephrostomy catheter to nephroureteral catheter, percutaneous via pre-existing nephrostomy tract, with ureteral stricture balloon dilation, including diagnostic nephrostogram and/or ureterogram when performed, imaging guidance (e.g., ultrasound and/or fluoroscopy) and all associated radiological supervision and interpretation E1 G2
AHA: 1Q,23

C7548 Exchange nephrostomy catheter, percutaneous, with ureteral stricture balloon dilation, including diagnostic nephrostogram and/or ureterogram when performed, imaging guidance (e.g., ultrasound and/or fluoroscopy) and all associated radiological supervision and interpretation E1 G2
AHA: 1Q,23

C7549 Change of ureterostomy tube or externally accessible ureteral stent via ileal conduit with ureteral stricture balloon dilation, including imaging guidance (e.g., ultrasound and/or fluoroscopy) and all associated radiological supervision and interpretation E1
AHA: 1Q,23

C7550 Cystourethroscopy, with biopsy(ies) with adjunctive blue light cystoscopy with fluorescent imaging agent E1 G2
AHA: 1Q,23

C7551 Excision of major peripheral nerve neuroma, except sciatic, with implantation of nerve end into bone or muscle G2
AHA: 1Q,23

C7552 Catheter placement in coronary artery(s) for coronary angiography, including intraprocedural injection(s) for coronary angiography, imaging supervision and interpretation; with catheter placement(s) in bypass graft(s) (internal mammary, free arterial, venous grafts) including intraprocedural injection(s) for bypass graft angiography and right heart catheterization with intravascular doppler velocity and/or pressure derived coronary flow reserve measurement (coronary vessel or graft) during coronary angiography including pharmacologically induced stress, initial vessel E1
AHA: 1Q,23

C7553 Catheter placement in coronary artery(s) for coronary angiography, including intraprocedural injection(s) for coronary angiography, imaging supervision and interpretation; with right and left heart catheterization including intraprocedural injection(s) for left ventriculography, when performed, catheter placement(s) in bypass graft(s) (internal mammary, free arterial, venous grafts) with bypass graft angiography with pharmacologic agent administration (e.g., inhaled nitric oxide, intravenous infusion of nitroprusside, dobutamine, milrinone, or other agent) including assessing hemodynamic measurements before, during, after and repeat pharmacologic agent administration, when performed E1
AHA: 1Q,23

C7554 Cystourethroscopy with adjunctive blue light cystoscopy with fluorescent imaging agent E1 G2
AHA: 1Q,23

C7555 Thyroidectomy, total or complete with parathyroid autotransplantation E1
AHA: 1Q,23

C7556 Bronchoscopy, rigid or flexible, with bronchial alveolar lavage and transendoscopic endobronchial ultrasound (EBUS) during bronchoscopic diagnostic or therapeutic intervention(s) for peripheral lesion(s), including fluoroscopic guidance, when performed E1 G2
AHA: 1Q,24

C7557 Catheter placement in coronary artery(s) for coronary angiography, including intraprocedural injection(s) for coronary angiography, imaging supervision and interpretation with left heart catheterization including intraprocedural injection(s) for left ventriculography, when performed and intraprocedural coronary fractional flow reserve (FFR) with 3D functional mapping of color-coded FFR values for the coronary tree, derived from coronary angiogram data, for real-time review and interpretation of possible atherosclerotic stenosis(es) intervention E1 G2
AHA: 1Q,24

~~**C7558** Catheter placement in coronary artery(s) for coronary angiography, including intraprocedural injection(s) for coronary angiography, imaging supervision and interpretation with right and left heart catheterization including intraprocedural injection(s) for left ventriculography, when performed, catheter placement(s) in bypass graft(s) (internal mammary, free arterial, venous grafts) with bypass graft angiography with pharmacologic agent administration (eg, inhaled nitric oxide, intravenous infusion of nitroprusside, dobutamine, milrinone, or other agent) including assessing hemodynamic measurements before, during, after and repeat pharmacologic agent administration, when performed~~

C7560 Endoscopic retrograde cholangiopancreatography (ERCP) with removal of foreign body(ies) or stent(s) from biliary/pancreatic duct(s) and endoscopic cannulation of papilla with direct visualization of pancreatic/common bile duct(s) E1 G2
AHA: 1Q,24

● **C7562** Catheter placement in coronary artery(ies) for coronary angiography, including intraprocedural injection(s) for coronary angiography, imaging supervision and interpretation; with right and left heart catheterization including intraprocedural injection(s) for left ventriculography, when performed with intraprocedural coronary fractional flow reserve (FFR) with 3D functional mapping of color-coded FFR values for the coronary tree, derived from coronary angiogram data, for real-time review and interpretation of possible atherosclerotic stenosis(es) intervention

● **C7563** Transluminal balloon angioplasty (except lower extremity artery(ies) for occlusive disease, intracranial, coronary, pulmonary, or dialysis circuit), open or percutaneous, including all imaging and radiological supervision and interpretation necessary to perform the angioplasty within the same artery, initial artery and all additional arteries

● **C7564** Percutaneous transluminal mechanical thrombectomy, vein(s), including intraprocedural pharmacological thrombolytic injections and fluoroscopic guidance with intravascular ultrasound (noncoronary vessel(s)) during diagnostic evaluation and/or therapeutic intervention, including radiological supervision and interpretation

● **C7565** Repair of anterior abdominal hernia(s) (i.e., epigastric, incisional, ventral, umbilical, spigelian), any approach (i.e., open, laparoscopic, robotic), recurrent, including implantation of mesh or other prosthesis when performed, total length of defect(s) less than 3 cm, reducible with removal of total or near total noninfected mesh or other prosthesis at the time of initial or recurrent anterior abdominal hernia repair or parastomal hernia repair

▲ **C7900** Service for diagnosis, evaluation, or treatment of a mental health or substance use disorder, 15-29 minutes, provided remotely by hospital staff who are licensed to provide mental health services under applicable state law(s), when the patient is in their home, and there is no associated professional service S
AHA: 1Q,23

▲ **C7901** Service for diagnosis, evaluation, or treatment of a mental health or substance use disorder, 30-60 minutes, provided remotely by hospital staff who are licensed to provided mental health services under applicable state law(s), when the patient is in their home, and there is no associated professional service S
AHA: 1Q,23

C7902 Service for diagnosis, evaluation, or treatment of a mental health or substance use disorder, each additional 15 minutes, provided remotely by hospital staff who are licensed to provide mental health services under applicable state law(s), when the patient is in their home, and there is no associated professional service (list separately in addition to code for primary service) N
AHA: 1Q,23

C7903 Group psychotherapy service for diagnosis, evaluation, or treatment of a mental health or substance use disorder provided remotely by hospital staff who are licensed to provide mental health services under applicable state law(s), when the patient is in their home, and there is no associated professional service S
AHA: 1Q,24

● **C8000** Support device, extravascular, for arteriovenous fistula (implantable) J7

● **C8001** 3D anatomical segmentation imaging for preoperative planning, data preparation and transmission, obtained from previous diagnostic computed tomographic or magnetic resonance examination of the same anatomy

● **C8002** Preparation of skin cell suspension autograft, automated, including all enzymatic processing and device components (do not report with manual suspension preparation)

● **C8003** Implantation of medial knee extraarticular implantable shock absorber spanning the knee joint from distal femur to proximal tibia, open, includes measurements, positioning and adjustments, with imaging guidance (e.g., fluoroscopy)

C8900 Magnetic resonance angiography with contrast, abdomen Q3 Z2 ⃠
CMS: 100-04,13,40.1.1; 100-04,13,40.1.2

C8901 Magnetic resonance angiography without contrast, abdomen Q3 Z2 ⃠
CMS: 100-04,13,40.1.1; 100-04,13,40.1.2

C8902 Magnetic resonance angiography without contrast followed by with contrast, abdomen Q3 Z2 ⃠
CMS: 100-04,13,40.1.1; 100-04,13,40.1.2

C8903 Magnetic resonance imaging with contrast, breast; unilateral Q3 Z2 ⃠

C8905 Magnetic resonance imaging without contrast followed by with contrast, breast; unilateral Q3 Z2 ⃠

C8906 Magnetic resonance imaging with contrast, breast; bilateral Q3 Z2 ⃠

C8908 Magnetic resonance imaging without contrast followed by with contrast, breast; bilateral Q3 Z2 ⃠

C8909 Magnetic resonance angiography with contrast, chest (excluding myocardium) Q3 Z2 ⃠
CMS: 100-04,13,40.1.1; 100-04,13,40.1.2

C8910 Magnetic resonance angiography without contrast, chest (excluding myocardium) Q3 Z2 ⃠
CMS: 100-04,13,40.1.1; 100-04,13,40.1.2

C8911 Magnetic resonance angiography without contrast followed by with contrast, chest (excluding myocardium) Q3 Z2 ⃠
CMS: 100-04,13,40.1.1; 100-04,13,40.1.2

C8912 Magnetic resonance angiography with contrast, lower extremity Q3 Z2 ⃠
CMS: 100-04,13,40.1.1; 100-04,13,40.1.2

C8913 Magnetic resonance angiography without contrast, lower extremity Q3 Z2 ⃠
CMS: 100-04,13,40.1.1; 100-04,13,40.1.2

C8914 Magnetic resonance angiography without contrast followed by with contrast, lower extremity Q3 Z2 ⃠
CMS: 100-04,13,40.1.1; 100-04,13,40.1.2

C8918 Magnetic resonance angiography with contrast, pelvis Q3 Z2 ⃠
CMS: 100-04,13,40.1.1; 100-04,13,40.1.2

C8919 Magnetic resonance angiography without contrast, pelvis Q3 Z2 ⃠
CMS: 100-04,13,40.1.1; 100-04,13,40.1.2

C8920 Magnetic resonance angiography without contrast followed by with contrast, pelvis Q3 Z2 ⃠
CMS: 100-04,13,40.1.1; 100-04,13,40.1.2

C8921 Transthoracic echocardiography (TTE) with contrast, or without contrast followed by with contrast, for congenital cardiac anomalies; complete S
CMS: 100-04,4,200.7.2

C8922 Transthoracic echocardiography (TTE) with contrast, or without contrast followed by with contrast, for congenital cardiac anomalies; follow-up or limited study S

C8923 Transthoracic echocardiography (TTE) with contrast, or without contrast followed by with contrast, real-time with image documentation (2D), includes M-mode recording, when performed, complete, without spectral or color doppler echocardiography S

C8924 Transthoracic echocardiography (TTE) with contrast, or without contrast followed by with contrast, real-time with image documentation (2D), includes M-mode recording when performed, follow-up or limited study S

C8925 Transesophageal echocardiography (TEE) with contrast, or without contrast followed by with contrast, real time with image documentation (2D) (with or without M-mode recording); including probe placement, image acquisition, interpretation and report S

C8926 Transesophageal echocardiography (TEE) with contrast, or without contrast followed by with contrast, for congenital cardiac anomalies; including probe placement, image acquisition, interpretation and report S

C8927 Transesophageal echocardiography (TEE) with contrast, or without contrast followed by with contrast, for monitoring purposes, including probe placement, real time (2D) image acquisition and interpretation leading to ongoing (continuous) assessment of (dynamically changing) cardiac pumping function and to therapeutic measures on an immediate time basis S

C8928 Transthoracic echocardiography (TTE) with contrast, or without contrast followed by with contrast, real-time with image documentation (2D), includes M-mode recording, when performed, during rest and cardiovascular stress test using treadmill, bicycle exercise and/or pharmacologically induced stress, with interpretation and report S

C8929 Transthoracic echocardiography (TTE) with contrast, or without contrast followed by with contrast, real-time with image documentation (2D), includes M-mode recording, when performed, complete, with spectral doppler echocardiography, and with color flow doppler echocardiography S

C8930 **Transthoracic echocardiography (TTE) with contrast, or without contrast followed by with contrast, real-time with image documentation (2D), includes M-mode recording, when performed, during rest and cardiovascular stress test using treadmill, bicycle exercise and/or pharmacologically induced stress, with interpretation and report; including performance of continuous electrocardiographic monitoring, with physician supervision** S

C8931 **Magnetic resonance angiography with contrast, spinal canal and contents** Q3 Z2

C8932 **Magnetic resonance angiography without contrast, spinal canal and contents** Q3 Z2

C8933 **Magnetic resonance angiography without contrast followed by with contrast, spinal canal and contents** Q3 Z2

C8934 **Magnetic resonance angiography with contrast, upper extremity** Q3 Z2

C8935 **Magnetic resonance angiography without contrast, upper extremity** Q3 Z2

C8936 **Magnetic resonance angiography without contrast followed by with contrast, upper extremity** Q3 Z2

C8937 **Computer-aided detection, including computer algorithm analysis of breast MRI image data for lesion detection/characterization, pharmacokinetic analysis, with further physician review for interpretation (list separately in addition to code for primary procedure)** N

C8957 **Intravenous infusion for therapy/diagnosis; initiation of prolonged infusion (more than 8 hours), requiring use of portable or implantable pump** S
CMS: 100-04,4,230.2

C9046 **Cocaine HCl nasal solution for topical administration, 1 mg** N N1
Use this code for Goprelto.
AHA: 1Q,23; 2Q,19

C9047 **Injection, caplacizumab-yhdp, 1 mg** K K2
Use this code for Cablivi.
AHA: 3Q,19

C9067 **Gallium Ga-68, Dotatoc, diagnostic, 0.01 mCi** N N1
AHA: 4Q,20

C9088 **Instillation, bupivacaine and meloxicam, 1 mg/0.03 mg** G K2
Use this code for Zynrelef.
AHA: 1Q,22

C9089 **Bupivacaine, collagen-matrix implant, 1 mg** N K2
Use this code for Xaracoll.
AHA: 1Q,22

C9101 **Injection, oliceridine, 0.1 mg** G K2
Use this code for Olinvyk.
AHA: 4Q,22

~~**C9113** **Injection, pantoprazole sodium, per vial**~~
To report, see ~J2470-J2471

C9143 **Cocaine HCl nasal solution (Numbrino), 1 mg** N N1
Use this code for cocaine HCl (Numbrino) manufactured by Lannett.
AHA: 1Q,23

C9144 **Injection, bupivacaine (Posimir), 1 mg** G K2
AHA: 1Q,23

C9145 **Injection, aprepitant, (Aponvie), 1 mg** G K2
Use this code for Aponvie.
AHA: 2Q,23

~~**C9150** **Xenon Xe-129 hyperpolarized gas, diagnostic, per study dose**~~
To report, see ~A9610

~~**C9159** **Injection, prothrombin complex concentrate (human), Balfaxar, per IU of Factor IX activity**~~
To report, see ~J7165

~~**C9160** **Injection, daxibotulinumtoxina-lanm, 1 unit**~~
To report, see ~J0589

~~**C9161** **Injection, aflibercept HD, 1 mg**~~
To report, see ~J0177

~~**C9162** **Injection, avacincaptad pegol, 0.1 mg**~~
To report, see ~J2782

~~**C9163** **Injection, talquetamab-tgvs, 0.25 mg**~~
To report, see ~J3055

~~**C9164** **Cantharidin for topical administration, 0.7%, single unit dose applicator (3.2 mg)**~~
To report, see ~J7354

~~**C9165** **Injection, elranatamab-bcmm, 1 mg**~~
To report, see ~J1323

~~**C9166** **Injection, secukinumab, IV, 1 mg**~~
To report, see ~J3247

~~**C9167** **Injection, ADAMTS13, recombinant-krhn, 10 IU**~~
To report, see ~J7171

~~**C9168** **Injection, mirikizumab-mrkz, 1 mg**~~

~~**C9169** **Injection, nogapendekin alfa inbakicept-pmln, for intravesical use, 1 mcg**~~

~~**C9170** **Injection, tarlatamab-dlle, 1 mg**~~

~~**C9171** **Injection, pegulicianine, 1 mg**~~

~~**C9172** **Injection, fidanacogene elaparvovec-dzkt, per therapeutic dose**~~

● **C9173** Injection, filgrastim-txid (Nypozi), biosimilar, 1 mcg

C9248 **Injection, clevidipine butyrate, 1 mg** N N1 ☑
Use this code for Cleviprex.

C9250 **Human plasma fibrin sealant, vapor-heated, solvent-detergent (Artiss), 2 ml** K K2 ☑

C9254 **Injection, lacosamide, 1 mg** N N1 ☑
Use this code for VIMPAT.

C9257 **Injection, bevacizumab, 0.25 mg** K K2 ☑
Use this code for Avastin.
CMS: 100-03,110.17

C9285 **Lidocaine 70 mg/tetracaine 70 mg, per patch** N N1 ☑
Use this code for SYNERA.

~~**C9290** **Injection, bupivacaine liposome, 1 mg**~~

C9293 **Injection, glucarpidase, 10 units** E ☑
Use this code for Voraxaze.

C9352 Microporous collagen implantable tube (NeuraGen Nerve Guide), per cm length N N1 ☑

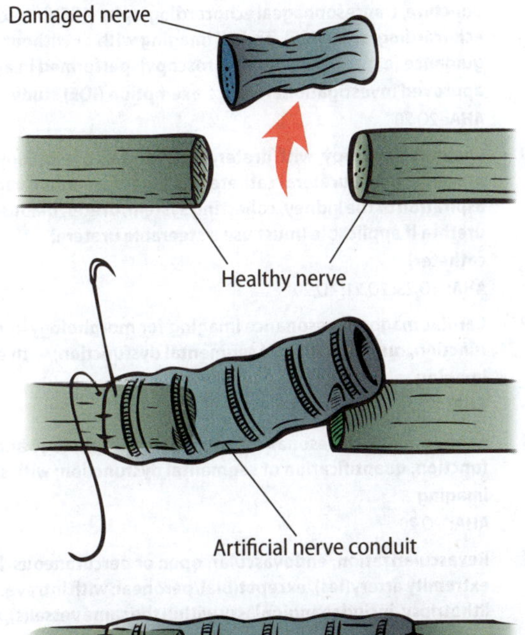

A synthetic "bridge" is affixed to each end of a severed nerve with sutures. This procedure is performed using an operating microscope

C9353 Microporous collagen implantable slit tube (NeuraWrap Nerve Protector), per cm length N N1 ☑

C9354 Acellular pericardial tissue matrix of nonhuman origin (Veritas), per sq cm N N1 ☑

C9355 Collagen nerve cuff (NeuroMatrix), per 0.5 cm length N N1 ☑

C9356 Tendon, porous matrix of cross-linked collagen and glycosaminoglycan matrix (TenoGlide Tendon Protector Sheet), per sq cm N N1 ☑

C9358 Dermal substitute, native, nondenatured collagen, fetal bovine origin (SurgiMend Collagen Matrix), per 0.5 sq cm N N1 ☑
AHA: 1Q,24

C9361 Collagen matrix nerve wrap (NeuroMend Collagen Nerve Wrap), per 0.5 cm length N N1 ☑

C9362 Porous purified collagen matrix bone void filler (Integra Mozaik Osteoconductive Scaffold Strip), per 0.5 cc N N1 ☑

C9363 Skin substitute (Integra Meshed Bilayer Wound Matrix), per sq cm N N1 ☑
CMS: 100-04,4,260.1; 100-04,4,260.1.1

C9364 Porcine implant, Permacol, per sq cm N N1 ☑

C9399 Unclassified drugs or biologicals A K7
CMS: 100-02,15,50.5; 100-04,17,90.3; 100-04,32,400; 100-04,32,400.1; 100-04,32,400.2; 100-04,32,400.2.1; 100-04,32,400.2.2; 100-04,32,400.2.3; 100-04,32,400.2.3.1; 100-04,32,400.2.4; 100-04,32,400.2.5; 100-04,32,400.3; 100-04,32,400.4; 100-04,32,412.1; 100-04,4,260.1; 100-04,4,260.1.1
AHA: 3Q,23

C9460 Injection, cangrelor, 1 mg K K2 ☑
Use this code for Kengreal.

C9462 Injection, delafloxacin, 1 mg E1
Use this code for Baxdela.

C9482 Injection, sotalol HCl, 1 mg K K2 ☑

C9488 Injection, conivaptan HCl, 1 mg K K2 ☑
Use this code for Vaprisol.

C9507 Fresh frozen plasma, high titer COVID-19 convalescent, frozen within 8 hours of collection, each unit R
AHA: 2Q,22

C9600 Percutaneous transcatheter placement of drug eluting intracoronary stent(s), with coronary angioplasty when performed; single major coronary artery or branch J J8
AHA: 1Q,24; 2Q,23; 4Q,21

C9601 Percutaneous transcatheter placement of drug-eluting intracoronary stent(s), with coronary angioplasty when performed; each additional branch of a major coronary artery (list separately in addition to code for primary procedure) N N1
AHA: 1Q,24; 2Q,23

C9602 Percutaneous transluminal coronary atherectomy, with drug eluting intracoronary stent, with coronary angioplasty when performed; single major coronary artery or branch J
AHA: 1Q,24; 2Q,23; 4Q,21

C9603 Percutaneous transluminal coronary atherectomy, with drug-eluting intracoronary stent, with coronary angioplasty when performed; each additional branch of a major coronary artery (list separately in addition to code for primary procedure) N
AHA: 1Q,24; 2Q,23

C9604 Percutaneous transluminal revascularization of or through coronary artery bypass graft (internal mammary, free arterial, venous), any combination of drug-eluting intracoronary stent, atherectomy and angioplasty, including distal protection when performed; single vessel J
AHA: 1Q,24; 2Q,23

C9605 Percutaneous transluminal revascularization of or through coronary artery bypass graft (internal mammary, free arterial, venous), any combination of drug-eluting intracoronary stent, atherectomy and angioplasty, including distal protection when performed; each additional branch subtended by the bypass graft (list separately in addition to code for primary procedure) N
AHA: 1Q,24; 2Q,23

C9606 Percutaneous transluminal revascularization of acute total/subtotal occlusion during acute myocardial infarction, coronary artery or coronary artery bypass graft, any combination of drug-eluting intracoronary stent, atherectomy and angioplasty, including aspiration thrombectomy when performed, single vessel C
CMS: 100-04,4,260.1; 100-04,4,260.1.1
AHA: 1Q,24; 2Q,23; 1Q,19

C9607 Percutaneous transluminal revascularization of chronic total occlusion, coronary artery, coronary artery branch, or coronary artery bypass graft, any combination of drug-eluting intracoronary stent, atherectomy and angioplasty; single vessel J
AHA: 1Q,24; 2Q,23; 4Q,21

C9608 Percutaneous transluminal revascularization of chronic total occlusion, coronary artery, coronary artery branch, or coronary artery bypass graft, any combination of drug-eluting intracoronary stent, atherectomy and angioplasty; each additional coronary artery, coronary artery branch, or bypass graft (list separately in addition to code for primary procedure) N
AHA: 1Q,24; 2Q,23

● **C9610** **Catheter, transluminal drug delivery with or without angioplasty, coronary, nonlaser (insertable)**

C9725 **Placement of endorectal intracavitary applicator for high intensity brachytherapy** T G2 ⃠

C9726 **Placement and removal (if performed) of applicator into breast for intraoperative radiation therapy, add-on to primary breast procedure** N N1

C9727 **Insertion of implants into the soft palate; minimum of three implants** J G2 ☑

C9728 **Placement of interstitial device(s) for radiation therapy/surgery guidance (e.g., fiducial markers, dosimeter), for other than the following sites (any approach): abdomen, pelvis, prostate, retroperitoneum, thorax, single or multiple** S G2

C9733 **Nonophthalmic fluorescent vascular angiography** Q2

AHA: 1Q,23

~~C9734~~ ~~**Focused ultrasound ablation/therapeutic intervention, other than uterine leiomyomata, with magnetic resonance (MR) guidance**~~

C9738 **Adjunctive blue light cystoscopy with fluorescent imaging agent (list separately in addition to code for primary procedure)** N N1

C9739 **Cystourethroscopy, with insertion of transprostatic implant; one to three implants** J J8

C9740 **Cystourethroscopy, with insertion of transprostatic implant; four or more implants** J J8

C9751 **Bronchoscopy, rigid or flexible, transbronchial ablation of lesion(s) by microwave energy, including fluoroscopic guidance, when performed, with computed tomography acquisition(s) and 3D rendering, computer-assisted, image-guided navigation, and endobronchial ultrasound (EBUS) guided transtracheal and/or transbronchial sampling (e.g., aspiration[s]/biopsy[ies]) and all mediastinal and/or hilar lymph node stations or structures and therapeutic intervention(s)** T

CMS: 100-04,4,260.1; 100-04,4,260.1.1

AHA: 1Q,19

C9756 **Intraoperative near-infrared fluorescence lymphatic mapping of lymph node(s) (sentinel or tumor draining) with administration of indocyanine green (ICG) (List separately in addition to code for primary procedure)** N

AHA: 1Q,21; 3Q,19

C9757 **Laminotomy (hemilaminectomy), with decompression of nerve root(s), including partial facetectomy, foraminotomy and excision of herniated intervertebral disc, and repair of annular defect with implantation of bone anchored annular closure device, including annular defect measurement, alignment and sizing assessment, and image guidance; 1 interspace, lumbar** J G2

AHA: 1Q,20

C9758 **Blind procedure for NYHA Class III/IV heart failure; transcatheter implantation of interatrial shunt including right heart catheterization, transesophageal echocardiography (TEE)/intracardiac echocardiography (ICE), and all imaging with or without guidance (e.g., ultrasound, fluoroscopy), performed in an approved investigational device exemption (IDE) study** T

C9759 **Transcatheter intraoperative blood vessel microinfusion(s) (e.g., intraluminal, vascular wall and/or perivascular) therapy, any vessel, including radiological supervision and interpretation, when performed** N N1

AHA: 2Q,20

C9760 **Nonrandomized, nonblinded procedure for NYHA Class II, III, IV heart failure; transcatheter implantation of interatrial shunt, including right and left heart catheterization, transeptal puncture, transesophageal echocardiography (TEE)/intracardiac echocardiography (ICE), and all imaging with or without guidance (e.g., ultrasound, fluoroscopy), performed in an approved investigational device exemption (IDE) study** T

AHA: 2Q,20

C9761 **Cystourethroscopy, with ureteroscopy and/or pyeloscopy, with lithotripsy, and ureteral catheterization for steerable vacuum aspiration of the kidney, collecting system, ureter, bladder, and urethra if applicable (must use a steerable ureteral catheter)** J G2

AHA: 1Q,23; 2Q,21; 4Q,20

C9762 **Cardiac magnetic resonance imaging for morphology and function, quantification of segmental dysfunction; with strain imaging** Q3 Z2

AHA: 2Q,20

C9763 **Cardiac magnetic resonance imaging for morphology and function, quantification of segmental dysfunction; with stress imaging** Q3 Z2

AHA: 2Q,20

C9764 **Revascularization, endovascular, open or percutaneous, lower extremity artery(ies), except tibial/peroneal; with intravascular lithotripsy, includes angioplasty within the same vessel(s), when performed** J J8

AHA: 2Q,20

C9765 **Revascularization, endovascular, open or percutaneous, lower extremity artery(ies), except tibial/peroneal; with intravascular lithotripsy, and transluminal stent placement(s), includes angioplasty within the same vessel(s), when performed** J J8

AHA: 2Q,20

C9766 **Revascularization, endovascular, open or percutaneous, lower extremity artery(ies), except tibial/peroneal; with intravascular lithotripsy and atherectomy, includes angioplasty within the same vessel(s), when performed** J J8

AHA: 2Q,20

C9767 **Revascularization, endovascular, open or percutaneous, lower extremity artery(ies), except tibial/peroneal; with intravascular lithotripsy and transluminal stent placement(s), and atherectomy, includes angioplasty within the same vessel(s), when performed** J J8

AHA: 2Q,20

C9768 **Endoscopic ultrasound-guided direct measurement of hepatic portosystemic pressure gradient by any method (list separately in addition to code for primary procedure)** N

AHA: 2Q,23; 4Q,20

~~C9769~~ ~~**Cystourethroscopy, with insertion of temporary prostatic implant/stent with fixation/anchor and incisional struts**~~

C9772 **Revascularization, endovascular, open or percutaneous, tibial/peroneal artery(ies), with intravascular lithotripsy, includes angioplasty within the same vessel(s), when performed** J J8

AHA: 1Q,21

C9773 **Revascularization, endovascular, open or percutaneous, tibial/peroneal artery(ies); with intravascular lithotripsy, and transluminal stent placement(s), includes angioplasty within the same vessel(s), when performed** J J8

AHA: 1Q,21

C9774 **Revascularization, endovascular, open or percutaneous, tibial/peroneal artery(ies); with intravascular lithotripsy and atherectomy, includes angioplasty within the same vessel(s), when performed** J J8

AHA: 1Q,21

C9775 Revascularization, endovascular, open or percutaneous, tibial/peroneal artery(ies); with intravascular lithotripsy and transluminal stent placement(s), and atherectomy, includes angioplasty within the same vessel(s), when performed J J8

AHA: 1Q,21

C9776 Intraoperative near-infrared fluorescence imaging of major extra-hepatic bile duct(s) (e.g., cystic duct, common bile duct and common hepatic duct) with intravenous administration of indocyanine green (ICG) (list separately in addition to code for primary procedure) N N1

AHA: 2Q,23; 1Q,22; 2Q,21

C9777 Esophageal mucosal integrity testing by electrical impedance, transoral, includes esophagoscopy or esophagogastroduodenoscopy J J8

AHA: 2Q,21

C9778 Colpopexy, vaginal; minimally invasive extraperitoneal approach (sacrospinous) J J8

AHA: 3Q,21

C9779 Endoscopic submucosal dissection (ESD), including endoscopy or colonoscopy, mucosal closure, when performed J

AHA: 3Q,23; 4Q,21

C9780 Insertion of central venous catheter through central venous occlusion via inferior and superior approaches (e.g., inside-out technique), including imaging guidance S

AHA: 4Q,21

C9781 Arthroscopy, shoulder, surgical; with implantation of subacromial spacer (e.g., balloon), includes debridement (e.g., limited or extensive), subacromial decompression, acromioplasty, and biceps tenodesis when performed J J8

AHA: 2Q,22

C9782 Blinded procedure for New York Heart Association (NYHA) Class II or III heart failure, or Canadian Cardiovascular Society (CCS) Class III or IV chronic refractory angina; transcatheter intramyocardial transplantation of autologous bone marrow cells (e.g., mononuclear) or placebo control, autologous bone marrow harvesting and preparation for transplantation, left heart catheterization including ventriculography, all laboratory services, and all imaging with or without guidance (e.g., transthoracic echocardiography, ultrasound, fluoroscopy), performed in an approved investigational device exemption (IDE) study T

AHA: 2Q,22

C9783 Blinded procedure for transcatheter implantation of coronary sinus reduction device or placebo control, including vascular access and closure, right heart catherization, venous and coronary sinus angiography, imaging guidance and supervision and interpretation when performed in an approved investigational device exemption (IDE) study J

AHA: 2Q,22

C9784 Gastric restrictive procedure, endoscopic sleeve gastroplasty, with esophagogastroduodenoscopy and intraluminal tube insertion, if performed, including all system and tissue anchoring components J

AHA: 3Q,23

C9785 Endoscopic outlet reduction, gastric pouch application, with endoscopy and intraluminal tube insertion, if performed, including all system and tissue anchoring components J

AHA: 3Q,23

~~**C9786** Echocardiography image post processing for computer aided detection of heart failure with preserved ejection fraction, including interpretation and report~~

~~**C9787** Gastric electrophysiology mapping with simultaneous patient symptom profiling~~

C9789 Instillation of antineoplastic pharmacologic/biologic agent into renal pelvis, any method, including all imaging guidance, including volumetric measurement if performed T G2

AHA: 4Q,23

~~**C9790** Histotripsy (i.e., nonthermal ablation via acoustic energy delivery) of malignant renal tissue, including image guidance~~

C9791 Magnetic resonance imaging with inhaled hyperpolarized xenon-129 contrast agent, chest, including preparation and administration of agent T

AHA: 4Q,23

C9792 Blinded or nonblinded procedure for symptomatic New York Heart Association (NYHA) Class II, III, IVA heart failure; transcatheter implantation of left atrial to coronary sinus shunt using jugular vein access, including all imaging necessary to intra procedurally map the coronary sinus for optimal shunt placement (e.g., transesophageal echocardiography (TTE), intracardiac echocardiography (ICE), fluoroscopy), performed under general anesthesia in an approved investigational device exemption (IDE) study S

AHA: 4Q,23

C9793 3D predictive model generation for preplanning of a cardiac procedure, using data from cardiac computed tomographic angiography with report S

AHA: 1Q,24

~~**C9794** Therapeutic radiology simulation-aided field setting; complex, including acquisition of PET and CT imaging data required for radiopharmaceutical-directed radiation therapy treatment planning (i.e., modeling)~~

To report, see ~G0562

~~**C9795** Stereotactic body radiation therapy, treatment delivery, per fraction to 1 or more lesions, including image guidance and real-time positron emissions-based delivery adjustments to 1 or more lesions, entire course not to exceed 5 fractions~~

To report, see ~G0563

● **C9796** Repair of enterocutaneous fistula small intestine or colon (excluding anorectal fistula) with plug (e.g., porcine small intestine submucosa [SIS]) J J8

AHA: 1Q,24

● **C9797** Vascular embolization or occlusion procedure with use of a pressure-generating catheter (e.g., one-way valve, intermittently occluding), inclusive of all radiological supervision and interpretation, intraprocedural roadmapping, and imaging guidance necessary to complete the intervention; for tumors, organ ischemia, or infarction J J8

AHA: 1Q,24

● **C9804** Elastomeric infusion pump (e.g., On-Q* pump with bolus), including catheter and all disposable system components, non-opioid medical device (must be a qualifying medicare non-opioid medical device for post-surgical pain relief in accordance with section 4135 of the caa, 2023)

● **C9806** Rotary peristaltic infusion pump (e.g., ambIT pump), including catheter and all disposable system components, nonopioid medical device (must be a qualifying Medicare nonopioid medical device for postsurgical pain relief in accordance with Section 4135 of the CAA, 2023)

● **C9807** Nerve stimulator, percutaneous, peripheral (e.g., sprint peripheral nerve stimulation system), including electrode and all disposable system components, nonopioid medical device (must be a qualifying Medicare nonopioid medical device for postsurgical pain relief in accordance with Section 4135 of the CAA, 2023)

● **C9808** **Nerve cryoablation probe (e.g., cryoICE, cryoSPHERE, cryoSPHERE MAX, cryo2), including probe and all disposable system components, nonopioid medical device (must be a qualifying Medicare nonopioid medical device for postsurgical pain relief in accordance with Section 4135 of the CAA, 2023)**

● **C9809** **Cryoablation needle (e.g., iovera system), including needle/tip and all disposable system components, nonopioid medical device (must be a qualifying Medicare nonopioid medical device for postsurgical pain relief in accordance with Section 4135 of the CAA, 2023)**

C9898 **Radiolabeled product provided during a hospital inpatient stay** N

CMS: 100-04,4,260.1; 100-04,4,260.1.1

C9899 **Implanted prosthetic device, payable only for inpatients who do not have inpatient coverage** A

● **C9901** **Endoscopic defect closure within the entire gastrointestinal tract, including upper endoscopy (including diagnostic, if performed) or colonoscopy (including diagnostic, if performed), with all system and tissue anchoring components**

AHA: 3Q,24

Durable Medical Equipment E0100-E8002

E codes include durable medical equipment such as canes, crutches, walkers, commodes, decubitus care, bath and toilet aids, hospital beds, oxygen and related respiratory equipment, monitoring equipment, pacemakers, patient lifts, safety equipment, restraints, traction equipment, fracture frames, wheelchairs, and artificial kidney machines.

Canes

E0100 **Cane, includes canes of all materials, adjustable or fixed, with tip** Y ♿ (NU, RR, UE)
White canes for the blind are not covered under Medicare.

E0105 **Cane, quad or three-prong, includes canes of all materials, adjustable or fixed, with tips** Y ♿ (NU, RR, UE)

Crutches

E0110 **Crutches, forearm, includes crutches of various materials, adjustable or fixed, pair, complete with tips and handgrips** Y ☑ ♿ (NU, RR, UE)

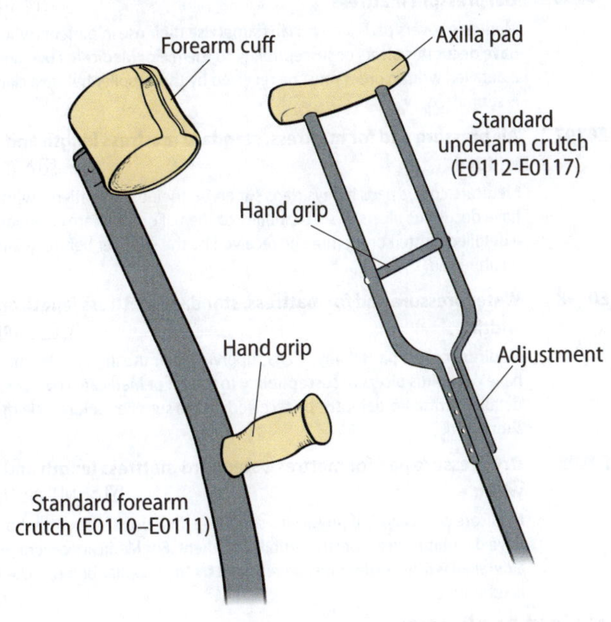

E0111 **Crutch, forearm, includes crutches of various materials, adjustable or fixed, each, with tip and handgrips** Y ☑ ♿ (NU, RR, UE)

E0112 **Crutches, underarm, wood, adjustable or fixed, pair, with pads, tips, and handgrips** Y ☑ ♿ (NU, RR, UE)

E0113 **Crutch, underarm, wood, adjustable or fixed, each, with pad, tip, and handgrip** Y ☑ ♿ (NU, RR, UE)

E0114 **Crutches, underarm, other than wood, adjustable or fixed, pair, with pads, tips, and handgrips** Y ☑ ♿ (NU, RR, UE)

E0116 **Crutch, underarm, other than wood, adjustable or fixed, with pad, tip, handgrip, with or without shock absorber, each** Y ☑ ♿ (NU, RR, UE)

E0117 **Crutch, underarm, articulating, spring assisted, each** Y ☑ ♿ (RR)

E0118 **Crutch substitute, lower leg platform, with or without wheels, each** E ☑
Medicare covers walkers if patient's ambulation is impaired.

Walkers

E0130 **Walker, rigid (pickup), adjustable or fixed height** Y ♿ (NU, RR, UE)
CMS: 100-04,36,50.15

E0135 **Walker, folding (pickup), adjustable or fixed height** Y ♿ (NU, RR, UE)
Medicare covers walkers if patient's ambulation is impaired.
CMS: 100-04,36,50.15

E0140 **Walker, with trunk support, adjustable or fixed height, any type** Y ♿ (RR)
CMS: 100-04,36,50.15

E0141 **Walker, rigid, wheeled, adjustable or fixed height** Y ♿ (NU, RR, UE)
Medicare covers walkers if patient's ambulation is impaired.
CMS: 100-04,36,50.15

E0143 **Walker, folding, wheeled, adjustable or fixed height** Y ♿ (NU, RR, UE)
Medicare covers walkers if patient's ambulation is impaired.
CMS: 100-04,36,50.15

E0144 **Walker, enclosed, four-sided framed, rigid or folding, wheeled with posterior seat** Y ♿ (RR)
CMS: 100-04,36,50.15

E0147 **Walker, heavy-duty, multiple braking system, variable wheel resistance** Y ♿ (NU, RR, UE)
Medicare covers safety roller walkers only in patients with severe neurological disorders or restricted use of one hand. In some cases, coverage will be extended to patients with a weight exceeding the limits of a standard wheeled walker.
CMS: 100-04,36,50.15

E0148 **Walker, heavy-duty, without wheels, rigid or folding, any type, each** Y ☑ ♿ (NU, RR, UE)
CMS: 100-04,36,50.15

E0149 **Walker, heavy-duty, wheeled, rigid or folding, any type** Y ♿ (RR)
CMS: 100-04,36,50.15

○ **E0152** **Walker, battery powered, wheeled, folding, adjustable or fixed height** E
AHA: 2Q,24

Attachments

E0153 **Platform attachment, forearm crutch, each** Y ☑ ♿ (NU, RR, UE)

E0154 **Platform attachment, walker, each** Y ☑ ♿ (NU, RR, UE)
CMS: 100-04,36,50.14; 100-04,36,50.15

E0155 **Wheel attachment, rigid pick-up walker, per pair** Y ☑ ♿ (NU, RR, UE)
CMS: 100-04,36,50.15

E0156 **Seat attachment, walker** Y ♿ (NU, RR, UE)
CMS: 100-04,36,50.14; 100-04,36,50.15

E0157 **Crutch attachment, walker, each** Y ☑ ♿ (NU, RR, UE)
CMS: 100-04,36,50.14; 100-04,36,50.15

E0158 **Leg extensions for walker, per set of four** Y ☑ ♿ (NU, RR, UE)
CMS: 100-04,36,50.14; 100-04,36,50.15

E0159 **Brake attachment for wheeled walker, replacement, each** Y ☑ ♿ (NU, RR, UE)
CMS: 100-04,36,50.15

Commodes

E0160 **Sitz type bath or equipment, portable, used with or without commode** Y ♿ (NU, RR, UE)
Medicare covers sitz baths if medical record indicates that the patient has an infection or injury of the perineal area and the sitz bath is prescribed by the physician.

E0161 **Sitz type bath or equipment, portable, used with or without commode, with faucet attachment(s)** Y ♿ (NU, RR, UE)
Medicare covers sitz baths if medical record indicates that the patient has an infection or injury of the perineal area and the sitz bath is prescribed by the physician.

E0162 **Sitz bath chair** Y ♿ (NU, RR, UE)
Medicare covers sitz baths if medical record indicates that the patient has an infection or injury of the perineal area and the sitz bath is prescribed by the physician.

E0163 **Commode chair, mobile or stationary, with fixed arms** Y ♿ (NU, RR, UE)
Medicare covers commodes for patients confined to their beds or rooms, for patients without indoor bathroom facilities, and to patients who cannot climb or descend the stairs necessary to reach the bathrooms in their homes.

E0165 **Commode chair, mobile or stationary, with detachable arms** Y ♿ (RR)
Medicare covers commodes for patients confined to their beds or rooms, for patients without indoor bathroom facilities, and to patients who cannot climb or descend the stairs necessary to reach the bathrooms in their homes.

E0167 **Pail or pan for use with commode chair, replacement only** Y ♿ (NU, RR, UE)
Medicare covers commodes for patients confined to their beds or rooms, for patients without indoor bathroom facilities, and to patients who cannot climb or descend the stairs necessary to reach the bathrooms in their homes.

E0168 **Commode chair, extra wide and/or heavy-duty, stationary or mobile, with or without arms, any type, each** Y ☑ ♿ (NU, RR, UE)

E0170 **Commode chair with integrated seat lift mechanism, electric, any type** Y ♿ (RR)

E0171 **Commode chair with integrated seat lift mechanism, nonelectric, any type** Y ♿ (RR)

E0172 **Seat lift mechanism placed over or on top of toilet, any type** E

E0175 **Footrest, for use with commode chair, each** Y ☑ ♿ (NU, RR, UE)

Decubitus Care Equipment

E0181 **Powered pressure reducing mattress overlay/pad, alternating, with pump, includes heavy-duty** Y ♿ (RR)
For Medicare coverage, a detailed written order must be received by the supplier before a claim is submitted.

E0182 **Pump for alternating pressure pad, for replacement only** Y ♿ (RR)
For Medicare coverage, a detailed written order must be received by the supplier before a claim is submitted.

E0183 **Powered pressure reducing underlay/pad, alternating, with pump, includes heavy duty** Y (RR)

E0184 **Dry pressure mattress** Y ♿ (NU, RR, UE)
For Medicare coverage, a detailed written order must be received by the supplier before a claim is submitted.

E0185 **Gel or gel-like pressure pad for mattress, standard mattress length and width** Y ♿ (NU, RR, UE)
For Medicare coverage, a detailed written order must be received by the supplier before a claim is submitted.

E0186 **Air pressure mattress** Y ♿ (RR)
For Medicare coverage, a detailed written order must be received by the supplier before a claim is submitted.

E0187 **Water pressure mattress** Y ♿ (RR)
For Medicare coverage, a detailed written order must be received by the supplier before a claim is submitted.

E0188 **Synthetic sheepskin pad** Y ♿ (NU, RR, UE)
For Medicare coverage, a detailed written order must be received by the supplier before a claim is submitted.

E0189 **Lambswool sheepskin pad, any size** Y ♿ (NU, RR, UE)
For Medicare coverage, a detailed written order must be received by the supplier before a claim is submitted.

E0190 **Positioning cushion/pillow/wedge, any shape or size, includes all components and accessories** E

E0191 **Heel or elbow protector, each** Y ☑ ♿ (NU, RR, UE)

E0193 **Powered air flotation bed (low air loss therapy)** Y ♿ (RR)

E0194 **Air fluidized bed** Y ♿ (RR)
An air fluidized bed is covered by Medicare if the patient has a stage 3 or stage 4 pressure sore and, without the bed, would require institutionalization. For Medicare coverage, a detailed written order must be received by the supplier before a claim is submitted.

E0196 **Gel pressure mattress** Y ♿ (RR)
Medicare covers pads if physicians supervise their use in patients who have decubitus ulcers or susceptibility to them. For Medicare coverage, a detailed written order must be received by the supplier before a claim is submitted.

E0197 **Air pressure pad for mattress, standard mattress length and width** Y ♿ (RR)
Medicare covers pads if physicians supervise their use in patients who have decubitus ulcers or susceptibility to them. For Medicare coverage, a detailed written order must be received by the supplier before a claim is submitted.

E0198 **Water pressure pad for mattress, standard mattress length and width** Y ♿ (RR)
Medicare covers pads if physicians supervise their use in patients who have decubitus ulcers or susceptibility to them.For Medicare coverage, a detailed written order must be received by the supplier before a claim is submitted.

E0199 **Dry pressure pad for mattress, standard mattress length and width** Y ♿ (NU, RR, UE)
Medicare covers pads if physicians supervise their use in patients who have decubitus ulcers or susceptibility to them. For Medicare coverage, a detailed written order must be received by the supplier before a claim is submitted.

Heat/Cold Application

E0200 **Heat lamp, without stand (table model), includes bulb, or infrared element** Y ♿ (NU, RR, UE)

E0202 **Phototherapy (bilirubin) light with photometer** Y ♿ (RR)

E0203 **Therapeutic lightbox, minimum 10,000 lux, table top model** E

E0205 **Heat lamp, with stand, includes bulb, or infrared element** Y ♿ (NU, RR, UE)

E0210 **Electric heat pad, standard** Y ♿ (NU, RR, UE)

E0215 **Electric heat pad, moist** Y ♿ (NU, RR, UE)

E0217 **Water circulating heat pad with pump** Y ♿ (NU, RR, UE)

E0218 **Fluid circulating cold pad with pump, any type** Y

E0221 **Infrared heating pad system** Y

E0225 **Hydrocollator unit, includes pads** Y ♿ (NU, RR, UE)

E0231 **Noncontact wound-warming device (temperature control unit, AC adapter and power cord) for use with warming card and wound cover** E

E0232 **Warming card for use with the noncontact wound-warming device and noncontact wound-warming wound cover** E

E0235 **Paraffin bath unit, portable (see medical supply code A4265 for paraffin)** Y ♿ (RR)

E0236 Pump for water circulating pad (RR)

E0239 Hydrocollator unit, portable (NU, RR, UE)

Bath and Toilet Aids

E0240 Bath/shower chair, with or without wheels, any size

E0241 Bathtub wall rail, each

E0242 Bathtub rail, floor base

E0243 Toilet rail, each

E0244 Raised toilet seat

E0245 Tub stool or bench

E0246 Transfer tub rail attachment

E0247 Transfer bench for tub or toilet with or without commode opening

E0248 Transfer bench, heavy-duty, for tub or toilet with or without commode opening

E0249 Pad for water circulating heat unit, for replacement only (NU, RR, UE)

Hospital Beds and Accessories

E0250 Hospital bed, fixed height, with any type side rails, with mattress (RR)

E0251 Hospital bed, fixed height, with any type side rails, without mattress (RR)

E0255 Hospital bed, variable height, hi-lo, with any type side rails, with mattress (RR)

E0256 Hospital bed, variable height, hi-lo, with any type side rails, without mattress (RR)

E0260 Hospital bed, semi-electric (head and foot adjustment), with any type side rails, with mattress (RR)

E0261 Hospital bed, semi-electric (head and foot adjustment), with any type side rails, without mattress (RR)

E0265 Hospital bed, total electric (head, foot, and height adjustments), with any type side rails, with mattress (RR)

E0266 Hospital bed, total electric (head, foot, and height adjustments), with any type side rails, without mattress (RR)

E0270 Hospital bed, institutional type includes: oscillating, circulating and Stryker frame, with mattress

E0271 Mattress, innerspring (NU, RR, UE)

CMS: 100-04,36,50.14

E0272 Mattress, foam rubber (NU, RR, UE)

CMS: 100-04,36,50.14

E0273 Bed board

E0274 Over-bed table

E0275 Bed pan, standard, metal or plastic (NU, RR, UE)

Reusable, autoclavable bedpans are covered by Medicare for bed-confined patients.

E0276 Bed pan, fracture, metal or plastic (NU, RR, UE)

Reusable, autoclavable bedpans are covered by Medicare for bed-confined patients.

E0277 Powered pressure-reducing air mattress (RR)

E0280 Bed cradle, any type (NU, RR, UE)

CMS: 100-04,36,50.14

E0290 Hospital bed, fixed height, without side rails, with mattress (RR)

E0291 Hospital bed, fixed height, without side rails, without mattress (RR)

E0292 Hospital bed, variable height, hi-lo, without side rails, with mattress (RR)

E0293 Hospital bed, variable height, hi-lo, without side rails, without mattress (RR)

E0294 Hospital bed, semi-electric (head and foot adjustment), without side rails, with mattress (RR)

E0295 Hospital bed, semi-electric (head and foot adjustment), without side rails, without mattress (RR)

E0296 Hospital bed, total electric (head, foot, and height adjustments), without side rails, with mattress (RR)

E0297 Hospital bed, total electric (head, foot, and height adjustments), without side rails, without mattress (RR)

E0300 Pediatric crib, hospital grade, fully enclosed, with or without top enclosure (RR)

E0301 Hospital bed, heavy-duty, extra wide, with weight capacity greater than 350 pounds, but less than or equal to 600 pounds, with any type side rails, without mattress (RR)

E0302 Hospital bed, extra heavy-duty, extra wide, with weight capacity greater than 600 pounds, with any type side rails, without mattress (RR)

E0303 Hospital bed, heavy-duty, extra wide, with weight capacity greater than 350 pounds, but less than or equal to 600 pounds, with any type side rails, with mattress (RR)

E0304 Hospital bed, extra heavy-duty, extra wide, with weight capacity greater than 600 pounds, with any type side rails, with mattress (RR)

E0305 Bedside rails, half-length (RR)

E0310 Bedside rails, full-length (NU, RR, UE)

CMS: 100-04,36,50.14

E0315 Bed accessory: board, table, or support device, any type

E0316 Safety enclosure frame/canopy for use with hospital bed, any type (RR)

E0325 Urinal; male, jug-type, any material (NU, RR, UE)

E0326 Urinal; female, jug-type, any material (NU, RR, UE)

E0328 Hospital bed, pediatric, manual, 360 degree side enclosures, top of headboard, footboard and side rails up to 24 in above the spring, includes mattress

E0329 Hospital bed, pediatric, electric or semi-electric, 360 degree side enclosures, top of headboard, footboard and side rails up to 24 in above the spring, includes mattress

E0350 Control unit for electronic bowel irrigation/evacuation system

E0352 Disposable pack (water reservoir bag, speculum, valving mechanism, and collection bag/box) for use with the electronic bowel irrigation/evacuation system

E0370 Air pressure elevator for heel

E0371 Nonpowered advanced pressure reducing overlay for mattress, standard mattress length and width (RR)

E0372 Powered air overlay for mattress, standard mattress length and width (RR)

E0373 Nonpowered advanced pressure reducing mattress (RR)

Oxygen and Related Respiratory Equipment

E0424 Stationary compressed gaseous oxygen system, rental; includes container, contents, regulator, flowmeter, humidifier, nebulizer, cannula or mask, and tubing Y ♿ (RR)

For the first claim filed for home oxygen equipment or therapy, submit a certificate of medical necessity that includes the oxygen flow rate, anticipated frequency and duration of oxygen therapy, and physician signature. Medicare accepts oxygen therapy as medically necessary in cases documenting any of the following: erythocythemia with a hematocrit greater than 56 percent; a P pulmonale on EKG; or dependent edema consistent with congestive heart failure.

CMS: 100-04,20,130.6; 100-04,20,30.6

E0425 Stationary compressed gas system, purchase; includes regulator, flowmeter, humidifier, nebulizer, cannula or mask, and tubing E

E0430 Portable gaseous oxygen system, purchase; includes regulator, flowmeter, humidifier, cannula or mask, and tubing E

E0431 Portable gaseous oxygen system, rental; includes portable container, regulator, flowmeter, humidifier, cannula or mask, and tubing Y ♿ (RR)

CMS: 100-04,20,130.6

E0433 Portable liquid oxygen system, rental; home liquefier used to fill portable liquid oxygen containers, includes portable containers, regulator, flowmeter, humidifier, cannula or mask and tubing, with or without supply reservoir and contents gauge Y ♿ (RR)

CMS: 100-04,20,130.6

E0434 Portable liquid oxygen system, rental; includes portable container, supply reservoir, humidifier, flowmeter, refill adaptor, contents gauge, cannula or mask, and tubing Y ♿ (RR)

CMS: 100-04,20,130.6

E0435 Portable liquid oxygen system, purchase; includes portable container, supply reservoir, flowmeter, humidifier, contents gauge, cannula or mask, tubing and refill adaptor E

E0439 Stationary liquid oxygen system, rental; includes container, contents, regulator, flowmeter, humidifier, nebulizer, cannula or mask, & tubing Y ♿ (RR)

CMS: 100-04,20,130.6

E0440 Stationary liquid oxygen system, purchase; includes use of reservoir, contents indicator, regulator, flowmeter, humidifier, nebulizer, cannula or mask, and tubing E

E0441 Stationary oxygen contents, gaseous, 1 month's supply = 1 unit Y ☑ ♿

CMS: 100-04,20,30.6

E0442 Stationary oxygen contents, liquid, 1 month's supply = 1 unit Y ☑ ♿

E0443 Portable oxygen contents, gaseous, 1 month's supply = 1 unit Y ☑ ♿

CMS: 100-04,20,30.6

E0444 Portable oxygen contents, liquid, 1 month's supply = 1 unit Y ☑ ♿

E0445 Oximeter device for measuring blood oxygen levels noninvasively N

E0446 Topical oxygen delivery system, not otherwise specified, includes all supplies and accessories A

E0447 Portable oxygen contents, liquid, 1 month's supply = 1 unit, prescribed amount at rest or nighttime exceeds 4 liters per minute (LPM) Y

E0455 Oxygen tent, excluding croup or pediatric tents Y

E0457 Chest shell (cuirass) E

E0459 Chest wrap E

E0462 Rocking bed, with or without side rails Y ♿ (RR)

E0465 Home ventilator, any type, used with invasive interface, (e.g., tracheostomy tube) Y ♿ (RR)

E0466 Home ventilator, any type, used with noninvasive interface, (e.g., mask, chest shell) Y ♿ (RR)

E0467 Home ventilator, multi-function respiratory device, also performs any or all of the additional functions of oxygen concentration, drug nebulization, aspiration, and cough stimulation, includes all accessories, components and supplies for all functions Y (RR)

● **E0468** Home ventilator, dual-function respiratory device, also performs additional function of cough stimulation, includes all accessories, components and supplies for all functions Y (RR)

AHA: 2Q,24

● **E0469** Lung expansion airway clearance, continuous high frequency oscillation, and nebulization device (RR)

E0470 Respiratory assist device, bi-level pressure capability, without backup rate feature, used with noninvasive interface, e.g., nasal or facial mask (intermittent assist device with continuous positive airway pressure device) Y ♿ (RR)

CMS: 100-03,240.4

E0471 Respiratory assist device, bi-level pressure capability, with back-up rate feature, used with noninvasive interface, e.g., nasal or facial mask (intermittent assist device with continuous positive airway pressure device) Y ♿ (RR)

CMS: 100-03,240.4

E0472 Respiratory assist device, bi-level pressure capability, with backup rate feature, used with invasive interface, e.g., tracheostomy tube (intermittent assist device with continuous positive airway pressure device) Y ♿ (RR)

CMS: 100-03,240.4

E0480 Percussor, electric or pneumatic, home model Y ♿ (RR)

E0481 Intrapulmonary percussive ventilation system and related accessories E

E0482 Cough stimulating device, alternating positive and negative airway pressure Y ♿ (RR)

E0483 High frequency chest wall oscillation system, with full anterior and/or posterior thoracic region receiving simultaneous external oscillation, includes all accessories and supplies, each Y ☑ ♿ (RR)

AHA: 4Q,22

E0484 Oscillatory positive expiratory pressure device, nonelectric, any type, each Y ☑ ♿ (NU, RR, UE)

E0485 Oral device/appliance used to reduce upper airway collapsibility, adjustable or nonadjustable, prefabricated, includes fitting and adjustment Y ♿ (NU, RR, UE)

E0486 Oral device/appliance used to reduce upper airway collapsibility, adjustable or nonadjustable, custom fabricated, includes fitting and adjustment Y ♿ (NU, RR, UE)

E0487 Spirometer, electronic, includes all accessories N

Oral Devices

E0490 Power source and control electronics unit for oral device/appliance for neuromuscular electrical stimulation of the tongue muscle, controlled by hardware remote E (RR)

AHA: 4Q,23

E0491 Oral device/appliance for neuromuscular electrical stimulation of the tongue muscle, used in conjunction with the power source and control electronics unit, controlled by hardware remote, 90-day supply E1
AHA: 4Q,23

E0492 Power source and control electronics unit for oral device/appliance for neuromuscular electrical stimulation of the tongue muscle, controlled by phone application E1

E0493 Oral device/appliance for neuromuscular electrical stimulation of the tongue muscle, used in conjunction with the power source and control electronics unit, controlled by phone application, 90-day supply E1

IPPB Machines

E0500 IPPB machine, all types, with built-in nebulization; manual or automatic valves; internal or external power source Y ♿ (RR)

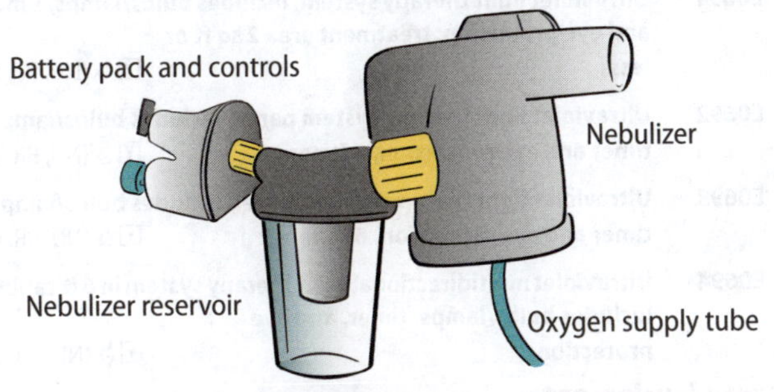

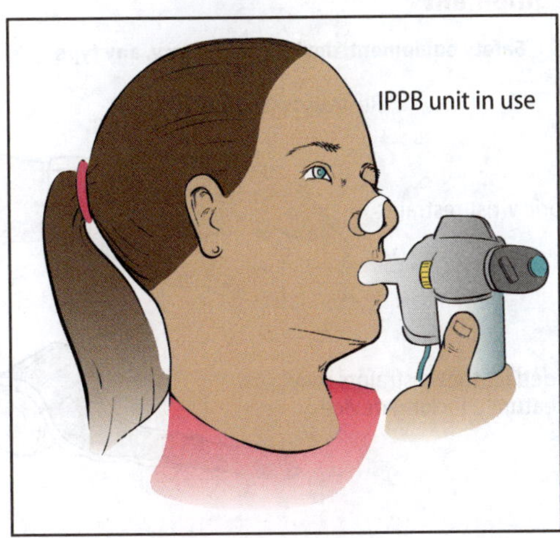

Obstructive Sleep Apnea Treatment

E0530 Electronic positional obstructive sleep apnea treatment, with sensor, includes all components and accessories, any type Y (RR)

Humidifiers/Compressors/Nebulizers

E0550 Humidifier, durable for extensive supplemental humidification during IPPB treatments or oxygen delivery Y ♿ (RR)

E0555 Humidifier, durable, glass or autoclavable plastic bottle type, for use with regulator or flowmeter Y

E0560 Humidifier, durable for supplemental humidification during IPPB treatment or oxygen delivery Y ♿ (NU, RR, UE)

E0561 Humidifier, nonheated, used with positive airway pressure device Y ♿ (NU, RR, UE)
CMS: 100-03,240.4; 100-04,36,50.14

E0562 Humidifier, heated, used with positive airway pressure device Y ♿ (NU, RR, UE)
CMS: 100-03,240.4; 100-04,36,50.14

E0565 Compressor, air power source for equipment which is not self-contained or cylinder driven Y ♿ (RR)

E0570 Nebulizer, with compressor Y ♿ (RR)

E0572 Aerosol compressor, adjustable pressure, light duty for intermittent use Y ♿ (RR)

E0574 Ultrasonic/electronic aerosol generator with small volume nebulizer Y ♿ (RR)

E0575 Nebulizer, ultrasonic, large volume Y ♿ (RR)

E0580 Nebulizer, durable, glass or autoclavable plastic, bottle type, for use with regulator or flowmeter Y ♿ (NU, RR, UE)

E0585 Nebulizer, with compressor and heater Y ♿ (RR)

Pumps and Vaporizers

E0600 Respiratory suction pump, home model, portable or stationary, electric Y ♿ (RR)

E0601 Continuous positive airway pressure (CPAP) device Y ♿ (RR)
CMS: 100-03,240.4

E0602 Breast pump, manual, any type M Y ♿ (NU, RR, UE)

E0603 Breast pump, electric (AC and/or DC), any type M N

E0604 Breast pump, hospital grade, electric (AC and/or DC), any type M A

E0605 Vaporizer, room type Y ♿ (NU, RR, UE)

E0606 Postural drainage board Y ♿ (RR)

Monitoring Devices

E0607 Home blood glucose monitor Y ♿ (NU, RR, UE)
Medicare covers home blood testing devices for diabetic patients when the devices are prescribed by the patients' physicians. Many commercial payers provide this coverage to noninsulin dependent diabetics as well.
CMS: 100-04,23,60.1

E0610 Pacemaker monitor, self-contained, (checks battery depletion, includes audible and visible check systems) Y ♿ (NU, RR, UE)

E0615 Pacemaker monitor, self-contained, checks battery depletion and other pacemaker components, includes digital/visible check systems Y ♿ (NU, RR, UE)

E0616 Implantable cardiac event recorder with memory, activator, and programmer N

E0617 External defibrillator with integrated electrocardiogram analysis Y ♿ (RR)

E0618 Apnea monitor, without recording feature Y ♿ (RR)

E0619 Apnea monitor, with recording feature Y ♿ (RR)

E0620 Skin piercing device for collection of capillary blood, laser, each Y ♿ (RR)

Patient Lifts

E0621 Sling or seat, patient lift, canvas or nylon Y ♿ (NU, RR, UE)

E0625 Patient lift, bathroom or toilet, not otherwise classified E1

E0627 Seat lift mechanism, electric, any type Y ♿ (NU, RR, UE)
CMS: 100-04,20,100; 100-04,20,130.2; 100-04,20,130.3; 100-04,20,130.4; 100-04,20,130.5

E0629 Seat lift mechanism, nonelectric, any type Y ♿ (NU, RR, UE)
CMS: 100-04,20,100; 100-04,20,130.2; 100-04,20,130.3; 100-04,20,130.4; 100-04,20,130.5

E0630 Patient lift, hydraulic or mechanical, includes any seat, sling, strap(s), or pad(s) Y ♿ (RR)

Durable Medical Equipment E0491 — E0630

E0635 Patient lift, electric, with seat or sling Y ♿ (RR)

E0636 Multipositional patient support system, with integrated lift, patient accessible controls Y ♿ (RR)

E0637 Combination sit-to-stand frame/table system, any size including pediatric, with seat lift feature, with or without wheels E

E0638 Standing frame/table system, one position (e.g., upright, supine or prone stander), any size including pediatric, with or without wheels E

E0639 Patient lift, moveable from room to room with disassembly and reassembly, includes all components/accessories E ♿ (RR)

E0640 Patient lift, fixed system, includes all components/accessories E ♿ (RR)

E0641 Standing frame/table system, multi-position (e.g., 3-way stander), any size including pediatric, with or without wheels E

E0642 Standing frame/table system, mobile (dynamic stander), any size including pediatric E

Compression Devices

E0650 Pneumatic compressor, nonsegmental home model Y ♿ (NU, RR, UE)

E0651 Pneumatic compressor, segmental home model without calibrated gradient pressure Y ♿ (NU, RR, UE)

E0652 Pneumatic compressor, segmental home model with calibrated gradient pressure Y ♿ (NU, RR, UE)

E0655 Nonsegmental pneumatic appliance for use with pneumatic compressor, half arm Y ♿ (NU, RR, UE)

E0656 Segmental pneumatic appliance for use with pneumatic compressor, trunk Y ♿ (RR)

E0657 Segmental pneumatic appliance for use with pneumatic compressor, chest Y ♿ (RR)

E0660 Nonsegmental pneumatic appliance for use with pneumatic compressor, full leg Y ♿ (NU, RR, UE)

E0665 Nonsegmental pneumatic appliance for use with pneumatic compressor, full arm Y ♿ (NU, RR, UE)

E0666 Nonsegmental pneumatic appliance for use with pneumatic compressor, half leg Y ♿ (NU, RR, UE)

E0667 Segmental pneumatic appliance for use with pneumatic compressor, full leg Y ♿ (NU, RR, UE)

E0668 Segmental pneumatic appliance for use with pneumatic compressor, full arm Y ♿ (NU, RR, UE)

E0669 Segmental pneumatic appliance for use with pneumatic compressor, half leg Y ♿ (NU, RR, UE)

E0670 Segmental pneumatic appliance for use with pneumatic compressor, integrated, two full legs and trunk Y ♿ (NU, RR, UE)

E0671 Segmental gradient pressure pneumatic appliance, full leg Y ♿ (NU, RR, UE)

E0672 Segmental gradient pressure pneumatic appliance, full arm Y ♿ (NU, RR, UE)

E0673 Segmental gradient pressure pneumatic appliance, half leg Y ♿ (NU, RR, UE)

E0675 Pneumatic compression device, high pressure, rapid inflation/deflation cycle, for arterial insufficiency (unilateral or bilateral system) Y ♿ (RR)

E0676 Intermittent limb compression device (includes all accessories), not otherwise specified Y

E0677 Nonpneumatic sequential compression garment, trunk Y (RR)
AHA: 2Q,23

E0678 Nonpneumatic sequential compression garment, full leg Y (RR)

E0679 Nonpneumatic sequential compression garment, half leg Y (RR)

E0680 Nonpneumatic compression controller with sequential calibrated gradient pressure Y (RR)

E0681 Nonpneumatic compression controller without calibrated gradient pressure Y (RR)

E0682 Nonpneumatic sequential compression garment, full arm Y (RR)

● **E0683** Nonpneumatic, nonsequential, peristaltic wave compression pump (RR)

Ultraviolet Light

E0691 Ultraviolet light therapy system, includes bulbs/lamps, timer and eye protection; treatment area 2 sq ft or less Y ♿ (NU, RR, UE)

E0692 Ultraviolet light therapy system panel, includes bulbs/lamps, timer and eye protection, 4 ft panel Y ♿ (NU, RR, UE)

E0693 Ultraviolet light therapy system panel, includes bulbs/lamps, timer and eye protection, 6 ft panel Y ♿ (NU, RR, UE)

E0694 Ultraviolet multidirectional light therapy system in 6 ft cabinet, includes bulbs/lamps, timer, and eye protection Y ♿ (NU, RR, UE)

Safety Equipment

E0700 Safety equipment, device or accessory, any type E

Restraints (E0710)

Fabric wrist restraint

Padded leather restraints may feature a locking device

Body restraint

Fabric gait belt for assistance in walking (E0700)

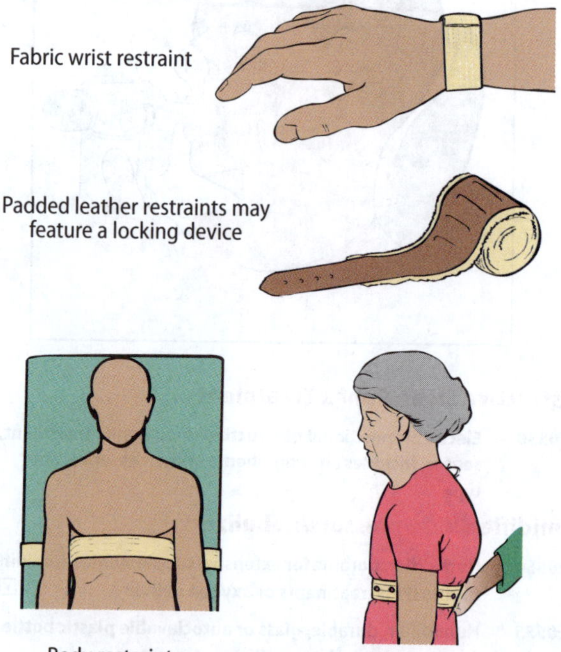

E0705 Transfer device, any type, each B ☑ ♿ (NU, RR, UE)

E0710 Restraints, any type (body, chest, wrist, or ankle) E

E0711 Upper extremity medical tubing/lines enclosure or covering device, restricts elbow range of motion E1
AHA: 2Q,23

Kegel Devices

● E0715 Intravaginal device intended to strengthen pelvic floor muscles during Kegel exercises

● E0716 Supplies and accessories for intravaginal device intended to strengthen pelvic floor muscles during Kegel exercises

Nerve Stimulators and Devices

E0720 Transcutaneous electrical nerve stimulation (TENS) device, two-lead, localized stimulation Y & (NU)
A Certificate of Medical Necessity is required for the purchase of a TENS. It is not required for rentals.
CMS: 100-03,10.2; 100-03,160.27; 100-03,160.7.1; 100-04,20,30.1.2

● E0721 Transcutaneous electrical nerve stimulator for nerves in the auricular region

E0730 Transcutaneous electrical nerve stimulation (TENS) device, four or more leads, for multiple nerve stimulation Y & (NU)
A Certificate of Medical Necessity is required for the purchase of a TENS. It is not required for rentals.
CMS: 100-03,10.2; 100-03,160.27; 100-03,160.7.1; 100-04,20,30.1.2

E0731 Form-fitting conductive garment for delivery of TENS or NMES (with conductive fibers separated from the patient's skin by layers of fabric) Y & (NU)
CMS: 100-03,10.2; 100-03,160.13

E0732 Cranial electrotherapy stimulation (CES) system, any type Y (RR)

E0733 Transcutaneous electrical nerve stimulator for electrical stimulation of the trigeminal nerve Y (RR)

E0734 External upper limb tremor stimulator of the peripheral nerves of the wrist Y (RR)

E0735 Noninvasive vagus nerve stimulator Y (RR)

● E0736 Transcutaneous tibial nerve stimulator A (RR)
AHA: 2Q,24

● E0737 Transcutaneous tibial nerve stimulator, controlled by phone application

● E0738 Upper extremity rehabilitation system providing active assistance to facilitate muscle re-education, includes microprocessor, all components and accessories A (RR)
AHA: 2Q,24

▲ E0739 Rehabilitation system with interactive interface providing active assistance in rehabilitation therapy, includes all components and accessories, motors, microprocessors, sensors A (RR)
AHA: 2Q,24

E0740 Nonimplanted pelvic floor electrical stimulator, complete system Y & (RR)

● E0743 External lower extremity nerve stimulator for restless legs syndrome, each (RR)

E0744 Neuromuscular stimulator for scoliosis Y & (RR)

E0745 Neuromuscular stimulator, electronic shock unit Y & (RR)

E0746 Electromyography (EMG), biofeedback device N
Biofeedback therapy is covered by Medicare only for re-education of specific muscles or for treatment of incapacitating muscle spasm or weakness.

E0747 Osteogenesis stimulator, electrical, noninvasive, other than spinal applications Y (NU, RR, UE)
Medicare covers noninvasive osteogenic stimulation for nonunion of long bone fractures, failed fusion, or congenital pseudoarthroses.

E0748 Osteogenesis stimulator, electrical, noninvasive, spinal applications Y (NU, RR, UE)
Medicare covers noninvasive osteogenic stimulation as an adjunct to spinal fusion surgery for patients at high risk of pseudoarthroses due to previously failed spinal fusion, or for those undergoing fusion of three or more vertebrae.

E0749 Osteogenesis stimulator, electrical, surgically implanted N (RR)
Medicare covers invasive osteogenic stimulation for nonunion of long bone fractures or as an adjunct to spinal fusion surgery for patients at high risk of pseudoarthroses due to previously failed spinal fusion, or for those undergoing fusion of three or more vertebrae.
CMS: 100-04,4,190

E0755 Electronic salivary reflex stimulator (intraoral/noninvasive) E1

E0760 Osteogenesis stimulator, low intensity ultrasound, noninvasive Y (NU, RR, UE)
CMS: 100-04,32,110.5

E0761 Nonthermal pulsed high frequency radiowaves, high peak power electromagnetic energy treatment device E1

E0762 Transcutaneous electrical joint stimulation device system, includes all accessories B & (RR)

E0764 Functional neuromuscular stimulation, transcutaneous stimulation of sequential muscle groups of ambulation with computer control, used for walking by spinal cord injured, entire system, after completion of training program Y (RR)

E0765 FDA approved nerve stimulator, with replaceable batteries, for treatment of nausea and vomiting Y & (NU, RR, UE)

E0766 Electrical stimulation device used for cancer treatment, includes all accessories, any type Y (RR)

● E0767 Intrabuccal, systemic delivery of amplitude-modulated, radiofrequency electromagnetic field device, for cancer treatment, includes all accessories

E0769 Electrical stimulation or electromagnetic wound treatment device, not otherwise classified B
CMS: 100-04,32,11.1

E0770 Functional electrical stimulator, transcutaneous stimulation of nerve and/or muscle groups, any type, complete system, not otherwise specified Y

Infusion Supplies

E0776 IV pole Y & (NU, RR, UE)

E0779 Ambulatory infusion pump, mechanical, reusable, for infusion 8 hours or greater Y & (RR)

E0780 Ambulatory infusion pump, mechanical, reusable, for infusion less than 8 hours Y & (NU)

E0781 Ambulatory infusion pump, single or multiple channels, electric or battery operated, with administrative equipment, worn by patient Y & (RR)

E0782 Infusion pump, implantable, nonprogrammable (includes all components, e.g., pump, catheter, connectors, etc.) N (NU, RR, UE)
CMS: 100-04,4,190

E0783 Infusion pump system, implantable, programmable (includes all components, e.g., pump, catheter, connectors, etc.) N (NU, RR, UE)
CMS: 100-04,4,190

E0784 External ambulatory infusion pump, insulin Y & (RR)
Covered by some commercial payers with preauthorization.

E0785 Implantable intraspinal (epidural/intrathecal) catheter used with implantable infusion pump, replacement N & (KF)
CMS: 100-04,4,190

E0786 Implantable programmable infusion pump, replacement (excludes implantable intraspinal catheter) N (NU, RR, UE)

E0787 External ambulatory infusion pump, insulin, dosage rate adjustment using therapeutic continuous glucose sensing E

E0791 Parenteral infusion pump, stationary, single, or multichannel Y ♿ (RR)

Traction Equipment

E0830 Ambulatory traction device, all types, each N

E0840 Traction frame, attached to headboard, cervical traction Y ♿ (NU, RR, UE)

E0849 Traction equipment, cervical, free-standing stand/frame, pneumatic, applying traction force to other than mandible Y ♿ (RR)

E0850 Traction stand, freestanding, cervical traction Y ♿ (NU, RR, UE)

E0855 Cervical traction equipment not requiring additional stand or frame Y ♿ (RR)

E0856 Cervical traction device, with inflatable air bladder(s) Y ♿ (RR)

E0860 Traction equipment, overdoor, cervical Y ♿ (NU, RR, UE)

E0870 Traction frame, attached to footboard, extremity traction (e.g., Buck's) Y ♿ (NU, RR, UE)

E0890 Traction frame, attached to footboard, pelvic traction Y ♿ (NU, RR, UE)

E0900 Traction stand, freestanding, pelvic traction (e.g., Buck's) Y ♿ (NU, RR, UE)

Orthopedic Devices

E0910 Trapeze bars, also known as Patient Helper, attached to bed, with grab bar Y ♿ (RR)

E0911 Trapeze bar, heavy-duty, for patient weight capacity greater than 250 pounds, attached to bed, with grab bar Y ♿ (RR)

E0912 Trapeze bar, heavy-duty, for patient weight capacity greater than 250 pounds, freestanding, complete with grab bar Y ♿ (RR)

E0920 Fracture frame, attached to bed, includes weights Y ♿ (RR)

E0930 Fracture frame, freestanding, includes weights Y ♿ (RR)

E0935 Continuous passive motion exercise device for use on knee only Y ♿ (RR)

E0936 Continuous passive motion exercise device for use other than knee E

E0940 Trapeze bar, freestanding, complete with grab bar Y ♿ (RR)

E0941 Gravity assisted traction device, any type Y ♿ (RR)

E0942 Cervical head harness/halter Y ♿ (NU, RR, UE)

E0944 Pelvic belt/harness/boot Y ♿ (NU, RR, UE)

E0945 Extremity belt/harness Y ♿ (NU, RR, UE)

E0946 Fracture, frame, dual with cross bars, attached to bed, (e.g., Balkan, four-poster) Y ♿ (RR)

E0947 Fracture frame, attachments for complex pelvic traction Y ♿ (NU, RR, UE)

E0948 Fracture frame, attachments for complex cervical traction Y ♿ (NU, RR, UE)

Wheelchair Accessories

E0950 Wheelchair accessory, tray, each Y ☑ ♿ (NU, RR, UE)

E0951 Heel loop/holder, any type, with or without ankle strap, each Y ☑ ♿ (NU, RR, UE)

E0952 Toe loop/holder, any type, each Y ☑ ♿ (NU, RR, UE)

E0953 Wheelchair accessory, lateral thigh or knee support, any type including fixed mounting hardware, each Y ♿ (NU, RR, UE)

E0954 Wheelchair accessory, foot box, any type, includes attachment and mounting hardware, each foot Y ♿ (NU, RR, UE)

E0955 Wheelchair accessory, headrest, cushioned, any type, including fixed mounting hardware, each Y ☑ ♿ (RR)

E0956 Wheelchair accessory, lateral trunk or hip support, any type, including fixed mounting hardware, each Y ☑ ♿ (NU, RR, UE)

E0957 Wheelchair accessory, medial thigh support, any type, including fixed mounting hardware, each Y ☑ ♿ (NU, RR, UE)

E0958 Manual wheelchair accessory, one-arm drive attachment, each Y ☑ ♿ (RR)

E0959 Manual wheelchair accessory, adapter for amputee, each B ☑ ♿ (NU, RR, UE)

E0960 Wheelchair accessory, shoulder harness/straps or chest strap, including any type mounting hardware Y ♿ (NU, RR, UE)

E0961 Manual wheelchair accessory, wheel lock brake extension (handle), each B ☑ ♿ (NU, RR, UE)

E0966 Manual wheelchair accessory, headrest extension, each B ☑ ♿ (NU, RR, UE)

E0967 Manual wheelchair accessory, hand rim with projections, any type, replacement only, each Y ☑ ♿ (NU, RR, UE)

E0968 Commode seat, wheelchair Y ♿ (RR)

E0969 Narrowing device, wheelchair Y ♿ (NU, RR, UE)

E0970 No. 2 footplates, except for elevating legrest E

See code(s): K0037, K0042

E0971 Manual wheelchair accessory, antitipping device, each B ☑ ♿ (NU, RR, UE)

E0973 Wheelchair accessory, adjustable height, detachable armrest, complete assembly, each B ☑ ♿ (NU, RR, UE)

E0974 Manual wheelchair accessory, antirollback device, each B ☑ ♿ (NU, RR, UE)

E0978 Wheelchair accessory, positioning belt/safety belt/pelvic strap, each B ☑ ♿ (NU, RR, UE)

E0980 Safety vest, wheelchair Y ♿ (NU, RR, UE)

E0981 Wheelchair accessory, seat upholstery, replacement only, each Y ☑ ♿ (NU, RR, UE)

E0982 Wheelchair accessory, back upholstery, replacement only, each Y ☑ ♿ (NU, RR, UE)

E0983 Manual wheelchair accessory, power add-on to convert manual wheelchair to motorized wheelchair, joystick control Y ♿ (RR)

E0984 Manual wheelchair accessory, power add-on to convert manual wheelchair to motorized wheelchair, tiller control Y ♿ (RR)

E0985 Wheelchair accessory, seat lift mechanism Y ♿ (RR)

E0986 Manual wheelchair accessory, push-rim activated power assist system Y ☑ ♿ (RR)

E0988 Manual wheelchair accessory, lever-activated, wheel drive, pair Y ☑ ♿ (RR)

E0990 Wheelchair accessory, elevating legrest, complete assembly, each B ☑ ♿ (NU, RR, UE)

E0992 Manual wheelchair accessory, solid seat insert B ♿ (NU, RR, UE)

E0994 Armrest, each Y ☑ ♿ (NU, RR, UE)

E0995 Wheelchair accessory, calf rest/pad, replacement only, each (NU, RR, UE)

E1002 Wheelchair accessory, power seating system, tilt only (RR)

E1003 Wheelchair accessory, power seating system, recline only, without shear reduction (RR)

E1004 Wheelchair accessory, power seating system, recline only, with mechanical shear reduction (RR)

E1005 Wheelchair accessory, power seating system, recline only, with power shear reduction (RR)

E1006 Wheelchair accessory, power seating system, combination tilt and recline, without shear reduction (RR)

E1007 Wheelchair accessory, power seating system, combination tilt and recline, with mechanical shear reduction (RR)

E1008 Wheelchair accessory, power seating system, combination tilt and recline, with power shear reduction (RR)

E1009 Wheelchair accessory, addition to power seating system, mechanically linked leg elevation system, including pushrod and legrest, each (NU, RR, UE)

E1010 Wheelchair accessory, addition to power seating system, power leg elevation system, including legrest, pair (RR)

E1011 Modification to pediatric size wheelchair, width adjustment package (not to be dispensed with initial chair) (NU, RR, UE)

E1012 Wheelchair accessory, addition to power seating system, center mount power elevating leg rest/platform, complete system, any type, each (RR)

E1014 Reclining back, addition to pediatric size wheelchair (RR)

E1015 Shock absorber for manual wheelchair, each (NU, RR, UE)

E1016 Shock absorber for power wheelchair, each (NU, RR, UE)

E1017 Heavy-duty shock absorber for heavy-duty or extra heavy-duty manual wheelchair, each (NU, RR, UE)

E1018 Heavy-duty shock absorber for heavy-duty or extra heavy-duty power wheelchair, each (NU, RR, UE)

E1020 Residual limb support system for wheelchair, any type (RR)

E1028 Wheelchair accessory, manual swingaway, retractable or removable mounting hardware for joystick, other control interface or positioning accessory (RR)

E1029 Wheelchair accessory, ventilator tray, fixed (RR)

E1030 Wheelchair accessory, ventilator tray, gimbaled (RR)

E1031 Rollabout chair, any and all types with castors 5 in or greater (RR)

E1035 Multi-positional patient transfer system, with integrated seat, operated by care giver, patient weight capacity up to and including 300 lbs (RR)
CMS: 100-02,15,110

E1036 Multi-positional patient transfer system, extra-wide, with integrated seat, operated by caregiver, patient weight capacity greater than 300 lbs (RR)

E1037 Transport chair, pediatric size (RR)

E1038 Transport chair, adult size, patient weight capacity up to and including 300 pounds (RR)

E1039 Transport chair, adult size, heavy-duty, patient weight capacity greater than 300 pounds (RR)

Wheelchairs

E1050 Fully-reclining wheelchair, fixed full-length arms, swing-away detachable elevating legrests (RR)

E1060 Fully-reclining wheelchair, detachable arms, desk or full-length, swing-away detachable elevating legrests (RR)

E1070 Fully-reclining wheelchair, detachable arms (desk or full-length) swing-away detachable footrest (RR)

E1083 Hemi-wheelchair, fixed full-length arms, swing-away detachable elevating legrest (RR)

E1084 Hemi-wheelchair, detachable arms desk or full-length arms, swing-away detachable elevating legrests (RR)

E1085 Hemi-wheelchair, fixed full-length arms, swing-away detachable footrests
See code(s): K0002

E1086 Hemi-wheelchair, detachable arms, desk or full-length, swing-away detachable footrests
See code(s): K0002

E1087 High strength lightweight wheelchair, fixed full-length arms, swing-away detachable elevating legrests (RR)

E1088 High strength lightweight wheelchair, detachable arms desk or full-length, swing-away detachable elevating legrests (RR)

E1089 High-strength lightweight wheelchair, fixed-length arms, swing-away detachable footrest
See code(s): K0004

E1090 High-strength lightweight wheelchair, detachable arms, desk or full-length, swing-away detachable footrests
See code(s): K0004

E1092 Wide heavy-duty wheel chair, detachable arms (desk or full-length), swing-away detachable elevating legrests (RR)

E1093 Wide heavy-duty wheelchair, detachable arms, desk or full-length arms, swing-away detachable footrests (RR)

E1100 Semi-reclining wheelchair, fixed full-length arms, swing-away detachable elevating legrests (RR)

E1110 Semi-reclining wheelchair, detachable arms (desk or full-length) elevating legrest (RR)

E1130 Standard wheelchair, fixed full-length arms, fixed or swing-away detachable footrests
See code(s): K0001

E1140 Wheelchair, detachable arms, desk or full-length, swing-away detachable footrests
See code(s): K0001

E1150 Wheelchair, detachable arms, desk or full-length swing-away detachable elevating legrests (RR)

E1160 Wheelchair, fixed full-length arms, swing-away detachable elevating legrests (RR)

E1161 Manual adult size wheelchair, includes tilt in space (RR)

E1170 Amputee wheelchair, fixed full-length arms, swing-away detachable elevating legrests (RR)

E1171 Amputee wheelchair, fixed full-length arms, without footrests or legrest (RR)

E1172 Amputee wheelchair, detachable arms (desk or full-length) without footrests or legrest (RR)

E1180 Amputee wheelchair, detachable arms (desk or full-length) swing-away detachable footrests (RR)

E1190 Amputee wheelchair, detachable arms (desk or full-length) swing-away detachable elevating legrests Y ♿ (RR)

E1195 Heavy-duty wheelchair, fixed full-length arms, swing-away detachable elevating legrests Y ♿ (RR)

E1200 Amputee wheelchair, fixed full-length arms, swing-away detachable footrest Y ♿ (RR)

E1220 Wheelchair; specially sized or constructed, (indicate brand name, model number, if any) and justification Y

E1221 Wheelchair with fixed arm, footrests Y ♿ (RR)

E1222 Wheelchair with fixed arm, elevating legrests Y ♿ (RR)

E1223 Wheelchair with detachable arms, footrests Y ♿ (RR)

E1224 Wheelchair with detachable arms, elevating legrests Y ♿ (RR)

E1225 Wheelchair accessory, manual semi-reclining back, (recline greater than 15 degrees, but less than 80 degrees), each Y ☑ ♿ (RR)

E1226 Wheelchair accessory, manual fully reclining back, (recline greater than 80 degrees), each B ☑ ♿ (NU, RR, UE)

See also K0028

E1227 Special height arms for wheelchair Y ♿ (NU, RR, UE)

E1228 Special back height for wheelchair Y ♿ (RR)

E1229 Wheelchair, pediatric size, not otherwise specified Y

E1230 Power operated vehicle (three- or four-wheel nonhighway), specify brand name and model number Y ♿ (NU, RR, UE)

Prior authorization is required by Medicare for this item.

E1231 Wheelchair, pediatric size, tilt-in-space, rigid, adjustable, with seating system Y ♿ (NU, RR, UE)

E1232 Wheelchair, pediatric size, tilt-in-space, folding, adjustable, with seating system Y ♿ (RR)

E1233 Wheelchair, pediatric size, tilt-in-space, rigid, adjustable, without seating system Y ♿ (RR)

E1234 Wheelchair, pediatric size, tilt-in-space, folding, adjustable, without seating system Y ♿ (RR)

E1235 Wheelchair, pediatric size, rigid, adjustable, with seating system Y ♿ (RR)

E1236 Wheelchair, pediatric size, folding, adjustable, with seating system Y ♿ (RR)

E1237 Wheelchair, pediatric size, rigid, adjustable, without seating system Y ♿ (RR)

E1238 Wheelchair, pediatric size, folding, adjustable, without seating system Y ♿ (RR)

E1239 Power wheelchair, pediatric size, not otherwise specified Y

E1240 Lightweight wheelchair, detachable arms, (desk or full-length) swing-away detachable, elevating legrest Y ♿ (RR)

E1250 Lightweight wheelchair, fixed full-length arms, swing-away detachable footrest E1

See code(s): K0003

E1260 Lightweight wheelchair, detachable arms (desk or full-length) swing-away detachable footrest E1

See code(s): K0003

E1270 Lightweight wheelchair, fixed full-length arms, swing-away detachable elevating legrests Y ♿ (RR)

E1280 Heavy-duty wheelchair, detachable arms (desk or full-length) elevating legrests Y ♿ (RR)

E1285 Heavy-duty wheelchair, fixed full-length arms, swing-away detachable footrest E1

See code(s): K0006

E1290 Heavy-duty wheelchair, detachable arms (desk or full-length) swing-away detachable footrest E1

See code(s): K0006

E1295 Heavy-duty wheelchair, fixed full-length arms, elevating legrest Y ♿ (RR)

E1296 Special wheelchair seat height from floor Y ♿ (NU, RR, UE)

E1297 Special wheelchair seat depth, by upholstery Y ♿ (NU, RR, UE)

E1298 Special wheelchair seat depth and/or width, by construction Y ♿ (NU, RR, UE)

Whirlpool - Equipment

E1300 Whirlpool, portable (overtub type) E1

E1301 Whirlpool tub, walk-in, portable E1

E1310 Whirlpool, nonportable (built-in type) Y ♿ (NU, RR, UE)

Additional Oxygen Related Equipment

E1352 Oxygen accessory, flow regulator capable of positive inspiratory pressure Y

E1353 Regulator Y ♿

E1354 Oxygen accessory, wheeled cart for portable cylinder or portable concentrator, any type, replacement only, each Y ☑

E1355 Stand/rack Y ♿

E1356 Oxygen accessory, battery pack/cartridge for portable concentrator, any type, replacement only, each Y ☑

E1357 Oxygen accessory, battery charger for portable concentrator, any type, replacement only, each Y ☑

E1358 Oxygen accessory, DC power adapter for portable concentrator, any type, replacement only, each Y ☑

E1372 Immersion external heater for nebulizer Y ♿ (NU, RR, UE)

E1390 Oxygen concentrator, single delivery port, capable of delivering 85 percent or greater oxygen concentration at the prescribed flow rate Y ♿ (RR)

CMS: 100-04,20,130.6

E1391 Oxygen concentrator, dual delivery port, capable of delivering 85 percent or greater oxygen concentration at the prescribed flow rate, each Y ☑ ♿ (RR)

CMS: 100-04,20,130.6

E1392 Portable oxygen concentrator, rental Y ♿ (RR)

CMS: 100-04,20,130.6

E1399 Durable medical equipment, miscellaneous Y

CMS: 100-04,20,30.9; 100-04,32,110.5

E1405 Oxygen and water vapor enriching system with heated delivery Y ♿ (RR)

CMS: 100-04,20,20; 100-04,20,20.4; 100-04,23,60.1

E1406 Oxygen and water vapor enriching system without heated delivery Y ♿ (RR)

CMS: 100-04,20,20; 100-04,20,20.4; 100-04,23,60.1

Artificial Kidney Machines and Accessories

E1500 Centrifuge, for dialysis A ⊘

E1510 Kidney, dialysate delivery system kidney machine, pump recirculating, air removal system, flowrate meter, power off, heater and temperature control with alarm, IV poles, pressure gauge, concentrate container A ⊘

E1520 Heparin infusion pump for hemodialysis A ⊘

Special Coverage Instructions | Noncovered by Medicare | Carrier Discretion | ☑ Quantity Alert | ● New Code | ○ Recycled/Reinstated | ▲ Revised Code

 A2-Z3 ASC | A-Y OPPS | CMS: IOM | AHA: Coding Clinic | ♿ DMEPOS Paid | ⊘ SNF Excluded | A Age | M Maternity

E1530 Air bubble detector for hemodialysis, each, replacement A ☑ ⊘

E1540 Pressure alarm for hemodialysis, each, replacement A ☑ ⊘

E1550 Bath conductivity meter for hemodialysis, each A ☑ ⊘

E1560 Blood leak detector for hemodialysis, each, replacement A ☑ ⊘

E1570 Adjustable chair, for ESRD patients A ⊘

E1575 Transducer protectors/fluid barriers, for hemodialysis, any size, per 10 A ☑ ⊘

E1580 Unipuncture control system for hemodialysis A ⊘

E1590 Hemodialysis machine A ⊘

E1592 Automatic intermittent peritoneal dialysis system A ⊘

E1594 Cycler dialysis machine for peritoneal dialysis A ⊘

E1600 Delivery and/or installation charges for hemodialysis equipment A ⊘

E1610 Reverse osmosis water purification system, for hemodialysis A ⊘

E1615 Deionizer water purification system, for hemodialysis A ⊘

E1620 Blood pump for hemodialysis, replacement A ⊘

E1625 Water softening system, for hemodialysis A ⊘

E1629 Tablo hemodialysis system for the billable dialysis service A

E1630 Reciprocating peritoneal dialysis system A ⊘

E1632 Wearable artificial kidney, each A ☑ ⊘

E1634 Peritoneal dialysis clamps, each B ☑

E1635 Compact (portable) travel hemodialyzer system A ⊘

E1636 Sorbent cartridges, for hemodialysis, per 10 A ☑ ⊘

E1637 Hemostats, each A ☑ ⊘

E1639 Scale, each A ☑ ⊘

E1699 Dialysis equipment, not otherwise specified A ⊘
CMS: 100-04,8,20

Jaw Motion Rehabilitation System and Accessories

E1700 Jaw motion rehabilitation system Y ♿ (RR)
Medicare jurisdiction: local contractor.

E1701 Replacement cushions for jaw motion rehabilitation system, package of 6 Y ☑ ♿
Medicare jurisdiction: local contractor.

E1702 Replacement measuring scales for jaw motion rehabilitation system, package of 200 Y ☑ ♿
Medicare jurisdiction: local contractor.

Flexion/Extension Device

▲ **E1800** Dynamic adjustable elbow extension and flexion device, includes soft interface material Y ♿ (RR)

E1801 Static progressive stretch elbow device, extension and/or flexion, with or without range of motion adjustment, includes all components and accessories Y ♿ (RR)

E1802 Dynamic adjustable forearm pronation/supination device, includes soft interface material Y ♿ (RR)

● **E1803** Dynamic adjustable elbow extension only device, includes soft interface material

● **E1804** Dynamic adjustable elbow flexion only device, includes soft interface material

▲ **E1805** Dynamic adjustable wrist extension and flexion device, includes soft interface material Y ♿ (RR)

E1806 Static progressive stretch wrist device, flexion and/or extension, with or without range of motion adjustment, includes all components and accessories Y ♿ (RR)

● **E1807** Dynamic adjustable wrist extension only device, includes soft interface material

● **E1808** Dynamic adjustable wrist flexion only device, includes soft interface material

▲ **E1810** Dynamic adjustable knee extension and flexion device, includes soft interface material Y ♿ (RR)

E1811 Static progressive stretch knee device, extension and/or flexion, with or without range of motion adjustment, includes all components and accessories Y ♿ (RR)

E1812 Dynamic knee, extension/flexion device with active resistance control Y ♿ (RR)

● **E1813** Dynamic adjustable knee extension only device, includes soft interface material

● **E1814** Dynamic adjustable knee flexion only device, includes soft interface material

▲ **E1815** Dynamic adjustable ankle extension and flexion device, includes soft interface material Y ♿ (RR)

E1816 Static progressive stretch ankle device, flexion and/or extension, with or without range of motion adjustment, includes all components and accessories Y ♿ (RR)

E1818 Static progressive stretch forearm pronation/supination device, with or without range of motion adjustment, includes all components and accessories Y ♿ (RR)

E1820 Replacement soft interface material, dynamic adjustable extension/flexion device Y ♿ (NU, RR, UE)

E1821 Replacement soft interface material/cuffs for bi-directional static progressive stretch device Y ♿ (NU, RR, UE)

● **E1822** Dynamic adjustable ankle extension only device, includes soft interface material

● **E1823** Dynamic adjustable ankle flexion only device, includes soft interface material

▲ **E1825** Dynamic adjustable finger extension and flexion device, includes soft interface material Y ♿ (RR)

● **E1826** Dynamic adjustable finger extension only device, includes soft interface material

● **E1827** Dynamic adjustable finger flexion only device, includes soft interface material

● **E1828** Dynamic adjustable toe extension only device, includes soft interface material

● **E1829** Dynamic adjustable toe flexion only device, includes soft interface material

▲ **E1830** Dynamic adjustable toe extension and flexion device, includes soft interface material Y ♿ (RR)

E1831 Static progressive stretch toe device, extension and/or flexion, with or without range of motion adjustment, includes all components and accessories Y ♿ (RR)

E1840 Dynamic adjustable shoulder flexion/abduction/rotation device, includes soft interface material Y ♿ (RR)

E1841 Static progressive stretch shoulder device, with or without range of motion adjustment, includes all components and accessories Y ♿ (RR)

Other Devices

E1902 Communication board, nonelectronic augmentative or alternative communication device [Y]

E1905 Virtual reality cognitive behavioral therapy device (CBT), including preprogrammed therapy software [A] (RR)
AHA: 2Q,23

E2000 Gastric suction pump, home model, portable or stationary, electric [Y] ♿ (RR)

▲ **E2001** Suction pump, home model, portable or stationary, electric, any type, for use with external urine and/or fecal management system [Y] (RR)
AHA: 2Q,24

E2100 Blood glucose monitor with integrated voice synthesizer [Y] ♿ (NU, RR, UE)

E2101 Blood glucose monitor with integrated lancing/blood sample [Y] ♿ (NU, RR, UE)

E2102 Adjunctive, nonimplanted continuous glucose monitor (CGM) or receiver [Y] (NU, RR, UE)

E2103 Nonadjunctive, nonimplanted continuous glucose monitor (CGM) or receiver [Y] (NU, RR, UE)

● **E2104** Home blood glucose monitor for use with integrated lancing/blood sample testing cartridge [A] (NU, RR, UE)
AHA: 2Q,24

E2120 Pulse generator system for tympanic treatment of inner ear endolymphatic fluid [Y] ♿ (RR)

DME Wheelchair Accessory

E2201 Manual wheelchair accessory, nonstandard seat frame, width greater than or equal to 20 in and less than 24 in [Y] ☑ ♿ (NU, RR, UE)

E2202 Manual wheelchair accessory, nonstandard seat frame width, 24-27 in [Y] ☑ ♿ (NU, RR, UE)

E2203 Manual wheelchair accessory, nonstandard seat frame depth, 20 to less than 22 in [Y] ☑ ♿ (NU, RR, UE)

E2204 Manual wheelchair accessory, nonstandard seat frame depth, 22 to 25 in [Y] ☑ ♿ (NU, RR, UE)

E2205 Manual wheelchair accessory, handrim without projections (includes ergonomic or contoured), any type, replacement only, each [Y] ☑ ♿ (NU, RR, UE)

E2206 Manual wheelchair accessory, wheel lock assembly, complete, replacement only, each [Y] ☑ ♿ (NU, RR, UE)

E2207 Wheelchair accessory, crutch and cane holder, each [Y] ☑ ♿ (NU, RR, UE)

E2208 Wheelchair accessory, cylinder tank carrier, each [Y] ☑ ♿ (NU, RR, UE)

E2209 Accessory, arm trough, with or without hand support, each [Y] ☑ ♿ (NU, RR, UE)

E2210 Wheelchair accessory, bearings, any type, replacement only, each [Y] ☑ ♿ (NU, RR, UE)

E2211 Manual wheelchair accessory, pneumatic propulsion tire, any size, each [Y] ☑ ♿ (NU, RR, UE)

E2212 Manual wheelchair accessory, tube for pneumatic propulsion tire, any size, each [Y] ☑ ♿ (NU, RR, UE)

E2213 Manual wheelchair accessory, insert for pneumatic propulsion tire (removable), any type, any size, each [Y] ☑ ♿ (NU, RR, UE)

E2214 Manual wheelchair accessory, pneumatic caster tire, any size, each [Y] ☑ ♿ (NU, RR, UE)

E2215 Manual wheelchair accessory, tube for pneumatic caster tire, any size, each [Y] ☑ ♿ (NU, RR, UE)

E2216 Manual wheelchair accessory, foam filled propulsion tire, any size, each [Y] ☑ ♿ (NU, RR, UE)

E2217 Manual wheelchair accessory, foam filled caster tire, any size, each [Y] ☑ ♿ (NU, RR, UE)

E2218 Manual wheelchair accessory, foam propulsion tire, any size, each [Y] ☑ ♿ (NU, RR, UE)

E2219 Manual wheelchair accessory, foam caster tire, any size, each [Y] ☑ ♿ (NU, RR, UE)

E2220 Manual wheelchair accessory, solid (rubber/plastic) propulsion tire, any size, replacement only, each [Y] ☑ ♿ (NU, RR, UE)

E2221 Manual wheelchair accessory, solid (rubber/plastic) caster tire (removable), any size, replacement only, each [Y] ☑ ♿ (NU, RR, UE)

E2222 Manual wheelchair accessory, solid (rubber/plastic) caster tire with integrated wheel, any size, replacement only, each [Y] ☑ ♿ (NU, RR, UE)

E2224 Manual wheelchair accessory, propulsion wheel excludes tire, any size, replacement only, each [Y] ☑ ♿ (NU, RR, UE)

E2225 Manual wheelchair accessory, caster wheel excludes tire, any size, replacement only, each [Y] ☑ ♿ (NU, RR, UE)

E2226 Manual wheelchair accessory, caster fork, any size, replacement only, each [Y] ☑ ♿ (NU, RR, UE)

E2227 Manual wheelchair accessory, gear reduction drive wheel, each [Y] ☑ ♿ (RR)

E2228 Manual wheelchair accessory, wheel braking system and lock, complete, each [Y] ☑ ♿ (RR)

E2230 Manual wheelchair accessory, manual standing system [Y]

E2231 Manual wheelchair accessory, solid seat support base (replaces sling seat), includes any type mounting hardware [Y] ♿ (NU, RR, UE)

E2291 Back, planar, for pediatric size wheelchair including fixed attaching hardware [Y]

E2292 Seat, planar, for pediatric size wheelchair including fixed attaching hardware [Y]

E2293 Back, contoured, for pediatric size wheelchair including fixed attaching hardware [Y]

E2294 Seat, contoured, for pediatric size wheelchair including fixed attaching hardware [Y]

E2295 Manual wheelchair accessory, for pediatric size wheelchair, dynamic seating frame, allows coordinated movement of multiple positioning features [Y]

● **E2298** Complex rehabilitative power wheelchair accessory, power seat elevation system, any type [Y] (RR)
AHA: 2Q,24

E2300 ~~Wheelchair accessory, power seat elevation system, any type~~

E2301 Wheelchair accessory, power standing system, any type [Y]

E2310 Power wheelchair accessory, electronic connection between wheelchair controller and one power seating system motor, including all related electronics, indicator feature, mechanical function selection switch, and fixed mounting hardware [Y] ♿ (RR)

E2311 Power wheelchair accessory, electronic connection between wheelchair controller and 2 or more power seating system motors, including all related electronics, indicator feature, mechanical function selection switch, and fixed mounting hardware [Y] ♿ (RR)

E2312 **Power wheelchair accessory, hand or chin control interface, mini-proportional remote joystick, proportional, including fixed mounting hardware** Y ♿ (RR)

E2313 **Power wheelchair accessory, harness for upgrade to expandable controller, including all fasteners, connectors and mounting hardware, each** Y ☑ ♿ (RR)

E2321 **Power wheelchair accessory, hand control interface, remote joystick, nonproportional, including all related electronics, mechanical stop switch, and fixed mounting hardware** Y ♿ (RR)

E2322 **Power wheelchair accessory, hand control interface, multiple mechanical switches, nonproportional, including all related electronics, mechanical stop switch, and fixed mounting hardware** Y ♿ (RR)

E2323 **Power wheelchair accessory, specialty joystick handle for hand control interface, prefabricated** Y ♿ (NU, RR, UE)

E2324 **Power wheelchair accessory, chin cup for chin control interface** Y ♿ (NU, RR, UE)

E2325 **Power wheelchair accessory, sip and puff interface, nonproportional, including all related electronics, mechanical stop switch, and manual swingaway mounting hardware** Y ♿ (RR)

E2326 **Power wheelchair accessory, breath tube kit for sip and puff interface** Y ♿ (RR)

E2327 **Power wheelchair accessory, head control interface, mechanical, proportional, including all related electronics, mechanical direction change switch, and fixed mounting hardware** Y ♿ (RR)

E2328 **Power wheelchair accessory, head control or extremity control interface, electronic, proportional, including all related electronics and fixed mounting hardware** Y ♿ (RR)

E2329 **Power wheelchair accessory, head control interface, contact switch mechanism, nonproportional, including all related electronics, mechanical stop switch, mechanical direction change switch, head array, and fixed mounting hardware** Y ♿ (RR)

E2330 **Power wheelchair accessory, head control interface, proximity switch mechanism, nonproportional, including all related electronics, mechanical stop switch, mechanical direction change switch, head array, and fixed mounting hardware** Y ♿ (RR)

E2331 **Power wheelchair accessory, attendant control, proportional, including all related electronics and fixed mounting hardware** Y

E2340 **Power wheelchair accessory, nonstandard seat frame width, 20-23 in** Y ☑ ♿ (NU, RR, UE)

E2341 **Power wheelchair accessory, nonstandard seat frame width, 24-27 in** Y ☑ ♿ (NU, RR, UE)

E2342 **Power wheelchair accessory, nonstandard seat frame depth, 20 or 21 in** Y ☑ ♿ (NU, RR, UE)

E2343 **Power wheelchair accessory, nonstandard seat frame depth, 22-25 in** Y ☑ ♿ (NU, RR, UE)

E2351 **Power wheelchair accessory, electronic interface to operate speech generating device using power wheelchair control interface** Y ♿ (NU, RR, UE)

E2358 **Power wheelchair accessory, group 34 nonsealed lead acid battery, each** Y ☑

E2359 **Power wheelchair accessory, group 34 sealed lead acid battery, each (e.g., gel cell, absorbed glass mat)** Y ♿ (NU, RR, UE)

E2360 **Power wheelchair accessory, 22 NF nonsealed lead acid battery, each** Y ☑ ♿ (NU, RR, UE)

E2361 **Power wheelchair accessory, 22 NF sealed lead acid battery, each (e.g., gel cell, absorbed glassmat)** Y ☑ ♿ (NU, RR, UE)

E2362 **Power wheelchair accessory, group 24 nonsealed lead acid battery, each** Y ☑ ♿ (NU, RR, UE)

E2363 **Power wheelchair accessory, group 24 sealed lead acid battery, each (e.g., gel cell, absorbed glassmat)** Y ☑ ♿ (NU, RR, UE)

E2364 **Power wheelchair accessory, U-1 nonsealed lead acid battery, each** Y ☑ ♿ (NU, RR, UE)

E2365 **Power wheelchair accessory, U-1 sealed lead acid battery, each (e.g., gel cell, absorbed glassmat)** Y ☑ ♿ (NU, RR, UE)

E2366 **Power wheelchair accessory, battery charger, single mode, for use with only one battery type, sealed or nonsealed, each** Y ☑ ♿ (NU, RR, UE)

E2367 **Power wheelchair accessory, battery charger, dual mode, for use with either battery type, sealed or nonsealed, each** Y ☑ ♿ (NU, RR, UE)

E2368 **Power wheelchair component, drive wheel motor, replacement only** Y ♿ (RR)

E2369 **Power wheelchair component, drive wheel gear box, replacement only** Y ♿ (RR)

E2370 **Power wheelchair component, integrated drive wheel motor and gear box combination, replacement only** Y ♿ (RR)

E2371 **Power wheelchair accessory, group 27 sealed lead acid battery, (e.g., gel cell, absorbed glassmat), each** Y ☑ ♿ (NU, RR, UE)

E2372 **Power wheelchair accessory, group 27 nonsealed lead acid battery, each** Y ☑ ♿ (NU, RR, UE)

E2373 **Power wheelchair accessory, hand or chin control interface, compact remote joystick, proportional, including fixed mounting hardware** Y ♿ (RR)

E2374 **Power wheelchair accessory, hand or chin control interface, standard remote joystick (not including controller), proportional, including all related electronics and fixed mounting hardware, replacement only** Y ♿ (RR)

E2375 **Power wheelchair accessory, nonexpandable controller, including all related electronics and mounting hardware, replacement only** Y ♿ (RR)

E2376 **Power wheelchair accessory, expandable controller, including all related electronics and mounting hardware, replacement only** Y ♿ (RR)

E2377 **Power wheelchair accessory, expandable controller, including all related electronics and mounting hardware, upgrade provided at initial issue** Y ♿ (RR)

E2378 **Power wheelchair component, actuator, replacement only** Y ♿ (RR)

E2381 **Power wheelchair accessory, pneumatic drive wheel tire, any size, replacement only, each** Y ☑ ♿ (NU, RR, UE)

E2382 **Power wheelchair accessory, tube for pneumatic drive wheel tire, any size, replacement only, each** Y ☑ ♿ (NU, RR, UE)

E2383 **Power wheelchair accessory, insert for pneumatic drive wheel tire (removable), any type, any size, replacement only, each** Y ☑ ♿ (NU, RR, UE)

E2384 **Power wheelchair accessory, pneumatic caster tire, any size, replacement only, each** Y ☑ ♿ (NU, RR, UE)

E2385 **Power wheelchair accessory, tube for pneumatic caster tire, any size, replacement only, each** Y ☑ ♿ (NU, RR, UE)

E2386 **Power wheelchair accessory, foam filled drive wheel tire, any size, replacement only, each** Y ☑ ♿ (NU, RR, UE)

E2387 Power wheelchair accessory, foam filled caster tire, any size, replacement only, each (NU, RR, UE)

E2388 Power wheelchair accessory, foam drive wheel tire, any size, replacement only, each (NU, RR, UE)

E2389 Power wheelchair accessory, foam caster tire, any size, replacement only, each (NU, RR, UE)

E2390 Power wheelchair accessory, solid (rubber/plastic) drive wheel tire, any size, replacement only, each (NU, RR, UE)

E2391 Power wheelchair accessory, solid (rubber/plastic) caster tire (removable), any size, replacement only, each (NU, RR, UE)

E2392 Power wheelchair accessory, solid (rubber/plastic) caster tire with integrated wheel, any size, replacement only, each (NU, RR, UE)

E2394 Power wheelchair accessory, drive wheel excludes tire, any size, replacement only, each (NU, RR, UE)

E2395 Power wheelchair accessory, caster wheel excludes tire, any size, replacement only, each (NU, RR, UE)

E2396 Power wheelchair accessory, caster fork, any size, replacement only, each (NU, RR, UE)

E2397 Power wheelchair accessory, lithium-based battery, each (NU, RR, UE)

E2398 Wheelchair accessory, dynamic positioning hardware for back (NU, RR, UE)

Wound Therapy

E2402 Negative pressure wound therapy electrical pump, stationary or portable (RR)

CMS: 100-02,7,40.1.2.8

Speech Generating Device

E2500 Speech generating device, digitized speech, using prerecorded messages, less than or equal to eight minutes recording time (NU, RR, UE)

E2502 Speech generating device, digitized speech, using prerecorded messages, greater than eight minutes but less than or equal to 20 minutes recording time (NU, RR, UE)

E2504 Speech generating device, digitized speech, using prerecorded messages, greater than 20 minutes but less than or equal to 40 minutes recording time (NU, RR, UE)

E2506 Speech generating device, digitized speech, using prerecorded messages, greater than 40 minutes recording time (NU, RR, UE)

E2508 Speech generating device, synthesized speech, requiring message formulation by spelling and access by physical contact with the device (NU, RR, UE)

E2510 Speech generating device, synthesized speech, permitting multiple methods of message formulation and multiple methods of device access (NU, RR, UE)

E2511 Speech generating software program, for personal computer or personal digital assistant (NU, RR, UE)

E2512 Accessory for speech generating device, mounting system (NU, RR, UE)

● **E2513** Accessory for speech generating device, electromyographic sensor (NU, RR, UE)

E2599 Accessory for speech generating device, not otherwise classified

Wheelchair Cushion

E2601 General use wheelchair seat cushion, width less than 22 in, any depth (NU, RR, UE)

E2602 General use wheelchair seat cushion, width 22 in or greater, any depth (NU, RR, UE)

E2603 Skin protection wheelchair seat cushion, width less than 22 in, any depth (NU, RR, UE)

E2604 Skin protection wheelchair seat cushion, width 22 in or greater, any depth (NU, RR, UE)

E2605 Positioning wheelchair seat cushion, width less than 22 in, any depth (NU, RR, UE)

E2606 Positioning wheelchair seat cushion, width 22 in or greater, any depth (NU, RR, UE)

E2607 Skin protection and positioning wheelchair seat cushion, width less than 22 in, any depth (NU, RR, UE)

E2608 Skin protection and positioning wheelchair seat cushion, width 22 in or greater, any depth (NU, RR, UE)

E2609 Custom fabricated wheelchair seat cushion, any size

E2610 Wheelchair seat cushion, powered

E2611 General use wheelchair back cushion, width less than 22 in, any height, including any type mounting hardware (NU, RR, UE)

E2612 General use wheelchair back cushion, width 22 in or greater, any height, including any type mounting hardware (NU, RR, UE)

E2613 Positioning wheelchair back cushion, posterior, width less than 22 in, any height, including any type mounting hardware (NU, RR, UE)

E2614 Positioning wheelchair back cushion, posterior, width 22 in or greater, any height, including any type mounting hardware (NU, RR, UE)

E2615 Positioning wheelchair back cushion, posterior-lateral, width less than 22 in, any height, including any type mounting hardware (NU, RR, UE)

E2616 Positioning wheelchair back cushion, posterior-lateral, width 22 in or greater, any height, including any type mounting hardware (NU, RR, UE)

E2617 Custom fabricated wheelchair back cushion, any size, including any type mounting hardware

E2619 Replacement cover for wheelchair seat cushion or back cushion, each (NU, RR, UE)

E2620 Positioning wheelchair back cushion, planar back with lateral supports, width less than 22 in, any height, including any type mounting hardware (NU, RR, UE)

E2621 Positioning wheelchair back cushion, planar back with lateral supports, width 22 in or greater, any height, including any type mounting hardware (NU, RR, UE)

E2622 Skin protection wheelchair seat cushion, adjustable, width less than 22 in, any depth (NU, RR, UE)

E2623 Skin protection wheelchair seat cushion, adjustable, width 22 in or greater, any depth (NU, RR, UE)

E2624 Skin protection and positioning wheelchair seat cushion, adjustable, width less than 22 in, any depth (NU, RR, UE)

E2625 Skin protection and positioning wheelchair seat cushion, adjustable, width 22 in or greater, any depth (NU, RR, UE)

Wheelchair Arm Support

E2626 Wheelchair accessory, shoulder elbow, mobile arm support attached to wheelchair, balanced, adjustable Y (NU, RR, UE)

E2627 Wheelchair accessory, shoulder elbow, mobile arm support attached to wheelchair, balanced, adjustable Rancho type Y (NU, RR, UE)

E2628 Wheelchair accessory, shoulder elbow, mobile arm support attached to wheelchair, balanced, reclining Y (NU, RR, UE)

E2629 Wheelchair accessory, shoulder elbow, mobile arm support attached to wheelchair, balanced, friction arm support (friction dampening to proximal and distal joints) Y (NU, RR, UE)

E2630 Wheelchair accessory, shoulder elbow, mobile arm support, monosuspension arm and hand support, overhead elbow forearm hand sling support, yoke type suspension support Y (NU, RR, UE)

E2631 Wheelchair accessory, addition to mobile arm support, elevating proximal arm Y (NU, RR, UE)

E2632 Wheelchair accessory, addition to mobile arm support, offset or lateral rocker arm with elastic balance control Y (NU, RR, UE)

E2633 Wheelchair accessory, addition to mobile arm support, supinator Y (NU, RR, UE)

Speech Volume Modulation System

E3000 Speech volume modulation system, any type, including all components and accessories Y (RR)

Gait Devices

● **E3200** Gait modulation system, rhythmic auditory stimulation, including restricted therapy software, all components and accessories, prescription only

E8000 Gait trainer, pediatric size, posterior support, includes all accessories and components E1

E8001 Gait trainer, pediatric size, upright support, includes all accessories and components E1

E8002 Gait trainer, pediatric size, anterior support, includes all accessories and components E1

Procedures/Professional Services (Temporary) G0008-G9999

The G codes are used to identify professional health care procedures and services that would otherwise be coded in CPT but for which there are no CPT codes. Please refer to your CPT book for possible alternate code(s).

Immunization Administration

G0008 Administration of influenza virus vaccine S

CMS: 100-02,12,40.11; 100-02,13,220; 100-02,13,220.1; 100-02,13,220.3; 100-02,15,50.4.4.2; 100-04,18,1.2; 100-04,18,10.2; 100-04,18,10.2.1; 100-04,18,10.2.2.1; 100-04,18,10.2.5.2; 100-04,18,10.3.1.1; 100-04,18,10.4; 100-04,18,10.4.1; 100-04,18,10.4.2; 100-04,18,10.4.3; 100-04,18,140.8; 1004-04,13,220.1

G0009 Administration of pneumococcal vaccine S

CMS: 100-02,12,40.11; 100-02,13,220; 100-02,13,220.1; 100-02,13,220.3; 100-02,15,50.4.4.2; 100-04,18,1.2; 100-04,18,10.2.1; 100-04,18,10.2.2.1; 100-04,18,10.2.5.2; 100-04,18,10.3.1.1; 100-04,18,10.4; 100-04,18,10.4.1; 100-04,18,10.4.2; 100-04,18,10.4.3; 100-04,18,140.8; 1004-04,13,220.1

G0010 Administration of hepatitis B vaccine S

CMS: 100-02,12,40.11; 100-02,13,220; 100-02,13,220.1; 100-02,13,220.3; 100-02,15,50.4.4.2; 100-04,18,1.2; 100-04,18,10.2.1; 100-04,18,10.2.2.1; 100-04,18,10.2.5.2; 100-04,18,10.3.1.1; 100-04,18,140.8; 1004-04,13,220.1

Pre-exposure Prophylaxis

G0011 Individual counseling for pre-exposure prophylaxis (PrEP) by physician or qualified health care professional (QHP) to prevent human immunodeficiency virus (HIV), includes HIV risk assessment (initial or continued assessment of risk), HIV risk reduction and medication adherence, 15 to 30 minutes B

AHA: 1Q,24

G0012 Injection of pre-exposure prophylaxis (PrEP) drug for HIV prevention, under skin or into muscle S

AHA: 1Q,24

G0013 Individual counseling for pre-exposure prophylaxis (PrEP) by clinical staff to prevent human immunodeficiency virus (HIV), includes: HIV risk assessment (initial or continued assessment of risk), HIV risk reduction and medication adherence S

AHA: 1Q,24

Psychotherapy Services

G0017 Psychotherapy for crisis furnished in an applicable site of service (any place of service at which the nonfacility rate for psychotherapy for crisis services applies, other than the office setting); first 60 minutes M

AHA: 1Q,24

G0018 Psychotherapy for crisis furnished in an applicable site of service (any place of service at which the nonfacility rate for psychotherapy for crisis services applies, other than the office setting); each additional 30 minutes (list separately in addition to code for primary service) M

AHA: 1Q,24

Community Health Integration Services

G0019 Community health integration services performed by certified or trained auxiliary personnel, including a community health worker, under the direction of a physician or other practitioner, 60 minutes per calendar month, in the following activities to address social determinants of health (SDOH) need(s) that are significantly limiting the ability to diagnose or treat problem(s) addressed in an initiating visit: S

— person-centered assessment, performed to better understand the individualized context of the intersection between the SDOH need(s) and the problem(s) addressed in the initiating visit;

— conducting a person-centered assessment to understand patient's life story, strengths, needs, goals, preferences and desired outcomes, including understanding cultural and linguistic factors and including unmet SDOH needs (that are not separately billed);

— facilitating patient-driven goal-setting and establishing an action plan;

— providing tailored support to the patient as needed to accomplish the practitioner's treatment plan;

— practitioner, home-, and community-based care coordination;

— coordinating receipt of needed services from health care practitioners, providers, and facilities, and from home- and community-based service providers, social service providers, and caregiver (if applicable);

— communication with practitioners, home- and community-based service providers, hospitals, and skilled nursing facilities (or other health care facilities) regarding the patient's psychosocial strengths and needs, functional deficits, goals, preferences, and desired outcomes, including cultural and linguistic factors;

— coordination of care transitions between and among health care practitioners and settings, including transitions involving referral to other clinicians;

— follow-up after an emergency department visit, or follow-up after discharges from hospitals, skilled nursing facilities or other health care facilities;

— facilitating access to community-based social services (e.g., housing, utilities, transportation, food assistance) to address the SDOH need(s);

— health education-helping the patient contextualize health education provided by the patient's treatment team with the patient's individual needs, goals, and preferences, in the context of the SDOH need(s), and educating the patient on how to best participate in medical decision-making;

— building patient self-advocacy skills, so that the patient can interact with members of the health care team and related community-based services addressing the SDOH need(s), in ways that are more likely to promote personalized and effective diagnosis or treatment;

— health care access/health system navigation; helping the patient access health care, including identifying appropriate practitioners or providers for clinical care and helping secure appointments with them;

— facilitating behavioral change as necessary for meeting diagnosis and treatment goals, including promoting patient motivation to participate in care and reach person-centered diagnosis or treatment goals;

— facilitating and providing social and emotional support to help the patient cope with the problem(s) addressed in the initiating visit, the SDOH need(s), and adjust daily routines to better meet diagnosis and treatment goals;

— leveraging lived experience when applicable to provide support, mentorship, or inspiration to meet treatment goals

AHA: 1Q,24

G0022 Community health integration services, each additional 30 minutes per calendar month (list separately in addition to G0019) N

AHA: 1Q,24

Principle Illness Navigation Services

G0023 **Principal illness navigation services by certified or trained auxiliary personnel under the direction of a physician or other practitioner, including a patient navigator, 60 minutes per calendar month, in the following activities:** S

— person-centered assessment, performed to better understand the individual context of the serious, high-risk condition;

— conducting a person-centered assessment to understand the patient's life story, strengths, needs, goals, preferences, and desired outcomes, including understanding cultural and linguistic factors and including unmet SDOH needs (that are not separately billed);

— facilitating patient-driven goal setting and establishing an action plan;

— providing tailored support as needed to accomplish the practitioner's treatment plan;

— identifying or referring patient (and caregiver or family, if applicable) to appropriate supportive services;

— practitioner, home, and community-based care coordination;

— coordinating receipt of needed services from health care practitioners, providers, and facilities, home- and community-based service providers, and caregiver (if applicable);

— communication with practitioners, home-, and community-based service providers, hospitals, and skilled nursing facilities (or other health care facilities) regarding the patient's psychosocial strengths and needs, functional deficits, goals, preferences, and desired outcomes, including cultural and linguistic factors;

— coordination of care transitions between and among health care practitioners and settings, including transitions involving referral to other clinicians, follow-up after an emergency department visit, or follow-up after discharges from hospitals, skilled nursing facilities, or other health care facilities;

— facilitating access to community-based social services (e.g., housing, utilities, transportation, food assistance) as need to address SDOH need(s);

— health education—helping the patient contextualize health education provided by the patient's treatment team with the patient's individual needs, goals, preferences, and SDOH need(s), and educating the patient (and caregiver if applicable) on how to best participate in medical decision-making;

— building patient self-advocacy skills, so that the patient can interact with members of the health care team and related community-based services (as needed), in ways that are more likely to promote personalized and effective treatment of their condition;

— health care access/health system navigation;

— helping the patient access health care, including identifying appropriate practitioners or providers for clinical care, and helping secure appointments with them;

— providing the patient with information/resources to consider participation in clinical trials or clinical research as applicable;

— facilitating behavioral change as necessary for meeting diagnosis and treatment goals, including promoting patient motivation to participate in care and reach person-centered diagnosis or treatment goals;

— facilitating and providing social and emotional support to help the patient cope with the condition, SDOH need(s), and adjust daily routines to better meet diagnosis and treatment goals;

— leverage knowledge of the serious, high-risk condition, and/or lived experience when applicable to provide support, mentorship, or inspiration to meet treatment goals

AHA: 1Q,24

G0024 **Principal illness navigation services, additional 30 minutes per calendar month (list separately in addition to G0023)** N

AHA: 1Q,24

Semen Analysis

G0027 **Semen analysis; presence and/or motility of sperm excluding Huhner** Q

Quality Measures

G0029 **Tobacco screening not performed or tobacco cessation intervention not provided during the measurement period or in the 6 months prior to the measurement period** M

G0030 **Patient screened for tobacco use and received tobacco cessation intervention during the measurement period or in the 6 months prior to the measurement period (counseling, pharmacotherapy, or both), if identified as a tobacco user** M

G0031 **Palliative care services given to patient any time during the measurement period** M

G0032 **Two or more antipsychotic prescriptions ordered for patients who had a diagnosis of schizophrenia, schizoaffective disorder, or bipolar disorder on or between January 1 of the year prior to the measurement period and the index prescription start date (IPSD) for antipsychotics** M

G0033 **Two or more benzodiazepine prescriptions ordered for patients who had a diagnosis of seizure disorders, rapid eye movement sleep behavior disorder, benzodiazepine withdrawal, ethanol withdrawal, or severe generalized anxiety disorder on or between January 1 of the year prior to the measurement period and the IPSD for benzodiazepines** M

G0034 **Patients receiving palliative care during the measurement period** M

G0035 **Patient has any emergency department encounter during the performance period with place of service indicator 23** M

G0036 **Patient or care partner decline assessment** M

G0037 **On date of encounter, patient is not able to participate in assessment or screening, including nonverbal patients, delirious, severely aphasic, severely developmentally delayed, severe visual or hearing impairment and for those patients, no knowledgeable informant available** M

G0038 **Clinician determines patient does not require referral** M

G0039 **Patient not referred, reason not otherwise specified** M

G0040 **Patient already receiving physical/occupational/speech/recreational therapy during the measurement period** M

G0041 **Patient and/or care partner decline referral** M

G0042 **Referral to physical, occupational, speech, or recreational therapy** M

G0043 **Patients with mechanical prosthetic heart valve** M

G0044 **Patients with moderate or severe mitral stenosis** M

G0045 **Clinical follow-up and MRS score assessed at 90 days following endovascular stroke intervention** M

G0046 **Clinical follow-up and MRS score not assessed at 90 days following endovascular stroke intervention** M

G0047 **Pediatric patient with minor blunt head trauma and PECARN prediction criteria are not assessed** M

G0048 **Patients who receive palliative care services any time during the intake period through the end of the measurement year** M

G0049 **With maintenance hemodialysis (in-center and home HD) for the complete reporting month** M

G0050 **Patients with a catheter that have limited life expectancy** M

G0051 **Patients under hospice care in the current reporting month** M

G0052 **Patients on peritoneal dialysis for any portion of the reporting month** M

G0053 **Advancing rheumatology patient care MIPS value pathways** M

G0054 **Coordinating stroke care to promote prevention and cultivate positive outcomes MIPS value pathways** M

G0055 **Advancing care for heart disease MIPS value pathways** M

G0057 Proposed adopting best practices and promoting patient safety within emergency medicine MIPS value pathways M

G0058 Improving care for lower extremity joint repair MIPS value pathways M

G0059 Patient safety and support of positive experiences with anesthesia MIPS value pathways M

G0060 Allergy/Immunology MIPS specialty set M

G0061 Anesthesiology MIPS specialty set M

G0062 Audiology MIPS specialty set M

G0063 Cardiology MIPS specialty set M

G0064 Certified Nurse Midwife MIPS specialty set M

G0065 Chiropractic Medicine MIPS specialty set M

G0066 Clinical Social Work MIPS specialty set M

G0067 Dentistry MIPS specialty set M

Professional Services

G0068 Professional services for the administration of anti-infective, pain management, chelation, pulmonary hypertension, inotropic, or other intravenous infusion drug or biological (excluding chemotherapy or other highly complex drug or biological) for each infusion drug administration calendar day in the individual's home, each 15 min A

CMS: 100-04,20,180; 100-04,32,411.3; 100-04,32,411.4; 100-04,32,411.5; 100-04,32,411.6

G0069 Professional services for the administration of subcutaneous immunotherapy or other subcutaneous infusion drug or biological for each infusion drug administration calendar day in the individual's home, each 15 min A

CMS: 100-04,20,180; 100-04,32,411.3; 100-04,32,411.4; 100-04,32,411.5; 100-04,32,411.6

G0070 Professional services for the administration of intravenous chemotherapy or other intravenous highly complex drug or biological infusion for each infusion drug administration calendar day in the individual's home, each 15 min A

CMS: 100-04,20,180; 100-04,32,411.3; 100-04,32,411.4; 100-04,32,411.5; 100-04,32,411.6

G0071 Payment for communication technology-based services for 5 minutes or more of a virtual (nonface-to-face) communication between a rural health clinic (RHC) or federally qualified health center (FQHC) practitioner and RHC or FQHC patient, or 5 minutes or more of remote evaluation of recorded video and/or images by an RHC or FQHC practitioner, occurring in lieu of an office visit; RHC or FQHC only A

CMS: 100-04,9,70.7

G0076 Brief (20 minutes) care management home visit for a new patient. For use only in a Medicare-approved CMMI model (services must be furnished within a beneficiary's home, domiciliary, rest home, assisted living and/or nursing facility) B

G0077 Limited (30 minutes) care management home visit for a new patient. For use only in a Medicare-approved CMMI model (services must be furnished within a beneficiary's home, domiciliary, rest home, assisted living and/or nursing facility) B

G0078 Moderate (45 minutes) care management home visit for a new patient. For use only in a Medicare-approved CMMI model (services must be furnished within a beneficiary's home, domiciliary, rest home, assisted living and/or nursing facility) B

G0079 Comprehensive (60 minutes) care management home visit for a new patient. For use only in a Medicare-approved CMMI model (services must be furnished within a beneficiary's home, domiciliary, rest home, assisted living and/or nursing facility) B

G0080 Extensive (75 minutes) care management home visit for a new patient. For use only in a Medicare-approved CMMI model (services must be furnished within a beneficiary's home, domiciliary, rest home, assisted living and/or nursing facility) B

G0081 Brief (20 minutes) care management home visit for an existing patient. For use only in a Medicare-approved CMMI model (services must be furnished within a beneficiary's home, domiciliary, rest home, assisted living and/or nursing facility) B

G0082 Limited (30 minutes) care management home visit for an existing patient. For use only in a Medicare-approved CMMI model (services must be furnished within a beneficiary's home, domiciliary, rest home, assisted living and/or nursing facility) B

G0083 Moderate (45 minutes) care management home visit for an existing patient. For use only in a Medicare-approved CMMI model (services must be furnished within a beneficiary's home, domiciliary, rest home, assisted living and/or nursing facility) B

G0084 Comprehensive (60 minutes) care management home visit for an existing patient. For use only in a Medicare-approved CMMI model (services must be furnished within a beneficiary's home, domiciliary, rest home, assisted living and/or nursing facility) B

G0085 Extensive (75 minutes) care management home visit for an existing patient. For use only in a Medicare-approved CMMI model (services must be furnished within a beneficiary's home, domiciliary, rest home, assisted living and/or nursing facility) B

G0086 Limited (30 minutes) care management home care plan oversight. For use only in a Medicare-approved CMMI model (services must be furnished within a beneficiary's home, domiciliary, rest home, assisted living and/or nursing facility) B

G0087 Comprehensive (60 minutes) care management home care plan oversight. For use only in a Medicare-approved CMMI model (services must be furnished within a beneficiary's home, domiciliary, rest home, assisted living and/or nursing facility) B

G0088 Professional services, initial visit, for the administration of anti-infective, pain management, chelation, pulmonary hypertension, inotropic, or other intravenous infusion drug or biological (excluding chemotherapy or other highly complex drug or biological) for each infusion drug administration calendar day in the individual's home, each 15 min A

CMS: 100-04,32,411.3; 100-04,32,411.4; 100-04,32,411.5; 100-04,32,411.6

G0089 Professional services, initial visit, for the administration of subcutaneous immunotherapy or other subcutaneous infusion drug or biological for each infusion drug administration calendar day in the individual's home, each 15 min A

CMS: 100-04,32,411.3; 100-04,32,411.4; 100-04,32,411.5; 100-04,32,411.6

G0090 Professional services, initial visit, for the administration of intravenous chemotherapy or other highly complex infusion drug or biological for each infusion drug administration calendar day in the individual's home, each 15 min A

CMS: 100-04,32,411.3; 100-04,32,411.4; 100-04,32,411.5; 100-04,32,411.6

Screening Services

G0101 **Cervical or vaginal cancer screening; pelvic and clinical breast examination** A S ⊘

G0101 can be reported with an E/M code when a separately identifiable E/M service was provided.

CMS: 100-02,13,220; 100-02,13,220.1; 100-03,210.2; 100-04,18,1.2; 1004-04,13,220.1

AHA: 2Q,24

G0102 **Prostate cancer screening; digital rectal examination** N ⊘

CMS: 100-02,13,220; 100-02,13,220.1; 100-02,13,220.3; 100-04,18,1.2; 100-04,18,50.3; 100-04,18,50.4

G0103 **Prostate cancer screening; prostate specific antigen test (PSA)** A

CMS: 100-04,18,1.2; 100-04,18,50.3

G0104 **Colorectal cancer screening; flexible sigmoidoscopy** T P3 ⊘

Medicare covers colorectal screening for cancer via flexible sigmoidoscopy once every four years for patients 45 years or older.

CMS: 100-02,15,280.2.2; 100-04,18,1.2; 100-04,18,60; 100-04,18,60.1; 100-04,18,60.1.1; 100-04,18,60.2; 100-04,18,60.2.1; 100-04,18,60.6; 100-04,18,60.7

G0105 **Colorectal cancer screening; colonoscopy on individual at high risk** T A2 ⊘

An individual with ulcerative enteritis or a history of a malignant neoplasm of the lower gastrointestinal tract is considered at high-risk for colorectal cancer, as defined by CMS.

CMS: 100-02,15,280.2.2; 100-04,12,30.1; 100-04,18,1.2; 100-04,18,60; 100-04,18,60.1; 100-04,18,60.1.1; 100-04,18,60.2; 100-04,18,60.2.1; 100-04,18,60.2.2; 100-04,18,60.6; 100-04,18,60.7; 100-04,18,60.8; 100-04,23,30.2; 100-04,4,250.18

AHA: 3Q,23; 4Q,22; 2Q,18

G0106 ~~**Colorectal cancer screening; alternative to G0104, screening sigmoidoscopy, barium enema**~~

G0108 **Diabetes outpatient self-management training services, individual, per 30 minutes** A ☑ ⊘

CMS: 100-02,13,220.3; 100-02,15,300; 100-02,15,300.2; 100-02,15,300.3; 100-02,15,300.4; 100-04,12,190.3; 100-04,12,190.3.6; 100-04,12,190.6; 100-04,12,190.6.1; 100-04,12,190.7; 100-04,18,1.2; 100-04,18,120.1; 100-04,4,300.6

AHA: 3Q,19

G0109 **Diabetes outpatient self-management training services, group session (two or more), per 30 minutes** A ☑ ⊘

CMS: 100-02,15,300.2; 100-02,15,300.3; 100-04,12,190.3; 100-04,12,190.3.6; 100-04,12,190.6; 100-04,12,190.6.1; 100-04,12,190.7; 100-04,18,1.2; 100-04,4,300.6

AHA: 3Q,19

G0117 **Glaucoma screening for high risk patients furnished by an optometrist or ophthalmologist** S ⊘

CMS: 100-02,13,220; 100-02,13,220.1; 100-02,13,220.3; 100-02,15,280.1; 100-04,18,1.2; 100-04,18,70.1.1; 1004-04,13,220.1

G0118 **Glaucoma screening for high risk patient furnished under the direct supervision of an optometrist or ophthalmologist** S ⊘

CMS: 100-02,13,220; 100-02,13,220.1; 100-02,13,220.3; 100-02,15,280.1; 100-04,18,1.2; 100-04,18,70.1.1; 1004-04,13,220.1

G0120 ~~**Colorectal cancer screening; alternative to G0105, screening colonoscopy, barium enema**~~

G0121 **Colorectal cancer screening; colonoscopy on individual not meeting criteria for high risk** T A2 ⊘

CMS: 100-02,15,280.2.2; 100-04,12,30.1; 100-04,18,1.2; 100-04,18,60; 100-04,18,60.1; 100-04,18,60.1.1; 100-04,18,60.2; 100-04,18,60.2.1; 100-04,18,60.2.2; 100-04,18,60.5; 100-04,18,60.6; 100-04,23,30.2; 100-04,4,250.18

AHA: 3Q,23; 4Q,22; 2Q,18

G0122 ~~**Colorectal cancer screening; barium enema**~~

G0123 **Screening cytopathology, cervical or vaginal (any reporting system), collected in preservative fluid, automated thin layer preparation, screening by cytotechnologist under physician supervision** A A

See also P3000-P3001.

CMS: 100-03,210.2.1; 100-04,18,1.2; 100-04,18,30.2.1; 100-04,18,30.5; 100-04,18,30.6

G0124 **Screening cytopathology, cervical or vaginal (any reporting system), collected in preservative fluid, automated thin layer preparation, requiring interpretation by physician** A B ⊘

See also P3000-P3001.

CMS: 100-03,210.2.1; 100-04,18,1.2; 100-04,18,30.2.1; 100-04,18,30.5; 100-04,18,30.6

Miscellaneous Services

G0127 **Trimming of dystrophic nails, any number** Q1 ⊘

CMS: 100-02,15,290

G0128 **Direct (face-to-face with patient) skilled nursing services of a registered nurse provided in a comprehensive outpatient rehabilitation facility, each 10 minutes beyond the first 5 minutes** B ☑ ⊘

CMS: 100-02,12,30.1; 100-02,12,40.8; 100-02,17,40.1.2; 100-04,39,30.6; 100-04,39,30.8; 100-04,5,100.3; 100-04,5,20.4

G0129 **Occupational therapy services requiring the skills of a qualified occupational therapist, furnished as a component of a partial hospitalization or intensive outpatient treatment program, per session (45 minutes or more)** P ☑

CMS: 100-04,4,260.1; 100-04,4,260.1.1

AHA: 1Q,24

G0130 **Single energy x-ray absorptiometry (SEXA) bone density study, one or more sites; appendicular skeleton (peripheral) (e.g., radius, wrist, heel)** S Z3

CMS: 100-04,18,1.2

G0136 **Administration of a standardized, evidence-based social determinants of health risk assessment tool, 5 to 15 minutes** S

CMS: 100-02,15,280.5.2; 100-04,18,140.9

AHA: 1Q,24

G0137 **Intensive outpatient services, weekly bundle, minimum of 9 services over a 7 contiguous day period, which can include:** A

— individual and group therapy with physicians or psychologists (or other mental health professionals to the extent authorized under state law);

— occupational therapy requiring the skills of a qualified occupational therapist;

— services of social workers, trained psychiatric nurses, and other staff trained to work with psychiatric patients;

— individualized activity therapies that are not primarily recreational or diversionary;

— family counseling (the primary purpose of which is treatment of the individual's condition);

— patient training and education (to the extent that training and educational activities are closely and clearly related to individual's care and treatment);

— diagnostic services;

— such other items and services (excluding meals and transportation) that are reasonable and necessary for the diagnosis or active treatment of the individual's condition, reasonably expected to improve or maintain the individual's condition and functional level, and to prevent relapse or hospitalization, and furnished pursuant to such guidelines relating to frequency and duration of services in accordance with a physician certification and plan of treatment (provision of the services by a Medicare-enrolled opioid treatment program) (List separately in addition to code for primary procedure)

CMS: 100-02,17,40.1.1; 100-04,39,30.2; 100-04,39,30.6; 100-04,39,30.6.1; 100-04,39,30.8; 100-04,39,30.9; 100-04,39,40; 100-04,39,40.2

AHA: 1Q,24

● **G0138** **IV infusion of cipaglucosidase alfa-atga, including provider/supplier acquisition and clinical supervision of oral administration of miglustat in preparation of receipt of cipaglucosidase alfa-atga** G

AHA: 2Q,24

G0140 **Principal illness navigation-peer support by certified or trained auxiliary personnel under the direction of a physician or other practitioner, including a certified peer specialist, 60 minutes per calendar month, in the following activities:** S

— person-centered interview, performed to better understand the individual context of the serious, high-risk condition;

— conducting a person-centered interview to understand the patient's life story, strengths, needs, goals, preferences, and desired outcomes, including understanding cultural and linguistic factors, and including unmet SDOH needs (that are not billed separately);

— facilitating patient-driven goal setting and establishing an action plan;

— providing tailored support as needed to accomplish the person-centered goals in the practitioner's treatment plan;

— identifying or referring patient (and caregiver or family, if applicable) to appropriate supportive services;

— practitioner, home-, and community-based care communication;

— assist the patient in communicating with their practitioners, home-, and community-based service providers, hospitals, and skilled nursing facilities (or other health care facilities) regarding the patient's psychosocial strengths and needs, goals, preferences, and desired outcomes, including cultural and linguistic factors;

— facilitating access to community-based social services (e.g., housing, utilities, transportation, food assistance) as needed to address SDOH need(s);

— health education-helping the patient contextualize health education provided by the patient's treatment team with the patient's individual needs, goals, preferences, and SDOH need(s), and educating the patient (and caregiver if applicable) on how to best participate in medical decision-making;

— building patient self-advocacy skills, so that the patient can interact with members of the health care team and related community-based services (as needed), in ways that are more likely to promote personalized and effective treatment of their condition;

— developing and proposing strategies to help meet person-centered treatment goals and supporting the patient in using chosen strategies to reach person-centered treatment goals;

— facilitating and providing social and emotional support to help the patient cope with the condition, SDOH need(s), and adjust daily routines to better meet person-centered diagnosis and treatment goals;

— leverage knowledge of the serious, high-risk condition and/or lived experience when applicable to provide support, mentorship, or inspiration to meet treatment goals

AHA: 1Q,24

G0141 **Screening cytopathology smears, cervical or vaginal, performed by automated system, with manual rescreening, requiring interpretation by physician** A B ⊘

CMS: 100-03,210.2.1; 100-04,18,1.2; 100-04,18,30.2.1; 100-04,18,30.5; 100-04,18,30.6

G0143 **Screening cytopathology, cervical or vaginal (any reporting system), collected in preservative fluid, automated thin layer preparation, with manual screening and rescreening by cytotechnologist under physician supervision** A A

CMS: 100-03,210.2.1; 100-04,18,1.2; 100-04,18,30.2.1; 100-04,18,30.5; 100-04,18,30.6

G0144 **Screening cytopathology, cervical or vaginal (any reporting system), collected in preservative fluid, automated thin layer preparation, with screening by automated system, under physician supervision** A A

CMS: 100-03,210.2.1; 100-04,18,30.2.1; 100-04,18,30.5; 100-04,18,30.6

G0145 **Screening cytopathology, cervical or vaginal (any reporting system), collected in preservative fluid, automated thin layer preparation, with screening by automated system and manual rescreening under physician supervision** A A

CMS: 100-03,210.2.1; 100-04,18,1.2; 100-04,18,30.2.1; 100-04,18,30.5; 100-04,18,30.6

G0146 **Principal illness navigation-peer support, additional 30 minutes per calendar month (list separately in addition to G0140)** N

CMS: 100-03,210.2.1; 100-04,18,30.2.1; 100-04,18,30.5; 100-04,18,30.6

AHA: 1Q,24

G0147 **Screening cytopathology smears, cervical or vaginal, performed by automated system under physician supervision** A A

CMS: 100-03,210.2.1; 100-04,18,1.2; 100-04,18,30.2.1; 100-04,18,30.5; 100-04,18,30.6

G0148 **Screening cytopathology smears, cervical or vaginal, performed by automated system with manual rescreening** A A

CMS: 100-03,210.2.1; 100-04,18,1.2; 100-04,18,30.2.1; 100-04,18,30.5; 100-04,18,30.6

G0151 **Services performed by a qualified physical therapist in the home health or hospice setting, each 15 minutes** B ☑

CMS: 100-01,3,30.3; 100-04,10,40.2; 100-04,11,10; 100-04,11,130.1; 100-04,11,30.3

G0152 **Services performed by a qualified occupational therapist in the home health or hospice setting, each 15 minutes** B ☑

CMS: 100-01,3,30.3; 100-04,10,40.2; 100-04,11,10; 100-04,11,130.1; 100-04,11,30.3

G0153 **Services performed by a qualified speech-language pathologist in the home health or hospice setting, each 15 minutes** B ☑

CMS: 100-01,3,30.3; 100-04,10,40.2; 100-04,11,10; 100-04,11,130.1; 100-04,11,30.3

G0155 **Services of clinical social worker in home health or hospice settings, each 15 minutes** B ☑

CMS: 100-01,3,30.3; 100-04,10,40.2; 100-04,11,10; 100-04,11,130.1; 100-04,11,30.3

G0156 **Services of home health/hospice aide in home health or hospice settings, each 15 minutes** B ☑

CMS: 100-01,3,30.3; 100-04,10,40.2; 100-04,11,10; 100-04,11,130.1; 100-04,11,30.3

G0157 **Services performed by a qualified physical therapist assistant in the home health or hospice setting, each 15 minutes** B ☑

CMS: 100-04,10,40.2; 100-04,11,10

G0158 **Services performed by a qualified occupational therapist assistant in the home health or hospice setting, each 15 minutes** B ☑

CMS: 100-04,10,40.2; 100-04,11,10

G0159 **Services performed by a qualified physical therapist, in the home health setting, in the establishment or delivery of a safe and effective physical therapy maintenance program, each 15 minutes** B ☑

CMS: 100-04,10,40.2

G0160 **Services performed by a qualified occupational therapist, in the home health setting, in the establishment or delivery of a safe and effective occupational therapy maintenance program, each 15 minutes** B ☑

CMS: 100-04,10,40.2

G0161 **Services performed by a qualified speech-language pathologist, in the home health setting, in the establishment or delivery of a safe and effective speech-language pathology maintenance program, each 15 minutes** B ☑

CMS: 100-04,10,40.2

G0162 Skilled services by a registered nurse (RN) for management and evaluation of the plan of care; each 15 minutes (the patient's underlying condition or complication requires an RN to ensure that essential nonskilled care achieves its purpose in the home health or hospice setting)
CMS: 100-04,10,40.2; 100-04,11,10

G0166 External counterpulsation, per treatment session
CMS: 100-04,32,130; 100-04,32,130.1

G0168 Wound closure utilizing tissue adhesive(s) only

G0175 Scheduled interdisciplinary team conference (minimum of three exclusive of patient care nursing staff) with patient present
CMS: 100-04,4,160

G0176 Activity therapy, such as music, dance, art or play therapies not for recreation, related to the care and treatment of patient's disabling mental health problems, per session (45 minutes or more)
CMS: 100-04,4,260.1; 100-04,4,260.1.1; 100-04,4,260.5

G0177 Training and educational services related to the care and treatment of patient's disabling mental health problems per session (45 minutes or more)
CMS: 100-04,4,260.1; 100-04,4,260.1.1

G0179 Physician or allowed practitioner re-certification for Medicare-covered home health services under a home health plan of care (patient not present), including contacts with home health agency and review of reports of patient status required by physicians and allowed practitioners to affirm the initial implementation of the plan of care
CMS: 100-02,7,30.5.4; 100-04,10,20.1.2; 100-04,12,180; 100-04,12,180.1

G0180 Physician or allowed practitioner certification for Medicare-covered home health services under a home health plan of care (patient not present), including contacts with home health agency and review of reports of patient status required by physicians or allowed practitioners to affirm the initial implementation of the plan of care
CMS: 100-02,7,30.5.4; 100-04,10,20.1.2; 100-04,12,180; 100-04,12,180.1

G0181 Physician or allowed practitioner supervision of a patient receiving Medicare-covered services provided by a participating home health agency (patient not present) requiring complex and multidisciplinary care modalities involving regular physician or allowed practitioner development and/or revision of care plans
CMS: 100-04,12,100.1.4; 100-04,12,180; 100-04,12,180.1

G0182 Physician supervision of a patient under a Medicare-approved hospice (patient not present) requiring complex and multidisciplinary care modalities involving regular physician development and/or revision of care plans, review of subsequent reports of patient status, review of laboratory and other studies, communication (including telephone calls) with other health care professionals involved in the patient's care, integration of new information into the medical treatment plan and/or adjustment of medical therapy, within a calendar month, 30 minutes or more
CMS: 100-04,11,40.1.3.1; 100-04,12,100.1.4; 100-04,12,180; 100-04,12,180.1

G0186 Destruction of localized lesion of choroid (for example, choroidal neovascularization); photocoagulation, feeder vessel technique (one or more sessions)

G0219 PET imaging whole body; melanoma for noncovered indications
CMS: 100-03,220.6.10; 100-03,220.6.12; 100-03,220.6.17; 100-03,220.6.3; 100-03,220.6.4; 100-03,220.6.6; 100-03,220.6.7; 100-04,13,60; 100-04,13,60.16

G0235 PET imaging, any site, not otherwise specified
CMS: 100-03,220.6.10; 100-03,220.6.12; 100-03,220.6.13; 100-03,220.6.17; 100-03,220.6.2; 100-03,220.6.3; 100-03,220.6.4; 100-03,220.6.5; 100-03,220.6.6; 100-03,220.6.7; 100-03,220.6.9; 100-04,13,60; 100-04,13,60.13; 100-04,13,60.14; 100-04,13,60.16; 100-04,13,60.17

G0237 Therapeutic procedures to increase strength or endurance of respiratory muscles, face-to-face, one-on-one, each 15 minutes (includes monitoring)
CMS: 100-02,12,30.1; 100-02,12,40.5

G0238 Therapeutic procedures to improve respiratory function, other than described by G0237, one-on-one, face-to-face, per 15 minutes (includes monitoring)
CMS: 100-02,12,30.1; 100-02,12,40.5

G0239 Therapeutic procedures to improve respiratory function or increase strength or endurance of respiratory muscles, two or more individuals (includes monitoring)
CMS: 100-02,12,30.1; 100-02,12,40.5

G0245 Initial physician evaluation and management of a diabetic patient with diabetic sensory neuropathy resulting in a loss of protective sensation (LOPS) which must include: (1) the diagnosis of LOPS, (2) a patient history, (3) a physical examination that consists of at least the following elements: (a) visual inspection of the forefoot, hindfoot, and toe web spaces, (b) evaluation of a protective sensation, (c) evaluation of foot structure and biomechanics, (d) evaluation of vascular status and skin integrity, and (e) evaluation and recommendation of footwear, and (4) patient education
CMS: 100-04,32,80.2; 100-04,32,80.3; 100-04,32,80.6; 100-04,32,80.8

G0246 Follow-up physician evaluation and management of a diabetic patient with diabetic sensory neuropathy resulting in a loss of protective sensation (LOPS) to include at least the following: (1) a patient history, (2) a physical examination that includes: (a) visual inspection of the forefoot, hindfoot, and toe web spaces, (b) evaluation of protective sensation, (c) evaluation of foot structure and biomechanics, (d) evaluation of vascular status and skin integrity, and (e) evaluation and recommendation of footwear, and (3) patient education
CMS: 100-03,70.2.1; 100-04,32,80; 100-04,32,80.2; 100-04,32,80.3; 100-04,32,80.6; 100-04,32,80.8

G0247 Routine foot care by a physician of a diabetic patient with diabetic sensory neuropathy resulting in a loss of protective sensation (LOPS) to include the local care of superficial wounds (i.e., superficial to muscle and fascia) and at least the following, if present: (1) local care of superficial wounds, (2) debridement of corns and calluses, and (3) trimming and debridement of nails
CMS: 100-03,70.2.1; 100-04,32,80; 100-04,32,80.2; 100-04,32,80.3; 100-04,32,80.6; 100-04,32,80.8

G0248 Demonstration, prior to initiation of home INR monitoring, for patient with either mechanical heart valve(s), chronic atrial fibrillation, or venous thromboembolism who meets Medicare coverage criteria, under the direction of a physician; includes: face-to-face demonstration of use and care of the INR monitor, obtaining at least one blood sample, provision of instructions for reporting home INR test results, and documentation of patient's ability to perform testing and report results
CMS: 100-03,190.11; 100-04,32,80

G0249 Provision of test materials and equipment for home INR monitoring of patient with either mechanical heart valve(s), chronic atrial fibrillation, or venous thromboembolism who meets Medicare coverage criteria; includes: provision of materials for use in the home and reporting of test results to physician; testing not occurring more frequently than once a week; testing materials, billing units of service include four tests V ☑
CMS: 100-03,190.11

G0250 Physician review, interpretation, and patient management of home INR testing for patient with either mechanical heart valve(s), chronic atrial fibrillation, or venous thromboembolism who meets Medicare coverage criteria; testing not occurring more frequently than once a week; billing units of service include four tests M ☑ ⊘
CMS: 100-03,190.11

G0252 PET imaging, full and partial-ring PET scanners only, for initial diagnosis of breast cancer and/or surgical planning for breast cancer (e.g., initial staging of axillary lymph nodes) E1
CMS: 100-03,220.6.10; 100-03,220.6.3; 100-04,13,60; 100-04,13,60.16

G0255 Current perception threshold/sensory nerve conduction test, (SNCT) per limb, any nerve E1

G0257 Unscheduled or emergency dialysis treatment for an ESRD patient in a hospital outpatient department that is not certified as an ESRD facility S
CMS: 100-04,4,200.2; 100-04,8,60.4.7

G0259 Injection procedure for sacroiliac joint; arthrography N

G0260 Injection procedure for sacroiliac joint; provision of anesthetic, steroid and/or other therapeutic agent, with or without arthrography T A2
AHA: 4Q,21

G0268 Removal of impacted cerumen (one or both ears) by physician on same date of service as audiologic function testing N ⊘

G0269 Placement of occlusive device into either a venous or arterial access site, postsurgical or interventional procedure (e.g., angioseal plug, vascular plug) N ⊘
AHA: 3Q,22

G0270 Medical nutrition therapy; reassessment and subsequent intervention(s) following second referral in same year for change in diagnosis, medical condition or treatment regimen (including additional hours needed for renal disease), individual, face-to-face with the patient, each 15 minutes A ☑ ⊘
CMS: 100-04,12,190.3; 100-04,12,190.6; 100-04,12,190.6.1; 100-04,12,190.7; 100-04,18,1.2
AHA: 3Q,19

G0271 Medical nutrition therapy, reassessment and subsequent intervention(s) following second referral in same year for change in diagnosis, medical condition, or treatment regimen (including additional hours needed for renal disease), group (two or more individuals), each 30 minutes A ☑ ⊘
CMS: 100-04,18,1.2

G0276 Blinded procedure for lumbar stenosis, percutaneous image-guided lumbar decompression (PILD) or placebo-control, performed in an approved coverage with evidence development (CED) clinical trial J G2
CMS: 100-03,150.13; 100-04,32,330.1; 100-04,32,330.2

G0277 Hyperbaric oxygen under pressure, full body chamber, per 30 minute interval S
CMS: 100-04,32,30.1

G0278 Iliac and/or femoral artery angiography, nonselective, bilateral or ipsilateral to catheter insertion, performed at the same time as cardiac catheterization and/or coronary angiography, includes positioning or placement of the catheter in the distal aorta or ipsilateral femoral or iliac artery, injection of dye, production of permanent images, and radiologic supervision and interpretation (List separately in addition to primary procedure) N N1 ⊘
AHA: 3Q,22

G0279 Diagnostic digital breast tomosynthesis, unilateral or bilateral (list separately in addition to 77065 or 77066) A
CMS: 100-04,18,20.2; 100-04,18,20.2.1; 100-04,18,20.2.2; 100-04,18,20.6

G0281 Electrical stimulation, (unattended), to one or more areas, for chronic Stage III and Stage IV pressure ulcers, arterial ulcers, diabetic ulcers, and venous stasis ulcers not demonstrating measurable signs of healing after 30 days of conventional care, as part of a therapy plan of care A
CMS: 100-02,15,220.4; 100-04,32,11.1; 100-04,5,10.3.2; 100-04,5,10.3.3

G0282 Electrical stimulation, (unattended), to one or more areas, for wound care other than described in G0281 E1
CMS: 100-04,32,11.1

G0283 Electrical stimulation (unattended), to one or more areas for indication(s) other than wound care, as part of a therapy plan of care A
CMS: 100-02,15,220.4; 100-04,5,10.3.2; 100-04,5,10.3.3

G0288 Reconstruction, computed tomographic angiography of aorta for surgical planning for vascular surgery N

G0289 Arthroscopy, knee, surgical, for removal of loose body, foreign body, debridement/shaving of articular cartilage (chondroplasty) at the time of other surgical knee arthroscopy in a different compartment of the same knee N ⊘
AHA: 4Q,20

G0293 Noncovered surgical procedure(s) using conscious sedation, regional, general, or spinal anesthesia in a Medicare qualifying clinical trial, per day Q1 ☑

G0294 Noncovered procedure(s) using either no anesthesia or local anesthesia only, in a Medicare qualifying clinical trial, per day Q1 ☑

G0295 Electromagnetic therapy, to one or more areas, for wound care other than described in G0329 or for other uses E1

G0296 Counseling visit to discuss need for lung cancer screening using low dose CT scan (LDCT) (service is for eligibility determination and shared decision making) S
CMS: 100-02,13,220; 100-02,13,220.1; 100-02,13,220.3; 100-04,18,1.2; 100-04,18,220; 100-04,18,220.1; 100-04,18,220.2; 100-04,18,220.3; 100-04,18,220.4; 100-04,18,220.5; 1004-04,13,220.1
AHA: 3Q,19

G0299 Direct skilled nursing services of a registered nurse (RN) in the home health or hospice setting, each 15 minutes B
CMS: 100-01,3,30.3; 100-04,10,40.2; 100-04,11,130.1; 100-04,11,30.3

G0300 Direct skilled nursing services of a licensed practical nurse (LPN) in the home health or hospice setting, each 15 minutes B
CMS: 100-01,3,30.3; 100-04,10,40.2; 100-04,11,130.1; 100-04,11,30.3

G0302 Preoperative pulmonary surgery services for preparation for LVRS, complete course of services, to include a minimum of 16 days of services S ☑

G0303 Preoperative pulmonary surgery services for preparation for LVRS, 10 to 15 days of services S ☑

G0304 Preoperative pulmonary surgery services for preparation for LVRS, 1 to 9 days of services S ☑

G0305 **Postdischarge pulmonary surgery services after LVRS, minimum of 6 days of services** S ☑

G0306 **Complete CBC, automated (HgB, HCT, RBC, WBC, without platelet count) and automated WBC differential count** Q
CMS: 100-02,11,20.2

G0307 **Complete CBC, automated (HgB, HCT, RBC, WBC; without platelet count)** Q
CMS: 100-02,11,20.2

G0310 **Immunization counseling by a physician or other qualified health care professional when the vaccine(s) is not administered on the same date of service, 5-15 minutes time (This code is used for Medicaid billing purposes)** E
AHA: 4Q,22

G0311 **Immunization counseling by a physician or other qualified health care professional when the vaccine(s) is not administered on the same date of service, 16-30 minutes time (This code is used for Medicaid billing purposes)** E
AHA: 4Q,22

G0312 **Immunization counseling by a physician or other qualified health care professional when the vaccine(s) is not administered on the same date of service for ages under 21, 5-15 minutes time (This code is used for Medicaid billing purposes)** E
AHA: 4Q,22

G0313 **Immunization counseling by a physician or other qualified health care professional when the vaccine(s) is not administered on the same date of service for ages under 21, 16-30 minutes time (This code is used for Medicaid billing purposes)** E
AHA: 4Q,22

G0314 **Immunization counseling by a physician or other qualified health care professional for COVID-19, ages under 21, 16-30 minutes time (This code is used for the Medicaid Early and Periodic Screening, Diagnostic, and Treatment Benefit [EPSDT])** E
AHA: 4Q,22

G0315 **Immunization counseling by a physician or other qualified health care professional for COVID-19, ages under 21, 5-15 minutes time (This code is used for the Medicaid Early and Periodic Screening, Diagnostic, and Treatment Benefit [EPSDT])** E
AHA: 4Q,22

G0316 **Prolonged hospital inpatient or observation care evaluation and management service(s) beyond the total time for the primary service (when the primary service has been selected using time on the date of the primary service); each additional 15 minutes by the physician or qualified healthcare professional, with or without direct patient contact (list separately in addition to CPT codes 99223, 99233, and 99236 for hospital inpatient or observation care evaluation and management services). (Do not report G0316 on the same date of service as other prolonged services for evaluation and management codes 99358, 99359, 99418, 99415, 99416). (Do not report G0316 for any time unit less than 15 minutes)** N
CMS: 100-04,12,30.6.15.3
AHA: 1Q,23

G0317 **Prolonged nursing facility evaluation and management service(s) beyond the total time for the primary service (when the primary service has been selected using time on the date of the primary service); each additional 15 minutes by the physician or qualified healthcare professional, with or without direct patient contact (list separately in addition to CPT codes 99306, 99310 for nursing facility evaluation and management services). (Do not report G0317 on the same date of service as other prolonged services for evaluation and management codes 99358, 99359, 99418). (Do not report G0317 for any time unit less than 15 minutes)** B
CMS: 100-04,12,30.6.13; 100-04,12,30.6.15.3

G0318 **Prolonged home or residence evaluation and management service(s) beyond the total time for the primary service (when the primary service has been selected using time on the date of the primary service); each additional 15 minutes by the physician or qualified healthcare professional, with or without direct patient contact (list separately in addition to CPT codes 99345, 99350 for home or residence evaluation and management services). (Do not report G0318 on the same date of service as other prolonged services for evaluation and management codes 99358, 99359, 99417). (Do not report G0318 for any time unit less than 15 minutes)** B
CMS: 100-04,12,30.6.15.3

G0320 **Home health services furnished using synchronous telemedicine rendered via a real-time two-way audio and video telecommunications system** A
CMS: 100-04,10,30.9; 100-04,10,40.2
AHA: 1Q,23

G0321 **Home health services furnished using synchronous telemedicine rendered via telephone or other real-time interactive audio-only telecommunications system** A
CMS: 100-04,10,30.9; 100-04,10,40.2
AHA: 1Q,23

G0322 **The collection of physiologic data digitally stored and/or transmitted by the patient to the home health agency (i.e., remote patient monitoring)** A
CMS: 100-04,10,40.2
AHA: 1Q,23

▲ **G0323** **Care management services for behavioral health conditions, at least 20 minutes of clinical psychologist, clinical social worker, mental health counselor, or marriage and family therapist time, per calendar month. (These services include the following required elements: initial assessment or follow-up monitoring, including the use of applicable validated rating scales; behavioral health care planning in relation to behavioral/psychiatric health problems, including revision for patients who are not progressing or whose status changes; facilitating and coordinating treatment such as psychotherapy, coordination with and/or referral to physicians and practitioners who are authorized by Medicare to prescribe medications and furnish E/M services, counseling and/or psychiatric consultation; and continuity of care with a designated member of the care team)** S
AHA: 1Q,24

G0327 **Colorectal cancer screening; blood-based biomarker** A
CMS: 100-02,15,280.2.2; 100-04,18,1.2; 100-04,18,60; 100-04,18,60.1; 100-04,18,60.1.1; 100-04,18,60.2; 100-04,18,60.2.1; 100-04,18,60.6; 100-04,18,60.7; 100-04,18,60.8
AHA: 3Q,21

G0328 **Colorectal cancer screening; fecal occult blood test, immunoassay, one to three simultaneous determinations** A
CMS: 100-02,15,280.2.2; 100-04,16,70.8; 100-04,18,1.2; 100-04,18,60; 100-04,18,60.1; 100-04,18,60.1.1; 100-04,18,60.2; 100-04,18,60.2.1; 100-04,18,60.6; 100-04,18,60.7
AHA: 3Q,23

G0329 **Electromagnetic therapy, to one or more areas for chronic Stage III and Stage IV pressure ulcers, arterial ulcers, diabetic ulcers and venous stasis ulcers not demonstrating measurable signs of healing after 30 days of conventional care as part of a therapy plan of care** A
CMS: 100-02,15,220.4; 100-04,32,11.2; 100-04,5,10.3.2; 100-04,5,10.3.3

G0330 **Facility services for dental rehabilitation procedure(s) performed on a patient who requires monitored anesthesia (e.g., general, intravenous sedation (monitored anesthesia care) and use of an operating room** J

G0333 **Pharmacy dispensing fee for inhalation drug(s); initial 30-day supply as a beneficiary** M

G0337 **Hospice evaluation and counseling services, preelection** B
CMS: 100-04,11,10

G0339 **Image guided robotic linear accelerator-based stereotactic radiosurgery, complete course of therapy in one session or first session of fractionated treatment** B ⊘

G0340 **Image guided robotic linear accelerator-based stereotactic radiosurgery, delivery including collimator changes and custom plugging, fractionated treatment, all lesions, per session, second through fifth sessions, maximum five sessions per course of treatment** B ⊘

G0341 **Percutaneous islet cell transplant, includes portal vein catheterization and infusion** C ⊘
CMS: 100-04,32,70

G0342 **Laparoscopy for islet cell transplant, includes portal vein catheterization and infusion** C ⊘
CMS: 100-04,32,70

G0343 **Laparotomy for islet cell transplant, includes portal vein catheterization and infusion** C ⊘
CMS: 100-04,32,70

G0372 **Physician service required to establish and document the need for a power mobility device** M ⊘
CMS: 100-04,12,30.6.15.4

Observation/Emergency Department Services

G0378 **Hospital observation service, per hour** N
CMS: 100-02,6,20.6; 100-04,01,50.3.2; 100-04,4,290.1; 100-04,4,290.2.2; 100-04,4,290.4.1; 100-04,4,290.4.2; 100-04,4,290.4.3; 100-04,4,290.5.1; 100-04,4,290.5.2; 100-04,4,290.5.3

G0379 **Direct admission of patient for hospital observation care** J
CMS: 100-02,6,20.6; 100-04,4,290.4.1; 100-04,4,290.4.2; 100-04,4,290.4.3; 100-04,4,290.5.1; 100-04,4,290.5.2; 100-04,4,290.5.3

G0380 **Level 1 hospital emergency department visit provided in a type B emergency department; (the ED must meet at least one of the following requirements: (1) it is licensed by the state in which it is located under applicable state law as an emergency room or emergency department; (2) it is held out to the public (by name, posted signs, advertising, or other means) as a place that provides care for emergency medical conditions on an urgent basis without requiring a previously scheduled appointment; or (3) during the calendar year immediately preceding the calendar year in which a determination under 42 CFR 489.24 is being made, based on a representative sample of patient visits that occurred during that calendar year, it provides at least one-third of all of its outpatient visits for the treatment of emergency medical conditions on an urgent basis without requiring a previously scheduled appointment)** J
CMS: 100-04,4,160

G0381 **Level 2 hospital emergency department visit provided in a type B emergency department; (the ED must meet at least one of the following requirements: (1) it is licensed by the state in which it is located under applicable state law as an emergency room or emergency department; (2) it is held out to the public (by name, posted signs, advertising, or other means) as a place that provides care for emergency medical conditions on an urgent basis without requiring a previously scheduled appointment; or (3) during the calendar year immediately preceding the calendar year in which a determination under 42 CFR 489.24 is being made, based on a representative sample of patient visits that occurred during that calendar year, it provides at least one-third of all of its outpatient visits for the treatment of emergency medical conditions on an urgent basis without requiring a previously scheduled appointment)** J
CMS: 100-04,4,160

G0382 **Level 3 hospital emergency department visit provided in a type B emergency department; (the ED must meet at least one of the following requirements: (1) it is licensed by the state in which it is located under applicable state law as an emergency room or emergency department; (2) it is held out to the public (by name, posted signs, advertising, or other means) as a place that provides care for emergency medical conditions on an urgent basis without requiring a previously scheduled appointment; or (3) during the calendar year immediately preceding the calendar year in which a determination under 42 CFR 489.24 is being made, based on a representative sample of patient visits that occurred during that calendar year, it provides at least one-third of all of its outpatient visits for the treatment of emergency medical conditions on an urgent basis without requiring a previously scheduled appointment)** J
CMS: 100-04,4,160

G0383 **Level 4 hospital emergency department visit provided in a type B emergency department; (the ED must meet at least one of the following requirements: (1) it is licensed by the state in which it is located under applicable state law as an emergency room or emergency department; (2) it is held out to the public (by name, posted signs, advertising, or other means) as a place that provides care for emergency medical conditions on an urgent basis without requiring a previously scheduled appointment; or (3) during the calendar year immediately preceding the calendar year in which a determination under 42 CFR 489.24 is being made, based on a representative sample of patient visits that occurred during that calendar year, it provides at least one-third of all of its outpatient visits for the treatment of emergency medical conditions on an urgent basis without requiring a previously scheduled appointment)** J
CMS: 100-04,4,160

G0384 **Level 5 hospital emergency department visit provided in a type B emergency department; (the ED must meet at least one of the following requirements: (1) it is licensed by the state in which it is located under applicable state law as an emergency room or emergency department; (2) it is held out to the public (by name, posted signs, advertising, or other means) as a place that provides care for emergency medical conditions on an urgent basis without requiring a previously scheduled appointment; or (3) during the calendar year immediately preceding the calendar year in which a determination under 42 CFR 489.24 is being made, based on a representative sample of patient visits that occurred during that calendar year, it provides at least one-third of all of its outpatient visits for the treatment of emergency medical conditions on an urgent basis without requiring a previously scheduled appointment)** J
CMS: 100-04,4,160; 100-04,4,290.5.1

Other Services

G0390 **Trauma response team associated with hospital critical care service** S
CMS: 100-04,4,160.1

Alcohol or Substance Abuse

G0396 **Alcohol and/or substance (other than tobacco) misuse structured assessment (e.g., audit, dast), and brief intervention 15 to 30 minutes** S ☑ ⊘
CMS: 100-04,12,190.3; 100-04,12,190.6; 100-04,12,190.6.1; 100-04,12,190.7; 100-04,4,200.6
AHA: 3Q,19

G0397 **Alcohol and/or substance (other than tobacco) misuse structured assessment (e.g., audit, dast), and intervention, greater than 30 minutes** S ☑ ⊘
CMS: 100-04,12,190.3; 100-04,12,190.6; 100-04,12,190.6.1; 100-04,12,190.7; 100-04,4,200.6
AHA: 3Q,19

Home Sleep Study

G0398 **Home sleep study test (HST) with type II portable monitor, unattended; minimum of 7 channels: EEG, EOG, EMG, ECG/heart rate, airflow, respiratory effort and oxygen saturation** S
CMS: 100-03,240.4

G0399 **Home sleep test (HST) with type III portable monitor, unattended; minimum of 4 channels: 2 respiratory movement/airflow, 1 ECG/heart rate and 1 oxygen saturation** S
CMS: 100-03,240.4

G0400 **Home sleep test (HST) with type IV portable monitor, unattended; minimum of 3 channels** S
CMS: 100-03,240.4

Initial Physical Exam

G0402 **Initial preventive physical examination; face-to-face visit, services limited to new beneficiary during the first 12 months of Medicare enrollment** V ⊘
CMS: 100-02,13,220; 100-02,13,220.1; 100-02,13,220.3; 100-04,12,100.1.1; 100-04,18,1.2; 100-04,18,140.6; 100-04,18,80; 100-04,18,80.1; 100-04,18,80.2; 100-04,18,80.3.3; 100-04,18,80.4; 1004-04,13,220.1

G0403 **Electrocardiogram, routine ECG with 12 leads; performed as a screening for the initial preventive physical examination with interpretation and report** M
CMS: 100-04,18,1.2; 100-04,18,80; 100-04,18,80.1; 100-04,18,80.2

G0404 **Electrocardiogram, routine ECG with 12 leads; tracing only, without interpretation and report, performed as a screening for the initial preventive physical examination** S
CMS: 100-04,18,1.2; 100-04,18,80; 100-04,18,80.1; 100-04,18,80.2; 100-04,18,80.3.3

G0405 **Electrocardiogram, routine ECG with 12 leads; interpretation and report only, performed as a screening for the initial preventive physical examination** B ⊘
CMS: 100-04,18,1.2; 100-04,18,80; 100-04,18,80.1; 100-04,18,80.2

Follow-up Telehealth

G0406 **Follow-up inpatient consultation, limited, physicians typically spend 15 minutes communicating with the patient via telehealth** B ⊘
CMS: 100-04,12,190.3; 100-04,12,190.3.1; 100-04,12,190.3.3; 100-04,12,190.3.5; 100-04,12,190.6; 100-04,12,190.6.1; 100-04,12,190.7
AHA: 3Q,19

G0407 **Follow-up inpatient consultation, intermediate, physicians typically spend 25 minutes communicating with the patient via telehealth** B ⊘
CMS: 100-04,12,190.3; 100-04,12,190.3.1; 100-04,12,190.3.3; 100-04,12,190.3.5; 100-04,12,190.6; 100-04,12,190.6.1; 100-04,12,190.7
AHA: 3Q,19

G0408 **Follow-up inpatient consultation, complex, physicians typically spend 35 minutes communicating with the patient via telehealth** B ⊘
CMS: 100-04,12,190.3; 100-04,12,190.3.1; 100-04,12,190.3.3; 100-04,12,190.3.5; 100-04,12,190.6; 100-04,12,190.6.1; 100-04,12,190.7
AHA: 3Q,19

Psychological Services

G0409 **Social work and psychological services, directly relating to and/or furthering the patient's rehabilitation goals, each 15 minutes, face-to-face; individual (services provided by a CORF qualified social worker or psychologist in a CORF)** B ☑
CMS: 100-02,12,30.1; 100-04,5,100.11; 100-04,5,100.4

G0410 **Group psychotherapy other than of a multiple-family group, in a partial hospitalization or intensive outpatient setting, approximately 45 to 50 minutes** P
CMS: 100-04,4,260.1; 100-04,4,260.1.1
AHA: 1Q,24

G0411 **Interactive group psychotherapy, in a partial hospitalization or intensive outpatient setting, approximately 45 to 50 minutes** P
CMS: 100-04,4,260.1; 100-04,4,260.1.1
AHA: 1Q,24

Fracture Care

G0412 **Open treatment of iliac spine(s), tuberosity avulsion, or iliac wing fracture(s), unilateral or bilateral for pelvic bone fracture patterns which do not disrupt the pelvic ring, includes internal fixation, when performed** C ⊘

G0413 **Percutaneous skeletal fixation of posterior pelvic bone fracture and/or dislocation, for fracture patterns which disrupt the pelvic ring, unilateral or bilateral, (includes ilium, sacroiliac joint and/or sacrum)** J ⊘

G0414 **Open treatment of anterior pelvic bone fracture and/or dislocation for fracture patterns which disrupt the pelvic ring, unilateral or bilateral, includes internal fixation when performed (includes pubic symphysis and/or superior/inferior rami)** C ⊘

G0415 **Open treatment of posterior pelvic bone fracture and/or dislocation, for fracture patterns which disrupt the pelvic ring, unilateral or bilateral, includes internal fixation, when performed (includes ilium, sacroiliac joint and/or sacrum)** C ⊘

Surgical Pathology

G0416 **Surgical pathology, gross and microscopic examinations, for prostate needle biopsy, any method** Q2
AHA: 2Q,22

Educational Services

G0420 **Face-to-face educational services related to the care of chronic kidney disease; individual, per session, per 1 hour** A ☑ ⊘
CMS: 100-02,15,200; 100-02,15,310; 100-02,15,310.1; 100-02,15,310.2; 100-02,15,310.4; 100-02,15,310.5; 100-04,12,190.3; 100-04,12,190.6; 100-04,12,190.6.1; 100-04,12,190.7
AHA: 3Q,19

G0421 **Face-to-face educational services related to the care of chronic kidney disease; group, per session, per 1 hour** A ☑ ⊘
CMS: 100-02,15,200; 100-02,15,310; 100-02,15,310.1; 100-02,15,310.2; 100-02,15,310.4; 100-02,15,310.5; 100-04,12,190.3; 100-04,12,190.6; 100-04,12,190.6.1; 100-04,12,190.7
AHA: 3Q,19

Cardiac and Pulmonary Rehabilitation

G0422 **Intensive cardiac rehabilitation; with or without continuous ECG monitoring with exercise, per session** S ☑ ⊘
CMS: 100-02,15,232; 100-04,32,140.2.2.1; 100-04,32,140.2.2.2; 100-04,32,140.3; 100-04,32,140.3.1; 100-08,15,4.2.8

G0423 **Intensive cardiac rehabilitation; with or without continuous ECG monitoring; without exercise, per session** S ☑ ⊘
CMS: 100-02,15,232; 100-04,32,140.2.2.1; 100-04,32,140.2.2.2; 100-04,32,140.3; 100-04,32,140.3.1; 100-08,15,4.2.8

Inpatient Telehealth

G0425 **Telehealth consultation, emergency department or initial inpatient, typically 30 minutes communicating with the patient via telehealth** B ☑ ⊘
CMS: 100-04,12,190.3; 100-04,12,190.3.1; 100-04,12,190.3.2; 100-04,12,190.6; 100-04,12,190.6.1; 100-04,12,190.7
AHA: 3Q,19

G0426 Telehealth consultation, emergency department or initial inpatient, typically 50 minutes communicating with the patient via telehealth B ☑ ⊘
CMS: 100-04,12,190.3; 100-04,12,190.3.1; 100-04,12,190.3.2; 100-04,12,190.6; 100-04,12,190.6.1; 100-04,12,190.7
AHA: 3Q,19

G0427 Telehealth consultation, emergency department or initial inpatient, typically 70 minutes or more communicating with the patient via telehealth B ☑ ⊘
CMS: 100-04,12,190.3; 100-04,12,190.3.1; 100-04,12,190.3.2; 100-04,12,190.6; 100-04,12,190.6.1; 100-04,12,190.7
AHA: 3Q,19

Defect Fillers

G0428 Collagen meniscus implant procedure for filling meniscal defects (e.g., CMI, collagen scaffold, Menaflex) E1
CMS: 100-03,150.12

G0429 Dermal filler injection(s) for the treatment of facial lipodystrophy syndrome (LDS) (e.g., as a result of highly active antiretroviral therapy) T P3
CMS: 100-03,250.5; 100-04,32,260.1; 100-04,32,260.2.1; 100-04,32,260.2.2

Laboratory Services

G0432 Infectious agent antibody detection by enzyme immunoassay (EIA) technique, HIV-1 and/or HIV-2, screening A
CMS: 100-03,190.14; 100-03,190.9; 100-03,210.7; 100-04,18,1.2; 100-04,18,130.1; 100-04,18,130.2; 100-04,18,130.3; 100-04,18,130.4; 100-04,18,130.5

G0433 Infectious agent antibody detection by enzyme-linked immunosorbent assay (ELISA) technique, HIV-1 and/or HIV-2, screening A
CMS: 100-03,190.14; 100-03,190.9; 100-03,210.7; 100-04,16,70.8; 100-04,18,1.2; 100-04,18,130.1; 100-04,18,130.2; 100-04,18,130.3; 100-04,18,130.4; 100-04,18,130.5

G0435 Infectious agent antibody detection by rapid antibody test, HIV-1 and/or HIV-2, screening A
CMS: 100-03,190.14; 100-03,190.9; 100-03,210.7; 100-04,18,1.2; 100-04,18,130.1; 100-04,18,130.2; 100-04,18,130.3; 100-04,18,130.4; 100-04,18,130.5

Counseling and Wellness Visit

G0438 Annual wellness visit; includes a personalized prevention plan of service (PPS), initial visit A
CMS: 100-02,13,220; 100-02,13,220.1; 100-02,13,220.3; 100-02,15,280.5; 100-02,15,280.5.1; 100-02,15,280.5.2; 100-04,12,100.1.1; 100-04,18,1.2; 100-04,18,140; 100-04,18,140.1; 100-04,18,140.5; 100-04,18,140.6; 100-04,18,140.8; 100-04,18,140.9; 100-04,4,200.11; 1004-04,13,220.1
AHA: 3Q,19

G0439 Annual wellness visit, includes a personalized prevention plan of service (PPS), subsequent visit A
CMS: 100-02,13,220; 100-02,13,220.1; 100-02,13,220.3; 100-02,15,280.5; 100-02,15,280.5.1; 100-02,15,280.5.2; 100-04,12,100.1.1; 100-04,18,1.2; 100-04,18,140; 100-04,18,140.1; 100-04,18,140.5; 100-04,18,140.6; 100-04,18,140.8; 100-04,18,140.9; 100-04,4,200.11; 1004-04,13,220.1
AHA: 3Q,19

Other Services

G0442 Annual alcohol misuse screening, 5 to 15 minutes S ☑
CMS: 100-03,210.8; 100-04,12,190.3; 100-04,12,190.6; 100-04,12,190.6.1; 100-04,12,190.7; 100-04,18,180; 100-04,18,180.1; 100-04,18,180.2; 100-04,18,180.3; 100-04,18,180.4; 100-04,18,180.5; 100-04,32,180.4; 100-04,32,180.5
AHA: 3Q,19

G0443 Brief face-to-face behavioral counseling for alcohol misuse, 15 minutes S ☑
CMS: 100-03,210.8; 100-04,12,190.3; 100-04,12,190.6; 100-04,12,190.6.1; 100-04,12,190.7; 100-04,18,180; 100-04,18,180.1; 100-04,18,180.2; 100-04,18,180.3; 100-04,18,180.4; 100-04,18,180.5; 100-04,32,180.4; 100-04,32,180.5
AHA: 3Q,19

G0444 Annual depression screening, 5 to 15 minutes S ☑
CMS: 100-04,12,190.3; 100-04,12,190.6; 100-04,12,190.6.1; 100-04,12,190.7; 100-04,18,190; 100-04,18,190.1; 100-04,18,190.2; 100-04,18,190.3; 100-04,18,190.5
AHA: 3Q,19

G0445 Semiannual high intensity behavioral counseling to prevent STIs, individual, face-to-face, includes education skills training & guidance on how to change sexual behavior S ☑
CMS: 100-03,210.10; 100-04,12,190.3; 100-04,12,190.6; 100-04,12,190.6.1; 100-04,12,190.7; 100-04,18,170.1; 100-04,18,170.2; 100-04,18,170.3; 100-04,18,170.4; 100-04,18,170.4.1; 100-04,18,170.5
AHA: 3Q,19

G0446 Annual, face-to-face intensive behavioral therapy for cardiovascular disease, individual, 15 minutes S ☑
CMS: 100-03,210.11; 100-04,12,190.3; 100-04,12,190.6; 100-04,12,190.6.1; 100-04,12,190.7; 100-04,18,160; 100-04,18,160.1; 100-04,18,160.2.1; 100-04,18,160.2.2; 100-04,18,160.3; 100-04,18,160.4; 100-04,18,160.5
AHA: 3Q,19

G0447 Face-to-face behavioral counseling for obesity, 15 minutes S ☑
CMS: 100-03,210.12; 100-04,12,190.3; 100-04,12,190.6; 100-04,12,190.6.1; 100-04,12,190.7; 100-04,18,1.2; 100-04,18,200; 100-04,18,200.1; 100-04,18,200.2; 100-04,18,200.3; 100-04,18,200.4; 100-04,18,200.5
AHA: 3Q,19

G0448 Insertion or replacement of a permanent pacing cardioverter-defibrillator system with transvenous lead(s), single or dual chamber with insertion of pacing electrode, cardiac venous system, for left ventricular pacing B
CMS: 100-04,32,270; 100-04,32,270.1; 100-04,32,270.2; 100-04,32,270.3

G0451 Development testing, with interpretation and report, per standardized instrument form Q3
CMS: 100-02,15,220.4; 100-04,5,10.3.2; 100-04,5,10.3.3

Molecular Pathology

G0452 Molecular pathology procedure; physician interpretation and report B

Neurophysiology Monitoring

G0453 Continuous intraoperative neurophysiology monitoring, from outside the operating room (remote or nearby), per patient, (attention directed exclusively to one patient) each 15 minutes (list in addition to primary procedure) N

Documentation and Preparation

G0454 Physician documentation of face-to-face visit for durable medical equipment determination performed by nurse practitioner, physician assistant or clinical nurse specialist B

G0455 Preparation with instillation of fecal microbiota by any method, including assessment of donor specimen T

Prostate Brachytherapy

G0458 Low dose rate (LDR) prostate brachytherapy services, composite rate B

Inpatient Telehealth Pharmacologic Management

G0459 Inpatient telehealth pharmacologic management, including prescription, use, and review of medication with no more than minimal medical psychotherapy B
CMS: 100-04,12,190.3; 100-04,12,190.6; 100-04,12,190.6.1; 100-04,12,190.7
AHA: 3Q,19

Other Wound/Ulcer Care

G0460 Autologous platelet rich plasma (PRP) or other blood-derived product for nondiabetic chronic wounds/ulcers (includes, as applicable: administration, dressings, phlebotomy, centrifugation or mixing, and all other preparatory procedures, per treatment) T
CMS: 100-03,270.3; 100-04,32,11.3.1; 100-04,32,11.3.2; 100-04,32,11.3.3; 100-04,32,11.3.4; 100-04,32,11.3.5; 100-04,32,11.3.6
AHA: 3Q,23; 3Q,22

Hospital Outpatient Visit

G0463 Hospital outpatient clinic visit for assessment and management of a patient J
CMS: 100-04,32,130.1; 100-04,4,160.2; 100-04,4,260.1; 100-04,4,260.1.1; 100-04,4,290.5.1; 100-04,4,290.5.3; 100-04,6,20.1.1.2; 100-04,6,30.4.1
AHA: 4Q,20; 2Q,20

Platelet Rich Plasma

G0465 Autologous platelet rich plasma (PRP) or other blood-derived product for diabetic chronic wounds/ulcers, using an FDA-cleared device for this indication, (includes, as applicable: administration, dressings, phlebotomy, centrifugation or mixing, and all other preparatory procedures, per treatment) T
CMS: 100-04,32,11.3.1; 100-04,32,11.3.2; 100-04,32,11.3.3; 100-04,32,11.3.4; 100-04,32,11.3.5; 100-04,32,11.3.6
AHA: 3Q,23; 3Q,22

Federally Qualified Health Center Visits

G0466 Federally qualified health center (FQHC) visit, new patient A
CMS: 100-04,9,60.6

G0467 Federally qualified health center (FQHC) visit, established patient A
CMS: 100-04,9,60.6

G0468 Federally qualified health center (FQHC) visit, initial preventive physical exam (IPPE) or annual wellness visit (AWV) A
CMS: 100-04,9,60.6

G0469 Federally qualified health center (FQHC) visit, mental health, new patient A
CMS: 100-04,9,60.6

G0470 Federally qualified health center (FQHC) visit, mental health, established patient A
CMS: 100-04,9,60.6

HHA and SNF Specimen Collection

G0471 Collection of venous blood by venipuncture or urine sample by catheterization from an individual in a skilled nursing facility (SNF) or by a laboratory on behalf of a home health agency (HHA) A
CMS: 100-04,16,60.1.2; 100-04,16,60.1.4

Hepatitis C Screening

G0472 Hepatitis C antibody screening for individual at high risk and other covered indication(s) A
CMS: 100-02,13,220; 100-02,13,220.1; 100-02,13,220.3; 100-03,210.13; 100-04,18,1.2; 100-04,18,210; 100-04,18,210.2; 100-04,18,210.3; 100-04,18,210.4; 1004-04,13,220.1

Behavioral Counseling

G0473 Face-to-face behavioral counseling for obesity, group (2-10), 30 minutes S
CMS: 100-04,18,1.2; 100-04,18,200.1; 100-04,18,200.2; 100-04,18,200.3; 100-04,18,200.4; 100-04,18,200.5

Screening Measures

G0475 HIV antigen/antibody, combination assay, screening A
CMS: 100-03,210.7; 100-04,18,130.1; 100-04,18,130.2; 100-04,18,130.3; 100-04,18,130.5

G0476 Infectious agent detection by nucleic acid (DNA or RNA); human papillomavirus HPV), high-risk types (e.g., 16, 18, 31, 33, 35, 39, 45, 51, 52, 56, 58, 59, 68) for cervical cancer screening, must be performed in addition to pap test A
CMS: 100-03,210.2.1; 100-04,18,30.2.1; 100-04,18,30.5; 100-04,18,30.6; 100-04,18,30.8; 100-04,18,30.9

Drug Testing

G0480 Drug test(s), definitive, utilizing (1) drug identification methods able to identify individual drugs and distinguish between structural isomers (but not necessarily stereoisomers), including, but not limited to, GC/MS (any type, single or tandem) and LC/MS (any type, single or tandem and excluding immunoassays (e.g., IA, EIA, ELISA, EMIT, FPIA) and enzymatic methods (e.g., alcohol dehydrogenase)), (2) stable isotope or other universally recognized internal standards in all samples (e.g., to control for matrix effects, interferences and variations in signal strength), and (3) method or drug-specific calibration and matrix-matched quality control material (e.g., to control for instrument variations and mass spectral drift); qualitative or quantitative, all sources, includes specimen validity testing, per day; 1-7 drug class(es), including metabolite(s) if performed Q
AHA: 2Q,22; 1Q,18

G0481 Drug test(s), definitive, utilizing (1) drug identification methods able to identify individual drugs and distinguish between structural isomers (but not necessarily stereoisomers), including, but not limited to, GC/MS (any type, single or tandem) and LC/MS (any type, single or tandem and excluding immunoassays (e.g., IA, EIA, ELISA, EMIT, FPIA) and enzymatic methods (e.g., alcohol dehydrogenase)), (2) stable isotope or other universally recognized internal standards in all samples (e.g., to control for matrix effects, interferences and variations in signal strength), and (3) method or drug-specific calibration and matrix-matched quality control material (e.g., to control for instrument variations and mass spectral drift); qualitative or quantitative, all sources, includes specimen validity testing, per day; 8-14 drug class(es), including metabolite(s) if performed Q
AHA: 2Q,22; 1Q,18

G0482 Drug test(s), definitive, utilizing (1) drug identification methods able to identify individual drugs and distinguish between structural isomers (but not necessarily stereoisomers), including, but not limited to, GC/MS (any type, single or tandem) and LC/MS (any type, single or tandem and excluding immunoassays (e.g., IA, EIA, ELISA, EMIT, FPIA) and enzymatic methods (e.g., alcohol dehydrogenase)), (2) stable isotope or other universally recognized internal standards in all samples (e.g., to control for matrix effects, interferences and variations in signal strength), and (3) method or drug-specific calibration and matrix-matched quality control material (e.g., to control for instrument variations and mass spectral drift); qualitative or quantitative, all sources, includes specimen validity testing, per day; 15-21 drug class(es), including metabolite(s) if performed Q
AHA: 2Q,22; 1Q,18

G0483 Drug test(s), definitive, utilizing (1) drug identification methods able to identify individual drugs and distinguish between structural isomers (but not necessarily stereoisomers), including, but not limited to, GC/MS (any type, single or tandem) and LC/MS (any type, single or tandem and excluding immunoassays (e.g., IA, EIA, ELISA, EMIT, FPIA) and enzymatic methods (e.g., alcohol dehydrogenase)), (2) stable isotope or other universally recognized internal standards in all samples (e.g., to control for matrix effects, interferences and variations in signal strength), and (3) method or drug-specific calibration and matrix-matched quality control material (e.g., to control for instrument variations and mass spectral drift); qualitative or quantitative, all sources, includes specimen validity testing, per day; 22 or more drug class(es), including metabolite(s) if performed Q
AHA: 2Q,22; 1Q,18

Home Health Nursing Visit

G0490 Face-to-face home health nursing visit by a rural health clinic (RHC) or federally qualified health center (FQHC) in an area with a shortage of home health agencies; (services limited to RN or LPN only) A

Dialysis Procedures

G0491 Dialysis procedure at a Medicare certified ESRD facility for acute kidney injury without ESRD B
CMS: 100-04,8,40; 100-04,8,50.2

G0492 Dialysis procedure with single evaluation by a physician or other qualified health care professional for acute kidney injury without ESRD B

Skilled Nursing Services

G0493 Skilled services of a registered nurse (RN) for the observation and assessment of the patient's condition, each 15 minutes (the change in the patient's condition requires skilled nursing personnel to identify and evaluate the patient's need for possible modification of treatment in the home health or hospice setting) B
CMS: 100-04,10,40.2

G0494 Skilled services of a licensed practical nurse (LPN) for the observation and assessment of the patient's condition, each 15 minutes (the change in the patient's condition requires skilled nursing personnel to identify and evaluate the patient's need for possible modification of treatment in the home health or hospice setting) B
CMS: 100-04,10,40.2

G0495 Skilled services of a registered nurse (RN), in the training and/or education of a patient or family member, in the home health or hospice setting, each 15 minutes B
CMS: 100-04,10,40.2

G0496 Skilled services of a licensed practical nurse (LPN), in the training and/or education of a patient or family member, in the home health or hospice setting, each 15 minutes B
CMS: 100-04,10,40.2

Chemotherapy Infusion

G0498 Chemotherapy administration, intravenous infusion technique; initiation of infusion in the office/clinic setting using office/clinic pump/supplies, with continuation of the infusion in the community setting (e.g., home, domiciliary, rest home or assisted living) using a portable pump provided by the office/clinic, includes follow up office/clinic visit at the conclusion of the infusion S

Hepatitis B Screening

G0499 Hepatitis B screening in nonpregnant, high-risk individual includes hepatitis B surface antigen (HBSAG), antibodies to HBSAG (anti-HBS) and antibodies to hepatitis B core antigen (anti-HBC), and is followed by a neutralizing confirmatory test, when performed, only for an initially reactive HBSAG result A
CMS: 100-03,1,210.6; 100-04,18,230; 100-04,18,230.1; 100-04,18,230.2; 100-04,18,230.3; 100-04,18,230.4

Moderate Sedation

G0500 Moderate sedation services provided by the same physician or other qualified health care professional performing a gastrointestinal endoscopic service that sedation supports, requiring the presence of an independent trained observer to assist in the monitoring of the patient's level of consciousness and physiological status; initial 15 minutes of intra-service time; patient age 5 years or older (additional time may be reported with 99153, as appropriate) N
CMS: 100-04,18,60.1.1

Mobility-Assistive Technology

G0501 Resource-intensive services for patients for whom the use of specialized mobility-assistive technology (such as adjustable height chairs or tables, patient lift, and adjustable padded leg supports) is medically necessary and used during the provision of an office/outpatient, evaluation and management visit (list separately in addition to primary service) N

Care Management Services

G0506 Comprehensive assessment of and care planning for patients requiring chronic care management services (list separately in addition to primary monthly care management service) N
AHA: 3Q,19

Telehealth Consultation

G0508 Telehealth consultation, critical care, initial, physicians typically spend 60 minutes communicating with the patient and providers via telehealth B
AHA: 3Q,19

G0509 Telehealth consultation, critical care, subsequent, physicians typically spend 50 minutes communicating with the patient and providers via telehealth B
AHA: 3Q,19

RHC or FQHC General Care Management

G0511 Rural health clinic or federally qualified health center (RHC or FQHC) only, general care management, 20 minutes or more of clinical staff time for chronic care management services or behavioral health integration services directed by an RHC or FQHC practitioner (physician, NP, PA, or CNM), per calendar month A
CMS: 100-02,13,230.2; 100-04,9,70.8

G0512 Rural health clinic or federally qualified health center (RHC/FQHC) only, psychiatric collaborative care model (psychiatric COCM), 60 minutes or more of clinical staff time for psychiatric COCM services directed by an RHC or FQHC practitioner (physician, NP, PA, or CNM) and including services furnished by a behavioral health care manager and consultation with a psychiatric consultant, per calendar month A
CMS: 100-02,13,230.2; 100-02,13,230.3; 100-04,9,70.8

Prolonged Services

G0513 Prolonged preventive service(s) (beyond the typical service time of the primary procedure), in the office or other outpatient setting requiring direct patient contact beyond the usual service; first 30 minutes (list separately in addition to code for preventive service) N
AHA: 3Q,19

G0514 Prolonged preventive service(s) (beyond the typical service time of the primary procedure), in the office or other outpatient setting requiring direct patient contact beyond the usual service; each additional 30 minutes (list separately in addition to code G0513 for additional 30 minutes of preventive service) N
AHA: 3Q,19

Drug Delivery Implants

G0516 Insertion of nonbiodegradable drug delivery implants, four or more (services for subdermal rod implant) Q1 N1

G0517 Removal of nonbiodegradable drug delivery implants, four or more (services for subdermal implants) Q1 N1

G0518 Removal with reinsertion, nonbiodegradable drug delivery implants, four or more (services for subdermal implants) Q1 N1

Quality Measures

● **G0519** Management of new patient-caregiver dyad with dementia, low complexity, for use in CMMI model
AHA: 3Q,24

Special Coverage Instructions | Noncovered by Medicare | Carrier Discretion | ☑ Quantity Alert | ● New Code | ○ Recycled/Reinstated | ▲ Revised Code

● **G0520** Management of new patient-caregiver dyad with dementia, moderate complexity, for use in CMMI model
AHA: 3Q,24

● **G0521** Management of new patient-caregiver dyad with dementia, high complexity, for use in CMMI model
AHA: 3Q,24

● **G0522** Management of a new patient with dementia, low complexity, for use in CMMI model
AHA: 3Q,24

● **G0523** Management of a new patient with dementia, moderate to high complexity, for use in CMMI model
AHA: 3Q,24

● **G0524** Management of established patient-caregiver dyad with dementia, low complexity, for use in CMMI model
AHA: 3Q,24

● **G0525** Management of established patient-caregiver dyad with dementia, moderate complexity, for use in CMMI model
AHA: 3Q,24

● **G0526** Management of established patient-caregiver dyad with dementia, high complexity, for use in CMMI model
AHA: 3Q,24

● **G0527** Management of established patient with dementia, low complexity, for use in CMMI model
AHA: 3Q,24

● **G0528** Management of established patient with dementia, moderate to high complexity, for use in CMMI model
AHA: 3Q,24

● **G0529** In-home respite care, 4-hour unit, for use in CMMI model
AHA: 3Q,24

● **G0530** Adult day center, 8-hour unit, for use in CMMI model
AHA: 3Q,24

● **G0531** Facility-based respite, 24-hour unit, for use in CMMI model
AHA: 3Q,24

Medicare-enrolled Opioid Treatment Services

● **G0532** Take-home supply of nasal nalmefene HCl; one carton of two, 2.7 mg per 0.1 ml nasal sprays (provision of the services by a Medicare-enrolled opioid treatment program); (list separately in addition to each primary code)

● **G0533** Medication assisted treatment, buprenorphine (injectable) administered on a weekly basis; weekly bundle including dispensing and/or administration, substance use counseling, individual and group therapy, and toxicology testing if performed (provision of the services by a Medicare-enrolled opioid treatment program)

● **G0534** Coordinated care and/or referral services, such as to adequate and accessible community resources to address unmet health-related social needs, including harm reduction interventions and recovery support services a patient needs and wishes to pursue, which significantly limit the ability to diagnose or treat an opioid use disorder; each additional 30 minutes of services (provision of the services by a Medicare-enrolled opioid treatment program); (list separately in addition to each primary code)

● **G0535** Patient navigational services, provided directly or by referral; including helping the patient to navigate health systems and identify care providers and supportive services, to build patient self advocacy and communication skills with care providers, and to promote patient-driven action plans and goals; each additional 30 minutes of services (provision of the services by a Medicare-enrolled opioid treatment program); (list separately in addition to each primary code)

● **G0536** Peer recovery support services, provided directly or by referral; including leveraging knowledge of the condition or lived experience to provide support, mentorship, or inspiration to meet MOUD treatment and recovery goals; conducting a person-centered interview to understand the patient's life story, strengths, needs, goals, preferences, and desired outcomes; developing and proposing strategies to help meet person-centered treatment goals; assisting the patient in locating or navigating recovery support services; each additional 30 minutes of services (provision of the services by a Medicare-enrolled opioid treatment program); (list separately in addition to each primary code)

Atherosclerotic Cardiovascular Disease Services

● **G0537** Administration of a standardized, evidence-based atherosclerotic cardiovascular disease (ASCVD) risk assessment, 5-15 minutes, not more often than every 12 months

● **G0538** Atherosclerotic cardiovascular disease (ASCVD) risk management services; clinical staff time; per calendar month

Caregiver Training

● **G0539** Caregiver training in behavior management/modification for caregiver(s) of patients with a mental or physical health diagnosis, administered by physician or other qualified health care professional (without the patient present), face-to-face; initial 30 minutes

● **G0540** Caregiver training in behavior management/modification for parent(s)/guardian(s)/caregiver(s) of patients with a mental or physical health diagnosis, administered by physician or other qualified health care professional (without the patient present), face-to-face; each additional 15 minutes

● **G0541** Caregiver training in direct care strategies and techniques to support care for patients with an ongoing condition or illness and to reduce complications (including, but not limited to, techniques to prevent decubitus ulcer formation, wound care, and infection control) (without the patient present), face-to-face; initial 30 minutes

● **G0542** Caregiver training in direct care strategies and techniques to support care for patients with an ongoing condition or illness and to reduce complications (including, but not limited to, techniques to prevent decubitus ulcer formation, wound care, and infection control) (without the patient present), face-to-face; each additional 15 minutes (list separately in addition to code for primary service) (use G0542 in conjunction with G0541)

● **G0543** Group caregiver training in direct care strategies and techniques to support care for patients with an ongoing condition or illness and to reduce complications (including, but not limited to, techniques to prevent decubitus ulcer formation, wound care, and infection control) (without the patient present), face-to-face with multiple sets of caregivers

Postdischarge Follow-up Contact

● **G0544** Post discharge telephonic follow-up contacts performed in conjunction with a discharge from the emergency department for behavioral health or other crisis encounter, 4 calls per calendar month

Visit Complexity

● **G0545** Visit complexity inherent to hospital inpatient or observation care associated with a confirmed or suspected infectious disease by an infectious diseases specialist, including disease transmission risk assessment and mitigation, public health investigation, analysis, testing, and complex antimicrobial therapy counseling and treatment (add-on code, list separately in addition to hospital inpatient or observation evaluation and management visit, initial, same day discharge, subsequent, or discharge)

Interprofessional Health Record Assessment/Management Services

● **G0546** **Interprofessional telephone/internet/electronic health record assessment and management service provided by a practitioner in a specialty whose covered services are limited by statute to services for the diagnosis and treatment of mental illness, including a verbal and written report to the patient's treating/requesting practitioner; 5-10 minutes of medical consultative discussion and review**

● **G0547** **Interprofessional telephone/internet/electronic health record assessment and management service provided by a practitioner in a specialty whose covered services are limited by statute to services for the diagnosis and treatment of mental illness, including a verbal and written report to the patient's treating/requesting practitioner; 11-20 minutes of medical consultative discussion and review**

● **G0548** **Interprofessional telephone/internet/electronic health record assessment and management service provided by a practitioner in a specialty whose covered services are limited by statute to services for the diagnosis and treatment of mental illness, including a verbal and written report to the patient's treating/requesting practitioner; 21-30 minutes of medical consultative discussion and review**

● **G0549** **Interprofessional telephone/internet/electronic health record assessment and management service provided by a practitioner in a specialty whose covered services are limited by statute to services for the diagnosis and treatment of mental illness, including a verbal and written report to the patient's treating/requesting practitioner; 31 or more minutes of medical consultative discussion and review**

● **G0550** **Interprofessional telephone/internet/electronic health record assessment and management service provided by a practitioner in a specialty whose covered services are limited by statute to services for the diagnosis and treatment of mental illness, including a written report to the patient's treating/requesting practitioner, 5 minutes or more of medical consultative time**

● **G0551** **Interprofessional telephone/internet/electronic health record referral service(s) provided by a treating/requesting practitioner in a specialty whose covered services are limited by statute to services for the diagnosis and treatment of mental illness, 30 minutes**

Digital Mental Health Treatment

● **G0552** **Supply of digital mental health treatment device and initial education and onboarding, per course of treatment that augments a behavioral therapy plan**

● **G0553** **First 20 minutes of monthly treatment management services directly related to the patient's therapeutic use of the digital mental health treatment (DMHT) device that augments a behavioral therapy plan, physician/other qualified health care professional time reviewing information related to the use of the DMHT device, including patient observations and patient specific inputs in a calendar month and requiring at least one interactive communication with the patient/caregiver during the calendar month**

● **G0554** **Each additional 20 minutes of monthly treatment management services directly related to the patient's therapeutic use of the digital mental health treatment (DMHT) device that augments a behavioral therapy plan, physician/other qualified health care professional time reviewing data generated from the DMHT device from patient observations and patient specific inputs in a calendar month and requiring at least one interactive communication with the patient/caregiver during the calendar month**

Home Pulmonary Artery Pressure Monitoring Supplies

● **G0555** **Provision of replacement patient electronics system (e.g., system pillow, handheld reader) for home pulmonary artery pressure monitoring**

Advanced Primary Care Management Services

● **G0556** **Advanced primary care management services for a patient with one chronic condition [expected to last at least 12 months, or until the death of the patient, which place the patient at significant risk of death, acute exacerbation/decompensation, or functional decline], or fewer, provided by clinical staff and directed by a physician or other qualified health care professional who is responsible for all primary care and serves as the continuing focal point for all needed health care services, per calendar month, with the following elements, as appropriate:**

— consent;
— inform patient:
- of availability of service;
- only one practitioner can furnish and be paid for service during a calendar month;
- right to stop services at any time (effective at end of the calendar month);
- cost sharing may apply;

— document in patient's medical record consent was obtained;
— initiation during a qualifying visit for new patients or patients not seen within 3 years;
— provide 24/7 access for urgent needs to care team/practitioner, including providing patients/caregivers with a way to contact health care professionals in practice to discuss urgent needs regardless of time of day or day of week;
— continuity of care with designated member of care team with whom patient is able to schedule successive routine appointments;
— deliver care in alternative ways to traditional office visits to best meet patient's needs, such as home visits and/or expanded hours;
— overall comprehensive care management;
— systematic needs assessment (medical and psychosocial);
— system-based approaches to ensure receipt of preventive services;
— medication reconciliation, management and oversight of self-management;
— development, implementation, revision, and maintenance of electronic patient-centered comprehensive care plan;
— care plan is available timely within and outside billing practice as appropriate to individuals involved in beneficiary's care, can be routinely accessed and updated by care team/practitioner, and copy of care plan to patient/caregiver;
— coordination of care transitions between and among health care providers and settings, including referrals to other clinicians and follow-up after emergency department visit, discharges from hospitals, skilled nursing facilities, or other health care facilities as applicable;
— ensure timely exchange of electronic health information with other practitioners and providers to support continuity of care;
— ensure timely follow-up communication (direct contact, telephone, electronic) with the patient and/or caregiver after emergency department visit, discharges from hospitals, skilled nursing facilities, or other health care facilities, within 7 calendar days of discharge, as clinically indicated;
— ongoing communication and coordinating receipt of needed services from practitioners, home- and community-based service providers, community-based social service providers, hospitals, and skilled nursing facilities (or other health care facilities), and document communication regarding patient's psychosocial strengths and needs, functional deficits, goals, preferences, and desired outcomes, including cultural and linguistic factors, in patient's medical record;
— enhanced opportunities for beneficiary and any caregiver to communicate with care team/practitioner regarding beneficiary's care through use of asynchronous non-face-to-face consultation methods other than telephone, such as secure messaging, email, internet, or patient portal, and other communication-technology based services, including remote evaluation of prerecorded patient information and interprofessional telephone/internet/EHR referral service(s), to maintain ongoing communication with patients, as appropriate;

— ensure access to patient-initiated digital communications that require clinical decision, such as virtual check-ins, digital online assessment and management, and E/M visits (or e-visits);
— analyze patient population data to identify gaps in care and offer additional interventions, as appropriate;
— risk stratify practice population based on defined diagnoses, claims, or other electronic data to identify and target services to patients;
— be assessed through performance measurement of primary care quality, total cost of care, and meaningful use of certified EHR technology

● **G0557** **Advanced primary care management services for a patient with multiple (two or more) chronic conditions expected to last at least 12 months, or until the death of the patient, which place the patient at significant risk of death, acute exacerbation/ decompensation, or functional decline, provided by clinical staff and directed by a physician or other qualified health care professional who is responsible for all primary care and serves as the continuing focal point for all needed health care services, per calendar month, with the following elements, as appropriate:**
— consent;
— inform patient:
- of availability of service;
- only one practitioner can furnish and be paid for service during a calendar month;
- right to stop services at any time (effective at end of the calendar month);
- cost sharing may apply;
— document in patient's medical record consent was obtained;
— initiation during a qualifying visit for new patients or patients not seen within 3 years;
— provide 24/7 access for urgent needs to care team/practitioner, including providing patients/caregivers with a way to contact health care professionals in practice to discuss urgent needs regardless of time of day or day of week;
— continuity of care with designated member of care team with whom patient is able to schedule successive routine appointments;
— deliver care in alternative ways to traditional office visits to best meet patient's needs, such as home visits and/or expanded hours;
— overall comprehensive care management;
— systematic needs assessment (medical and psychosocial);
— system-based approaches to ensure receipt of preventive services;
— medication reconciliation, management and oversight of self-management;
— development, implementation, revision, and maintenance of an electronic patient-centered comprehensive care plan;
— care plan is available timely within and outside billing practice as appropriate to individuals involved in beneficiary's care, can be routinely accessed and updated by care team/practitioner, and copy of care plan to patient/caregiver;
— coordination of care transitions between and among health care providers and settings, including referrals to other clinicians and follow-up after emergency department visit, discharges from hospitals, skilled nursing facilities, or other health care facilities as applicable;
— ensure timely exchange of electronic health information with other practitioners and providers to support continuity of care;
— ensure timely follow-up communication (direct contact, telephone, electronic) with the patient and/or caregiver after emergency department visit, discharges from hospitals, skilled nursing facilities, or other health care facilities, within 7 calendar days of discharge, as clinically indicated;
— ongoing communication and coordinating receipt of needed services from practitioners, home- and community-based service providers, community-based social service providers, hospitals, and skilled nursing facilities (or other health care facilities), and document communication regarding patient's psychosocial strengths and needs, functional deficits, goals, preferences, and desired outcomes, including cultural and linguistic factors, in patient's medical record;
— enhanced opportunities for beneficiary and any caregiver to communicate with care team/practitioner regarding beneficiary's care through use of asynchronous non-face-to-face consultation methods other than telephone, such as secure messaging, email, internet, or patient portal, and other communication-technology based services, including remote evaluation of prerecorded patient information and interprofessional telephone/internet/EHR referral service(s), to maintain ongoing communication with patients, as appropriate;
— ensure access to patient-initiated digital communications that require clinical decision, such as virtual check-ins, digital online assessment and management, and E/M visits (or e-visits);
— analyze patient population data to identify gaps in care and offer additional interventions, as appropriate;
— risk stratify practice population based on defined diagnoses, claims, or other electronic data to identify and target services to patients;
— be assessed through performance measurement of primary care quality, total cost of care, and meaningful use of certified EHR technology

● **G0558** **Advanced primary care management services for a patient that is a qualified Medicare beneficiary with multiple (two or more) chronic conditions expected to last at least 12 months, or until the death of the patient, which place the patient at significant risk of death, acute exacerbation/decompensation, or functional decline, provided by clinical staff and directed by a physician or other qualified health care professional who is responsible for all primary care and serves as the continuing focal point for all needed health care services, per calendar month, with the following elements, as appropriate:**
— consent;
— inform patient:
- of availability of service;
- only one practitioner can furnish and be paid for service during a calendar month;
- right to stop services at any time (effective at end of the calendar month);
- cost sharing may apply;
— document in patient's medical record consent was obtained;
— initiation during a qualifying visit for new patients or patients not seen within 3 years;
— provide 24/7 access for urgent needs to care team/practitioner, including providing patients/caregivers with a way to contact health care professionals in practice to discuss urgent needs regardless of time of day or day of week;
— continuity of care with designated member of care team with whom patient is able to schedule successive routine appointments;
— deliver care in alternative ways to traditional office visits to best meet patient's needs, such as home visits and/or expanded hours;
— overall comprehensive care management;
— systematic needs assessment (medical and psychosocial);
— system-based approaches to ensure receipt of preventive services;— medication reconciliation, management and oversight of self-management;
— development, implementation, revision, and maintenance of an electronic patient-centered comprehensive care plan;
— care plan is available timely within and outside billing practice as appropriate to individuals involved in beneficiary's care, can be routinely accessed and updated by care team/practitioner, and copy of care plan to patient/caregiver;
— coordination of care transitions between and among health care providers and settings, including referrals to other clinicians and follow-up after an emergency department visit, discharges from hospitals, skilled nursing facilities, or other health care facilities as applicable;
— ensure timely exchange of electronic health information with other practitioners and providers to support continuity of care;
— ensure timely follow-up communication (direct contact, telephone, electronic) with the patient and/or caregiver after emergency department visit, discharges from hospitals, skilled nursing facilities, or other health care facilities, within 7 calendar days of discharge, as clinically indicated;
— ongoing communication and coordinating receipt of needed services from practitioners, home- and community-based service providers, community-based social service providers, hospitals, and skilled nursing facilities (or other health care facilities), and document communication regarding patient's psychosocial strengths and needs, functional deficits, goals, preferences, and desired outcomes, including cultural and linguistic factors, in patient's medical record;
— enhanced opportunities for beneficiary and any caregiver to communicate with care team/practitioner regarding beneficiary's care through use of asynchronous non-face-to-face consultation methods

other than telephone, such as secure messaging, email, internet, or patient portal, and other communication-technology based services, including remote evaluation of prerecorded patient information and interprofessional telephone/internet/EHR referral service(s), to maintain ongoing communication with patients, as appropriate;
— ensure access to patient-initiated digital communications that require clinical decision, such as virtual check-ins, digital online assessment and management, and E/M visits (or e-visits);
— analyze patient population data to identify gaps in care and offer additional interventions, as appropriate;
— risk stratify practice population based on defined diagnoses, claims, or other electronic data to identify and target services to patients;
— be assessed through performance measurement of primary care quality, total cost of care, and meaningful use of certified EHR technology

Postoperative follow-up Visit Complexity

● **G0559** **Postoperative follow-up visit complexity inherent to evaluation and management services addressing surgical procedure(s), provided by a physician or qualified health care professional who is not the practitioner who performed the procedure (or in the same group practice) and is of the same or of a different specialty than the practitioner who performed the procedure, within the 90-day global period of the procedure(s), once per 90-day global period, when there has not been a formal transfer of care and requires the following required elements, when possible and applicable:**
— reading available surgical note to understand relative success of procedure, anatomy affected, and potential complications that could have arisen due to unique circumstances of patient's operation;
— research procedure to determine expected postoperative course and potential complications (in case of doing a postop for a procedure outside specialty);
— evaluate and physically examine patient to determine whether postoperative course is progressing appropriately;
— communicate with practitioner who performed procedure if any questions or concerns arise (list separately in addition to office/outpatient evaluation and management visit, new or established)

Safety Planning Interventions

● **G0560** **Safety planning interventions, each 20 minutes personally performed by the billing practitioner, including assisting the patient in the identification of the following personalized elements of a safety plan:**
— recognizing warning signs of impending suicidal or substance use-related crisis;
— employing internal coping strategies;
— utilizing social contacts and social settings as means of distraction from suicidal thoughts or risky substance use;
— utilizing family members, significant others, caregivers, and/or friends to help resolve crisis;
— contacting mental health or substance use disorder professionals or agencies;
— making environment safe

Tympanostomy

● **G0561** **Tympanostomy with local or topical anesthesia and insertion of a ventilating tube when performed with tympanostomy tube delivery device, unilateral (list separately in addition to 69433) (do not use in conjunction with 0583T)**

Imaging Services

● **G0562** **Therapeutic radiology simulation-aided field setting; complex, including acquisition of PET and CT imaging data required for radiopharmaceutical-directed radiation therapy treatment planning (i.e., modeling)**

● **G0563** **Stereotactic body radiation therapy, treatment delivery, per fraction to 1 or more lesions, including image guidance and real-time positron emissions-based delivery adjustments to 1 or more lesions, entire course not to exceed 5 fractions**

Interstitial Glucose Sensor, Implantable

● **G0564** **Creation of subcutaneous pocket with insertion of 365 day implantable interstitial glucose sensor, including system activation and patient training**

● **G0565** **Removal of implantable interstitial glucose sensor with creation of subcutaneous pocket at different anatomic site and insertion of new 365 day implantable sensor, including system activation**

Drug Test(s)

G0659 **Drug test(s), definitive, utilizing drug identification methods able to identify individual drugs and distinguish between structural isomers (but not necessarily stereoisomers), including but not limited to GC/MS (any type, single or tandem) and LC/MS (any type, single or tandem), excluding immunoassays (e.g., IA, EIA, ELISA, EMIT, FPIA) and enzymatic methods (e.g., alcohol dehydrogenase), performed without method or drug-specific calibration, without matrix-matched quality control material, or without use of stable isotope or other universally recognized internal standard(s) for each drug, drug metabolite or drug class per specimen; qualitative or quantitative, all sources, includes specimen validity testing, per day, any number of drug classes** Q
AHA: 2Q,22

Quality Measures

G0913 **Improvement in visual function achieved within 90 days following cataract surgery** M

G0914 **Patient care survey was not completed by patient** M

G0915 **Improvement in visual function not achieved within 90 days following cataract surgery** M

G0916 **Satisfaction with care achieved within 90 days following cataract surgery** M

G0917 **Patient care survey was not completed by patient** M

G0918 **Satisfaction with care not achieved within 90 days following cataract surgery** M

Clinical Decision Support Mechanism

G1001 **Clinical Decision Support Mechanism eviCore, as defined by the Medicare Appropriate Use Criteria Program** E

G1002 **Clinical Decision Support Mechanism MedCurrent, as defined by the Medicare Appropriate Use Criteria Program** E

G1003 **Clinical Decision Support Mechanism Medicalis, as defined by the Medicare Appropriate Use Criteria Program** E

G1004 **Clinical Decision Support Mechanism National Decision Support Company, as defined by the Medicare Appropriate Use Criteria Program** E

G1007 **Clinical Decision Support Mechanism AIM Specialty Health, as defined by the Medicare Appropriate Use Criteria Program** E

G1008 **Clinical Decision Support Mechanism Cranberry Peak, as defined by the Medicare Appropriate Use Criteria Program** E

G1010 **Clinical Decision Support Mechanism Stanson, as defined by the Medicare Appropriate Use Criteria Program** E

G1011 **Clinical Decision Support Mechanism, qualified tool not otherwise specified, as defined by the Medicare Appropriate Use Criteria Program** E

G1012 **Clinical Decision Support Mechanism AgileMD, as defined by the Medicare Appropriate Use Criteria Program** E

G1013 **Clinical Decision Support Mechanism EvidenceCare ImagingCare, as defined by the Medicare Appropriate Use Criteria Program** E

G1014 **Clinical Decision Support Mechanism InveniQA Semantic Answers in Medicine, as defined by the Medicare Appropriate Use Criteria Program** E

G1015 Clinical Decision Support Mechanism Reliant Medical Group, as defined by the Medicare Appropriate Use Criteria Program E

G1016 Clinical Decision Support Mechanism Speed of Care, as defined by the Medicare Appropriate Use Criteria Program E

G1017 Clinical Decision Support Mechanism HealthHelp, as defined by the Medicare Appropriate Use Criteria Program E

G1018 Clinical Decision Support Mechanism INFINX, as defined by the Medicare Appropriate Use Criteria Program E

G1019 Clinical Decision Support Mechanism LogicNets, as defined by the Medicare Appropriate Use Criteria Program E

G1020 Clinical Decision Support Mechanism Curbside Clinical Augmented Workflow, as defined by the Medicare Appropriate Use Criteria Program E

G1021 Clinical Decision Support Mechanism EHealthLine Clinical Decision Support Mechanism, as defined by the Medicare Appropriate Use Criteria Program E

G1022 Clinical Decision Support Mechanism Intermountain Clinical Decision Support Mechanism, as defined by the Medicare Appropriate Use Criteria Program E

G1023 Clinical Decision Support Mechanism Persivia Clinical Decision Support, as defined by the Medicare Appropriate Use Criteria Program E

G1024 Clinical decision support mechanism Radrite, as defined by the Medicare Appropriate Use Criteria Program E

Patient-Month Quality Measures

G1025 Patient-months where there are more than one Medicare capitated payment (MCP) provider listed for the month M

G1026 The number of adult patient-months in the denominator who were on maintenance hemodialysis using a catheter continuously for 3 months or longer under the care of the same practitioner or group partner as of the last hemodialysis session of the reporting month M

G1027 The number of adult patient-months in the denominator who were on maintenance hemodialysis under the care of the same practitioner or group partner as of the last hemodialysis session of the reporting month using a catheter continuously for less than 3 months M

Nasal Naloxone

G1028 Take-home supply of nasal naloxone; 2-pack of 8 mg per 0.1 ml nasal spray (provision of the services by a Medicare-enrolled Opioid Treatment Program); list separately in addition to code for primary procedure A

CMS: 100-02,17,20; 100-02,17,40.1.1; 100-04,39,30.6.1

Convulsive Therapy Procedure

G2000 Blinded administration of convulsive therapy procedure, either electroconvulsive therapy (ECT, current covered gold standard) or magnetic seizure therapy (MST, noncovered experimental therapy), performed in an approved IDE-based clinical trial, per treatment session S

Assessments, Evaluations, and CMMI Home Visits

G2001 Brief (20 minutes) in-home visit for a new patient postdischarge. For use only in a Medicare-approved CMMI model. (Services must be furnished within a beneficiary's home, domiciliary, rest home, assisted living and/or nursing facility within 90 days following discharge from an inpatient facility and no more than nine times.) B

G2002 Limited (30 minutes) in-home visit for a new patient postdischarge. For use only in a Medicare-approved CMMI model. (Services must be furnished within a beneficiary's home, domiciliary, rest home, assisted living and/or nursing facility within 90 days following discharge from an inpatient facility and no more than nine times.) B

G2003 Moderate (45 minutes) in-home visit for a new patient postdischarge. For use only in a Medicare-approved CMMI model. (Services must be furnished within a beneficiary's home, domiciliary, rest home, assisted living and/or nursing facility within 90 days following discharge from an inpatient facility and no more than nine times.) B

G2004 Comprehensive (60 minutes) in-home visit for a new patient postdischarge. For use only in a Medicare-approved CMMI model. (Services must be furnished within a beneficiary's home, domiciliary, rest home, assisted living and/or nursing facility within 90 days following discharge from an inpatient facility and no more than nine times.) B

G2005 Extensive (75 minutes) in-home visit for a new patient postdischarge. For use only in a Medicare-approved CMMI model. (Services must be furnished within a beneficiary's home, domiciliary, rest home, assisted living and/or nursing facility within 90 days following discharge from an inpatient facility and no more than nine times.) B

G2006 Brief (20 minutes) in-home visit for an existing patient postdischarge. For use only in a Medicare-approved CMMI model. (Services must be furnished within a beneficiary's home, domiciliary, rest home, assisted living and/or nursing facility within 90 days following discharge from an inpatient facility and no more than nine times.) B

G2007 Limited (30 minutes) in-home visit for an existing patient postdischarge. For use only in a Medicare-approved CMMI model. (Services must be furnished within a beneficiary's home, domiciliary, rest home, assisted living and/or nursing facility within 90 days following discharge from an inpatient facility and no more than nine times.) B

G2008 Moderate (45 minutes) in-home visit for an existing patient postdischarge. For use only in a Medicare-approved CMMI model. (Services must be furnished within a beneficiary's home, domiciliary, rest home, assisted living and/or nursing facility within 90 days following discharge from an inpatient facility and no more than nine times.) B

G2009 Comprehensive (60 minutes) in-home visit for an existing patient postdischarge. For use only in a Medicare-approved CMMI model. (Services must be furnished within a beneficiary's home, domiciliary, rest home, assisted living and/or nursing facility within 90 days following discharge from an inpatient facility and no more than nine times.) B

G2010 Remote evaluation of recorded video and/or images submitted by an established patient (e.g., store and forward), including interpretation with follow-up with the patient within 24 business hours, not originating from a related E/M service provided within the previous 7 days nor leading to an E/M service or procedure within the next 24 hours or soonest available appointment B

G2011 Alcohol and/or substance (other than tobacco) misuse structured assessment (e.g., audit, dast), and brief intervention, 5-14 minutes S

G2012 Brief communication technology-based service, e.g., virtual check-in, by a physician or other qualified health care professional who can report evaluation and management services, provided to an established patient, not originating from a related E/M service provided within the previous 7 days nor leading to an E/M service or procedure within the next 24 hours or soonest available appointment; 5-10 minutes of medical discussion

G2013 Extensive (75 minutes) in-home visit for an existing patient postdischarge. For use only in a Medicare-approved CMMI model. (Services must be furnished within a beneficiary's home, domiciliary, rest home, assisted living and/or nursing facility within 90 days following discharge from an inpatient facility and no more than nine times.) B

G2014 Limited (30 minutes) care plan oversight. For use only in a Medicare-approved CMMI model. (Services must be furnished within a beneficiary's home, domiciliary, rest home, assisted living and/or nursing facility within 90 days following discharge from an inpatient facility and no more than nine times.) B

G2015 Comprehensive (60 minutes) home care plan oversight. For use only in a Medicare-approved CMMI model. (Services must be furnished within a beneficiary's home, domiciliary, rest home, assisted living and/or nursing facility within 90 days following discharge from an inpatient facility.) B

Treatment in Place

G2020 Services for high intensity clinical services associated with the initial engagement and outreach of beneficiaries assigned to the SIP component of the PCF model (do not bill with chronic care management codes) A

AHA: 2Q,21

G2021 Health care practitioners rendering treatment in place (TIP) E1

G2022 A model participant (ambulance supplier/provider), the beneficiary refuses services covered under the model (transport to an alternate destination/treatment in place) E1

Telehealth Distant Site Service

G2025 Payment for a telehealth distant site service furnished by a Rural Health Clinic (RHC) or Federally Qualified Health Center (FQHC) only A

AHA: 2Q,20

Medication Assisted Treatment and Other Services

G2067 Medication assisted treatment, methadone; weekly bundle including dispensing and/or administration, substance use counseling, individual and group therapy, and toxicology testing, if performed (provision of the services by a Medicare-enrolled opioid treatment program) A

CMS: 100-02,17,20; 100-02,17,40.1.1; 100-02,17,40.1.2; 100-04,26,10.5; 100-04,39,30.6; 100-04,39,30.6.1; 100-04,39,30.7; 100-04,39,30.8; 100-04,39,30.9; 100-04,39,40; 100-04,39,40.2; 100-04,39,50; 100-04,39,50.1

G2068 Medication assisted treatment, buprenorphine (oral); weekly bundle including dispensing and/or administration, substance use counseling, individual and group therapy, and toxicology testing if performed (provision of the services by a Medicare-enrolled opioid treatment program) A

CMS: 100-02,17,20; 100-02,17,40.1.1; 100-02,17,40.1.2; 100-04,26,10.5; 100-04,39,30.6; 100-04,39,30.6.1; 100-04,39,30.7; 100-04,39,30.8; 100-04,39,30.9; 100-04,39,40; 100-04,39,40.2; 100-04,39,50; 100-04,39,50.1

▲ **G2069** Medication assisted treatment, buprenorphine (injectable) administered on a monthly basis; bundle including dispensing and/or administration, substance use counseling, individual and group therapy, and toxicology testing if performed (provision of the services by a Medicare-enrolled opioid treatment program) A

CMS: 100-02,17,20; 100-02,17,40.1.1; 100-02,17,40.1.2; 100-04,26,10.5; 100-04,39,30.6; 100-04,39,30.6.1; 100-04,39,30.7; 100-04,39,30.8; 100-04,39,30.9; 100-04,39,40; 100-04,39,40.2; 100-04,39,50; 100-04,39,50.1

~~**G2070** Medication assisted treatment, buprenorphine (implant insertion); weekly bundle including dispensing and/or administration, substance use counseling, individual and group therapy, and toxicology testing if performed (provision of the services by a Medicare-enrolled opioid treatment program)~~

~~**G2071** Medication assisted treatment, buprenorphine (implant removal); weekly bundle including dispensing and/or administration, substance use counseling, individual and group therapy, and toxicology testing if performed (provision of the services by a Medicare-enrolled opioid treatment program)~~

~~**G2072** Medication assisted treatment, buprenorphine (implant insertion and removal); weekly bundle including dispensing and/or administration, substance use counseling, individual and group therapy, and toxicology testing if performed (provision of the services by a Medicare-enrolled opioid treatment program)~~

G2073 Medication assisted treatment, naltrexone; weekly bundle including dispensing and/or administration, substance use counseling, individual and group therapy, and toxicology testing if performed (provision of the services by a Medicare-enrolled opioid treatment program) A

CMS: 100-02,17,20; 100-02,17,40.1.1; 100-02,17,40.1.2; 100-04,26,10.5; 100-04,39,30.6; 100-04,39,30.6.1; 100-04,39,30.7; 100-04,39,30.8; 100-04,39,30.9; 100-04,39,40; 100-04,39,40.2; 100-04,39,50; 100-04,39,50.1

G2074 Medication assisted treatment, weekly bundle not including the drug, including substance use counseling, individual and group therapy, and toxicology testing if performed (provision of the services by a Medicare-enrolled opioid treatment program) A

CMS: 100-02,17,20; 100-02,17,40.1.1; 100-02,17,40.1.2; 100-04,26,10.5; 100-04,39,30.2; 100-04,39,30.3; 100-04,39,30.6; 100-04,39,30.6.1; 100-04,39,30.7; 100-04,39,30.8; 100-04,39,30.9; 100-04,39,40; 100-04,39,40.2; 100-04,39,50; 100-04,39,50.1

G2075 Medication assisted treatment, medication not otherwise specified; weekly bundle including dispensing and/or administration, substance use counseling, individual and group therapy, and toxicology testing, if performed (provision of the services by a Medicare-enrolled opioid treatment program) A

CMS: 100-02,17,20; 100-02,17,40.1.1; 100-02,17,40.1.2; 100-04,26,10.5; 100-04,39,30.4; 100-04,39,30.6; 100-04,39,30.6.1; 100-04,39,30.7; 100-04,39,30.8; 100-04,39,30.9; 100-04,39,40; 100-04,39,40.2; 100-04,39,50; 100-04,39,50.1

▲ **G2076** Intake activities, including initial medical examination that is conducted by an appropriately licensed practitioner and preparation of a care plan, which may be informed by administration of a standardized, evidence-based social determinants of health risk assessment to identify unmet health-related social needs, and that includes the patient's goals and mutually agreed-upon actions for the patient to meet those goals, including harm reduction interventions; the patient's needs and goals in the areas of education, vocational training, and employment; and the medical and psychiatric, psychosocial, economic, legal, housing, and other recovery support services that a patient needs and wishes to pursue, conducted by an appropriately licensed/credentialed personnel (provision of the services by a Medicare-enrolled opioid treatment program); list separately in addition to each primary code A

CMS: 100-02,17,20; 100-02,17,40.1.1; 100-02,17,40.1.2; 100-04,26,10.5; 100-04,39,30.6; 100-04,39,30.6.1; 100-04,39,30.7; 100-04,39,30.8; 100-04,39,30.9; 100-04,39,40; 100-04,39,40.2; 100-04,39,50; 100-04,39,50.1

▲ **G2077** Periodic assessment; assessing periodically by an OTP practitioner and includes a review of MOUD dosing, treatment response, other substance use disorder treatment needs, responses and patient-identified goals, and other relevant physical and psychiatric treatment needs and goals; assessment may be informed by administration of a standardized, evidence-based social determinants of health risk assessment to identify unmet health-related social needs, or the need and interest for harm reduction interventions and recovery support services (provision of the services by a Medicare-enrolled opioid treatment program); list separately in addition to each primary code A

CMS: 100-02,17,20; 100-02,17,40.1.1; 100-02,17,40.1.2; 100-04,26,10.5; 100-04,39,30.6; 100-04,39,30.6.1; 100-04,39,30.7; 100-04,39,30.8; 100-04,39,30.9; 100-04,39,40; 100-04,39,40.2; 100-04,39,50; 100-04,39,50.1

G2078 Take home supply of methadone; up to 7 additional day supply (provision of the services by a Medicare-enrolled opioid treatment program); list separately in addition to code for primary procedure A
CMS: 100-02,17,20; 100-02,17,40.1.1; 100-02,17,40.1.2; 100-04,26,10.5; 100-04,39,30.6; 100-04,39,30.6.1; 100-04,39,30.7; 100-04,39,30.8; 100-04,39,30.9; 100-04,39,40; 100-04,39,40.2; 100-04,39,50; 100-04,39,50.1

G2079 Take home supply of buprenorphine (oral); up to 7 additional day supply (provision of the services by a Medicare-enrolled opioid treatment program); list separately in addition to code for primary procedure A
CMS: 100-02,17,20; 100-02,17,40.1.1; 100-02,17,40.1.2; 100-04,26,10.5; 100-04,39,30.6; 100-04,39,30.6.1; 100-04,39,30.7; 100-04,39,30.8; 100-04,39,30.9; 100-04,39,40; 100-04,39,40.2; 100-04,39,50; 100-04,39,50.1

G2080 Each additional 30 minutes of counseling in a week of medication assisted treatment, (provision of the services by a Medicare-enrolled opioid treatment program); list separately in addition to code for primary procedure A
CMS: 100-02,17,20; 100-02,17,40.1.1; 100-02,17,40.1.2; 100-04,26,10.5; 100-04,39,30.5; 100-04,39,30.6; 100-04,39,30.6.1; 100-04,39,30.7; 100-04,39,30.8; 100-04,39,30.9; 100-04,39,40; 100-04,39,40.2; 100-04,39,50; 100-04,39,50.1

G2081 Patients age 66 and older in institutional special needs plans (SNP) or residing in long-term care with a POS code 32, 33, 34, 54 or 56 for more than 90 consecutive days during the measurement period A M

G2082 Office or other outpatient visit for the evaluation and management of an established patient that requires the supervision of a physician or other qualified health care professional and provision of up to 56 mg of esketamine nasal self administration, includes 2 hours post administration observation S

G2083 Office or other outpatient visit for the evaluation and management of an established patient that requires the supervision of a physician or other qualified health care professional and provision of greater than 56 mg esketamine nasal self administration, includes 2 hours post administration observation S

G2086 Office-based treatment for opioid use disorder, including development of the treatment plan, care coordination, individual therapy and group therapy and counseling; at least 70 minutes in the first calendar month S
AHA: 1Q,20

G2087 Office-based treatment for opioid use disorder, including care coordination, individual therapy and group therapy and counseling; at least 60 minutes in a subsequent calendar month S
AHA: 1Q,20

G2088 Office-based treatment for opioid use disorder, including care coordination, individual therapy and group therapy and counseling; each additional 30 minutes beyond the first 120 minutes (list separately in addition to code for primary procedure) N
AHA: 1Q,20

G2090 Patients 66 years of age and older with at least one claim/encounter for frailty during the measurement period and a dispensed medication for dementia during the measurement period or the year prior to the measurement period A M

▲ **G2091** Patients 66 years of age and older with at least one claim/encounter for frailty during the measurement period and an advanced illness diagnosis during the measurement period or the year prior to the measurement period A M

G2092 Angiotensin converting enzyme (ACE) inhibitor or angiotensin receptor blocker (ARB) or angiotensin receptor-neprilysin inhibitor (ARNI) therapy prescribed or currently being taken M

G2093 Documentation of medical reason(s) for not prescribing ACE inhibitor or ARB or ARNI therapy (e.g., hypotensive patients who are at immediate risk of cardiogenic shock, hospitalized patients who have experienced marked azotemia, allergy, intolerance, other medical reasons) M

G2094 Documentation of patient reason(s) for not prescribing ACE inhibitor or ARB or ARNI therapy (e.g., patient declined, other patient reasons) M

G2096 Angiotensin converting enzyme (ACE) inhibitor or angiotensin receptor blocker (ARB) or angiotensin receptor-neprilysin inhibitor (ARNI) therapy was not prescribed, reason not given M

G2097 Episodes where the patient had a competing diagnosis on or within 3 days after the episode date (e.g., intestinal infection, pertussis, bacterial infection, Lyme disease, otitis media, acute sinusitis, chronic sinusitis, infection of the adenoids, prostatitis, cellulitis, mastoiditis, or bone infections, acute lymphadenitis, impetigo, skin staph infections, pneumonia/gonococcal infections, venereal disease (syphilis, chlamydia, inflammatory diseases [female reproductive organs]), infections of the kidney, cystitis or UTI) M

G2098 Patients 66 years of age and older with at least one claim/encounter for frailty during the measurement period and a dispensed medication for dementia during the measurement period or the year prior to the measurement period A M

▲ **G2099** Patients 66 years of age and older with at least one claim/encounter for frailty during the measurement period and an advanced illness diagnosis during the measurement period or the year prior to the measurement period A M

G2100 Patients 66 years of age and older with at least one claim/encounter for frailty during the measurement period and a dispensed medication for dementia during the measurement period or the year prior to the measurement period A M

▲ **G2101** Patients 66 years of age and older with at least one claim/encounter for frailty during the measurement period and an advanced illness diagnosis during the measurement period or the year prior to the measurement period A M

G2105 Patient age 66 or older in institutional special needs plans (SNP) or residing in long-term care with POS code 32, 33, 34, 54 or 56 for more than 90 consecutive days during the measurement period A M

G2106 Patients 66 years of age and older with at least one claim/encounter for frailty during the measurement period and a dispensed medication for dementia during the measurement period or the year prior to the measurement period A M

▲ **G2107** Patients 66 years of age and older with at least one claim/encounter for frailty during the measurement period and an advanced illness diagnosis during the measurement period or the year prior to the measurement period A M

G2112 Patient receiving <=5 mg daily prednisone (or equivalent), or RA activity is worsening, or glucocorticoid use is for less than 6 months M

G2113 Patient receiving >5 mg daily prednisone (or equivalent) for longer than 6 months, and improvement or no change in disease activity M

G2115 Patients 66 - 80 years of age with at least one claim/encounter for frailty during the measurement period and a dispensed medication for dementia during the measurement period or the year prior to the measurement period A M

▲**G2116** Patients 66 - 80 years of age with at least one claim/encounter for frailty during the measurement period and an advanced illness diagnosis during the measurement period or the year prior to the measurement period A M

G2118 Patients 81 years of age and older with at least one claim/encounter for frailty during the measurement period A M

G2121 Depression, anxiety, apathy, and psychosis assessed M

G2122 Depression, anxiety, apathy, and psychosis not assessed M

G2125 Patients 81 years of age and older with at least one claim/encounter for frailty during the six months prior to the measurement period through December 31 of the measurement period A M

▲**G2126** Patients 66-80 years of age with at least one claim/encounter for frailty during the measurement period and an advanced illness diagnosis during the measurement period or the year prior to the measurement period A M

G2127 Patients 66 - 80 years of age with at least one claim/encounter for frailty during the measurement period and a dispensed medication for dementia during the measurement period or the year prior to the measurement period A M

G2128 Documentation of medical reason(s) for not on a daily aspirin or other antiplatelet (e.g., history of gastrointestinal bleed, intracranial bleed, blood disorders, idiopathic thrombocytopenic purpura (ITP), gastric bypass or documentation of active anticoagulant use during the measurement period) M

G2129 Procedure related BP's not taken during an outpatient visit. Examples include same day surgery, ambulatory service center, GI, lab, dialysis, infusion center, chemotherapy M

G2136 Back pain measured by the visual analog scale (VAS) or numeric pain scale at 3 months (6 to 20 weeks) postoperatively was less than or equal to 3.0 or back pain measured by the visual analog scale (VAS) or numeric pain scale within 3 months preoperatively and at 3 months (6 to 20 weeks) postoperatively demonstrated an improvement of 5.0 points or greater M

G2137 Back pain measured by the visual analog scale (VAS) or numeric pain scale at 3 months (6 to 20 weeks) postoperatively was greater than 3.0 and back pain measured by the visual analog scale (VAS) or numeric pain scale within 3 months preoperatively and at 3 months (6 to 20 weeks) postoperatively demonstrated improvement of less than 5.0 points M

AHA: 1Q,24

G2138 Back pain as measured by the visual analog scale (VAS) or numeric pain scale at 1 year (9 to 15 months) postoperatively was less than or equal to 3.0 or back pain measured by the visual analog scale (VAS) or numeric pain scale within 3 months preoperatively and at 1 year (9 to 15 months) postoperatively demonstrated an improvement of 5.0 points or greater M

G2139 Back pain measured by the visual analog scale (VAS) or numeric pain scale at 1 year (9 to 15 months) postoperatively was greater than 3.0 and back pain measured by the visual analog scale (VAS) or numeric pain scale within 3 months preoperatively and at 1 year (9 to 15 months) postoperatively demonstrated improvement of less than 5.0 points M

AHA: 1Q,24

G2140 Leg pain measured by the visual analog scale (VAS) or numeric pain scale at 3 months (6 to 20 weeks) postoperatively was less than or equal to 3.0 or leg pain measured by the visual analog scale (VAS) or numeric pain scale within 3 months preoperatively and at 3 months (6 to 20 weeks) postoperatively demonstrated an improvement of 5.0 points or greater M

AHA: 2Q,21

G2141 Leg pain measured by the visual analog scale (VAS) or numeric pain scale at 3 months (6 to 20 weeks) postoperatively was greater than 3.0 and leg pain measured by the visual analog scale (VAS) or numeric pain scale within 3 months preoperatively and at 3 months (6 to 20 weeks) postoperatively demonstrated improvement of less than 5.0 points M

AHA: 1Q,24

G2142 Functional status measured by the Oswestry Disability Index (ODI version 2.1a) at 1 year (9 to 15 months) postoperatively was less than or equal to 22 or functional status measured by the ODI version 2.1a within 3 months preoperatively and at 1 year (9 to 15 months) postoperatively demonstrated an improvement of 30 points or greater M

G2143 Functional status measured by the Oswestry Disability Index (ODI version 2.1a) at 1 year (9 to 15 months) postoperatively was greater than 22 and functional status measured by the ODI version 2.1a within 3 months preoperatively and at 1 year (9 to 15 months) postoperatively demonstrated an improvement of less than 30 points M

G2144 Functional status measured by the Oswestry Disability Index (ODI version 2.1a) at 3 months (6 to 20 weeks) postoperatively was less than or equal to 22 or functional status measured by the ODI version 2.1a within 3 months preoperatively and at 3 months (6 to 20 weeks) postoperatively demonstrated an improvement of 30 points or greater M

G2145 Functional status measured by the Oswestry Disability Index (ODI version 2.1a) at 3 months (6 to 20 weeks) postoperatively was greater than 22 and functional status measured by the ODI version 2.1a within 3 months preoperatively and at 3 months (6 to 20 weeks) postoperatively demonstrated an improvement of less than 30 points M

G2146 Leg pain as measured by the visual analog scale (VAS) or numeric pain scale at 1 year (9 to 15 months) postoperatively was less than or equal to 3.0 or leg pain measured by the visual analog scale (VAS) or numeric pain scale within 3 months preoperatively and at 1 year (9 to 15 months) postoperatively demonstrated an improvement of 5.0 points or greater M

G2147 Leg pain measured by the visual analog scale (VAS) or numeric pain scale at 1 year (9 to 15 months) postoperatively was greater than 3.0 and leg pain measured by the visual analog scale (VAS) or numeric pain scale within 3 months preoperatively and at 1 year (9 to 15 months) postoperatively demonstrated improvement of less than 5.0 points M

AHA: 1Q,24

G2148 Multimodal pain management was used M

G2149 Documentation of medical reason(s) for not using multimodal pain management (e.g., allergy to multiple classes of analgesics, intubated patient, hepatic failure, patient reports no pain during PACU stay, other medical reason(s)) M

G2150 Multimodal pain management was not used M

G2151 Documentation stating patient has a diagnosis of a degenerative neurological condition such as ALS, MS, or Parkinson's diagnosed at any time before or during the episode of care M

G2152 Residual score for the neck impairment successfully calculated and the score was equal to zero (0) or greater than zero (> 0) M

G2167 Residual score for the neck impairment successfully calculated and the score was less than zero (< 0) M

Home Health

G2168 Services performed by a physical therapist assistant in the home health setting in the delivery of a safe and effective physical therapy maintenance program, each 15 minutes B

CMS: 100-04,10,40.2

Special Coverage Instructions | Noncovered by Medicare | Carrier Discretion | ☑ Quantity Alert | ● New Code | ○ Recycled/Reinstated | ▲ Revised Code

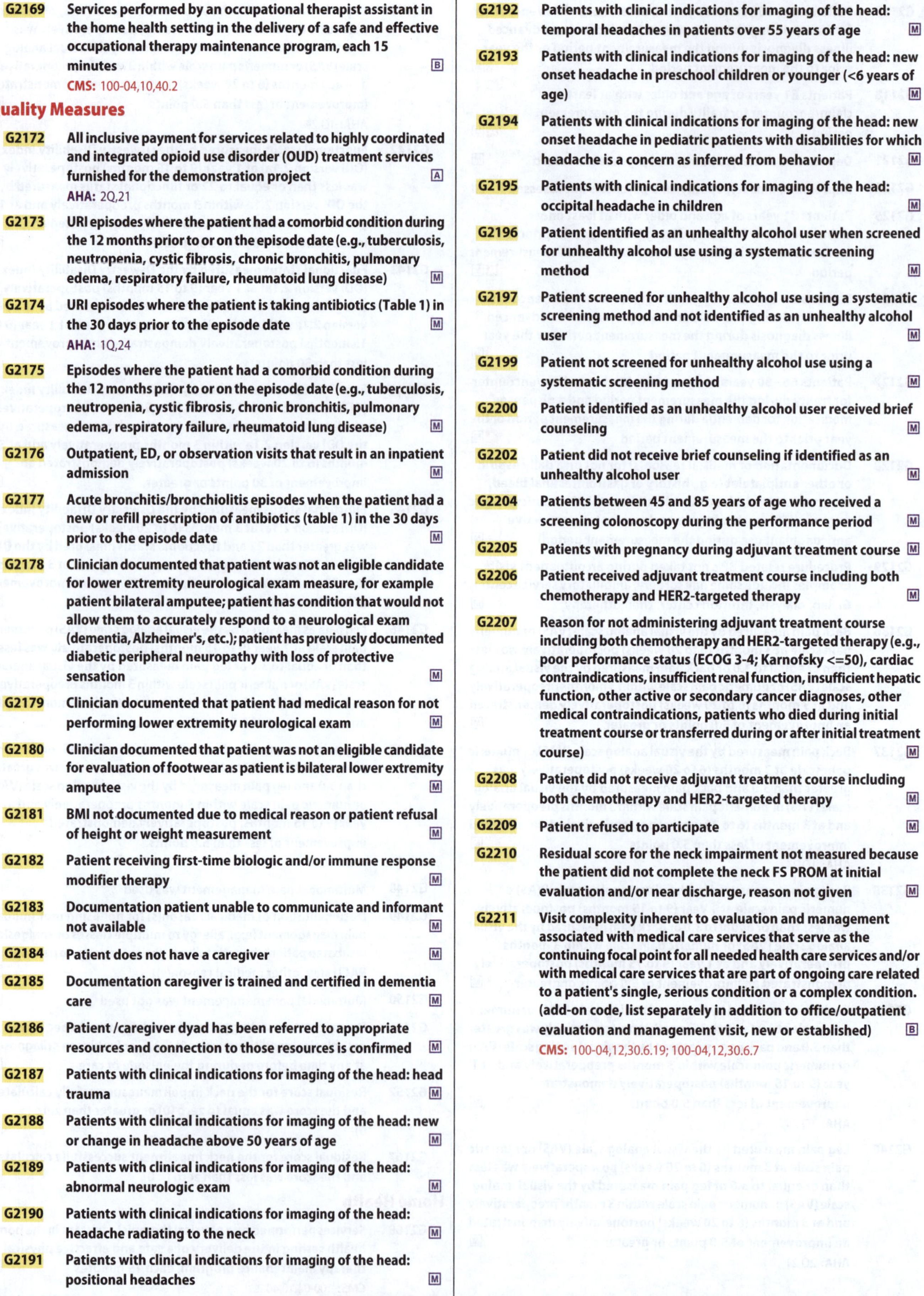

G2169 Services performed by an occupational therapist assistant in the home health setting in the delivery of a safe and effective occupational therapy maintenance program, each 15 minutes B
CMS: 100-04,10,40.2

Quality Measures

G2172 All inclusive payment for services related to highly coordinated and integrated opioid use disorder (OUD) treatment services furnished for the demonstration project A
AHA: 2Q,21

G2173 URI episodes where the patient had a comorbid condition during the 12 months prior to or on the episode date (e.g., tuberculosis, neutropenia, cystic fibrosis, chronic bronchitis, pulmonary edema, respiratory failure, rheumatoid lung disease) M

G2174 URI episodes where the patient is taking antibiotics (Table 1) in the 30 days prior to the episode date M
AHA: 1Q,24

G2175 Episodes where the patient had a comorbid condition during the 12 months prior to or on the episode date (e.g., tuberculosis, neutropenia, cystic fibrosis, chronic bronchitis, pulmonary edema, respiratory failure, rheumatoid lung disease) M

G2176 Outpatient, ED, or observation visits that result in an inpatient admission M

G2177 Acute bronchitis/bronchiolitis episodes when the patient had a new or refill prescription of antibiotics (table 1) in the 30 days prior to the episode date M

G2178 Clinician documented that patient was not an eligible candidate for lower extremity neurological exam measure, for example patient bilateral amputee; patient has condition that would not allow them to accurately respond to a neurological exam (dementia, Alzheimer's, etc.); patient has previously documented diabetic peripheral neuropathy with loss of protective sensation M

G2179 Clinician documented that patient had medical reason for not performing lower extremity neurological exam M

G2180 Clinician documented that patient was not an eligible candidate for evaluation of footwear as patient is bilateral lower extremity amputee M

G2181 BMI not documented due to medical reason or patient refusal of height or weight measurement M

G2182 Patient receiving first-time biologic and/or immune response modifier therapy M

G2183 Documentation patient unable to communicate and informant not available M

G2184 Patient does not have a caregiver M

G2185 Documentation caregiver is trained and certified in dementia care M

G2186 Patient /caregiver dyad has been referred to appropriate resources and connection to those resources is confirmed M

G2187 Patients with clinical indications for imaging of the head: head trauma M

G2188 Patients with clinical indications for imaging of the head: new or change in headache above 50 years of age M

G2189 Patients with clinical indications for imaging of the head: abnormal neurologic exam M

G2190 Patients with clinical indications for imaging of the head: headache radiating to the neck M

G2191 Patients with clinical indications for imaging of the head: positional headaches M

G2192 Patients with clinical indications for imaging of the head: temporal headaches in patients over 55 years of age M

G2193 Patients with clinical indications for imaging of the head: new onset headache in preschool children or younger (<6 years of age) M

G2194 Patients with clinical indications for imaging of the head: new onset headache in pediatric patients with disabilities for which headache is a concern as inferred from behavior M

G2195 Patients with clinical indications for imaging of the head: occipital headache in children M

G2196 Patient identified as an unhealthy alcohol user when screened for unhealthy alcohol use using a systematic screening method M

G2197 Patient screened for unhealthy alcohol use using a systematic screening method and not identified as an unhealthy alcohol user M

G2199 Patient not screened for unhealthy alcohol use using a systematic screening method M

G2200 Patient identified as an unhealthy alcohol user received brief counseling M

G2202 Patient did not receive brief counseling if identified as an unhealthy alcohol user M

G2204 Patients between 45 and 85 years of age who received a screening colonoscopy during the performance period M

G2205 Patients with pregnancy during adjuvant treatment course M

G2206 Patient received adjuvant treatment course including both chemotherapy and HER2-targeted therapy M

G2207 Reason for not administering adjuvant treatment course including both chemotherapy and HER2-targeted therapy (e.g., poor performance status (ECOG 3-4; Karnofsky <=50), cardiac contraindications, insufficient renal function, insufficient hepatic function, other active or secondary cancer diagnoses, other medical contraindications, patients who died during initial treatment course or transferred during or after initial treatment course) M

G2208 Patient did not receive adjuvant treatment course including both chemotherapy and HER2-targeted therapy M

G2209 Patient refused to participate M

G2210 Residual score for the neck impairment not measured because the patient did not complete the neck FS PROM at initial evaluation and/or near discharge, reason not given M

G2211 Visit complexity inherent to evaluation and management associated with medical care services that serve as the continuing focal point for all needed health care services and/or with medical care services that are part of ongoing care related to a patient's single, serious condition or a complex condition. (add-on code, list separately in addition to office/outpatient evaluation and management visit, new or established) B
CMS: 100-04,12,30.6.19; 100-04,12,30.6.7

G2212 Prolonged office or other outpatient evaluation and management service(s) beyond the maximum required time of the primary procedure which has been selected using total time on the date of the primary service; each additional 15 minutes by the physician or qualified healthcare professional, with or without direct patient contact (list separately in addition to CPT codes 99205, 99215, 99483 for office or other outpatient evaluation and management services.) (Do not report G2212 on the same date of service as codes 99358, 99359, 99415, 99416). (Do not report G2212 for any time unit less than 15 minutes) N
CMS: 100-04,12,30.6.15.1; 100-04,12,30.6.15.2; 100-04,12,30.6.15.3; 100-04,12,30.6.18

G2213 Initiation of medication for the treatment of opioid use disorder in the emergency department setting, including assessment, referral to ongoing care, and arranging access to supportive services (list separately in addition to code for primary procedure) N

G2214 Initial or subsequent psychiatric collaborative care management, first 30 minutes in a month of behavioral health care manager activities, in consultation with a psychiatric consultant, and directed by the treating physician or other qualified health care professional S

G2215 Take home supply of nasal naloxone; 2-pack of 4 mg per 0.1 ml nasal spray (provision of the services by a Medicare-enrolled Opioid Treatment Program); list separately in addition to code for primary procedure A
CMS: 100-02,17,20; 100-02,17,40.1.1; 100-02,17,40.1.2; 100-04,39,30.6; 100-04,39,30.6.1; 100-04,39,30.7; 100-04,39,30.8; 100-04,39,40

G2216 Take home supply of injectable naloxone (provision of the services by a Medicare-enrolled opioid treatment program); list separately in addition to code for primary procedure A
CMS: 100-02,17,20; 100-02,17,40.1.1; 100-02,17,40.1.2; 100-04,39,30.6; 100-04,39,30.6.1; 100-04,39,30.7; 100-04,39,30.8; 100-04,39,40

G2250 Remote assessment of recorded video and/or images submitted by an established patient (e.g., store and forward), including interpretation with follow-up with the patient within 24 business hours, not originating from a related service provided within the previous 7 days nor leading to a service or procedure within the next 24 hours or soonest available appointment A

G2251 Brief communication technology-based service, e.g. virtual check-in, by a qualified health care professional who cannot report evaluation and management services, provided to an established patient, not originating from a related service provided within the previous 7 days nor leading to a service or procedure within the next 24 hours or soonest available appointment; 5-10 minutes of clinical discussion A

G2252 Brief communication technology-based service, e.g. virtual check-in, by a physician or other qualified health care professional who can report evaluation and management services, provided to an established patient, not originating from a related EM service provided within the previous 7 days nor leading to an EM service or procedure within the next 24 hours or soonest available appointment; 11-20 minutes of medical discussion A

Chronic Pain Management

G3002 Chronic pain management and treatment, monthly bundle including, diagnosis; assessment and monitoring; administration of a validated pain rating scale or tool; the development, implementation, revision, and/or maintenance of a person-centered care plan that includes strengths, goals, clinical needs, and desired outcomes; overall treatment management; facilitation and coordination of any necessary behavioral health treatment; medication management; pain and health literacy counseling; any necessary chronic pain related crisis care; and ongoing communication and care coordination between relevant practitioners furnishing care e.g., physical therapy and occupational therapy, complementary and integrative approaches, and community-based care, as appropriate. Requires initial face-to-face visit at least 30 minutes provided by a physician or other qualified health professional; first 30 minutes personally provided by physician or other qualified health care professional, per calendar month. (When using G3002, 30 minutes must be met or exceeded) M

G3003 Each additional 15 minutes of chronic pain management and treatment by a physician or other qualified health care professional, per calendar month. (List separately in addition to code for G3002. When using G3003, 15 minutes must be met or exceeded) M

MIPS Specialty Sets

G4000 Dermatology MIPS specialty set M

G4001 Diagnostic Radiology MIPS specialty set M

G4002 Electrophysiology Cardiac Specialist MIPS specialty set M

G4003 Emergency Medicine MIPS specialty set M

G4004 Endocrinology MIPS specialty set M

G4005 Family Medicine MIPS specialty set M

G4006 Gastroenterology MIPS specialty set M

G4007 General Surgery MIPS specialty set M

G4008 Geriatrics MIPS specialty set M

G4009 Hospitalists MIPS specialty set M

G4010 Infectious Disease MIPS specialty set M

G4011 Internal Medicine MIPS specialty set M

G4012 Interventional Radiology MIPS specialty set M

G4013 Mental/behavioral and Psychiatry MIPS specialty set M

G4014 Nephrology MIPS specialty set M

G4015 Neurology MIPS specialty set M

G4016 Neurosurgical MIPS specialty set M

G4017 Nutrition/Dietician MIPS specialty set M

G4018 Obstetrics/Gynecology MIPS specialty set M

G4019 Oncology/Hematology MIPS specialty set M

G4020 Ophthalmology/Optometry MIPS specialty set M

G4021 Orthopedic surgery MIPS specialty set M

G4022 Otolaryngology MIPS specialty set M

G4023 Pathology MIPS specialty set M

G4024 Pediatrics MIPS specialty set M

G4025 Physical Medicine MIPS specialty set M

G4026 Physical Therapy/Occupational Therapy MIPS specialty set M

G4027 Plastic Surgery MIPS specialty set M

G4028 Podiatry MIPS specialty set M

G4029 Preventive Medicine MIPS specialty set M

G4030 Pulmonology MIPS specialty set M

G4031 Radiation Oncology MIPS specialty set M

G4032 Rheumatology MIPS specialty set M

G4033 Skilled Nursing Facility MIPS specialty set M

G4034 Speech Language Pathology MIPS specialty set M

G4035 Thoracic Surgery MIPS specialty set M

G4036 Urgent Care MIPS specialty set M

G4037 Urology MIPS specialty set M

G4038 Vascular Surgery MIPS specialty set M

Radiation Therapy

G6001 Ultrasonic guidance for placement of radiation therapy fields B

G6002 Stereoscopic x-ray guidance for localization of target volume for the delivery of radiation therapy B

G6003 Radiation treatment delivery, single treatment area, single port or parallel opposed ports, simple blocks or no blocks: up to 5 mev B

G6004 Radiation treatment delivery, single treatment area, single port or parallel opposed ports, simple blocks or no blocks: 6-10 mev B

G6005 Radiation treatment delivery, single treatment area, single port or parallel opposed ports, simple blocks or no blocks: 11-19 mev B

G6006 Radiation treatment delivery, single treatment area, single port or parallel opposed ports, simple blocks or no blocks: 20 mev or greater B

G6007 Radiation treatment delivery, two separate treatment areas, three or more ports on a single treatment area, use of multiple blocks: up to 5 mev B

G6008 Radiation treatment delivery, two separate treatment areas, three or more ports on a single treatment area, use of multiple blocks: 6-10 mev B

G6009 Radiation treatment delivery, two separate treatment areas, three or more ports on a single treatment area, use of multiple blocks: 11-19 mev B

G6010 Radiation treatment delivery, two separate treatment areas, three or more ports on a single treatment area, use of multiple blocks: 20 mev or greater B

G6011 Radiation treatment delivery, three or more separate treatment areas, custom blocking, tangential ports, wedges, rotational beam, compensators, electron beam; up to 5 mev B

G6012 Radiation treatment delivery, three or more separate treatment areas, custom blocking, tangential ports, wedges, rotational beam, compensators, electron beam; 6-10 mev B

G6013 Radiation treatment delivery, three or more separate treatment areas, custom blocking, tangential ports, wedges, rotational beam, compensators, electron beam; 11-19 mev B

G6014 Radiation treatment delivery, three or more separate treatment areas, custom blocking, tangential ports, wedges, rotational beam, compensators, electron beam; 20 mev or greater B

G6015 Intensity modulated treatment delivery, single or multiple fields/arcs, via narrow spatially and temporally modulated beams, binary, dynamic MLC, per treatment session B

G6016 Compensator-based beam modulation treatment delivery of inverse planned treatment using three or more high resolution (milled or cast) compensator, convergent beam modulated fields, per treatment session B

G6017 Intra-fraction localization and tracking of target or patient motion during delivery of radiation therapy (e.g., 3D positional tracking, gating, 3D surface tracking), each fraction of treatment B

Quality Measures

G8395 Left ventricular ejection fraction (LVEF) ≥ 40% or documentation as normal or mildly depressed left ventricular systolic function M

G8396 Left ventricular ejection fraction (LVEF) not performed or documented M

G8397 Dilated macular or fundus exam performed, including documentation of the presence or absence of macular edema and level of severity of retinopathy M

G8399 Patient with documented results of a central dual-energy x-ray absorptiometry (DXA) ever being performed M

G8400 Patient with central dual-energy x-ray absorptiometry (DXA) results not documented, reason not given M

G8404 Lower extremity neurological exam performed and documented M

G8405 Lower extremity neurological exam not performed M

G8410 Footwear evaluation performed and documented M

G8415 Footwear evaluation was not performed M

G8416 Clinician documented that patient was not an eligible candidate for footwear evaluation measure M

G8417 BMI is documented above normal parameters and a follow-up plan is documented M

G8418 BMI is documented below normal parameters and a follow-up plan is documented M

G8419 BMI documented outside normal parameters, no follow-up plan documented, no reason given M

G8420 BMI is documented within normal parameters and no follow-up plan is required M

G8421 BMI not documented and no reason is given M

G8427 Eligible clinician attests to documenting in the medical record they obtained, updated, or reviewed the patient's current medications M

G8428 Current list of medications not documented as obtained, updated, or reviewed by the eligible clinician, reason not given M

G8430 Documentation of a medical reason(s) for not documenting, updating, or reviewing the patient's current medications list (e.g., patient is in an urgent or emergent medical situation) M

G8431 Screening for depression is documented as being positive and a follow-up plan is documented M

G8432 Depression screening not documented, reason not given M

G8433 Screening for depression not completed, documented patient or medical reason M

G8450 Beta-blocker therapy prescribed M

G8451 Beta-blocker therapy for LVEF <=40% not prescribed for reasons documented by the clinician (e.g., low blood pressure, fluid overload, asthma, patients recently treated with an intravenous positive inotropic agent, allergy, intolerance, other medical reasons, patient declined, other patient reasons) M

G8452 Beta-blocker therapy not prescribed

G8465 High or very high risk of recurrence of prostate cancer

G8473 Angiotensin converting enzyme (ACE) inhibitor or angiotensin receptor blocker (ARB) therapy prescribed

G8474 Angiotensin converting enzyme (ACE) inhibitor or angiotensin receptor blocker (ARB) therapy not prescribed for reasons documented by the clinician (e.g., allergy, intolerance, pregnancy, renal failure due to ACE inhibitor, diseases of the aortic or mitral valve, other medical reasons) or (e.g., patient declined, other patient reasons)
AHA: 1Q,24

G8475 Angiotensin converting enzyme (ACE) inhibitor or angiotensin receptor blocker (ARB) therapy not prescribed, reason not given

G8476 Most recent blood pressure has a systolic measurement of < 140 mm Hg and a diastolic measurement of < 90 mm Hg

G8477 Most recent blood pressure has a systolic measurement of >=140 mm Hg and/or a diastolic measurement of >=90 mm Hg

G8478 Blood pressure measurement not performed or documented, reason not given

G8482 ~~Influenza immunization administered or previously received~~

G8483 ~~Influenza immunization was not administered for reasons documented by clinician (e.g., patient allergy or other medical reasons, patient declined or other patient reasons, vaccine not available or other system reasons)~~

G8484 ~~Influenza immunization was not administered, reason not given~~

G8510 Screening for depression is documented as negative, a follow-up plan is not required

G8511 Screening for depression documented as positive, follow-up plan not documented, reason not given

G8535 Elder maltreatment screen not documented; documentation that patient is not eligible for the elder maltreatment screen at the time of the encounter related to one of the following reasons: (1) patient refuses to participate in the screening and has reasonable decisional capacity for self-protection, or (2) patient is in an urgent or emergent situation where time is of the essence and to delay treatment to perform the screening would jeopardize the patient's health status
AHA: 1Q,24

G8536 No documentation of an elder maltreatment screen, reason not given

G8539 Functional outcome assessment documented as positive using a standardized tool and a care plan based on identified deficiencies is documented within 2 days of the functional outcome assessment

G8540 Functional outcome assessment not documented as being performed, documentation the patient is not eligible for a functional outcome assessment using a standardized tool at the time of the encounter

G8541 Functional outcome assessment using a standardized tool, not documented, reason not given

G8542 Functional outcome assessment using a standardized tool is documented; no functional deficiencies identified, care plan not required

G8543 Documentation of a positive functional outcome assessment using a standardized tool; care plan not documented within 2 days of assessment, reason not given

G8559 Patient referred to a physician (preferably a physician with training in disorders of the ear) for an otologic evaluation

G8560 Patient has a history of active drainage from the ear within the previous 90 days

G8561 Patient is not eligible for the referral for otologic evaluation for patients with a history of active drainage measure

G8562 Patient does not have a history of active drainage from the ear within the previous 90 days

G8563 Patient not referred to a physician (preferably a physician with training in disorders of the ear) for an otologic evaluation, reason not given

G8564 Patient was referred to a physician (preferably a physician with training in disorders of the ear) for an otologic evaluation, reason not specified)

G8565 Verification and documentation of sudden or rapidly progressive hearing loss

G8566 Patient is not eligible for the "referral for otologic evaluation for sudden or rapidly progressive hearing loss" measure

G8567 Patient does not have verification and documentation of sudden or rapidly progressive hearing loss

G8568 Patient was not referred to a physician (preferably a physician with training in disorders of the ear) for an otologic evaluation, reason not given

G8569 Prolonged postoperative intubation (> 24 hrs) required

G8570 Prolonged postoperative intubation (> 24 hrs) not required

G8575 Developed postoperative renal failure or required dialysis

G8576 No postoperative renal failure/dialysis not required

▲ **G8577** Re-exploration required due to mediastinal bleeding with or without tamponade, unplanned coronary artery intervention (native, vessel, graft, or both), valve dysfunction, aortic reintervention, or other cardiac reason

▲ **G8578** Re-exploration not required due to mediastinal bleeding with or without tamponade, unplanned coronary artery intervention (native, vessel, graft, or both), valve dysfunction, aortic reintervention, or other cardiac reason

G8598 Aspirin or another antiplatelet therapy used

G8599 Aspirin or another antiplatelet therapy not used, reason not given

G8600 IV tPA initiated within 3 hours (≤ 180 minutes) of time last known well

G8601 IV thrombolytic therapy not initiated within 4.5 hours (<= 270 minutes) of time last known well for reasons documented by clinician (e.g., patient enrolled in clinical trial for stroke, patient admitted for elective carotid intervention)
AHA: 1Q,24

G8602 IV tPA not initiated within 3 hours (≤ 180 minutes) of time last known well, reason not given

G8633 Pharmacologic therapy (other than minerals/vitamins) for osteoporosis prescribed

G8635 Pharmacologic therapy for osteoporosis was not prescribed, reason not given

G8647 Residual score for the knee impairment successfully calculated and the score was equal to zero (0) or greater than zero (> 0)

G8648 Residual score for the knee impairment successfully calculated and the score was less than zero (< 0)

G8650 Residual score for the knee impairment not measured because the patient did not complete the LEPF PROM at initial evaluation and/or near discharge, reason not given

G8651 Residual score for the hip impairment successfully calculated and the score was equal to zero (0) or greater than zero (> 0) M ☑

G8652 Residual score for the hip impairment successfully calculated and the score was less than zero (< 0) M ☑

G8654 Residual score for the hip impairment not measured because the patient did not complete the LEPF PROM at initial evaluation and/or near discharge, reason not given M

G8655 Risk-adjusted functional status change residual score for the foot or ankle successfully calculated and the score was equal to zero (0) or greater than zero (> 0) M ☑

G8656 Residual score for the lower leg, foot or ankle impairment successfully calculated and the score was less than zero (< 0) M ☑

G8658 Residual score for the lower leg, foot or ankle impairment not measured because the patient did not complete the LEPF PROM at initial evaluation and/or near discharge, reason not given M

G8659 Residual score for the low back impairment successfully calculated and the score was equal to zero (0) or greater than zero (> 0) M ☑

G8660 Residual score for the low back impairment successfully calculated and the score was less than zero (< 0) M ☑

G8661 Risk-adjusted functional status change residual score for the low back impairment not measured because the patient did not complete the FS status survey near discharge, patient not appropriate M

G8662 Residual score for the low back impairment not measured because the patient did not complete the low back FS PROM at initial evaluation and/or near discharge, reason not given M

G8663 Residual score for the shoulder impairment successfully calculated and the score was equal to zero (0) or greater than zero (> 0) M ☑

G8664 Residual score for the shoulder impairment successfully calculated and the score was less than zero (< 0) M ☑

G8666 Residual score for the shoulder impairment not measured because the patient did not complete the shoulder FS PROM at initial evaluation and/or near discharge, reason not given M

G8667 Residual score for the elbow, wrist or hand impairment successfully calculated and the score was equal to zero (0) or greater than zero (> 0) M ☑

G8668 Residual score for the elbow, wrist or hand impairment successfully calculated and the score was less than zero (< 0) M ☑

G8670 Residual score for the elbow, wrist or hand impairment not measured because the patient did not complete the elbow/wrist/hand FS PROM at initial evaluation and/or near discharge, reason not given M

▲ **G8694** Current or prior left ventricular ejection fraction (LVEF) < = 40% or documentation of moderate or severe LVSD M ☑

G8708 Patient not prescribed antibiotic M

G8709 URI episodes when the patient had competing diagnoses on or three days after the episode date (e.g., intestinal infection, pertussis, bacterial infection, Lyme disease, otitis media, acute sinusitis, acute pharyngitis, acute tonsillitis, chronic sinusitis, infection of the pharynx/larynx/tonsils/adenoids, prostatitis, cellulitis, mastoiditis, or bone infections, acute lymphadenitis, impetigo, skin staph infections, pneumonia/gonococcal infections, venereal disease (syphilis, chlamydia, inflammatory diseases [female reproductive organs]), infections of the kidney, cystitis or UTI, and acne) M

G8710 Patient prescribed antibiotic M

G8711 Prescribed antibiotic on or within 3 days after the episode date M

G8712 Antibiotic not prescribed or dispensed M

G8721 PT category (primary tumor), PN category (regional lymph nodes), and histologic grade were documented in pathology report M

G8722 Documentation of medical reason(s) for not including the PT category, the PN category or the histologic grade in the pathology report (e.g., re-excision without residual tumor; noncarcinomasanal canal) M

G8723 Specimen site is other than anatomic location of primary tumor M

G8724 PT category, PN category and histologic grade were not documented in the pathology report, reason not given M

G8733 Elder maltreatment screen documented as positive and a follow-up plan is documented M

G8734 Elder maltreatment screen documented as negative, follow-up is not required M

G8735 Elder maltreatment screen documented as positive, follow-up plan not documented, reason not given M

G8749 Absence of signs of melanoma (tenderness, jaundice, localized neurologic signs such as weakness, or any other sign suggesting systemic spread) or absence of symptoms of melanoma (cough, dyspnea, pain, paresthesia, or any other symptom suggesting the possibility of systemic spread of melanoma) M

G8752 Most recent systolic blood pressure < 140 mm Hg M ☑

G8753 Most recent systolic blood pressure ≥ 140 mm Hg M ☑

G8754 Most recent diastolic blood pressure < 90 mm Hg M ☑

G8755 Most recent diastolic blood pressure ≥ 90 mm Hg M ☑

G8756 No documentation of blood pressure measurement, reason not given M

G8783 Normal blood pressure reading documented, follow-up not required M

G8785 Blood pressure reading not documented, reason not given M

G8797 Specimen site other than anatomic location of esophagus M

G8798 Specimen site other than anatomic location of prostate M

G8806 Performance of trans-abdominal or trans-vaginal ultrasound and pregnancy location documented A M

G8807 Transabdominal or transvaginal ultrasound not performed for reasons documented by clinician (e.g., patient has a documented intrauterine pregnancy [IUP]) A M

AHA: 1Q,24

G8808 Transabdominal or transvaginal ultrasound not performed, reason not given A M

G8815 Documented reason in the medical records for why the statin therapy was not prescribed (i.e., lower extremity bypass was for a patient with nonartherosclerotic disease) M

G8816 Statin medication prescribed at discharge M

G8817 Statin therapy not prescribed at discharge, reason not given M

G8826 Patient discharged to home no later than postoperative day #2 following EVAR M

G8833 Patient not discharged to home by postoperative day #2 following EVAR M

G8834 Patient discharged to home no later than postoperative day #2 following CEA M

G8838 Patient not discharged to home by postoperative day #2 following CEA M

G8839 Sleep apnea symptoms assessed, including presence or absence of snoring and daytime sleepiness M

G8840 Documentation of reason(s) for not documenting an assessment of sleep symptoms (e.g., patient didn't have initial daytime sleepiness, patient visited between initial testing and initiation of therapy) M

G8841 Sleep apnea symptoms not assessed, reason not given M

▲G8842 Apnea hypopnea index (AHI), respiratory disturbance index (RDI) or respiratory event index (REI) documented or measured within 2 months after initial evaluation for suspected obstructive sleep apnea M

▲G8843 Documentation of reason(s) for not measuring an apnea hypopnea index (AHI), a respiratory disturbance index (RDI), or a respiratory event index (REI) within 2 months after initial evaluation for suspected obstructive sleep apnea (e.g., medical, neurological, or psychiatric disease that prohibits successful completion of a sleep study, patients for whom a sleep study would present a bigger risk than benefit or would pose an undue burden, dementia, patients previously diagnosed with OSA and severity assessed by another provider, patients who decline AHI/RDI/REI measurement, patients who had a financial reason for not completing testing, test was ordered but not completed, patients decline because their insurance (payer) does not cover the expense) M

▲G8844 Apnea hypopnea index (AHI), respiratory disturbance index (RDI), or respiratory event index (REI) not documented or measured within 2 months after initial evaluation for suspected obstructive sleep apnea, reason not given M

G8845 Positive airway pressure therapy prescribed M

G8846 Moderate or severe obstructive sleep apnea (apnea hypopnea index (AHI) or respiratory disturbance index (RDI) of 15 or greater) M ☑

G8849 Documentation of reason(s) for not prescribing positive airway pressure therapy (e.g., patient unable to tolerate, alternative therapies use, patient declined, financial, insurance coverage) M

G8850 Positive airway pressure therapy not prescribed, reason not given M

G8851 Adherence to therapy was assessed at least annually through an objective informatics system or through self-reporting (if objective reporting is not available, documented) M
AHA: 1Q,24

G8854 Documentation of reason(s) for not objectively reporting adherence to evidence-based therapy (e.g., patients who have been diagnosed with a terminal or advanced disease with an expected life span of less than 6 months, patients who decline therapy, patients who do not return for follow-up at least annually, patients unable to access/afford therapy, patient's insurance will not cover therapy) M
AHA: 1Q,24

G8855 Adherence to therapy was not assessed at least annually through an objective informatics system or through self-reporting (if objective reporting is not available), reason not given M
AHA: 1Q,24

G8856 Referral to a physician for an otologic evaluation performed M

G8857 Patient is not eligible for the referral for otologic evaluation measure (e.g., patients who are already under the care of a physician for acute or chronic dizziness) M

G8858 Referral to a physician for an otologic evaluation not performed, reason not given M

G8863 Patients not assessed for risk of bone loss, reason not given M

G8864 Pneumococcal vaccine administered or previously received M

G8865 Documentation of medical reason(s) for not administering or previously receiving pneumococcal vaccine (e.g., patient allergic reaction, potential adverse drug reaction) M

G8866 Documentation of patient reason(s) for not administering or previously receiving pneumococcal vaccine (e.g., patient refusal) M

G8867 Pneumococcal vaccine not administered or previously received, reason not given M

G8869 Patient has documented immunity to hepatitis B and initiating anti-TNF therapy M

G8875 Clinician diagnosed breast cancer preoperatively by a minimally invasive biopsy method M

G8876 Documentation of reason(s) for not performing minimally invasive biopsy to diagnose breast cancer preoperatively (e.g., lesion too close to skin, implant, chest wall, etc., lesion could not be adequately visualized for needle biopsy, patient condition prevents needle biopsy [weight, breast thickness, etc.], duct excision without imaging abnormality, prophylactic mastectomy, reduction mammoplasty, excisional biopsy performed by another physician) M

G8877 Clinician did not attempt to achieve the diagnosis of breast cancer preoperatively by a minimally invasive biopsy method, reason not given M

G8878 Sentinel lymph node biopsy procedure performed M

G8880 Documentation of reason(s) sentinel lymph node biopsy not performed (e.g., reasons could include but not limited to: noninvasive cancer, incidental discovery of breast cancer on prophylactic mastectomy, incidental discovery of breast cancer on reduction mammoplasty, preoperative biopsy proven lymph node (LN) metastases, inflammatory carcinoma, Stage III locally advanced cancer, recurrent invasive breast cancer, clinically node positive after neoadjuvant systemic therapy, patient refusal after informed consent, patient with significant age, comorbidities, or limited life expectancy and favorable tumor; adjuvant systemic therapy unlikely to change) M

G8881 Stage of breast cancer is greater than T1N0M0 or T2N0M0 M

G8882 Sentinel lymph node biopsy procedure not performed, reason not given M

G8907 Patient documented not to have experienced any of the following events: a burn prior to discharge; a fall within the facility; wrong site/side/patient/procedure/implant event; or a hospital transfer or hospital admission upon discharge from the facility M

G8908 Patient documented to have received a burn prior to discharge M

G8909 Patient documented not to have received a burn prior to discharge M

G8910 Patient documented to have experienced a fall within ASC M

G8911 Patient documented not to have experienced a fall within ASC M

G8912 Patient documented to have experienced a wrong site, wrong side, wrong patient, wrong procedure or wrong implant event M

G8913 Patient documented not to have experienced a wrong site, wrong side, wrong patient, wrong procedure or wrong implant event M

G8914 Patient documented to have experienced a hospital transfer or hospital admission upon discharge from ASC M

G8915 Patient documented not to have experienced a hospital transfer or hospital admission upon discharge from ASC M

G8916 Patient with preoperative order for IV antibiotic surgical site infection (SSI) prophylaxis, antibiotic initiated on time M

G8917 Patient with preoperative order for IV antibiotic surgical site infection (SSI) prophylaxis, antibiotic not initiated on time M

G8918 Patient without preoperative order for IV antibiotic surgical site infection (SSI) prophylaxis M

▲ **G8923** Current or prior left ventricular ejection fraction (LVEF) <= 40% or documentation of moderately or severely depressed left ventricular systolic function M

G8924 Spirometry results documented (FEV1/FVC < 70%) M

▲ **G8934** Current or prior left ventricular ejection fraction (LVEF) <=40% or documentation of moderately or severely depressed left ventricular systolic function M

G8935 Clinician prescribed angiotensin converting enzyme (ACE) inhibitor or angiotensin receptor blocker (ARB) therapy M

G8936 Clinician documented that patient was not an eligible candidate for angiotensin converting enzyme (ACE) inhibitor or angiotensin receptor blocker (ARB) therapy (e.g., allergy, intolerance, pregnancy, renal failure due to ACE inhibitor, diseases of the aortic or mitral valve, other medical reasons) or (e.g., patient declined, other patient reasons) M
AHA: 1Q,24

G8937 Clinician did not prescribe angiotensin converting enzyme (ACE) inhibitor or angiotensin receptor blocker (ARB) therapy, reason not given M

G8942 Functional outcome assessment using a standardized tool is documented within the previous 30 days and a care plan, based on identified deficiencies is documented within 2 days of the functional outcome assessment M
AHA: 1Q,24

G8944 AJCC melanoma cancer stage 0 through IIC melanoma M

G8946 Minimally invasive biopsy method attempted but not diagnostic of breast cancer (e.g., high risk lesion of breast such as atypical ductal hyperplasia, lobular neoplasia, atypical lobular hyperplasia, lobular carcinoma in situ, atypical columnar hyperplasia, flat epithelial atypia, radial scar, complex sclerosing lesion, papillary lesion, or any lesion with spindle cells) M

G8950 Elevated or hypertensive blood pressure reading documented, and the indicated follow-up is documented M

G8952 Elevated or hypertensive blood pressure reading documented, indicated follow-up not documented, reason not given M

G8955 Most recent assessment of adequacy of volume management documented M

G8956 Patient receiving maintenance hemodialysis in an outpatient dialysis facility M

G8958 Assessment of adequacy of volume management not documented, reason not given M

G8961 Cardiac stress imaging test primarily performed on low-risk surgery patient for preoperative evaluation within 30 days preceding this surgery M

G8962 Cardiac stress imaging test performed on patient for any reason including those who did not have low risk surgery or test that was performed more than 30 days preceding low risk surgery M

G8965 ~~Cardiac stress imaging test primarily performed on low CHD risk patient for initial detection and risk assessment~~

G8966 ~~Cardiac stress imaging test performed on symptomatic or higher than low CHD risk patient or for any reason other than initial detection and risk assessment~~

G8967 FDA-approved oral anticoagulant is prescribed M

G8968 Documentation of medical reason(s) for not prescribing an FDA-approved anticoagulant (e.g., present or planned atrial appendage occlusion or ligation or patient being currently enrolled in a clinical trial related to AF/atrial flutter treatment) M
AHA: 1Q,24

G8969 Documentation of patient reason(s) for not prescribing an oral anticoagulant that is FDA-approved for the prevention of thromboembolism (e.g., patient preference for not receiving anticoagulation) M

G8970 No risk factors or one moderate risk factor for thromboembolism M

Coordinated Care

G9001 Coordinated care fee, initial rate B

G9002 Coordinated care fee B

G9003 Coordinated care fee, risk adjusted high, initial B

G9004 Coordinated care fee, risk adjusted low, initial B

G9005 Coordinated care fee risk adjusted maintenance B

G9006 Coordinated care fee, home monitoring B

G9007 Coordinated care fee, scheduled team conference B

G9008 Coordinated care fee, physician coordinated care oversight services B

G9009 Coordinated care fee, risk adjusted maintenance, Level 3 B

G9010 Coordinated care fee, risk adjusted maintenance, Level 4 B

G9011 Coordinated care fee, risk adjusted maintenance, Level 5 B

G9012 Other specified case management service not elsewhere classified B

Demonstration Project

G9013 ESRD demo basic bundle Level I E

G9014 ESRD demo expanded bundle including venous access and related services E

G9016 Smoking cessation counseling, individual, in the absence of or in addition to any other evaluation and management service, per session (6-10 minutes) [demo project code only] E ☑
CMS: 100-03,210.4.1

● **G9037** Interprofessional telephone/internet/electronic health record clinical question/request for specialty recommendations by a treating/requesting physician or other qualified health care professional for the care of the patient (i.e., not for professional education or scheduling) and may include subsequent follow up on the specialist's recommendations; 30 minutes
AHA: 3Q,24

● **G9038** Co-management services with the following elements: new diagnosis or acute exacerbation and stabilization of existing condition; condition which may benefit from joint care planning; condition for which specialist is taking a co-management role; condition expected to last at least 3 months; comprehensive care plan established, implemented, revised or monitored in partnership with co-managing clinicians; ongoing communication and care coordination between co-managing clinicians furnishing care
AHA: 3Q,24

G9050 Oncology; primary focus of visit; work-up, evaluation, or staging at the time of cancer diagnosis or recurrence (for use in a Medicare-approved demonstration project) E1

G9051 Oncology; primary focus of visit; treatment decision-making after disease is staged or restaged, discussion of treatment options, supervising/coordinating active cancer-directed therapy or managing consequences of cancer-directed therapy (for use in a Medicare-approved demonstration project) E1

G9052 Oncology; primary focus of visit; surveillance for disease recurrence for patient who has completed definitive cancer-directed therapy and currently lacks evidence of recurrent disease; cancer-directed therapy might be considered in the future (for use in a Medicare-approved demonstration project) E1

G9053 Oncology; primary focus of visit; expectant management of patient with evidence of cancer for whom no cancer-directed therapy is being administered or arranged at present; cancer-directed therapy might be considered in the future (for use in a Medicare-approved demonstration project) E1

G9054 Oncology; primary focus of visit; supervising, coordinating or managing care of patient with terminal cancer or for whom other medical illness prevents further cancer treatment; includes symptom management, end-of-life care planning, management of palliative therapies (for use in a Medicare-approved demonstration project) E1

G9055 Oncology; primary focus of visit; other, unspecified service not otherwise listed (for use in a Medicare-approved demonstration project) E1

G9056 Oncology; practice guidelines; management adheres to guidelines (for use in a Medicare-approved demonstration project) E1

G9057 Oncology; practice guidelines; management differs from guidelines as a result of patient enrollment in an institutional review board-approved clinical trial (for use in a Medicare-approved demonstration project) E1

G9058 Oncology; practice guidelines; management differs from guidelines because the treating physician disagrees with guideline recommendations (for use in a Medicare-approved demonstration project) E1

G9059 Oncology; practice guidelines; management differs from guidelines because the patient, after being offered treatment consistent with guidelines, has opted for alternative treatment or management, including no treatment (for use in a Medicare-approved demonstration project) E1

G9060 Oncology; practice guidelines; management differs from guidelines for reason(s) associated with patient comorbid illness or performance status not factored into guidelines (for use in a Medicare-approved demonstration project) E1

G9061 Oncology; practice guidelines; patient's condition not addressed by available guidelines (for use in a Medicare-approved demonstration project) E1

G9062 Oncology; practice guidelines; management differs from guidelines for other reason(s) not listed (for use in a Medicare-approved demonstration project) E1

G9063 Oncology; disease status; limited to nonsmall cell lung cancer; extent of disease initially established as Stage I (prior to neoadjuvant therapy, if any) with no evidence of disease progression, recurrence, or metastases (for use in a Medicare-approved demonstration project) M

G9064 Oncology; disease status; limited to nonsmall cell lung cancer; extent of disease initially established as Stage II (prior to neoadjuvant therapy, if any) with no evidence of disease progression, recurrence, or metastases (for use in a Medicare-approved demonstration project) M

G9065 Oncology; disease status; limited to nonsmall cell lung cancer; extent of disease initially established as Stage III a (prior to neoadjuvant therapy, if any) with no evidence of disease progression, recurrence, or metastases (for use in a Medicare-approved demonstration project) M

G9066 Oncology; disease status; limited to nonsmall cell lung cancer; Stage III B-IV at diagnosis, metastatic, locally recurrent, or progressive (for use in a Medicare-approved demonstration project) M

G9067 Oncology; disease status; limited to nonsmall cell lung cancer; extent of disease unknown, staging in progress, or not listed (for use in a Medicare-approved demonstration project) M

G9068 Oncology; disease status; limited to small cell and combined small cell/nonsmall cell; extent of disease initially established as limited with no evidence of disease progression, recurrence, or metastases (for use in a Medicare-approved demonstration project) M

G9069 Oncology; disease status; small cell lung cancer, limited to small cell and combined small cell/nonsmall cell; extensive Stage at diagnosis, metastatic, locally recurrent, or progressive (for use in a Medicare-approved demonstration project) M

G9070 Oncology; disease status; small cell lung cancer, limited to small cell and combined small cell/nonsmall; extent of disease unknown, staging in progress, or not listed (for use in a Medicare-approved demonstration project) M

G9071 Oncology; disease status; invasive female breast cancer (does not include ductal carcinoma in situ); adenocarcinoma as predominant cell type; Stage I or Stage IIA-IIB; or T3, N1, M0; and ER and/or PR positive; with no evidence of disease progression, recurrence, or metastases (for use in a Medicare-approved demonstration project) M

G9072 Oncology; disease status; invasive female breast cancer (does not include ductal carcinoma in situ); adenocarcinoma as predominant cell type; Stage I, or Stage IIA-IIB; or T3, N1, M0; and ER and PR negative; with no evidence of disease progression, recurrence, or metastases (for use in a Medicare-approved demonstration project) M

G9073 Oncology; disease status; invasive female breast cancer (does not include ductal carcinoma in situ); adenocarcinoma as predominant cell type; Stage IIIA-IIIB; and not T3, N1, M0; and ER and/or PR positive; with no evidence of disease progression, recurrence, or metastases (for use in a Medicare-approved demonstration project) M

G9074 Oncology; disease status; invasive female breast cancer (does not include ductal carcinoma in situ); adenocarcinoma as predominant cell type; Stage IIIA-IIIB; and not T3, N1, M0; and ER and PR negative; with no evidence of disease progression, recurrence, or metastases (for use in a Medicare-approved demonstration project) M

G9075 Oncology; disease status; invasive female breast cancer (does not include ductal carcinoma in situ); adenocarcinoma as predominant cell type; M1 at diagnosis, metastatic, locally recurrent, or progressive (for use in a Medicare-approved demonstration project) M

G9077 Oncology; disease status; prostate cancer, limited to adenocarcinoma as predominant cell type; T1-T2c and Gleason 2-7 and PSA < or equal to 20 at diagnosis with no evidence of disease progression, recurrence, or metastases (for use in a Medicare-approved demonstration project) M

G9078 Oncology; disease status; prostate cancer, limited to adenocarcinoma as predominant cell type; T2 or T3a Gleason 8-10 or PSA > 20 at diagnosis with no evidence of disease progression, recurrence, or metastases (for use in a Medicare-approved demonstration project) M

G9079 Oncology; disease status; prostate cancer, limited to adenocarcinoma as predominant cell type; T3b-T4, any N; any T, N1 at diagnosis with no evidence of disease progression, recurrence, or metastases (for use in a Medicare-approved demonstration project) M

G9080 Oncology; disease status; prostate cancer, limited to adenocarcinoma; after initial treatment with rising PSA or failure of PSA decline (for use in a Medicare-approved demonstration project) M

G9083 Oncology; disease status; prostate cancer, limited to adenocarcinoma; extent of disease unknown, staging in progress, or not listed (for use in a Medicare-approved demonstration project) M

G9084 Oncology; disease status; colon cancer, limited to invasive cancer, adenocarcinoma as predominant cell type; extent of disease initially established as T1-3, N0, M0 with no evidence of disease progression, recurrence or metastases (for use in a Medicare-approved demonstration project) M

G9085 Oncology; disease status; colon cancer, limited to invasive cancer, adenocarcinoma as predominant cell type; extent of disease initially established as T4, N0, M0 with no evidence of disease progression, recurrence, or metastases (for use in a Medicare-approved demonstration project) M

G9086 Oncology; disease status; colon cancer, limited to invasive cancer, adenocarcinoma as predominant cell type; extent of disease initially established as T1-4, N1-2, M0 with no evidence of disease progression, recurrence, or metastases (for use in a Medicare-approved demonstration project) M

G9087 Oncology; disease status; colon cancer, limited to invasive cancer, adenocarcinoma as predominant cell type; M1 at diagnosis, metastatic, locally recurrent, or progressive with current clinical, radiologic, or biochemical evidence of disease (for use in a Medicare-approved demonstration project) M

G9088 Oncology; disease status; colon cancer, limited to invasive cancer, adenocarcinoma as predominant cell type; M1 at diagnosis, metastatic, locally recurrent, or progressive without current clinical, radiologic, or biochemical evidence of disease (for use in a Medicare-approved demonstration project) M

G9089 Oncology; disease status; colon cancer, limited to invasive cancer, adenocarcinoma as predominant cell type; extent of disease unknown, staging in progress or not listed (for use in a Medicare-approved demonstration project) M

G9090 Oncology; disease status; rectal cancer, limited to invasive cancer, adenocarcinoma as predominant cell type; extent of disease initially established as T1-2, N0, M0 (prior to neoadjuvant therapy, if any) with no evidence of disease progression, recurrence, or metastases (for use in a Medicare-approved demonstration project) M

G9091 Oncology; disease status; rectal cancer, limited to invasive cancer, adenocarcinoma as predominant cell type; extent of disease initially established as T3, N0, M0 (prior to neoadjuvant therapy, if any) with no evidence of disease progression, recurrence, or metastases (for use in a Medicare-approved demonstration project) M

G9092 Oncology; disease status; rectal cancer, limited to invasive cancer, adenocarcinoma as predominant cell type; extent of disease initially established as T1-3, N1-2, M0 (prior to neoadjuvant therapy, if any) with no evidence of disease progression, recurrence or metastases (for use in a Medicare-approved demonstration project) M

G9093 Oncology; disease status; rectal cancer, limited to invasive cancer, adenocarcinoma as predominant cell type; extent of disease initially established as T4, any N, M0 (prior to neoadjuvant therapy, if any) with no evidence of disease progression, recurrence, or metastases (for use in a Medicare-approved demonstration project) M

G9094 Oncology; disease status; rectal cancer, limited to invasive cancer, adenocarcinoma as predominant cell type; M1 at diagnosis, metastatic, locally recurrent, or progressive (for use in a Medicare-approved demonstration project) M

G9095 Oncology; disease status; rectal cancer, limited to invasive cancer, adenocarcinoma as predominant cell type; extent of disease unknown, staging in progress or not listed (for use in a Medicare-approved demonstration project) M

G9096 Oncology; disease status; esophageal cancer, limited to adenocarcinoma or squamous cell carcinoma as predominant cell type; extent of disease initially established as T1-T3, N0-N1 or NX (prior to neoadjuvant therapy, if any) with no evidence of disease progression, recurrence, or metastases (for use in a Medicare-approved demonstration project) M

G9097 Oncology; disease status; esophageal cancer, limited to adenocarcinoma or squamous cell carcinoma as predominant cell type; extent of disease initially established as T4, any N, M0 (prior to neoadjuvant therapy, if any) with no evidence of disease progression, recurrence, or metastases (for use in a Medicare-approved demonstration project) M

G9098 Oncology; disease status; esophageal cancer, limited to adenocarcinoma or squamous cell carcinoma as predominant cell type; M1 at diagnosis, metastatic, locally recurrent, or progressive (for use in a Medicare-approved demonstration project) M

G9099 Oncology; disease status; esophageal cancer, limited to adenocarcinoma or squamous cell carcinoma as predominant cell type; extent of disease unknown, staging in progress, or not listed (for use in a Medicare-approved demonstration project) M

G9100 Oncology; disease status; gastric cancer, limited to adenocarcinoma as predominant cell type; post R0 resection (with or without neoadjuvant therapy) with no evidence of disease recurrence, progression, or metastases (for use in a Medicare-approved demonstration project) M

G9101 Oncology; disease status; gastric cancer, limited to adenocarcinoma as predominant cell type; post R1 or R2 resection (with or without neoadjuvant therapy) with no evidence of disease progression, or metastases (for use in a Medicare-approved demonstration project) M

G9102 Oncology; disease status; gastric cancer, limited to adenocarcinoma as predominant cell type; clinical or pathologic M0, unresectable with no evidence of disease progression, or metastases (for use in a Medicare-approved demonstration project) M

G9103 Oncology; disease status; gastric cancer, limited to adenocarcinoma as predominant cell type; clinical or pathologic M1 at diagnosis, metastatic, locally recurrent, or progressive (for use in a Medicare-approved demonstration project) M

G9104 Oncology; disease status; gastric cancer, limited to adenocarcinoma as predominant cell type; extent of disease unknown, staging in progress, or not listed (for use in a Medicare-approved demonstration project) M

G9105 Oncology; disease status; pancreatic cancer, limited to adenocarcinoma as predominant cell type; post R0 resection without evidence of disease progression, recurrence, or metastases (for use in a Medicare-approved demonstration project) M

G9106 Oncology; disease status; pancreatic cancer, limited to adenocarcinoma; post R1 or R2 resection with no evidence of disease progression, or metastases (for use in a Medicare-approved demonstration project) M

G9107 Oncology; disease status; pancreatic cancer, limited to adenocarcinoma; unresectable at diagnosis, M1 at diagnosis, metastatic, locally recurrent, or progressive (for use in a Medicare-approved demonstration project) M

G9108 Oncology; disease status; pancreatic cancer, limited to adenocarcinoma; extent of disease unknown, staging in progress, or not listed (for use in a Medicare-approved demonstration project) M

G9109 Oncology; disease status; head and neck cancer, limited to cancers of oral cavity, pharynx and larynx with squamous cell as predominant cell type; extent of disease initially established as T1-T2 and N0, M0 (prior to neoadjuvant therapy, if any) with no evidence of disease progression, recurrence, or metastases (for use in a Medicare-approved demonstration project) M

G9110 Oncology; disease status; head and neck cancer, limited to cancers of oral cavity, pharynx and larynx with squamous cell as predominant cell type; extent of disease initially established as T3-4 and/or N1-3, M0 (prior to neoadjuvant therapy, if any) with no evidence of disease progression, recurrence, or metastases (for use in a Medicare-approved demonstration project) M

G9111 Oncology; disease status; head and neck cancer, limited to cancers of oral cavity, pharynx and larynx with squamous cell as predominant cell type; M1 at diagnosis, metastatic, locally recurrent, or progressive (for use in a Medicare-approved demonstration project) M

G9112 Oncology; disease status; head and neck cancer, limited to cancers of oral cavity, pharynx and larynx with squamous cell as predominant cell type; extent of disease unknown, staging in progress, or not listed (for use in a Medicare-approved demonstration project) M

G9113 Oncology; disease status; ovarian cancer, limited to epithelial cancer; pathologic Stage IA-B (Grade 1) without evidence of disease progression, recurrence, or metastases (for use in a Medicare-approved demonstration project) M

G9114 Oncology; disease status; ovarian cancer, limited to epithelial cancer; pathologic Stage IA-B (Grade 2-3); or Stage IC (all grades); or Stage II; without evidence of disease progression, recurrence, or metastases (for use in a Medicare-approved demonstration project) M

G9115 Oncology; disease status; ovarian cancer, limited to epithelial cancer; pathologic Stage III-IV; without evidence of progression, recurrence, or metastases (for use in a Medicare-approved demonstration project) M

G9116 Oncology; disease status; ovarian cancer, limited to epithelial cancer; evidence of disease progression, or recurrence, and/or platinum resistance (for use in a Medicare-approved demonstration project) M

G9117 Oncology; disease status; ovarian cancer, limited to epithelial cancer; extent of disease unknown, staging in progress, or not listed (for use in a Medicare-approved demonstration project) M

G9123 Oncology; disease status; chronic myelogenous leukemia, limited to Philadelphia chromosome positive and/or BCR-ABL positive; chronic phase not in hematologic, cytogenetic, or molecular remission (for use in a Medicare-approved demonstration project) M

G9124 Oncology; disease status; chronic myelogenous leukemia, limited to Philadelphia chromosome positive and /or BCR-ABL positive; accelerated phase not in hematologic cytogenetic, or molecular remission (for use in a Medicare-approved demonstration project) M

G9125 Oncology; disease status; chronic myelogenous leukemia, limited to Philadelphia chromosome positive and/or BCR-ABL positive; blast phase not in hematologic, cytogenetic, or molecular remission (for use in a Medicare-approved demonstration project) M

G9126 Oncology; disease status; chronic myelogenous leukemia, limited to Philadelphia chromosome positive and/or BCR-ABL positive; in hematologic, cytogenetic, or molecular remission (for use in a Medicare-approved demonstration project) M

G9128 Oncology; disease status; limited to multiple myeloma, systemic disease; smoldering, Stage I (for use in a Medicare-approved demonstration project) M

G9129 Oncology; disease status; limited to multiple myeloma, systemic disease; Stage II or higher (for use in a Medicare-approved demonstration project) M

G9130 Oncology; disease status; limited to multiple myeloma, systemic disease; extent of disease unknown, staging in progress, or not listed (for use in a Medicare-approved demonstration project) M

G9131 Oncology; disease status; invasive female breast cancer (does not include ductal carcinoma in situ); adenocarcinoma as predominant cell type; extent of disease unknown, staging in progress, or not listed (for use in a Medicare-approved demonstration project) M

G9132 Oncology; disease status; prostate cancer, limited to adenocarcinoma; hormone-refractory/androgen-independent (e.g., rising PSA on antiandrogen therapy or postorchiectomy); clinical metastases (for use in a Medicare-approved demonstration project) M

G9133 Oncology; disease status; prostate cancer, limited to adenocarcinoma; hormone-responsive; clinical metastases or M1 at diagnosis (for use in a Medicare-approved demonstration project) M

G9134 Oncology; disease status; non-Hodgkin's lymphoma, any cellular classification; Stage I, II at diagnosis, not relapsed, not refractory (for use in a Medicare-approved demonstration project) M

G9135 Oncology; disease status; non-Hodgkin's lymphoma, any cellular classification; Stage III, IV, not relapsed, not refractory (for use in a Medicare-approved demonstration project) M

G9136 Oncology; disease status; non-Hodgkin's lymphoma, transformed from original cellular diagnosis to a second cellular classification (for use in a Medicare-approved demonstration project) M

Procedures/Professional Services (Temporary) G9103 — G9136

G9137 Oncology; disease status; non-Hodgkin's lymphoma, any cellular classification; relapsed/refractory (for use in a Medicare-approved demonstration project) M

G9138 Oncology; disease status; non-Hodgkin's lymphoma, any cellular classification; diagnostic evaluation, stage not determined, evaluation of possible relapse or nonresponse to therapy, or not listed (for use in a Medicare-approved demonstration project) M

G9139 Oncology; disease status; chronic myelogenous leukemia, limited to Philadelphia chromosome positive and/or BCR-ABL positive; extent of disease unknown, staging in progress, not listed (for use in a Medicare-approved demonstration project) M

G9140 Frontier Extended Stay Clinic demonstration; for a patient stay in a clinic approved for the CMS demonstration project; the following measures should be present: the stay must be equal to or greater than 4 hours; weather or other conditions must prevent transfer or the case falls into a category of monitoring and observation cases that are permitted by the rules of the demonstration; there is a maximum Frontier Extended Stay Clinic (FESC) visit of 48 hours, except in the case when weather or other conditions prevent transfer; payment is made on each period up to 4 hours, after the first 4 hours A ☑

Warfarin Testing

G9143 Warfarin responsiveness testing by genetic technique using any method, any number of specimen(s) N

CMS: 100-03,90.1; 100-04,32,250.1; 100-04,32,250.2; 100-04,32,250.3

Outpatient IV Insulin TX

G9147 Outpatient Intravenous Insulin Treatment (OIVIT) either pulsatile or continuous, by any means, guided by the results of measurements for: respiratory quotient; and/or, urine urea nitrogen (UUN); and/or, arterial, venous or capillary glucose; and/or potassium concentration E

CMS: 100-03,40.7; 100-04,4,320.1; 100-04,4,320.2

Quality Assurance

G9148 National Committee for Quality Assurance-Level 1 Medical Home M

G9149 National Committee for Quality Assurance-Level 2 Medical Home M

G9150 National Committee for Quality Assurance-Level 3 Medical Home M

G9151 MAPCP Demonstration-state provided services M

G9152 MAPCP Demonstration-Community Health Teams M

G9153 MAPCP Demonstration-Physician Incentive Pool M

Wheelchair Evaluation

G9156 Evaluation for wheelchair requiring face-to-face visit with physician M

Monitor

G9157 Transesophageal Doppler used for cardiac monitoring B

CMS: 100-04,32,310; 100-04,32,310.2; 100-04,32,310.3

BPCI Services

G9187 Bundled payments for care improvement initiative home visit for patient assessment performed by a qualified health care professional for individuals not considered homebound including, but not limited to, assessment of safety, falls, clinical status, fluid status, medication reconciliation/management, patient compliance with orders/plan of care, performance of activities of daily living, appropriateness of care setting; (for use only in the Medicare-approved bundled payments for care improvement initiative); may not be billed for a 30-day period covered by a transitional care management code E

Miscellaneous Quality Measures

G9188 Beta-blocker therapy not prescribed, reason not given M

G9189 Beta-blocker therapy prescribed or currently being taken M

G9190 Documentation of medical reason(s) for not prescribing beta-blocker therapy (e.g., allergy, intolerance, other medical reasons) M

G9191 Documentation of patient reason(s) for not prescribing beta-blocker therapy (e.g., patient declined, other patient reasons) M

G9212 DSM-IVTM criteria for major depressive disorder documented at the initial evaluation M

G9213 DSM-IV-TR criteria for major depressive disorder not documented at the initial evaluation, reason not otherwise specified M

G9223 Pneumocystis jiroveci pneumonia prophylaxis prescribed within 3 months of low CD4+ cell count below 500 cells/mm3 or a CD4 percentage below 15% M

G9225 Foot exam was not performed, reason not given M

G9226 Foot examination performed (includes examination through visual inspection, sensory exam with 10-g monofilament plus testing any one of the following: vibration using 128-Hz tuning fork, pinprick sensation, ankle reflexes, or vibration perception threshold, and pulse exam; report when all of the three components are completed) M

G9227 Functional outcome assessment documented, care plan not documented, documentation the patient is not eligible for a care plan at the time of the encounter M

G9228 Chlamydia, gonorrhea and syphilis screening results documented (report when results are present for all of the three screenings) M

G9230 Chlamydia, gonorrhea, and syphilis not screened, reason not given M

G9231 Documentation of end stage renal disease (ESRD), dialysis, renal transplant before or during the measurement period or pregnancy during the measurement period M

G9242 Documentation of viral load equal to or greater than 200 copies/ml or viral load not performed M

G9243 Documentation of viral load less than 200 copies/ml M

▲ **G9246** Patient did not have two eligible encounters at least 90 days apart or one eligible encounter and one HIV viral load test at least 90 days apart M

▲ **G9247** Patient had two eligible encounters at least 90 days apart or one eligible encounter and one HIV viral load test at least 90 days apart M

▲ **G9254** Documentation of patient discharged to home later than postoperative day 2 following CEA or CAS M

▲ **G9255** Documentation of patient discharged to home no later than postoperative day 2 following CEA or CAS M

G9273 Blood pressure has a systolic value of < 140 and a diastolic value of < 90 M

G9274 Blood pressure has a systolic value of = 140 and a diastolic value of = 90 or systolic value < 140 and diastolic value = 90 or systolic value = 140 and diastolic value < 90 M

G9275 Documentation that patient is a current nontobacco user M

G9276 Documentation that patient is a current tobacco user M

G9277 Documentation that the patient is on daily aspirin or antiplatelet or has documentation of a valid contraindication or exception to aspirin/antiplatelet; contraindications/exceptions include anticoagulant use, allergy to aspirin or antiplatelets, history of gastrointestinal bleed and bleeding disorder. Additionally, the following exceptions documented by the physician as a reason for not taking daily aspirin or antiplatelet are acceptable (use of nonsteroidal anti-inflammatory agents, documented risk for drug interaction, uncontrolled hypertension defined as > 180 systolic or > 110 diastolic or gastroesophageal reflux) M

G9278 Documentation that the patient is not on daily aspirin or antiplatelet regimen M

G9279 Pneumococcal screening performed and documentation of vaccination received prior to discharge M

G9280 Pneumococcal vaccination not administered prior to discharge, reason not specified M

G9281 Screening performed and documentation that vaccination not indicated/patient refusal M

G9282 Documentation of medical reason(s) for not reporting the histological type or NSCLC-NOS classification with an explanation (e.g., biopsy taken for other purposes in a patient with a history of nonsmall cell lung cancer or other documented medical reasons) M

G9283 Nonsmall cell lung cancer biopsy and cytology specimen report documents classification into specific histologic type or classified as NSCLC-NOS with an explanation M

G9284 Nonsmall cell lung cancer biopsy and cytology specimen report does not document classification into specific histologic type or classified as NSCLC-NOS with an explanation M

G9285 Specimen site other than anatomic location of lung or is not classified as nonsmall cell lung cancer M

G9286 Antibiotic regimen prescribed within 10 days after onset of symptoms M

G9287 Antibiotic regimen not prescribed within 10 days after onset of symptoms M

G9288 Documentation of medical reason(s) for not reporting the histological type or NSCLC-NOS classification with an explanation (e.g., a solitary fibrous tumor in a person with a history of nonsmall cell carcinoma or other documented medical reasons) M

G9289 Nonsmall cell lung cancer biopsy and cytology specimen report documents classification into specific histologic type or classified as NSCLC-NOS with an explanation M

G9290 Nonsmall cell lung cancer biopsy and cytology specimen report does not document classification into specific histologic type or classified as NSCLC-NOS with an explanation M

G9291 Specimen site other than anatomic location of lung, is not classified as nonsmall cell lung cancer or classified as NSCLC-NOS M

G9292 Documentation of medical reason(s) for not reporting PT category and a statement on thickness and ulceration and for PT1, mitotic rate (e.g., negative skin biopsies in a patient with a history of melanoma or other documented medical reasons) M

G9293 Pathology report does not include the PT category and a statement on thickness and ulceration and for PT1, mitotic rate M

G9294 Pathology report includes the PT category and a statement on thickness and ulceration and for PT1, mitotic rate M

G9295 Specimen site other than anatomic cutaneous location M

G9296 Patients with documented shared decision-making including discussion of conservative (nonsurgical) therapy (e.g., NSAIDs, analgesics, weight loss, exercise, injections) prior to the procedure M

G9297 Shared decision-making including discussion of conservative (nonsurgical) therapy (e.g., NSAIDs, analgesics, weight loss, exercise, injections) prior to the procedure, not documented, reason not given M

G9298 Patients who are evaluated for venous thromboembolic and cardiovascular risk factors within 30 days prior to the procedure (e.g., history of DVT, PE, MI, arrhythmia and stroke) M

G9299 Patients who are not evaluated for venous thromboembolic and cardiovascular risk factors within 30 days prior to the procedure (e.g., history of DVT, PE, MI, arrhythmia and stroke, reason not given) M

G9305 Intervention for presence of leak of endoluminal contents through an anastomosis not required M

G9306 Intervention for presence of leak of endoluminal contents through an anastomosis required M

G9307 No return to the operating room for a surgical procedure, for complications of the principal operative procedure, within 30 days of the principal operative procedure M

G9308 Unplanned return to the operating room for a surgical procedure, for complications of the principal operative procedure, within 30 days of the principal operative procedure M

G9309 No unplanned hospital readmission within 30 days of principal procedure M

G9310 Unplanned hospital readmission within 30 days of principal procedure M

G9311 No surgical site infection M

G9312 Surgical site infection M

G9313 Amoxicillin, with or without clavulanate, not prescribed as first line antibiotic at the time of diagnosis for documented reason M

G9314 Amoxicillin, with or without clavulanate, not prescribed as first line antibiotic at the time of diagnosis, reason not given M

G9315 Amoxicillin, with or without clavulanate, prescribed as a first line antibiotic at the time of diagnosis M

G9316 Documentation of patient-specific risk assessment with a risk calculator based on multi-institutional clinical data, the specific risk calculator used, and communication of risk assessment from risk calculator with the patient or family M

G9317 Documentation of patient-specific risk assessment with a risk calculator based on multi-institutional clinical data, the specific risk calculator used, and communication of risk assessment from risk calculator with the patient or family not completed M

G9318 Imaging study named according to standardized nomenclature M

G9319 Imaging study not named according to standardized nomenclature, reason not given M

▲ G9321 Count of previous CT (any type of CT) and cardiac nuclear medicine (myocardial perfusion or infarct-avid imaging) studies documented in the 12-month period prior to the current study M

▲ G9322 Count of previous CT and cardiac nuclear medicine (myocardial perfusion or infarct-avid imaging) studies not documented in the 12-month period prior to the current study, reason not given M

G9341 Search conducted for prior patient CT studies completed at nonaffiliated external health care facilities or entities within the past 12-months and are available through a secure, authorized, media-free, shared archive prior to an imaging study being performed M

G9342 Search not conducted prior to an imaging study being performed for prior patient CT studies completed at nonaffiliated external health care facilities or entities within the past 12 months and are available through a secure, authorized, media-free, shared archive, reason not given M

G9344 Due to system reasons search not conducted for DICOM format images for prior patient CT imaging studies completed at nonaffiliated external health care facilities or entities within the past 12 months that are available through a secure, authorized, media-free, shared archive (e.g., nonaffiliated external health care facilities or entities does not have archival abilities through a shared archival system) M

G9345 Follow-up recommendations documented according to recommended guidelines for incidentally detected pulmonary nodules (e.g., follow-up CT imaging studies needed or that no follow-up is needed) based at a minimum on nodule size and patient risk factors M

G9347 Follow-up recommendations not documented according to recommended guidelines for incidentally detected pulmonary nodules, reason not given M

G9352 More than one CT scan of the paranasal sinuses ordered or received within 90 days after the date of diagnosis, reason not given M

G9355 Elective delivery (without medical indication) by Cesarean birth or induction of labor not performed (<39 weeks of gestation) M

G9356 Elective delivery (without medical indication) by Cesarean birth or induction of labor performed (<39 weeks of gestation) M

G9357 Post-partum screenings, evaluations and education performed M

G9358 Post-partum screenings, evaluations and education not performed M

G9361 Medical indication for delivery by Cesarean birth or induction of labor (<39 weeks of gestation) [documentation of reason(s) for elective delivery (e.g., hemorrhage and placental complications, hypertension, preeclampsia and eclampsia, rupture of membranes (premature or prolonged), maternal conditions complicating pregnancy/delivery, fetal conditions complicating pregnancy/delivery, late pregnancy, prior uterine surgery, or participation in clinical trial)] M

G9364 Sinusitis caused by, or presumed to be caused by, bacterial infection M

G9367 At least two orders for high risk medications from the same drug class M

G9368 At least two orders for high risk medications from the same drug class not ordered M

G9380 Patient offered assistance with end of life issues or existing end of life plan was reviewed or updated during the measurement period M
AHA: 1Q,24

G9382 Patient not offered assistance with end of life issues or existing end of life plan was not reviewed or updated during the measurement period M
AHA: 1Q,24

G9383 Patient received screening for HCV infection within the 12 month reporting period M

G9384 Documentation of medical reason(s) for not receiving annual screening for HCV infection (e.g., decompensated cirrhosis indicating advanced disease [i.e., ascites, esophageal variceal bleeding, hepatic encephalopathy], hepatocellular carcinoma, waitlist for organ transplant, limited life expectancy, other medical reasons) M

G9385 Documentation of patient reason(s) for not receiving annual screening for HCV infection (e.g., patient declined, other patient reasons) M

G9386 Screening for HCV infection not received within the twelve-month reporting period, reason not given M

G9393 Patient with an initial PHQ-9 score greater than nine who achieves remission at twelve months as demonstrated by a twelve-month (+/- 30 days) PHQ-9 score of less than five M

G9394 Patient who had a diagnosis of bipolar disorder or personality disorder, death, permanent nursing home resident or receiving hospice or palliative care any time during the measurement or assessment period M

G9395 Patient with an initial PHQ-9 score greater than nine who did not achieve remission at twelve months as demonstrated by a twelve-month (+/- 30 days) PHQ-9 score greater than or equal to five M

G9396 Patient with an initial PHQ-9 score greater than nine who was not assessed for remission at twelve months (+/- 30 days) M

G9402 ~~Patient received follow-up within 30 days after discharge~~

G9403 ~~Clinician documented reason patient was not able to complete 30-day follow-up from acute inpatient setting discharge (e.g., patient death prior to follow-up visit, patient noncompliant for visit follow-up)~~

G9404 ~~Patient did not receive follow-up within 30 days after discharge~~

G9405 ~~Patient received follow-up within 7 days after discharge~~

G9406 ~~Clinician documented reason patient was not able to complete 7-day follow-up from acute inpatient setting discharge (i.e., patient death prior to follow-up visit, patient noncompliance for visit follow-up)~~

G9407 ~~Patient did not receive follow-up within 7 days after discharge~~

G9408 Patients with cardiac tamponade and/or pericardiocentesis occurring within 30 days M

G9409 Patients without cardiac tamponade and/or pericardiocentesis occurring within 30 days M

G9410 Patient admitted within 180 days, status post CIED implantation, replacement, or revision with an infection requiring device removal or surgical revision M

G9411 Patient not admitted within 180 days, status post CIED implantation, replacement, or revision with an infection requiring device removal or surgical revision M

G9412 Patient admitted within 180 days, status post CIED implantation, replacement, or revision with an infection requiring device removal or surgical revision M

G9413 Patient not admitted within 180 days, status post CIED implantation, replacement, or revision with an infection requiring device removal or surgical revision M

G9414 Patient had one dose of meningococcal vaccine (serogroups A, C, W, Y) on or between the patient's 11th and 13th birthdays M

G9415 Patient did not have one dose of meningococcal vaccine (serogroups A, C, W, Y) on or between the patient's 11th and 13th birthdays M

G9416 Patient had one tetanus, diphtheria toxoids and acellular pertussis vaccine (TDaP) on or between the patient's 10th and 13th birthdays M

G9417 Patient did not have one tetanus, diphtheria toxoids and acellular pertussis vaccine (TDaP) on or between the patient's 10th and 13th birthdays M

G9418 Primary nonsmall cell lung cancer lung biopsy and cytology specimen report documents classification into specific histologic type following IASLC guidance or classified as NSCLC-NOS with an explanation M

G9419 Documentation of medical reason(s) for not including the histological type or NSCLC-NOS classification with an explanation (e.g. specimen insufficient or non-diagnostic, specimen does not contain cancer, or other documented medical reasons) M

G9420 Specimen site other than anatomic location of lung or is not classified as primary nonsmall cell lung cancer M

G9421 Primary nonsmall cell lung cancer lung biopsy and cytology specimen report does not document classification into specific histologic type or histologic type does not follow IASLC guidance or is classified as NSCLC-NOS but without an explanation M

G9422 Primary lung carcinoma resection report documents PT category, PN category and for nonsmall cell lung cancer, histologic type (e.g., squamous cell carcinoma, adenocarcinoma and not NSCLC-NOS) M

G9423 Documentation of medical reason for not including PT category, PN category and histologic type (for patient with appropriate exclusion criteria [e.g., metastatic disease, benign tumors, malignant tumors other than carcinomas, inadequate surgical specimens]) M

G9424 Specimen site other than anatomic location of lung, or classified as NSCLC-NOS M

G9425 Primary lung carcinoma resection report does not document PT category, PN category and for nonsmall cell lung cancer, histologic type (e.g., squamous cell carcinoma, adenocarcinoma) M

G9426 Improvement in median time from ED arrival to initial ED oral or parenteral pain medication administration performed for ED admitted patients M

G9427 Improvement in median time from ED arrival to initial ED oral or parenteral pain medication administration not performed for ED admitted patients M

G9428 Pathology report includes the PT category, thickness, ulceration and mitotic rate, peripheral and deep margin status and presence or absence of microsatellitosis for invasive tumors M

G9429 Documentation of medical reason(s) for not including PT category, thickness, ulceration and mitotic rate, peripheral and deep margin status and presence or absence of microsatellitosis for invasive tumors (e.g., negative skin biopsies, insufficient tissue, or other documented medical reasons) M

G9430 Specimen site other than anatomic cutaneous location M

G9431 Pathology report does not include the PT category, thickness, ulceration and mitotic rate, peripheral and deep margin status and presence or absence of microsatellitosis for invasive tumors M

G9432 Asthma well-controlled based on the ACT, C-ACT, ACQ, or ATAQ score and results documented M

G9434 Asthma not well-controlled based on the ACT, C-ACT, ACQ, or ATAQ score, or specified asthma control tool not used, reason not given M

G9452 Documentation of medical reason(s) for not receiving HCV antibody test due to limited life expectancy M
AHA: 1Q,24

G9455 Patient underwent abdominal imaging with ultrasound, contrast enhanced CT or contrast MRI for HCC M

G9456 Documentation of medical or patient reason(s) for not ordering or performing screening for HCC. Medical reason: comorbid medical conditions with expected survival < 5 years, hepatic decompensation and not a candidate for liver transplantation, or other medical reasons; patient reasons: patient declined or other patient reasons (e.g., cost of tests, time related to accessing testing equipment) M

G9457 Patient did not undergo abdominal imaging and did not have a documented reason for not undergoing abdominal imaging in the submission period M

G9458 ~~Patient documented as tobacco user and received tobacco cessation intervention (must include at least one of the following: advice given to quit smoking or tobacco use, counseling on the benefits of quitting smoking or tobacco use, assistance with or referral to external smoking or tobacco cessation support programs, or current enrollment in smoking or tobacco use cessation program) if identified as a tobacco user~~

G9459 ~~Currently a tobacco nonuser~~

G9460 ~~Tobacco assessment or tobacco cessation intervention not performed, reason not given~~

G9468 Patient not receiving corticosteroids greater than or equal to 10 mg/day of prednisone equivalents for 60 or greater consecutive days or a single prescription equating to 600 mg prednisone or greater for all fills M

G9470 Patients not receiving corticosteroids greater than or equal to 10 mg/day of prednisone equivalents for 60 or greater consecutive days or a single prescription equating to 600 mg prednisone or greater for all fills M

G9471 Within the past 2 years, central dual-energy x-ray absorptiometry (DXA) not ordered or documented M

Hospice Services

G9473 Services performed by chaplain in the hospice setting, each 15 minutes B

G9474 Services performed by dietary counselor in the hospice setting, each 15 minutes B

G9475 Services performed by other counselor in the hospice setting, each 15 minutes B

G9476 Services performed by volunteer in the hospice setting, each 15 minutes B

G9477 Services performed by care coordinator in the hospice setting, each 15 minutes B

G9478 Services performed by other qualified therapist in the hospice setting, each 15 minutes B

G9479 Services performed by qualified pharmacist in the hospice setting, each 15 minutes B

Medicare Care Choice Model Program

G9480 Admission to Medicare Care Choice Model Program (MCCM) B

CMS Innovation Center Demonstration Project

G9481 Remote in-home visit for the evaluation and management of a new patient for use only in a Medicare-approved CMS Innovation Center Demonstration Project, which requires these three key components: a problem focused history; a problem focused examination; straightforward medical decision making, furnished in real time using interactive audio and video technology. Counseling and coordination of care with other physicians, other qualified health care professionals or agencies are provided consistent with the nature of the problem(s) and the needs of the patient or the family or both. Usually, the presenting problem(s) are self limited or minor. Typically, 10 minutes are spent with the patient or family or both via real time, audio and video intercommunications technology B

G9482 Remote in-home visit for the evaluation and management of a new patient for use only in a Medicare-approved CMS Innovation Center Demonstration Project, which requires these three key components: an expanded problem focused history; an expanded problem focused examination; straightforward medical decision making, furnished in real time using interactive audio and video technology. Counseling and coordination of care with other physicians, other qualified health care professionals or agencies are provided consistent with the nature of the problem(s) and the needs of the patient or the family or both. Usually, the presenting problem(s) are of low to moderate severity. Typically, 20 minutes are spent with the patient or family or both via real time, audio and video intercommunications technology B

G9483 Remote in-home visit for the evaluation and management of a new patient for use only in a Medicare-approved CMS Innovation Center Demonstration Project, which requires these three key components: a detailed history; a detailed examination; medical decision making of low complexity, furnished in real time using interactive audio and video technology. Counseling and coordination of care with other physicians, other qualified health care professionals or agencies are provided consistent with the nature of the problem(s) and the needs of the patient or the family or both. Usually, the presenting problem(s) are of moderate severity. Typically, 30 minutes are spent with the patient or family or both via real time, audio and video intercommunications technology B

G9484 Remote in-home visit for the evaluation and management of a new patient for use only in a Medicare-approved CMS Innovation Center Demonstration Project, which requires these three key components: a comprehensive history; a comprehensive examination; medical decision making of moderate complexity, furnished in real time using interactive audio and video technology. Counseling and coordination of care with other physicians, other qualified health care professionals or agencies are provided consistent with the nature of the problem(s) and the needs of the patient or the family or both. Usually, the presenting problem(s) are of moderate to high severity. Typically, 45 minutes are spent with the patient or family or both via real time, audio and video intercommunications technology B

G9485 Remote in-home visit for the evaluation and management of a new patient for use only in a Medicare-approved CMS Innovation Center Demonstration Project, which requires these three key components: a comprehensive history; a comprehensive examination; medical decision making of high complexity, furnished in real time using interactive audio and video technology. Counseling and coordination of care with other physicians, other qualified health care professionals or agencies are provided consistent with the nature of the problem(s) and the needs of the patient or the family or both. Usually, the presenting problem(s) are of moderate to high severity. Typically, 60 minutes are spent with the patient or family or both via real time, audio and video intercommunications technology B

G9486 Remote in-home visit for the evaluation and management of an established patient for use only in a Medicare-approved CMS Innovation Center Demonstration Project, which requires at least two of the following three key components: a problem focused history; a problem focused examination; straightforward medical decision making, furnished in real time using interactive audio and video technology. Counseling and coordination of care with other physicians, other qualified health care professionals or agencies are provided consistent with the nature of the problem(s) and the needs of the patient or the family or both. Usually, the presenting problem(s) are self limited or minor. Typically, 10 minutes are spent with the patient or family or both via real time, audio and video intercommunications technology B

G9487 Remote in-home visit for the evaluation and management of an established patient for use only in a Medicare-approved CMS Innovation Center Demonstration Project, which requires at least two of the following three key components: an expanded problem focused history; an expanded problem focused examination; medical decision making of low complexity, furnished in real time using interactive audio and video technology. Counseling and coordination of care with other physicians, other qualified health care professionals or agencies are provided consistent with the nature of the problem(s) and the needs of the patient or the family or both. Usually, the presenting problem(s) are of low to moderate severity. Typically, 15 minutes are spent with the patient or family or both via real time, audio and video intercommunications technology B

G9488 Remote in-home visit for the evaluation and management of an established patient for use only in a Medicare-approved CMS Innovation Center Demonstration Project, which requires at least two of the following three key components: a detailed history; a detailed examination; medical decision making of moderate complexity, furnished in real time using interactive audio and video technology. Counseling and coordination of care with other physicians, other qualified health care professionals or agencies are provided consistent with the nature of the problem(s) and the needs of the patient or the family or both. Usually, the presenting problem(s) are of moderate to high severity. Typically, 25 minutes are spent with the patient or family or both via real time, audio and video intercommunications technology B

G9489 Remote in-home visit for the evaluation and management of an established patient for use only in a Medicare-approved CMS Innovation Center Demonstration Project, which requires at least two of the following three key components: a comprehensive history; a comprehensive examination; medical decision making of high complexity, furnished in real time using interactive audio and video technology. Counseling and coordination of care with other physicians, other qualified health care professionals or agencies are provided consistent with the nature of the problem(s) and the needs of the patient or the family or both. Usually, the presenting problem(s) are of moderate to high severity. Typically, 40 minutes are spent with the patient or family or both via real time, audio and video intercommunications technology B

G9490 CMS Innovation Center Models, home visit for patient assessment performed by clinical staff for an individual not considered homebound, including, but not necessarily limited to patient assessment of clinical status, safety/fall prevention, functional status/ambulation, medication reconciliation/management, compliance with orders/plan of care, performance of activities of daily living, and ensuring beneficiary connections to community and other services. (For use only in Medicare-approved CMS Innovation Center Models); may not be billed for a 30 day period covered by a transitional care management code B

Quality Measures

G9497 Received instruction from the anesthesiologist or proxy prior to the day of surgery to abstain from smoking on the day of surgery M

G9498 Antibiotic regimen prescribed M

G9500 Radiation exposure indices documented in final report for procedure using fluoroscopy M

G9501 Radiation exposure indices not documented in final report for procedure using fluoroscopy, reason not given M

G9502 Documentation of medical reason for not performing foot exam (i.e., patients who have had either a bilateral amputation above or below the knee, or both a left and right amputation above or below the knee before or during the measurement period) M

G9504 Documented reason for not assessing hepatitis B virus (HBV) status (e.g., patient not initiating anti-TNF therapy, patient declined) prior to initiating anti-TNF therapy M

G9505 Antibiotic regimen prescribed within 10 days after onset of symptoms for documented medical reason M

G9507 Documentation that the patient is on a statin medication or has documentation of a valid contraindication or exception to statin medications; contraindications/exceptions that can be defined by diagnosis codes include pregnancy during the measurement period, active liver disease, rhabdomyolysis, end stage renal disease on dialysis and heart failure; provider documented contraindications/exceptions include breastfeeding during the measurement period, woman of child-bearing age not actively taking birth control, allergy to statin, drug interaction (HIV protease inhibitors, nefazodone, cyclosporine, gemfibrozil, and danazol) and intolerance (with supporting documentation of trying a statin at least once within the last 5 years or diagnosis codes for myostitis or toxic myopathy related to drugs) M

G9508 Documentation that the patient is not on a statin medication M

G9509 Adult patients 18 years of age or older with major depression or dysthymia who reached remission at twelve months as demonstrated by a twelve-month (+/-60 days) PHQ-9 or PHQ-9M score of less than 5 M

G9510 Adult patients 18 years of age or older with major depression or dysthymia who did not reach remission at 12 months as demonstrated by a 12 month (+/-60 days) PHQ-9 or PHQ-9M score of less than 5. Either PHQ-9 or PHQ-9M score was not assessed or is greater than or equal to 5 M

G9511 Index PHQ-9 or PHQ-9M score greater than 9 documented during the twelve-month denominator identification period M

G9512 Individual had a PDC of 0.8 or greater M

G9513 Individual did not have a PDC of 0.8 or greater M

G9514 Patient required a return to the operating room within 90 days of surgery M

G9515 Patient did not require a return to the operating room within 90 days of surgery M

G9516 Patient achieved an improvement in visual acuity, from their preoperative level, within 90 days of surgery M

G9517 Patient did not achieve an improvement in visual acuity, from their preoperative level, within 90 days of surgery, reason not given M

G9518 Documentation of active injection drug use M

G9519 Patient achieves final refraction (spherical equivalent) +/- 1.0 diopters of their planned refraction within 90 days of surgery M

G9520 Patient does not achieve final refraction (spherical equivalent) +/- 1.0 diopters of their planned refraction within 90 days of surgery M

G9521 Total number of emergency department visits and inpatient hospitalizations less than two in the past 12 months M

G9522 Total number of emergency department visits and inpatient hospitalizations equal to or greater than two in the past 12 months or patient not screened, reason not given M

Blunt Head Trauma

G9529 Patient with minor blunt head trauma had an appropriate indication(s) for a head CT M

G9530 Patient presented with a minor blunt head trauma and had a head CT ordered for trauma by an emergency care provider M

G9531 Patient has documentation of ventricular shunt, brain tumor, multisystem trauma, or is currently taking an antiplatelet medication including: abciximab, anagrelide, cangrelor, cilostazol, clopidogrel, dipyridamole, eptifibatide, prasugrel, ticlopidine, ticagrelor, tirofiban, or vorapaxar M

G9533 Patient with minor blunt head trauma did not have an appropriate indication(s) for a head CT M

Miscellaneous Quality Measures

G9537 Imaging needed as part of a clinical trial; or other clinician ordered the study M

G9539 Intent for potential removal at time of placement M

G9540 Patient alive 3 months post procedure M

G9541 Filter removed within 3 months of placement M

G9542 Documented reassessment for the appropriateness of filter removal within 3 months of placement M

G9543 Documentation of at least two attempts to reach the patient to arrange a clinical reassessment for the appropriateness of filter removal within 3 months of placement M

Procedures/Professional Services (Temporary)

G9489 — G9543

G9544 Patients that do not have the filter removed, documented reassessment for the appropriateness of filter removal, or documentation of at least two attempts to reach the patient to arrange a clinical reassessment for the appropriateness of filter removal within 3 months of placement M

G9547 Cystic renal lesion that is simple appearing (Bosniak I or II), or adrenal lesion less than or equal to 1.0 cm or adrenal lesion greater than 1.0 cm but less than or equal to 4.0 cm classified as likely benign by unenhanced CT or washout protocol CT, or MRI with in- and opposed-phase sequences or other equivalent institutional imaging protocols M

G9548 Final reports for imaging studies stating no follow up imaging is recommended M

G9549 Documentation of medical reason(s) that follow up imaging is indicated (e.g., patient has lymphadenopathy, signs of metastasis or an active diagnosis or history of cancer, and other medical reason(s)) M

G9550 Final reports for imaging studies with follow-up imaging recommended, or final reports that do not include a specific recommendation of no follow-up M

G9551 Final reports for imaging studies without an incidentally found lesion noted M

G9552 Incidental thyroid nodule < 1.0 cm noted in report M

G9553 Prior thyroid disease diagnosis M

G9554 Final reports for CT, CTA, MRI or MRA of the chest or neck with follow-up imaging recommended M

G9555 Documentation of medical reason(s) for recommending follow up imaging (e.g., patient has multiple endocrine neoplasia, patient has cervical lymphadenopathy, other medical reason(s)) M

G9556 Final reports for CT, CTA, MRI or MRA of the chest or neck with follow-up imaging not recommended M

G9557 Final reports for CT, CTA, MRI or MRA studies of the chest or neck without an incidentally found thyroid nodule < 1.0 cm noted or no nodule found M

Stroke Therapy

G9580 Door to puncture time of 90 minutes or less M

G9582 Door to puncture time of greater than 90 minutes, no reason given M

Blunt Head Trauma

G9593 Pediatric patient with minor blunt head trauma classified as low risk according to the PECARN prediction rules M

G9594 Patient presented with a minor blunt head trauma and had a head CT ordered for trauma by an emergency care provider M

G9595 Patient has documentation of ventricular shunt, brain tumor, or coagulopathy M

G9597 Pediatric patient with minor blunt head trauma not classified as low risk according to the PECARN prediction rules M

Aortic Aneurysm

G9598 Aortic aneurysm 5.5-5.9 cm maximum diameter on centerline formatted CT or minor diameter on axial formatted CT M

G9599 Aortic aneurysm 6.0 cm or greater maximum diameter on centerline formatted CT or minor diameter on axial formatted CT M

Patient Survey

G9603 Patient survey score improved from baseline following treatment M

G9604 Patient survey results not available M

G9605 Patient survey score did not improve from baseline following treatment M

Intraoperative Cystoscopy

G9606 Intraoperative cystoscopy performed to evaluate for lower tract injury M

G9607 Documented medical reasons for not performing intraoperative cystoscopy (e.g., urethral pathology precluding cystoscopy, any patient who has a congenital or acquired absence of the urethra) or in the case of patient death M

G9608 Intraoperative cystoscopy not performed to evaluate for lower tract injury M

Aspirin/Antiplatelet Therapy

G9609 Documentation of an order for antiplatelet agents M

G9610 Documentation of medical reason(s) in the patient's record for not ordering antiplatelet agents M

G9611 Order for antiplatelet agents was not documented in the patient's record, reason not given M

Uterine Malignancy Screening

Alcohol Use

G9621 Patient identified as an unhealthy alcohol user when screened for unhealthy alcohol use using a systematic screening method and received brief counseling M

G9622 Patient not identified as an unhealthy alcohol user when screened for unhealthy alcohol use using a systematic screening method M

G9624 Patient not screened for unhealthy alcohol use using a systematic screening method or patient did not receive brief counseling if identified as an unhealthy alcohol user M

Bladder/Ureter Injury

G9625 Patient sustained bladder injury at the time of surgery or discovered subsequently up to 30 days post-surgery M

G9626 Documented medical reason for not reporting bladder injury (e.g., gynecologic or other pelvic malignancy documented, concurrent surgery involving bladder pathology, injury that occurs during urinary incontinence procedure, patient death from nonmedical causes not related to surgery, patient died during procedure without evidence of bladder injury) M

G9627 Patient did not sustain bladder injury at the time of surgery nor discovered subsequently up to 30 days post-surgery M

G9628 Patient sustained bowel injury at the time of surgery or discovered subsequently up to 30 days post-surgery M

G9629 Documented medical reasons for not reporting bowel injury (e.g., gynecologic or other pelvic malignancy documented, planned (e.g., not due to an unexpected bowel injury) resection and/or re-anastomosis of bowel, or patient death from nonmedical causes not related to surgery, patient died during procedure without evidence of bowel injury) M

G9630 Patient did not sustain a bowel injury at the time of surgery nor discovered subsequently up to 30 days post-surgery M

Quality Measures

G9637 Final reports with documentation of one or more dose reduction techniques (e.g., automated exposure control, adjustment of the mA and/or kV according to patient size, use of iterative reconstruction technique) M

G9638 Final reports without documentation of one or more dose reduction techniques (e.g., automated exposure control, adjustment of the mA and/or kV according to patient size, use of iterative reconstruction technique) M

G9642 Current smoker (e.g., cigarette, cigar, pipe, e-cigarette or marijuana) M

G9643 Elective surgery M

G9644 Patients who abstained from smoking prior to anesthesia on the day of surgery or procedure M

G9645 Patients who did not abstain from smoking prior to anesthesia on the day of surgery or procedure M

G9646 Patients with 90 day MRS score of 0 to 2 M

G9648 Patients with 90 day MRS score greater than 2 M

Psoriasis Therapy

G9649 Psoriasis assessment tool documented meeting any one of the specified benchmarks (e.g., (PGA; 5-point or 6-point scale), body surface area (BSA), psoriasis area and severity index (PASI) and/or dermatology life quality index (DLQI)) M

G9651 Psoriasis assessment tool documented not meeting any one of the specified benchmarks (e.g., (PGA; 5-point or 6-point scale), body surface area (BSA), psoriasis area and severity index (PASI) and/or dermatology life quality index (DLQI)) or psoriasis assessment tool not documented M

Anesthesia Services

G9654 Monitored anesthesia care (MAC) M

G9655 A transfer of care protocol or handoff tool/checklist that includes the required key handoff elements is used M

G9656 Patient transferred directly from anesthetizing location to PACU or other non-ICU location M

G9658 A transfer of care protocol or handoff tool/checklist that includes the required key handoff elements is not used M

Reason for Colonoscopy

▲ **G9659** Patients greater than or equal to 86 years of age who underwent a screening colonoscopy and did not have a history of colorectal cancer or other valid medical reason for the colonoscopy, including: iron deficiency anemia, lower gastrointestinal bleeding, familial adenomatous polyposis, lynch syndrome (i.e., hereditary non-polyposis colorectal cancer), inflammatory bowel disease (i.e., Crohn's disease or ulcerative colitis), abnormal finding of gastrointestinal tract, weight loss, or changes in bowel habits M

▲ **G9660** Documentation of medical reason(s) for a colonoscopy performed on a patient greater than or equal to 86 years of age (e.g., iron deficiency anemia, lower gastrointestinal bleeding, familial history of adenomatous polyposis, lynch syndrome (i.e., hereditary non-polyposis colorectal cancer), inflammatory bowel disease (i.e., Crohn's disease or ulcerative colitis), abnormal finding of gastrointestinal tract, weight loss, or changes in bowel habits) M

G9661 Patients greater than or equal to 86 years of age who received a colonoscopy for an assessment of signs/symptoms of GI tract illness, and/or because the patient meets high risk criteria, and/or to follow-up on previously diagnosed advanced lesions M

Statin Therapy

G9662 Previously diagnosed or have a diagnosis of clinical ASCVD, including ASCVD procedure M

G9663 Any LDL-C laboratory result >= 190 mg/dl M

G9664 Patients who are currently statin therapy users or received an order (prescription) for statin therapy M

G9665 Patients who are not currently statin therapy users or did not receive an order (prescription) for statin therapy M

Cardiovascular Measures

G9674 Patients with clinical ASCVD diagnosis M

G9675 Patients who have ever had a fasting or direct laboratory result of LDL-C = 190 mg/dl M

G9676 Patients aged 40 to 75 years at the beginning of the measurement period with type 1 or type 2 diabetes and with an ldl-c result of 70-189 mg/dl recorded as the highest fasting or direct laboratory test result in the measurement year or during the two years prior to the beginning of the measurement period M

Nursing Facility Care

G9679 Onsite acute care treatment of a nursing facility resident with pneumonia. May only be billed once per day per beneficiary B

G9680 Onsite acute care treatment of a nursing facility resident with CHF. May only be billed once per day per beneficiary B

G9681 Onsite acute care treatment of a nursing facility resident with COPD or asthma. May only be billed once per day per beneficiary B

G9682 Onsite acute care treatment of a nursing facility resident with a skin infection. May only be billed once per day per beneficiary B

G9683 Facility service(s) for the onsite acute care treatment of a nursing facility resident with fluid or electrolyte disorder. (May only be billed once per day per beneficiary.) This service is for a demonstration project B

G9684 Onsite acute care treatment of a nursing facility resident for a UTI. May only be billed once per day per beneficiary B

G9685 Physician service or other qualified health care professional for the evaluation and management of a beneficiary's acute change in condition in a nursing facility. This service is for a demonstration project M

Other Quality Measures

G9687 Hospice services provided to patient any time during the measurement period M

G9688 Patients using hospice services any time during the measurement period M

G9689 Patient admitted for performance of elective carotid intervention M

G9690 Patient receiving hospice services any time during the measurement period M

G9691 Patient had hospice services any time during the measurement period M

G9692 Hospice services received by patient any time during the measurement period M

G9693 Patient use of hospice services any time during the measurement period M

G9694 Hospice services utilized by patient any time during the measurement period M

G9695 Long-acting inhaled bronchodilator prescribed M

G9696 Documentation of medical reason(s) for not prescribing a long-acting inhaled bronchodilator (e.g., patient intolerance or history of side effects) M

AHA: 1Q,24

G9698 Documentation of system reason(s) for not prescribing a long-acting inhaled bronchodilator (e.g., cost of treatment or lack of insurance) M
AHA: 1Q,24

G9699 Long-acting inhaled bronchodilator not prescribed, reason not otherwise specified M

G9700 Patients who use hospice services any time during the measurement period M

G9702 Patients who use hospice services any time during the measurement period M

G9703 Episodes where the patient is taking antibiotics (Table 1) in the 30 days prior to the episode date M
AHA: 1Q,24

G9704 AJCC breast cancer Stage I: T1 mic or T1a documented M

G9705 AJCC breast cancer Stage I: T1b (tumor > 0.5 cm but <= 1 cm in greatest dimension) documented M

G9706 Low (or very low) risk of recurrence, prostate cancer M

~~G9707 Patient received hospice services any time during the measurement period~~

G9708 Women who had a bilateral mastectomy or who have a history of a bilateral mastectomy or for whom there is evidence of a right and a left unilateral mastectomy M

G9709 Hospice services used by patient any time during the measurement period M

G9710 Patient was provided hospice services any time during the measurement period M

G9711 Patients with a diagnosis or past history of total colectomy or colorectal cancer M

G9712 Documentation of medical reason(s) for prescribing or dispensing antibiotic (e.g., intestinal infection, pertussis, bacterial infection, lyme disease, otitis media, acute sinusitis, acute pharyngitis, acute tonsillitis, chronic sinusitis, infection of the pharynx/larynx/tonsils/adenoids, prostatitis, cellulitis/mastoiditis/bone infections, acute lymphadenitis, impetigo, skin staph infections, pneumonia, gonococcal infections/venereal disease (syphilis, chlamydia, inflammatory diseases [female reproductive organs]), infections of the kidney, cystitis/UTI, acne, HIV disease/asymptomatic HIV, cystic fibrosis, disorders of the immune system, malignancy neoplasms, chronic bronchitis, emphysema, bronchiectasis, extrinsic allergic alveolitis, chronic airway obstruction, chronic obstructive asthma, pneumoconiosis and other lung disease due to external agents, other diseases of the respiratory system, and tuberculosis M

G9713 Patients who use hospice services any time during the measurement period M

G9714 Patient is using hospice services any time during the measurement period M

G9716 BMI is documented as being outside of normal parameters, follow-up plan is not completed for documented medical reason M

G9717 Documentation stating the patient has had a diagnosis of bipolar disorder M
AHA: 1Q,24

G9719 Patient is not ambulatory, bed ridden, immobile, confined to chair, wheelchair bound, dependent on helper pushing wheelchair, independent in wheelchair or minimal help in wheelchair M

G9720 Hospice services for patient occurred any time during the measurement period M

G9721 Patient not ambulatory, bed ridden, immobile, confined to chair, wheelchair bound, dependent on helper pushing wheelchair, independent in wheelchair or minimal help in wheelchair M

G9722 Documented history of renal failure or baseline serum creatinine >= 4.0 mg/dl; renal transplant recipients are not considered to have preoperative renal failure, unless, since transplantation the CR has been or is 4.0 or higher M

G9723 Hospice services for patient received any time during the measurement period M

G9724 Patients who had documentation of use of anticoagulant medications overlapping the measurement year M

G9726 Patient refused to participate M

G9727 Patient unable to complete the LEPF PROM at initial evaluation and/or discharge due to blindness, illiteracy, severe mental incapacity or language incompatibility and an adequate proxy is not available M

G9728 Patient refused to participate M

G9729 Patient unable to complete the LEPF PROM at initial evaluation and/or discharge due to blindness, illiteracy, severe mental incapacity or language incompatibility and an adequate proxy is not available M

G9730 Patient refused to participate M

G9731 Patient unable to complete the LEPF PROM at initial evaluation and/or discharge due to blindness, illiteracy, severe mental incapacity or language incompatibility and an adequate proxy is not available M

G9732 Patient refused to participate M

G9733 Patient unable to complete the low back FS PROM at initial evaluation and/or discharge due to blindness, illiteracy, severe mental incapacity or language incompatibility and an adequate proxy is not available M

G9734 Patient refused to participate M

G9735 Patient unable to complete the shoulder FS PROM at initial evaluation and/or discharge due to blindness, illiteracy, severe mental incapacity or language incompatibility and an adequate proxy is not available M

G9736 Patient refused to participate M

G9737 Patient unable to complete the elbow/wrist/hand FS PROM at initial evaluation and/or discharge due to blindness, illiteracy, severe mental incapacity or language incompatibility and an adequate proxy is not available M

G9740 Hospice services given to patient any time during the measurement period M

G9741 Patients who use hospice services any time during the measurement period M

G9744 Patient not eligible due to active diagnosis of hypertension M

G9745 Documented reason for not screening or recommending a follow-up for high blood pressure M

G9746 Patient has mitral stenosis or prosthetic heart valves or patient has transient or reversible cause of AF (e.g., pneumonia, hyperthyroidism, pregnancy, cardiac surgery) M

~~G9751 Patient died at any time during the 24-month measurement period~~

G9752 Emergency surgery M

G9753 Documentation of medical reason for not conducting a search for DICOM format images for prior patient CT imaging studies completed at nonaffiliated external healthcare facilities or entities within the past 12 months that are available through a secure, authorized, media-free, shared archive (e.g., trauma, acute myocardial infarction, stroke, aortic aneurysm where time is of the essence) M

G9754 A finding of an incidental pulmonary nodule M

G9755 Documentation of medical reason(s) for not including a recommended interval and modality for follow-up or for no follow-up, and source of recommendations (e.g., patients with unexplained fever, immunocompromised patients who are at risk for infection) M

G9756 Surgical procedures that included the use of silicone oil M

G9757 Surgical procedures that included the use of silicone oil M

G9758 Patient in hospice at any time during the measurement period M

G9760 ~~Patients who use hospice services any time during the measurement period~~

G9761 Patients who use hospice services any time during the measurement period M

G9762 Patient had at least two HPV vaccines (with at least 146 days between the two) or three HPV vaccines on or between the patient's 9th and 13th birthdays M

G9763 Patient did not have at least two HPV vaccines (with at least 146 days between the two) or three HPV vaccines on or between the patient's 9th and 13th birthdays M

G9764 Patient has been treated with a systemic medication for psoriasis vulgaris M

G9765 Documentation that the patient declined change in medication or alternative therapies were unavailable, has documented contraindications, or has not been treated with a systemic medication for at least six consecutive months (e.g., experienced adverse effects or lack of efficacy with all other therapy options) in order to achieve better disease control as measured by PGA, BSA, PASI, or DLQI M

G9766 Patients who are transferred from one institution to another with a known diagnosis of CVA for endovascular stroke treatment M

G9767 Hospitalized patients with newly diagnosed CVA considered for endovascular stroke treatment M

G9768 Patients who utilize hospice services any time during the measurement period M

G9769 Patient had a bone mineral density test in the past two years or received osteoporosis medication or therapy in the past 12 months M

G9770 Peripheral nerve block (PNB) M

G9771 At least one body temperature measurement equal to or greater than 35.5 degrees Celsius (or 95.9 degrees Fahrenheit) achieved within the 30 minutes immediately before or 15 minutes immediately after anesthesia end time M
AHA: 1Q,24

G9772 Documentation of medical reason(s) for not achieving at least one body temperature measurement equal to or greater than 35.5 degrees Celsius (or 95.9 degrees Fahrenheit) within the 30 minutes immediately before or 15 minutes immediately after anesthesia end time (e.g., emergency cases, intentional hypothermia, etc.) M
AHA: 1Q,24

G9773 At least one body temperature measurement equal to or greater than 35.5 degrees Celsius (or 95.9 degrees Fahrenheit) not achieved within the 30 minutes immediately before or 15 minutes immediately after anesthesia end time, reason not given M
AHA: 1Q,24

G9775 Patient received at least two prophylactic pharmacologic antiemetic agents of different classes preoperatively and/or intraoperatively M

G9776 Documentation of medical reason for not receiving at least two prophylactic pharmacologic antiemetic agents of different classes preoperatively and/or intraoperatively (e.g., intolerance or other medical reason) M

G9777 Patient did not receive at least two prophylactic pharmacologic antiemetic agents of different classes preoperatively and/or intraoperatively M

G9779 Patients who are breastfeeding at any time during the performance period M
AHA: 1Q,24

G9780 Patients who have a diagnosis of rhabdomyolysis at any time during the performance period M
AHA: 1Q,24

G9781 Documentation of medical reason(s) for not currently being a statin therapy user or receiving an order (prescription) for statin therapy (e.g., patients with statin-associated muscle symptoms or an allergy to statin medication therapy, patients who are receiving palliative or hospice care, patients with active liver disease or hepatic disease or insufficiency, patients with end stage renal disease [ESRD], or other medical reasons) M

G9782 History of or active diagnosis of familial hypercholesterolemia M

G9784 Pathologists/dermatopathologists providing a second opinion on a biopsy M

G9785 Pathology report diagnosing cutaneous basal cell carcinoma, squamous cell carcinoma, or melanoma (to include in situ disease) sent from the pathologist/dermatopathologist to the biopsying clinician for review within 7 days from the time when the tissue specimen was received by the pathologist M

G9786 Pathology report diagnosing cutaneous basal cell carcinoma, squamous cell carcinoma, or melanoma (to include in situ disease) was not sent from the pathologist/dermatopathologist to the biopsying clinician for review within 7 days from the time when the tissue specimen was received by the pathologist M

G9787 Patient alive as of the last day of the measurement year M

G9788 Most recent BP is less than or equal to 140/90 mm Hg M

G9789 Blood pressure recorded during inpatient stays, emergency room visits, or urgent care visits M

G9790 Most recent BP is greater than 140/90 mm Hg, or blood pressure not documented M

G9791 Most recent tobacco status is tobacco free M

G9792 Most recent tobacco status is not tobacco free M

G9793 Patient is currently on a daily aspirin or other antiplatelet M

G9794 Documentation of medical reason(s) for not on a daily aspirin or other antiplatelet (e.g., history of gastrointestinal bleed, intracranial bleed, idiopathic thrombocytopenic purpura (ITP), gastric bypass or documentation of active anticoagulant use during the measurement period) M

G9795 Patient is not currently on a daily aspirin or other antiplatelet M

G9796 Patient is currently on a statin therapy M

G9797 Patient is not on a statin therapy M

G9805 Patients who use hospice services any time during the measurement period M

G9806 Patients who received cervical cytology or an HPV test M

G9807 Patients who did not receive cervical cytology or an HPV test M

G9812 Patient died including all deaths occurring during the hospitalization in which the operation was performed, even if after 30 days, and those deaths occurring after discharge from the hospital, but within 30 days of the procedure M

G9813 Patient did not die within 30 days of the procedure or during the index hospitalization M

G9818 Documentation of sexual activity M

G9819 Patients who use hospice services any time during the measurement period M

G9820 Documentation of a chlamydia screening test with proper follow-up M

G9821 No documentation of a chlamydia screening test with proper follow-up M

G9822 Patients who had an endometrial ablation procedure during the 12 months prior to the index date (exclusive of the index date) M

G9823 Endometrial sampling or hysteroscopy with biopsy and results documented during the 12 months prior to the index date (exclusive of the index date) of the endometrial ablation M

G9824 Endometrial sampling or hysteroscopy with biopsy and results not documented during the 12 months prior to the index date (exclusive of the index date) of the endometrial ablation M

G9830 HER2/neu positive M

G9831 AJCC Stage at breast cancer diagnosis = II or III M

G9832 AJCC Stage at breast cancer diagnosis = I (Ia or Ib) and T-Stage at breast cancer diagnosis does not equal = T1, T1a, T1b M

G9838 Patient has metastatic disease at diagnosis M

G9839 Anti-EGFR monoclonal antibody therapy M

G9840 RAS (KRAS and NRAS) gene mutation testing performed before initiation of anti-EGFR MoAb M

G9841 RAS (KRAS and NRAS) gene mutation testing not performed before initiation of anti-EGFR MoAb M

G9842 Patient has metastatic disease at diagnosis M

G9843 RAS (KRAS or NRAS) gene mutation M

G9844 Patient did not receive anti-EGFR monoclonal antibody therapy M

G9845 Patient received anti-EGFR monoclonal antibody therapy M

G9846 Patients who died from cancer M

G9847 Patient received systemic cancer-directed therapy in the last 14 days of life M

G9848 Patient did not receive systemic cancer-directed therapy in the last 14 days of life M

G9858 Patient enrolled in hospice M

G9859 Patients who died from cancer M

G9860 Patient spent less than three days in hospice care M

G9861 Patient spent greater than or equal to three days in hospice care M

G9862 Documentation of medical reason(s) for not recommending at least a 10 year follow-up interval (e.g., inadequate prep, familial or personal history of colonic polyps, patient had no adenoma and age is = 66 years old, or life expectancy < 10 years old, other medical reasons) M

G9868 Receipt and analysis of remote, asynchronous images for dermatologic and/or ophthalmologic evaluation, for use only in a Medicare-approved CMMI model, less than 10 minutes B
AHA: 2Q,21

G9869 Receipt and analysis of remote, asynchronous images for dermatologic and/or ophthalmologic evaluation, for use only in a Medicare-approved CMMI model, 10 to 20 minutes B
AHA: 2Q,21

G9870 Receipt and analysis of remote, asynchronous images for dermatologic and/or ophthalmologic evaluation, for use only in a Medicare-approved CMMI model, more than 20 minutes B
AHA: 2Q,21

G9873 First Medicare Diabetes Prevention Program (MDPP) core session was attended by an MDPP beneficiary under the MDPP Expanded Model (EM). A core session is an MDPP service that: (1) is furnished by an MDPP supplier during months 1 through 6 of the MDPP services period; (2) is approximately 1 hour in length; and (3) adheres to a CDC-approved DPP curriculum for core sessions M

G9874 Four total Medicare Diabetes Prevention Program (MDPP) core sessions were attended by an MDPP beneficiary under the MDPP Expanded Model (EM). A core session is an MDPP service that: (1) is furnished by an MDPP supplier during months 1 through 6 of the MDPP services period; (2) is approximately 1 hour in length; and (3) adheres to a CDC-approved DPP curriculum for core sessions M

G9875 Nine total Medicare Diabetes Prevention Program (MDPP) core sessions were attended by an MDPP beneficiary under the MDPP Expanded Model (EM). A core session is an MDPP service that: (1) is furnished by an MDPP supplier during months 1 through 6 of the MDPP services period; (2) is approximately 1 hour in length; and (3) adheres to a CDC-approved DPP curriculum for core sessions M

G9876 Two Medicare Diabetes Prevention Program (MDPP) core maintenance sessions (MS) were attended by an MDPP beneficiary in months (mo) 7-9 under the MDPP Expanded Model (EM). A core maintenance session is an MDPP service that: (1) is furnished by an MDPP supplier during months 7 through 12 of the MDPP services period; (2) is approximately 1 hour in length; and (3) adheres to a CDC-approved DPP curriculum for maintenance sessions. The beneficiary did not achieve at least 5% weight loss (WL) from his/her baseline weight, as measured by at least one in-person weight measurement at a core maintenance session in months 7-9 M

G9877 Two Medicare Diabetes Prevention Program (MDPP) core maintenance sessions (MS) were attended by an MDPP beneficiary in months (mo) 10-12 under the MDPP Expanded Model (EM). A core maintenance session is an MDPP service that: (1) is furnished by an MDPP supplier during months 7 through 12 of the MDPP services period; (2) is approximately 1 hour in length; and (3) adheres to a CDC-approved DPP curriculum for maintenance sessions. The beneficiary did not achieve at least 5% weight loss (WL) from his/her baseline weight, as measured by at least one in-person weight measurement at a core maintenance session in months 10-12 M

G9878 Two Medicare Diabetes Prevention Program (MDPP) core maintenance sessions (MS) were attended by an MDPP beneficiary in months (mo) 7-9 under the MDPP Expanded Model (EM). A core maintenance session is an MDPP service that: (1) is furnished by an MDPP supplier during months 7 through 12 of the MDPP services period; (2) is approximately 1 hour in length; and (3) adheres to a CDC-approved DPP curriculum for maintenance sessions. The beneficiary achieved at least 5% weight loss (WL) from his/her baseline weight, as measured by at least one in-person weight measurement at a core maintenance session in months 7-9 M

G9879 Two Medicare Diabetes Prevention Program (MDPP) core maintenance sessions (MS) were attended by an MDPP beneficiary in months (mo) 10-12 under the MDPP Expanded Model (EM). A core maintenance session is an MDPP service that: (1) is furnished by an MDPP supplier during months 7 through 12 of the MDPP services period; (2) is approximately 1 hour in length; and (3) adheres to a CDC-approved DPP curriculum for maintenance sessions. The beneficiary achieved at least 5% weight loss (WL) from his/her baseline weight, as measured by at least one in-person weight measurement at a core maintenance session in months 10-12 M

G9880 The MDPP beneficiary achieved at least 5% weight loss (WL) from his/her baseline weight in months 1-12 of the MDPP services period under the MDPP Expanded Model (EM). This is a one-time payment available when a beneficiary first achieves at least 5% weight loss from baseline as measured by an in-person weight measurement at a core session or core maintenance session M

G9881 The MDPP beneficiary achieved at least 9% weight loss (WL) from his/her baseline weight in months 1-24 under the MDPP Expanded Model (EM). This is a one-time payment available when a beneficiary first achieves at least 9% weight loss from baseline as measured by an in-person weight measurement at a core session, core maintenance session, or ongoing maintenance session M

G9882 Two Medicare Diabetes Prevention Program (MDPP) ongoing maintenance sessions (MS) were attended by an MDPP beneficiary in months (mo) 13-15 under the MDPP Expanded Model (EM). An ongoing maintenance session is an MDPP service that: (1) is furnished by an MDPP supplier during months 13 through 24 of the MDPP services period; (2) is approximately 1 hour in length; and (3) adheres to a CDC-approved DPP curriculum for maintenance sessions. The beneficiary maintained at least 5% weight loss (WL) from his/her baseline weight, as measured by at least one in-person weight measurement at an ongoing maintenance session in months 13-15 M

G9883 Two Medicare Diabetes Prevention Program (MDPP) ongoing maintenance sessions (MS) were attended by an MDPP beneficiary in months (mo) 16-18 under the MDPP Expanded Model (EM). An ongoing maintenance session is an MDPP service that: (1) is furnished by an MDPP supplier during months 13 through 24 of the MDPP services period; (2) is approximately 1 hour in length; and (3) adheres to a CDC-approved DPP curriculum for maintenance sessions. The beneficiary maintained at least 5% weight loss (WL) from his/her baseline weight, as measured by at least one in-person weight measurement at an ongoing maintenance session in months 16-18 M

G9884 Two Medicare Diabetes Prevention Program (MDPP) ongoing maintenance sessions (MS) were attended by an MDPP beneficiary in months (mo) 19-21 under the MDPP Expanded Model (EM). An ongoing maintenance session is an MDPP service that: (1) is furnished by an MDPP supplier during months 13 through 24 of the MDPP services period; (2) is approximately 1 hour in length; and (3) adheres to a CDC-approved DPP curriculum for maintenance sessions. The beneficiary maintained at least 5% weight loss (WL) from his/her baseline weight, as measured by at least one in-person weight measurement at an ongoing maintenance session in months 19-21 M

G9885 Two Medicare Diabetes Prevention Program (MDPP) ongoing maintenance sessions (MS) were attended by an MDPP beneficiary in months (mo) 22-24 under the MDPP Expanded Model (EM). An ongoing maintenance session is an MDPP service that: (1) is furnished by an MDPP supplier during months 13 through 24 of the MDPP services period; (2) is approximately 1 hour in length; and (3) adheres to a CDC-approved DPP curriculum for maintenance sessions. The beneficiary maintained at least 5% weight loss (WL) from his/her baseline weight, as measured by at least one in-person weight measurement at an ongoing maintenance session in months 22-24 M

Behavioral Counseling

● **G9886** Behavioral counseling for diabetes prevention, in-person, group, 60 minutes M

AHA: 1Q,24

● **G9887** Behavioral counseling for diabetes prevention, distance learning, 60 minutes M

AHA: 1Q,24

Other Quality Measure

● **G9888** Maintenance 5% WL from baseline weight in months 7-12 M

AHA: 1Q,24

G9890 Bridge Payment: A one-time payment for the first Medicare Diabetes Prevention Program (MDPP) core session, core maintenance session, or ongoing maintenance session furnished by an MDPP supplier to an MDPP beneficiary during months 1-24 of the MDPP Expanded Model (EM) who has previously received MDPP services from a different MDPP supplier under the MDPP Expanded Model. A supplier may only receive one bridge payment per MDPP beneficiary M

G9891 MDPP session reported as a line-item on a claim for a payable MDPP Expanded Model (EM) HCPCS code for a session furnished by the billing supplier under the MDPP Expanded Model and counting toward achievement of the attendance performance goal for the payable MDPP Expanded Model HCPCS code. (This code is for reporting purposes only) M

G9892 ~~Documentation of patient reason(s) for not performing a dilated macular examination~~

G9893 ~~Dilated macular exam was not performed, reason not otherwise specified~~

G9894 Androgen deprivation therapy prescribed/administered in combination with external beam radiotherapy to the prostate M

G9895 Documentation of medical reason(s) for not prescribing/administering androgen deprivation therapy in combination with external beam radiotherapy to the prostate (e.g., salvage therapy) M

G9896 Documentation of patient reason(s) for not prescribing/administering androgen deprivation therapy in combination with external beam radiotherapy to the prostate M

G9897 Patients who were not prescribed/administered androgen deprivation therapy in combination with external beam radiotherapy to the prostate, reason not given M

G9898 Patients age 66 or older in institutional special needs plans (SNP) or residing in long-term care with POS code 32, 33, 34, 54, or 56 for more than 90 consecutive days during the measurement period M

G9899 Screening, diagnostic, film, digital or digital breast tomosynthesis (3D) mammography results documented and reviewed M

G9900 Screening, diagnostic, film, digital or digital breast tomosynthesis (3D) mammography results were not documented and reviewed, reason not otherwise specified M

G9901 Patient age 66 or older in institutional special needs plans (SNP) or residing in long-term care with POS code 32, 33, 34, 54, or 56 for more than 90 consecutive days during the measurement period M

G9902 Patient screened for tobacco use and identified as a tobacco user M

G9903 Patient screened for tobacco use and identified as a tobacco nonuser M

G9905 Patient not screened for tobacco use M

G9906 Patient identified as a tobacco user received tobacco cessation intervention during the measurement period or in the 6 months prior to the measurement period (counseling and/or pharmacotherapy) M

G9908 Patient identified as tobacco user did not receive tobacco cessation intervention during the measurement period or in the 6 months prior to the measurement period (counseling and/or pharmacotherapy) M

G9910 Patients age 66 or older in institutional special needs plans (SNP) or residing in long-term care with POS code 32, 33, 34, 54 or 56 for more than 90 consecutive days during the measurement period M

G9911 Clinically node negative (T1N0M0 or T2N0M0) invasive breast cancer before or after neoadjuvant systemic therapy M

G9912 Hepatitis B virus (HBV) status assessed and results interpreted prior to initiating anti-TNF (tumor necrosis factor) therapy M

G9913 Hepatitis B virus (HBV) status not assessed and results interpreted prior to initiating anti-TNF (tumor necrosis factor) therapy, reason not otherwise specified M

G9914 Patient initiated an anti-TNF agent M
AHA: 1Q,24

G9915 No record of HBV results documented M

G9916 Functional status performed once in the last 12 months M

G9917 Documentation of advanced stage dementia and caregiver knowledge is limited M

G9918 Functional status not performed, reason not otherwise specified M

G9919 ~~Screening performed and positive and provision of recommendations~~

G9920 ~~Screening performed and negative~~

G9921 ~~No screening performed, partial screening performed or positive screen without recommendations and reason is not given or otherwise specified~~

G9922 Safety concerns screen provided and if positive then documented mitigation recommendations M

G9923 Safety concerns screen provided and negative M

G9925 Safety concerns screening not provided, reason not otherwise specified M

G9926 Safety concerns screening positive screen is without provision of mitigation recommendations, including but not limited to referral to other resources M

G9928 FDA-approved anticoagulant not prescribed, reason not given M

G9929 Patient with transient or reversible cause of AF (e.g., pneumonia, hyperthyroidism, pregnancy, cardiac surgery) M

G9930 Patients who are receiving comfort care only M

G9931 Documentation of CHA2DS2-VASc risk score of 0 or 1 for men; or 0, 1, or 2 for women M

G9938 Patients aged 66 or older in institutional special needs plans (SNP) or residing in long-term care with POS code 32, 33, 34, 54, or 56 for more than 90 consecutive days during the 6 months prior to the measurement period through December 31 of the measurement period M
AHA: 1Q,24

G9939 Pathologist(s)/dermatopathologist(s) is the same clinician who performed the biopsy M

G9940 Documentation of medical reason(s) for not on a statin (e.g., pregnancy, in vitro fertilization, clomiphene Rx, ESRD, cirrhosis, muscular pain and disease during the measurement period or prior year) M

G9943 Back pain was not measured by the visual analog scale (VAS) or numeric pain scale at three months (6 to 20 weeks) postoperatively M

G9945 Patient had cancer, acute fracture or infection related to the lumbar spine or patient had neuromuscular, idiopathic or congenital lumbar scoliosis M

G9946 Back pain was not measured by the visual analog scale (VAS) or numeric pain scale at one year (9 to 15 months) postoperatively M

G9949 Leg pain was not measured by the visual analog scale (VAS) or numeric pain scale at three months (6 to 20 weeks) postoperatively M

G9954 Patient exhibits 2 or more risk factors for postoperative vomiting M

G9955 Cases in which an inhalational anesthetic is used only for induction M

G9956 Patient received combination therapy consisting of at least two prophylactic pharmacologic antiemetic agents of different classes preoperatively and/or intraoperatively M

G9957 Documentation of medical reason for not receiving combination therapy consisting of at least two prophylactic pharmacologic antiemetic agents of different classes preoperatively and/or intraoperatively (e.g., intolerance or other medical reason) M

G9958 Patient did not receive combination therapy consisting of at least two prophylactic pharmacologic antiemetic agents of different classes preoperatively and/or intraoperatively M

G9959 Systemic antimicrobials not prescribed M

G9960 Documentation of medical reason(s) for prescribing systemic antimicrobials M

G9961 Systemic antimicrobials prescribed M

G9962 Embolization endpoints are documented separately for each embolized vessel and ovarian artery angiography or embolization performed in the presence of variant uterine artery anatomy M

G9963 Embolization endpoints are not documented separately for each embolized vessel or ovarian artery angiography or embolization not performed in the presence of variant uterine artery anatomy M

G9964 Patient received at least one well-child visit with a PCP during the performance period M

G9965 Patient did not receive at least one well-child visit with PCP during the performance period M

G9968 Patient was referred to another clinician or specialist during the measurement period M

G9969 Clinician who referred the patient to another clinician received a report from the clinician to whom the patient was referred M

G9970 Clinician who referred the patient to another clinician did not receive a report from the clinician to whom the patient was referred M

G9974 ~~Dilated macular exam performed, including documentation of the presence or absence of macular thickening or geographic atrophy or hemorrhage and the level of macular degeneration severity~~

G9975 ~~Documentation of medical reason(s) for not performing a dilated macular examination~~

G9978 Remote in-home visit for the evaluation and management of a new patient for use only in a Medicare-approved Bundled Payments for Care Improvement Advanced (BPCI Advanced) model episode of care, which requires these three key components: a problem focused history; a problem focused examination; straightforward medical decision making, furnished in real time using interactive audio and video technology. Counseling and coordination of care with other physicians, other qualified health care professionals or agencies are provided consistent with the nature of the problem(s) and the needs of the patient or the family or both. Usually, the presenting problem(s) are self limited or minor. Typically, 10 minutes are spent with the patient or family or both via real time, audio and video intercommunications technology B

G9979 Remote in-home visit for the evaluation and management of a new patient for use only in a Medicare-approved Bundled Payments for Care Improvement Advanced (BPCI Advanced) model episode of care, which requires these three key components: an expanded problem focused history; an expanded problem focused examination; straightforward medical decision making, furnished in real time using interactive audio and video technology. Counseling and coordination of care with other physicians, other qualified health care professionals or agencies are provided consistent with the nature of the problem(s) and the needs of the patient or the family or both. Usually, the presenting problem(s) are of low to moderate severity. Typically, 20 minutes are spent with the patient or family or both via real time, audio and video intercommunications technology B

G9980 Remote in-home visit for the evaluation and management of a new patient for use only in a Medicare-approved Bundled Payments for Care Improvement Advanced (BPCI Advanced) model episode of care, which requires these three key components: a detailed history; a detailed examination; medical decision making of low complexity, furnished in real time using interactive audio and video technology. Counseling and coordination of care with other physicians, other qualified health care professionals or agencies are provided consistent with the nature of the problem(s) and the needs of the patient or the family or both. Usually, the presenting problem(s) are of moderate severity. Typically, 30 minutes are spent with the patient or family or both via real time, audio and video intercommunications technology B

G9981 Remote in-home visit for the evaluation and management of a new patient for use only in a Medicare-approved Bundled Payments for Care Improvement Advanced (BPCI Advanced) model episode of care, which requires these three key components: a comprehensive history; a comprehensive examination; medical decision making of moderate complexity, furnished in real time using interactive audio and video technology. Counseling and coordination of care with other physicians, other qualified health care professionals or agencies are provided consistent with the nature of the problem(s) and the needs of the patient or the family or both. Usually, the presenting problem(s) are of moderate to high severity. Typically, 45 minutes are spent with the patient or family or both via real time, audio and video intercommunications technology B

G9982 Remote in-home visit for the evaluation and management of a new patient for use only in a Medicare-approved Bundled Payments for Care Improvement Advanced (BPCI Advanced) model episode of care, which requires these three key components: a comprehensive history; a comprehensive examination; medical decision making of high complexity, furnished in real time using interactive audio and video technology. Counseling and coordination of care with other physicians, other qualified health care professionals or agencies are provided consistent with the nature of the problem(s) and the needs of the patient or the family or both. Usually, the presenting problem(s) are of moderate to high severity. Typically, 60 minutes are spent with the patient or family or both via real time, audio and video intercommunications technology B

G9983 Remote in-home visit for the evaluation and management of an established patient for use only in a Medicare-approved Bundled Payments for Care Improvement Advanced (BPCI Advanced) model episode of care, which requires at least two of the following three key components: a problem focused history; a problem focused examination; straightforward medical decision making, furnished in real time using interactive audio and video technology. Counseling and coordination of care with other physicians, other qualified health care professionals or agencies are provided consistent with the nature of the problem(s) and the needs of the patient or the family or both. Usually, the presenting problem(s) are self limited or minor. Typically, 10 minutes are spent with the patient or family or both via real time, audio and video intercommunications technology B

G9984 Remote in-home visit for the evaluation and management of an established patient for use only in a Medicare-approved Bundled Payments for Care Improvement Advanced (BPCI Advanced) model episode of care, which requires at least two of the following three key components: an expanded problem focused history; an expanded problem focused examination; medical decision making of low complexity, furnished in real time using interactive audio and video technology. Counseling and coordination of care with other physicians, other qualified health care professionals or agencies are provided consistent with the nature of the problem(s) and the needs of the patient or the family or both. Usually, the presenting problem(s) are of low to moderate severity. Typically, 15 minutes are spent with the patient or family or both via real time, audio and video intercommunications technology B

G9985 Remote in-home visit for the evaluation and management of an established patient for use only in a Medicare-approved Bundled Payments for Care Improvement Advanced (BPCI Advanced) model episode of care, which requires at least two of the following three key components: a detailed history; a detailed examination; medical decision making of moderate complexity, furnished in real time using interactive audio and video technology. Counseling and coordination of care with other physicians, other qualified health care professionals or agencies are provided consistent with the nature of the problem(s) and the needs of the patient or the family or both. Usually, the presenting problem(s) are of moderate to high severity. Typically, 25 minutes are spent with the patient or family or both via real time, audio and video intercommunications technology B

G9986 Remote in-home visit for the evaluation and management of an established patient for use only in a Medicare-approved Bundled Payments for Care Improvement Advanced (BPCI Advanced) model episode of care, which requires at least two of the following three key components: a comprehensive history; a comprehensive examination; medical decision making of high complexity, furnished in real time using interactive audio and video technology. Counseling and coordination of care with other physicians, other qualified health care professionals or agencies are provided consistent with the nature of the problem(s) and the needs of the patient or the family or both. Usually, the presenting problem(s) are of moderate to high severity. Typically, 40 minutes are spent with the patient or family or both via real time, audio and video intercommunications technology B

G9987 Bundled Payments for Care Improvement Advanced (BPCI Advanced) model home visit for patient assessment performed by clinical staff for an individual not considered homebound, including, but not necessarily limited to patient assessment of clinical status, safety/fall prevention, functional status/ambulation, medication reconciliation/management, compliance with orders/plan of care, performance of activities of daily living, and ensuring beneficiary connections to community and other services; for use only for a BPCI Advanced model episode of care; may not be billed for a 30-day period covered by a transitional care management code B

G9988 Palliative care services provided to patient any time during the measurement period M

G9990 ~~Patient did not receive any pneumococcal conjugate or polysaccharide vaccine on or after their 19th birthday and before the end of the measurement period~~

G9991 ~~Patient received any pneumococcal conjugate or polysaccharide vaccine on or after their 19th birthday and before the end of the measurement period~~

G9992 Palliative care services used by patient any time during the measurement period M

G9993 Patient was provided palliative care services any time during the measurement period M

G9994 Patient is using palliative care services any time during the measurement period M

G9996 Documentation stating the patient has received or is currently receiving palliative or hospice care M

G9997 Documentation of patient pregnancy anytime during the measurement period prior to and including the current encounter M

G9998 Documentation of medical reason(s) for an interval of less than 3 years since the last colonoscopy (e.g., last colonoscopy incomplete, last colonoscopy had inadequate prep, piecemeal removal of adenomas, or sessile serrated polyps >= 20 mm in size, last colonoscopy found greater than 10 adenomas, lower gastrointestinal bleeding, or patient at high risk for colon cancer due to underlying medical history [i.e., Crohn's disease, ulcerative colitis, personal or family history of colon cancer, hereditary colorectal cancer syndromes])

AHA: 1Q,24

▲ **G9999** Documentation of system reason(s) for an interval of less than 3 years since the last colonoscopy (e.g., unable to locate previous colonoscopy report, patient cannot provide precise date or details from previous colonoscopy, previous colonoscopy report was incomplete) M

Alcohol and Drug Abuse Treatment Services H0001-H2041

The H codes are used by those state Medicaid agencies that are mandated by state law to establish separate codes for identifying mental health services that include alcohol and drug treatment services.

H0001 Alcohol and/or drug assessment

H0002 Behavioral health screening to determine eligibility for admission to treatment program

H0003 Alcohol and/or drug screening; laboratory analysis of specimens for presence of alcohol and/or drugs

H0004 Behavioral health counseling and therapy, per 15 minutes ☑

H0005 Alcohol and/or drug services; group counseling by a clinician

H0006 Alcohol and/or drug services; case management

H0007 Alcohol and/or drug services; crisis intervention (outpatient)

H0008 Alcohol and/or drug services; subacute detoxification (hospital inpatient)

H0009 Alcohol and/or drug services; acute detoxification (hospital inpatient)

H0010 Alcohol and/or drug services; subacute detoxification (residential addiction program inpatient)

H0011 Alcohol and/or drug services; acute detoxification (residential addiction program inpatient)

H0012 Alcohol and/or drug services; subacute detoxification (residential addiction program outpatient)

H0013 Alcohol and/or drug services; acute detoxification (residential addiction program outpatient)

H0014 Alcohol and/or drug services; ambulatory detoxification

H0015 Alcohol and/or drug services; intensive outpatient (treatment program that operates at least 3 hours/day and at least 3 days/week and is based on an individualized treatment plan), including assessment, counseling; crisis intervention, and activity therapies or education

H0016 Alcohol and/or drug services; medical/somatic (medical intervention in ambulatory setting)

H0017 Behavioral health; residential (hospital residential treatment program), without room and board, per diem ☑

H0018 Behavioral health; short-term residential (nonhospital residential treatment program), without room and board, per diem ☑

H0019 Behavioral health; long-term residential (nonmedical, nonacute care in a residential treatment program where stay is typically longer than 30 days), without room and board, per diem ☑

H0020 Alcohol and/or drug services; methadone administration and/or service (provision of the drug by a licensed program)

H0021 Alcohol and/or drug training service (for staff and personnel not employed by providers)

H0022 Alcohol and/or drug intervention service (planned facilitation)

H0023 Behavioral health outreach service (planned approach to reach a targeted population)

H0024 Behavioral health prevention information dissemination service (one-way direct or nondirect contact with service audiences to affect knowledge and attitude)

H0025 Behavioral health prevention education service (delivery of services with target population to affect knowledge, attitude and/or behavior)

H0026 Alcohol and/or drug prevention process service, community-based (delivery of services to develop skills of impactors)

H0027 Alcohol and/or drug prevention environmental service (broad range of external activities geared toward modifying systems in order to mainstream prevention through policy and law)

H0028 Alcohol and/or drug prevention problem identification and referral service (e.g., student assistance and employee assistance programs), does not include assessment

H0029 Alcohol and/or drug prevention alternatives service (services for populations that exclude alcohol and other drug use e.g., alcohol free social events)

H0030 Behavioral health hotline service

H0031 Mental health assessment, by nonphysician

H0032 Mental health service plan development by nonphysician

H0033 Oral medication administration, direct observation

H0034 Medication training and support, per 15 minutes ☑

H0035 Mental health partial hospitalization, treatment, less than 24 hours ☑

H0036 Community psychiatric supportive treatment, face-to-face, per 15 minutes ☑

H0037 Community psychiatric supportive treatment program, per diem ☑

H0038 Self-help/peer services, per 15 minutes ☑

H0039 Assertive community treatment, face-to-face, per 15 minutes ☑

H0040 Assertive community treatment program, per diem ☑

H0041 Foster care, child, nontherapeutic, per diem A ☑

H0042 Foster care, child, nontherapeutic, per month A ☑

H0043 Supported housing, per diem ☑

H0044 Supported housing, per month ☑

H0045 Respite care services, not in the home, per diem ☑

H0046 Mental health services, not otherwise specified

H0047 Alcohol and/or other drug abuse services, not otherwise specified

H0048 Alcohol and/or other drug testing: collection and handling only, specimens other than blood

H0049 Alcohol and/or drug screening

H0050 Alcohol and/or drug services, brief intervention, per 15 minutes ☑

● **H0051** Traditional healing service E1
AHA: 2Q,24

● **H0052** Missing and murdered indigenous persons (MMIP) mental health and clinical care

● **H0053** Historical trauma (HT) mental health and clinical care for indigenous persons

H1000 Prenatal care, at-risk assessment M

H1001 Prenatal care, at-risk enhanced service; antepartum management M

H1002 Prenatal care, at risk enhanced service; care coordination M

H1003 Prenatal care, at-risk enhanced service; education M

H1004 Prenatal care, at-risk enhanced service; follow-up home visit M

H1005 Prenatal care, at-risk enhanced service package (includes H1001-H1004) M

H1010 Nonmedical family planning education, per session ☑

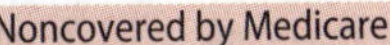
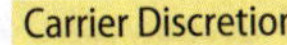
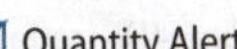
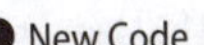
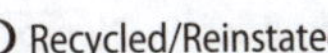
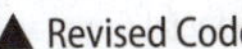

Alcohol and Drug Abuse Treatment Services

H1011 — H2041

H1011 Family assessment by licensed behavioral health professional for state defined purposes

H2000 Comprehensive multidisciplinary evaluation

H2001 Rehabilitation program, per 1/2 day ☑

H2010 Comprehensive medication services, per 15 minutes ☑

H2011 Crisis intervention service, per 15 minutes ☑

H2012 Behavioral health day treatment, per hour ☑

H2013 Psychiatric health facility service, per diem ☑

H2014 Skills training and development, per 15 minutes ☑

H2015 Comprehensive community support services, per 15 minutes ☑

H2016 Comprehensive community support services, per diem ☑

H2017 Psychosocial rehabilitation services, per 15 minutes ☑

H2018 Psychosocial rehabilitation services, per diem ☑

H2019 Therapeutic behavioral services, per 15 minutes ☑

H2020 Therapeutic behavioral services, per diem ☑

H2021 Community-based wrap-around services, per 15 minutes ☑

H2022 Community-based wrap-around services, per diem ☑

H2023 Supported employment, per 15 minutes ☑

H2024 Supported employment, per diem ☑

H2025 Ongoing support to maintain employment, per 15 minutes ☑

H2026 Ongoing support to maintain employment, per diem ☑

H2027 Psychoeducational service, per 15 minutes ☑

H2028 Sexual offender treatment service, per 15 minutes ☑

H2029 Sexual offender treatment service, per diem ☑

H2030 Mental health clubhouse services, per 15 minutes ☑

H2031 Mental health clubhouse services, per diem ☑

H2032 Activity therapy, per 15 minutes ☑

H2033 Multisystemic therapy for juveniles, per 15 minutes ☑

H2034 Alcohol and/or drug abuse halfway house services, per diem ☑

H2035 Alcohol and/or other drug treatment program, per hour ☑

H2036 Alcohol and/or other drug treatment program, per diem ☑

H2037 Developmental delay prevention activities, dependent child of client, per 15 minutes A ☑

H2038 Skills training and development, per diem ☑

H2040 Coordinated specialty care, team-based, for first episode psychosis, per month
AHA: 4Q,23

H2041 Coordinated specialty care, team-based, for first episode psychosis, per encounter
AHA: 4Q,23

J Codes Drugs J0120-J8499

J codes include drugs that ordinarily cannot be self-administered, chemotherapy drugs, immunosuppressive drugs, inhalation solutions, and other miscellaneous drugs and solutions.

Miscellaneous Drugs

J0120 **Injection, tetracycline, up to 250 mg** N N1 ☑

J0121 **Injection, omadacycline, 1 mg** K K2
Use this code for Nuzyra.
AHA: 4Q,19

J0122 **Injection, eravacycline, 1 mg** K K2
Use this code for Xerava.
AHA: 4Q,19

J0129 **Injection, abatacept, 10 mg (code may be used for Medicare when drug administered under the direct supervision of a physician, not for use when drug is self-administered)** K K2 ☑
Use this code for Orencia.
CMS: 100-02,15,50.5

J0130 **Injection abciximab, 10 mg** N N1 ☑
Use this code for ReoPro.

J0131 **Injection, acetaminophen, not otherwise specified, 10 mg** N N1 ☑
AHA: 1Q,23; 4Q,18

J0132 **Injection, acetylcysteine, 100 mg** N N1 ☑
Use this code for Acetadote.

J0133 **Injection, acyclovir, 5 mg** N N1 ☑
Use this code for Zovirax.
CMS: 100-04,20,180; 100-04,32,411.3

▲ **J0134** **Injection, acetaminophen (Fresenius Kabi), not therapeutically equivalent to J0131, 10 mg** K K2
Use this code for acetaminophen manufactured by Fresenius Kabi.
AHA: 1Q,23

J0135 ~~Injection, adalimumab, 20 mg~~

▲ **J0136** **Injection, acetaminophen (B. Braun), not therapeutically equivalent to J0131, 10 mg** K K2
Use this code for acetaminophen manufactured by B. Braun.
AHA: 1Q,23

▲ **J0137** **Injection, acetaminophen (Hikma), not therapeutically equivalent to J0131, 10 mg** K K2
Use this code for acetaminophen manufactured by Hikma.
AHA: 3Q,23

● **J0138** **Injection, acetaminophen 10 mg and ibuprofen 3 mg**
Use this code for Combogesic.

● **J0139** **Injection, adalimumab, 1 mg**
Use this code for Humira.

J0153 **Injection, adenosine, 1 mg (not to be used to report any adenosine phosphate compounds)** N N1 ☑
Use this code for Adenocard, Adenoscan.

J0171 **Injection, adrenalin, epinephrine, 0.1 mg** N N1 ☑

J0172 **Injection, aducanumab-avwa, 2 mg** K K2
Use this code for Aduhelm.
AHA: 1Q,22

▲ **J0173** **Injection, epinephrine (Belcher), not therapeutically equivalent to J0171, 0.1 mg** K K2
Use this code for epinephrine manufactured by Belcher.
AHA: 1Q,23

J0174 **Injection, lecanemab-irmb, 1 mg** G K2
Use this code for Leqembi.
CMS: 100-04,32,412.1
AHA: 3Q,23

● **J0175** **Injection, donanemab-azbt, 2 mg** K2
Use this code for Kisunla.

● **J0177** **Injection, aflibercept HD, 1 mg** G K2
Use this code for Eylea HD.
AHA: 2Q,24

J0178 **Injection, aflibercept, 1 mg** K K2 ☑
Use this code for Eylea.

J0179 **Injection, brolucizumab-dbll, 1 mg** K K2
Use this code for Beovu.
AHA: 1Q,20

J0180 **Injection, agalsidase beta, 1 mg** K K2 ☑
Use this code for Fabrazyme.

J0184 **Injection, amisulpride, 1 mg** G K2
Use this code for Barhemsys.
AHA: 1Q,24

J0185 **Injection, aprepitant, 1 mg** K K2
Use this code for Cinvanti.
AHA: 1Q,19; 4Q,18

J0190 **Injection, biperiden lactate, per 5 mg** E1 ☑

J0200 **Injection, alatrofloxacin mesylate, 100 mg** E1 ☑

J0202 **Injection, alemtuzumab, 1 mg** K K2 ☑
Use this code for Lemtrada.

J0205 **Injection, alglucerase, per 10 units** E1 ☑
Use this code for Ceredase.

J0206 **Injection, allopurinol sodium, 1 mg** K K2
AHA: 3Q,23

J0207 **Injection, amifostine, 500 mg** E1 ☑
Use this code for Ethyol.

▲ **J0208** **Injection, sodium thiosulfate (Pedmark), 100 mg** G K2
AHA: 2Q,24; 2Q,23

● **J0209** **Injection, sodium thiosulfate (Hope), 100 mg** N
Use this code for sodium thiosulfate manufactured by Hope.
AHA: 2Q,24

J0210 **Injection, methyldopate HCl, up to 250 mg** E1 ☑
Use this code for Aldomet.

● **J0211** **Injection, sodium nitrite 3 mg and sodium thiosulfate 125 mg (Nithiodote)** K2
AHA: 3Q,24

J0215 **Injection, alefacept, 0.5 mg** E1 ☑
Use this for Amevive.

J0216 **Injection, alfentanil HCl, 500 mcg** N N1
AHA: 3Q,23

J0217 **Injection, velmanase alfa-tycv, 1 mg** G K2
Use this code for Lamzede.
AHA: 1Q,24

J0218 **Injection, olipudase alfa-rpcp, 1 mg** G K2
Use this code for Xenpozyme.
AHA: 2Q,23

J0219 **Injection, avalglucosidase alfa-ngpt, 4 mg** G K2
Use this code for Nexviazyme.
AHA: 2Q,22

J0220 **Injection, alglucosidase alfa, 10 mg, not otherwise specified** K K2 ☑
Use this code for Myozyme.

J0221 **Injection, alglucosidase alfa, (Lumizyme), 10 mg** K K2 ☑

J0222 **Injection, patisiran, 0.1 mg** K K2
Use this code for Onpattro.
AHA: 4Q,19

J0223 **Injection, givosiran, 0.5 mg** K K2
Use this code for Givlaari.
AHA: 2Q,20

J0224 **Injection, lumasiran, 0.5 mg** K K2
AHA: 3Q,21

J0225 **Injection, vutrisiran, 1 mg** G K2
AHA: 1Q,23

J0248 **Injection, remdesivir, 1 mg** G
AHA: 1Q,22

J0256 **Injection, alpha 1-proteinase inhibitor (human), not otherwise specified, 10 mg** K K2 ☑
Use this code for Aralast, Aralast NP, Prolastin C, Zemaira.

J0257 **Injection, alpha 1 proteinase inhibitor (human), (GLASSIA), 10 mg** K K2 ☑

J0270 **Injection, alprostadil, 1.25 mcg (code may be used for Medicare when drug administered under the direct supervision of a physician, not for use when drug is self-administered)** B ☑
Use this code for Alprostadil, Caverject, Edex, Prostin VR Pediatric.

J0275 **Alprostadil urethral suppository (code may be used for Medicare when drug administered under the direct supervision of a physician, not for use when drug is self-administered)** B ☑
Use this code for Muse.

J0278 **Injection, amikacin sulfate, 100 mg** N N1 ☑
Use this code for Amikin.

J0280 **Injection, aminophylline, up to 250 mg** N N1 ☑

J0282 **Injection, amiodarone HCl, 30 mg** N N1 ☑
Use this code for Cordarone IV.

J0283 **Injection, amiodarone HCl (Nexterone), 30 mg** E
AHA: 1Q,23

J0285 **Injection, amphotericin B, 50 mg** N N1 ☑
Use this for Amphocin, Fungizone.
CMS: 100-04,20,180; 100-04,32,411.3

J0287 **Injection, amphotericin B lipid complex, 10 mg** K K2 ☑
Use this code for Abelcet.
CMS: 100-04,20,180; 100-04,32,411.3

J0288 **Injection, amphotericin B cholesteryl sulfate complex, 10 mg** E ☑
Use this code for Amphotec.
CMS: 100-04,20,180; 100-04,32,411.3

J0289 **Injection, amphotericin B liposome, 10 mg** K K2 ☑
Use this code for Ambisome.
CMS: 100-04,20,180; 100-04,32,411.3

J0290 **Injection, ampicillin sodium, 500 mg** N N1 ☑

J0291 **Injection, plazomicin, 5 mg** K K2
Use this code for Zemdri.
AHA: 4Q,19

J0295 **Injection, ampicillin sodium/sulbactam sodium, per 1.5 g** N N1 ☑
Use this code for Unasyn.

J0300 **Injection, amobarbital, up to 125 mg** K K2 ☑
Use this code for Amytal.

J0330 **Injection, succinylcholine chloride, up to 20 mg** N N1 ☑
Use this code for Anectine, Quelicin.

J0348 **Injection, anidulafungin, 1 mg** N N1 ☑
Use this code for Eraxis.

J0349 **Injection, rezafungin, 1 mg** G K2
Use this code for Rezzayo.
AHA: 4Q,23

J0350 **Injection, anistreplase, per 30 units** E ☑
Use this code for Eminase.

J0360 **Injection, hydralazine HCl, up to 20 mg** N N1 ☑

J0364 **Injection, apomorphine HCl, 1 mg** E ☑
Use this code for Apokyn.
CMS: 100-02,15,50.5

J0365 **Injection, aprotinin, 10,000 kiu** E ☑
Use this code for Trasylol.

J0380 **Injection, metaraminol bitartrate, per 10 mg** E ☑
Use this code for Aramine.

J0390 **Injection, chloroquine HCl, up to 250 mg** N N1 ☑
Use this code for Aralen.

J0391 **Injection, artesunate, 1 mg** K K2
AHA: 1Q,24

J0395 **Injection, arbutamine HCl, 1 mg** E ☑

J0400 **Injection, aripiprazole, intramuscular, 0.25 mg** N N1 ☑
Use this code for Abilify.

▲ **J0401** **Injection, aripiprazole (Abilify Maintena), 1 mg** K K2 ☑
Use this code for the Abilify Maintena kit.
AHA: 3Q,24; 4Q,18

J0402 **Injection, aripiprazole (Abilify Asimtufii), 1 mg** G K2
AHA: 1Q,24

J0456 **Injection, azithromycin, 500 mg** N N1 ☑
Use this code for Zithromax.

J0457 **Injection, aztreonam, 100 mg** K K2
Use this code for Azactam.
AHA: 3Q,23

J0461 **Injection, atropine sulfate, 0.01 mg** N N1 ☑
Use this code for AtroPen.

J0470 **Injection, dimercaprol, per 100 mg** K K2 ☑
Use this code for BAL.

J0475 **Injection, baclofen, 10 mg** K K2 ☑
Use this code for Lioresal, Gablofen.

J0476 **Injection, baclofen, 50 mcg for intrathecal trial** N N1 ☑
Use this code for Lioresal, Gablofen.

J0480 **Injection, basiliximab, 20 mg** K K2 ☑
Use this code for Simulect.

J0485 **Injection, belatacept, 1 mg** K K2 ☑
Use this code for Nulojix.

J0490 **Injection, belimumab, 10 mg** K K2 ☑
Use this code for BENLYSTA.

J0491 **Injection, anifrolumab-fnia, 1 mg** G K2
Use this code for Saphnello.
AHA: 2Q,22

J0500 **Injection, dicyclomine HCl, up to 20 mg** N N1 ☑
Use this code for Bentyl.

J0515 **Injection, benztropine mesylate, per 1 mg** N N1 ☑
Use this code for Cogentin.

J0517 **Injection, benralizumab, 1 mg** K K2
Use this code for Fasenra.
AHA: 1Q,19; 4Q,18

J0520 **Injection, bethanechol chloride, Myotonachol or Urecholine, up to 5 mg** E ☑

J0558 **Injection, penicillin G benzathine and penicillin G procaine, 100,000 units** K K2 ☑
Use this code for Bicillin CR, Bicillin CR 900/300, Bicillin CR Tubex.

J0561 **Injection, penicillin G benzathine, 100,000 units** K K2 ☑

J0565 **Injection, bezlotoxumab, 10 mg** K K2
Use this code for Zinplava.

J0567 **Injection, cerliponase alfa, 1 mg** E1
Use this code for Brineura.
AHA: 1Q,19; 4Q,18

~~**J0570** **Buprenorphine implant, 74.2 mg**~~

J0571 **Buprenorphine, oral, 1 mg** E1 ☑
Use this code for Subutex.

J0572 **Buprenorphine/naloxone, oral, less than or equal to 3 mg buprenorphine** E1 ☑
Use this code for Bunavail, Suboxone, Zubsolv.

J0573 **Buprenorphine/naloxone, oral, greater than 3 mg, but less than or equal to 6 mg buprenorphine** E1 ☑
Use this code for Bunavail, Suboxone, Zubsolv.

J0574 **Buprenorphine/naloxone, oral, greater than 6 mg, but less than or equal to 10 mg buprenorphine** E1 ☑
Use this code for Bunavail, Suboxone.

J0575 **Buprenorphine/naloxone, oral, greater than 10 mg buprenorphine** E1 ☑
Use this code for Suboxone.

~~**J0576** **Injection, buprenorphine extended-release (Brixadi), 1 mg**~~
To report, see ~J0577-J0578

● **J0577** **Injection, buprenorphine extended-release (Brixadi), less than or equal to 7 days of therapy** G K2
AHA: 2Q,24

● **J0578** **Injection, buprenorphine extended-release (Brixadi), greater than 7 days and up to 28 days of therapy** G K2
AHA: 2Q,24

J0583 **Injection, bivalirudin, 1 mg** N N1 ☑
Use this code for Angiomax.

J0584 **Injection, burosumab-twza, 1 mg** K K2
Use this code for Crysvita.
CMS: 100-04,4,260.1; 100-04,4,260.1.1
AHA: 1Q,19; 4Q,18

J0585 **Injection, onabotulinumtoxinA, 1 unit** K K2 ☑
Use this code for Botox, Botox Cosmetic.
AHA: 2Q,21; 4Q,18

J0586 **Injection, abobotulinumtoxinA, 5 units** K K2 ☑
Use this code for Dysport.

J0587 **Injection, rimabotulinumtoxinB, 100 units** K K2 ☑
Use this code for Myobloc.

J0588 **Injection, incobotulinumtoxinA, 1 unit** K K2 ☑
Use this code for XEOMIN.

● **J0589** **Injection, daxibotulinumtoxina-lanm, 1 unit** G K2
Use this code for Daxxify.
AHA: 2Q,24

J0591 **Injection, deoxycholic acid, 1 mg** E1
Use this code for Kybella.
AHA: 2Q,20

J0592 **Injection, buprenorphine HCl, 0.1 mg** N N1 ☑
Use this code for Buprenex.

J0593 **Injection, lanadelumab-flyo, 1 mg (code may be used for Medicare when drug administered under direct supervision of a physician, not for use when drug is self-administered)** E1
Use this code for Takhzyro.
AHA: 4Q,19

J0594 **Injection, busulfan, 1 mg** K K2 ☑
Use this code for Busulfex.

J0595 **Injection, butorphanol tartrate, 1 mg** N N1 ☑
Use this code for Stadol.

J0596 **Injection, C1 esterase inhibitor (recombinant), Ruconest, 10 units** K K2 ☑
CMS: 100-02,15,50.5

J0597 **Injection, C1 esterase inhibitor (human), Berinert, 10 units** K K2 ☑

J0598 **Injection, C1 esterase inhibitor (human), Cinryze, 10 units** K K2 ☑

J0599 **Injection, C1 esterase inhibitor (human), (Haegarda), 10 units** E1
AHA: 1Q,19; 4Q,18

J0600 **Injection, edetate calcium disodium, up to 1,000 mg** K K2 ☑
Use this code for Calcium Disodium Versenate, Calcium EDTA.

● **J0601** **Sevelamer carbonate (Renvela or therapeutically equivalent), oral, 20 mg (for ESRD on dialysis)**

● **J0602** **Sevelamer carbonate (Renvela or therapeutically equivalent), oral, powder, 20 mg (for ESRD on dialysis)**

● **J0603** **Sevelamer HCl (Renagel or therapeutically equivalent), oral, 20 mg (for ESRD on dialysis)**

J0604 **Cinacalcet, oral, 1 mg, (for ESRD on dialysis)** B
Use this code for Sensipar.

● **J0605** **Sucroferric oxyhydroxide, oral, 5 mg (for ESRD on dialysis)**
Use this code for Velphoro.

J0606 **Injection, etelcalcetide, 0.1 mg** K K2
Use this code for Parsabiv.

● **J0607** **Lanthanum carbonate, oral, 5 mg (for ESRD on dialysis)**
Use this code for Fosrenol.

● **J0608** **Lanthanum carbonate, oral, powder, 5 mg, not therapeutically equivalent to J0607 (for ESRD on dialysis)**

● **J0609** **Ferric citrate, oral, 3 mg ferric iron, (for ESRD on dialysis)**

▲ **J0612** **Injection, calcium gluconate, not otherwise specified, 10 mg** K K2
AHA: 2Q,24; 2Q,23

▲ **J0613** **Injection, calcium gluconate (WG Critical Care), not therapeutically equivalent to J0612, 10 mg** K K2
Use this code for calcium gluconate manufactured by WG Critical Care.
AHA: 2Q,24; 2Q,23

● **J0615** **Calcium acetate, oral, 23 mg (for ESRD on dialysis)**
Use this code for Phoslo.

J0620 **Injection, calcium glycerophosphate and calcium lactate, per 10 ml** N N1 ☑

J0630 **Injection, calcitonin salmon, up to 400 units** K K2 ☑
Use this code for Calcimar, Miacalcin.
CMS: 100-04,10,90.1

J0636 **Injection, calcitriol, 0.1 mcg** N N1 ☑
Use this code for Calcijex.

J0637 **Injection, caspofungin acetate, 5 mg** N N1 ☑
Use this code for Cancidas.

Drugs Administered Other Than Oral Method

J0558 — J0637

J0638 Injection, canakinumab, 1 mg K K2 ☑
Use this code for ILARIS.

J0640 Injection, leucovorin calcium, per 50 mg N N1 ☑

J0641 Injection, levoleucovorin, not otherwise specified, 0.5 mg K K2 ☑
AHA: 4Q,19; 4Q,18

J0642 Injection, levoleucovorin (Khapzory), 0.5 mg K K2
AHA: 1Q,20; 4Q,19

● **J0650** Injection, levothyroxine sodium, not otherwise specified, 10 mcg N
AHA: 2Q,24

▲ **J0651** Injection, levothyroxine sodium (Fresenius Kabi), not therapeutically equivalent to J0650, 10 mcg K K2
Use this code for levothyroxine sodium manufactured by Fresenius Kabi.
AHA: 2Q,24

▲ **J0652** Injection, levothyroxine sodium (Hikma), not therapeutically equivalent to J0650, 10 mcg K K2
Use this code for levothyroxine sodium manufactured by Hikma.
AHA: 2Q,24

J0665 Injection, bupivicaine, not otherwise specified, 0.5 mg K K2
AHA: 3Q,23

● **J0666** Injection, bupivacaine liposome, 1 mg
Use this code for Exparel.

J0670 Injection, mepivacaine HCl, per 10 ml N N1 ☑
Use this code for Carbocaine, Polocaine, Isocaine HCl, Scandonest

● **J0687** Injection, cefazolin sodium (WG Critical Care), not therapeutically equivalent to J0690, 500 mg K2
AHA: 3Q,24

J0688 Injection, cefazolin sodium (Hikma), not therapeutically equivalent to J0690, 500 mg N N1
AHA: 1Q,24

J0689 Injection, cefazolin sodium (Baxter), not therapeutically equivalent to J0690, 500 mg K K2
Use this code for cefazolin sodium manufactured by Baxter.
AHA: 1Q,23

J0690 Injection, cefazolin sodium, 500 mg N N1 ☑

J0691 Injection, lefamulin, 1 mg K K2
Use this code for Xenleta.
AHA: 2Q,20

J0692 Injection, cefepime HCl, 500 mg N N1 ☑

J0694 Injection, cefoxitin sodium, 1 g N N1 ☑

J0695 Injection, ceftolozane 50 mg and tazobactam 25 mg K K2 ☑
Use this code for Zerbaxa.

J0696 Injection, ceftriaxone sodium, per 250 mg N N1 ☑

J0697 Injection, sterile cefuroxime sodium, per 750 mg N N1 ☑

J0698 Injection, cefotaxime sodium, per g N N1 ☑

J0699 Injection, cefiderocol, 10 mg K K2
Use this code for Fetroja.
AHA: 4Q,21

J0701 Injection, cefepime HCl (Baxter), not therapeutically equivalent to Maxipime, 500 mg K K2
Use this code for cefepime HCl manufactured by Baxter.
AHA: 1Q,23

J0702 Injection, betamethasone acetate 3 mg and betamethasone sodium phosphate 3 mg N N1 ☑
AHA: 3Q,24; 4Q,18

J0703 Injection, cefepime HCl (B. Braun), not therapeutically equivalent to Maxipime, 500 mg K K2
Use this code for cefepime HCl manufactured by B. Braun.

J0706 Injection, caffeine citrate, 5 mg N N1 ☑

J0710 Injection, cephapirin sodium, up to 1 g E1 ☑

J0712 Injection, ceftaroline fosamil, 10 mg K K2 ☑

J0713 Injection, ceftazidime, per 500 mg N N1 ☑

J0714 Injection, ceftazidime and avibactam, 0.5 g/0.125 g K K2 ☑
Use this code for Avycaz.

J0715 Injection, ceftizoxime sodium, per 500 mg N N1 ☑

J0716 Injection, Centruroides immune f(ab)2, up to 120 mg K K2 ☑
Use this code for Anascorp.

J0717 Injection, certolizumab pegol, 1 mg (code may be used for Medicare when drug administered under the direct supervision of a physician, not for use when drug is self-administered) K K2 ☑
CMS: 100-02,15,50.5

J0720 Injection, chloramphenicol sodium succinate, up to 1 g N N1 ☑

J0725 Injection, chorionic gonadotropin, per 1,000 USP units N N1 ☑
CMS: 100-02,15,50.5

J0735 Injection, clonidine HCl, 1 mg N N1 ☑

J0736 Injection, clindamycin phosphate, 300 mg K K2
AHA: 3Q,23

J0737 Injection, clindamycin phosphate (Baxter), not therapeutically equivalent to J0736, 300 mg K K2
Use this code for clindamycin phosphate manufactured by Baxter.
AHA: 3Q,23

J0739 Injection, cabotegravir, 1 mg, FDA-approved prescription, only for use as HIV pre-exposure prophylaxis (not for use as treatment for HIV) A
Use this code for Apretude.
AHA: 3Q,22

J0740 Injection, cidofovir, 375 mg K K2 ☑

J0741 Injection, cabotegravir and rilpivirine, 2 mg/3 mg G K2
Use this code for Cabenuva.
AHA: 4Q,21

J0742 Injection, imipenem 4 mg, cilastatin 4 mg and relebactam 2 mg K K2
Use this code for Recarbrio.
AHA: 2Q,20

J0743 Injection, cilastatin sodium; imipenem, per 250 mg N N1 ☑

J0744 Injection, ciprofloxacin for intravenous infusion, 200 mg N N1 ☑

J0745 Injection, codeine phosphate, per 30 mg N N1 ☑

J0750 Emtricitabine 200 mg and tenofovir disoproxil fumarate 300 mg, oral, FDA-approved prescription, only for use as HIV pre-exposure prophylaxis (not for use as treatment of HIV) A
Use this code for Truvada for PReP.
AHA: 1Q,24

J0751 Emtricitabine 200 mg and tenofovir alafenamide 25 mg, oral, FDA-approved prescription, only for use as HIV pre-exposure prophylaxis (not for use as treatment of HIV) A
Use this code for Descovy for PReP.
AHA: 1Q,24

J0770 Injection, colistimethate sodium, up to 150 mg N N1 ☑

J0775 **Injection, collagenase, clostridium histolyticum, 0.01 mg** K K2 ☑

J0780 **Injection, prochlorperazine, up to 10 mg** N N1 ☑

J0791 **Injection, crizanlizumab-tmca, 5 mg** K K2
Use this code for ADAKVEO.
AHA: 2Q,20

J0795 **Injection, corticorelin ovine triflutate, 1 mcg** E1 ☑

J0799 **FDA-approved prescription drug, only for use as HIV pre-exposure prophylaxis (not for use as treatment of HIV), not otherwise classified** A
AHA: 1Q,24

J0801 **Injection, corticotropin (Acthar Gel), up to 40 units** K K2
AHA: 4Q,23

J0802 **Injection, corticotropin (ANI), up to 40 units** K K2
Use this code for corticotropin manufactured by ANI.
AHA: 4Q,23

J0834 **Injection, cosyntropin, 0.25 mg** N N1 ☑
Use this code for Cortrosyn.

J0840 **Injection, crotalidae polyvalent immune fab (ovine), up to 1 g** K K2 ☑

J0841 **Injection, crotalidae immune F(ab')2 (equine), 120 mg** K K2
Use this code for Anavip.
CMS: 100-04,4,260.1; 100-04,4,260.1.1
AHA: 1Q,19; 4Q,18

J0850 **Injection, cytomegalovirus immune globulin intravenous (human), per vial** K K2 ☑

○ **J0870** **Injection, imetelstat, 1 mg**
Use this code for Rytelo.

● **J0872** **Injection, daptomycin (Xellia), unrefrigerated, not therapeutically equivalent to J0878 or J0873, 1 mg** K2
AHA: 3Q,24

▲ **J0873** **Injection, daptomycin (Xellia), not therapeutically equivalent to J0878 or J0872, 1 mg** N N1
AHA: 3Q,24; 1Q,24

J0874 **Injection, daptomycin (Baxter), not therapeutically equivalent to J0878, 1 mg** E1
AHA: 4Q,23

J0875 **Injection, dalbavancin, 5 mg** K K2 ☑
Use this code for Dalvance.

J0877 **Injection, daptomycin (Hospira), not therapeutically equivalent to J0878, 1 mg** K K2
Use this code for daptomycin manufactured by Hospira.
AHA: 1Q,23

J0878 **Injection, daptomycin, 1 mg** N1 ☑
Use this code for Cubicin.

J0879 **Injection, difelikefalin, 0.1 mcg, (for ESRD on dialysis)** N N1
Use this code for Korsuva.
AHA: 2Q,22

J0881 **Injection, darbepoetin alfa, 1 mcg (non-ESRD use)** K K2 ☑
Use this code for Aranesp.
CMS: 100-03,110.21; 100-04,17,80.12

J0882 **Injection, darbepoetin alfa, 1 mcg (for ESRD on dialysis)** K K2 ☑ ⦸
Use this code for Aranesp.
CMS: 100-04,8,60.4; 100-04,8,60.4.1; 100-04,8,60.4.2; 100-04,8,60.4.5.1; 100-04,8,60.4.6.3; 100-04,8,60.4.6.4; 100-04,8,60.4.6.5

J0883 **Injection, argatroban, 1 mg (for non-ESRD use)** K K2 ☑

J0884 **Injection, argatroban, 1 mg (for ESRD on dialysis)** K K2 ☑

J0885 **Injection, epoetin alfa, (for non-ESRD use), 1000 units** K K2 ☑
Use this code for Epogen/Procrit.
CMS: 100-03,110.21; 100-04,17,80.12

J0887 **Injection, epoetin beta, 1 mcg, (for ESRD on dialysis)** K K2 ☑
Use this code for Mircera.

J0888 **Injection, epoetin beta, 1 mcg, (for non-ESRD use)** N K2 ☑
Use this code for Mircera.

J0889 **Daprodustat, oral, 1 mg, (for ESRD on dialysis)** E1
Use this code for Jesduvroq.
AHA: 4Q,23

J0890 **Injection, peginesatide, 0.1 mg (for ESRD on dialysis)** E1 ☑
Use this code for Omontys.
CMS: 100-04,8,60.4; 100-04,8,60.4.1; 100-04,8,60.4.2; 100-04,8,60.4.5.1; 100-04,8,60.4.7

J0891 **Injection, argatroban (Accord), not therapeutically equivalent to J0883, 1 mg (for non-ESRD use)** K K2
Use this code for argatroban manufactured by Accord; for non-ESRD use.
AHA: 1Q,23

J0892 **Injection, argatroban (Accord), not therapeutically equivalent to J0884, 1 mg (for ESRD on dialysis)** K K2
Use this code for argatroban manufactured by Accord; for patients on ESRD dialysis.
AHA: 1Q,23

▲ **J0893** **Injection, decitabine (Sun Pharma), not therapeutically equivalent to J0894, 1 mg** K K2
Use this code for decitabine manufactured by Sun Pharma.
AHA: 1Q,23

J0894 **Injection, decitabine, 1 mg** N N1 ☑ ⦸
Use this code for Dacogen.

J0895 **Injection, deferoxamine mesylate, 500 mg** N N1 ☑
Use this code for Desferal.
CMS: 100-04,20,180; 100-04,32,411.3

J0896 **Injection, luspatercept-aamt, 0.25 mg** K K2
Use this code for REBLOZYL.
AHA: 2Q,20

J0897 **Injection, denosumab, 1 mg** K K2 ☑
Use this code for XGEVA, Prolia.
CMS: 100-04,10,90.1

J0898 **Injection, argatroban (AuroMedics), not therapeutically equivalent to J0883, 1 mg (for non-ESRD use)** K K2
Use this code for argatroban manufactured by AuroMedics; for non-ESRD use.
AHA: 1Q,23

J0899 **Injection, argatroban (AuroMedics), not therapeutically equivalent to J0884, 1 mg (for ESRD on dialysis)** K K2
Use this code for argatroban manufactured by AuroMedics; for patients on ESRD dialysis.
AHA: 1Q,23

● **J0901** **Vadadustat, oral, 1 mg (for ESRD on dialysis)**
Use this code for Vafseo.

● **J0911** **Instillation, taurolidine 1.35 mg and heparin sodium 100 units (central venous catheter lock for adult patients receiving chronic hemodialysis)** K2
Use this code for DefenCath.
AHA: 3Q,24

J0945 **Injection, brompheniramine maleate, per 10 mg** E1 ☑

J1000 **Injection, depo-estradiol cypionate, up to 5 mg** N N1 ☑
Use this code for depGynogen, Depogen, Estradiol Cypionate.

● **J1010** **Injection, methylprednisolone acetate, 1 mg** N
Use this code for Depo-Medrol.
AHA: 2Q,24

J1020 ~~**Injection, methylprednisolone acetate, 20 mg**~~
To report, see ~J1010

J1030 ~~**Injection, methylprednisolone acetate, 40 mg**~~
To report, see ~J1010

J1040 ~~**Injection, methylprednisolone acetate, 80 mg**~~
To report, see ~J1010

J1050 **Injection, medroxyprogesterone acetate, 1 mg** N N1 ☑

J1071 **Injection, testosterone cypionate, 1 mg** N N1 ☑
Use this code for Depo-testostrone.

J1094 **Injection, dexamethasone acetate, 1 mg** N N1 ☑
Use this code for Cortastat LA, Dalalone L.A., Dexamethasone Acetate Anhydrous, Dexone LA.

J1095 **Injection, dexamethasone 9%, intraocular, 1 mcg** N N1
AHA: 1Q,19; 4Q,18

J1096 **Dexamethasone, lacrimal ophthalmic insert, 0.1 mg** N K2
Use this code for Dextenza.
AHA: 4Q,19

J1097 **Phenylephrine 10.16 mg/ml and ketorolac 2.88 mg/ml ophthalmic irrigation solution, 1 ml** N K2
Use this code for Omidria.
AHA: 4Q,19

J1100 **Injection, dexamethasone sodium phosphate, 1 mg** N N1 ☑
Use this code for Cortastat, Dalalone, Decaject, Dexone, Solurex, Adrenocort, Primethasone, Dexasone, Dexim, Medidex, Spectro-Dex.

J1105 **Dexmedetomidine, oral, 1 mcg** K K2
Use this code for Igalmi.
AHA: 1Q,24

J1110 **Injection, dihydroergotamine mesylate, per 1 mg** N N1 ☑
Use this code for D.H.E. 45.

J1120 **Injection, acetazolamide sodium, up to 500 mg** N N1 ☑
Use this code for Diamox.

J1130 **Injection, diclofenac sodium, 0.5 mg** N N1 ☑
Use this code for Dyloject.

J1160 **Injection, digoxin, up to 0.5 mg** N N1 ☑
Use this code for Lanoxin.

J1162 **Injection, digoxin immune fab (ovine), per vial** K K2 ☑
Use this code for Digibind, Digifab.

J1165 **Injection, phenytoin sodium, per 50 mg** N N1 ☑
Use this code for Dilantin.

J1170 ~~**Injection, hydromorphone, up to 4 mg**~~

● **J1171** **Injection, hydromorphone, 0.1 mg**
Use this code for Dilaudid, Dilaudid-HP.

J1180 **Injection, dyphylline, up to 500 mg** E1 ☑

J1190 **Injection, dexrazoxane HCl, per 250 mg** K K2 ☑
Use this code for Zinecard.

J1200 **Injection, diphenhydramine HCl, up to 50 mg** N N1 ☑
Use this code for Benadryl, Benahist 10, Benahist 50, Benoject-10, Benoject-50, Bena-D 10, Bena-D 50, Nordryl, Dihydrex, Diphenacen-50, Hyrexin-50, Truxadryl, Wehdryl.

J1201 **Injection, cetirizine HCl, 0.5 mg** K K2
Use this code for Quzytiir.
AHA: 2Q,20

● **J1202** **Miglustat, oral, 65 mg** E1
Use this code for Opfolda.
AHA: 2Q,24

● **J1203** **Injection, cipaglucosidase alfa-atga, 5 mg** K K2
Use this code for Pombiliti.
AHA: 2Q,24

J1205 **Injection, chlorothiazide sodium, per 500 mg** N N1 ☑
Use this code for Diuril Sodium.

J1212 **Injection, DMSO, dimethyl sulfoxide, 50%, 50 ml** K K2 ☑
Use this code for Rimso 50. DMSO is covered only as a treatment of interstitial cystitis.

J1230 **Injection, methadone HCl, up to 10 mg** N N1 ☑
Use this code for Dolophine HCl.

J1240 **Injection, dimenhydrinate, up to 50 mg** N N1 ☑
Use this code for Dramamine, Dinate, Dommanate, Dramanate, Dramilin, Dramocen, Dramoject, Dymenate, Hydrate, Marmine, Wehamine.

J1245 **Injection, dipyridamole, per 10 mg** N N1 ☑
Use this code for Persantine IV.

J1250 **Injection, dobutamine HCl, per 250 mg** N N1 ☑
CMS: 100-04,20,180; 100-04,32,411.3

J1260 **Injection, dolasetron mesylate, 10 mg** N N1 ☑
Use this code for Anzemet.

J1265 **Injection, dopamine HCl, 40 mg** N N1 ☑
CMS: 100-04,20,180; 100-04,32,411.3

J1267 **Injection, doripenem, 10 mg** E1 ☑
Use this code for Doribax.

J1270 **Injection, doxercalciferol, 1 mcg** N N1 ☑
Use this code for Hectorol.

J1290 **Injection, ecallantide, 1 mg** K K2 ☑
Use this code for KALBITOR.

J1300 **Injection, eculizumab, 10 mg** K K2 ☑
Use this code for Soliris.

J1301 **Injection, edaravone, 1 mg** K K2
Use this code for Radicava.
AHA: 1Q,19; 4Q,18

J1302 **Injection, sutimlimab-jome, 10 mg** G K2
Use this code for Enjaymo.
AHA: 4Q,22

J1303 **Injection, ravulizumab-cwvz, 10 mg** K K2
Use this code for Ultomiris.
AHA: 4Q,19

J1304 **Injection, tofersen, 1 mg** G K2
Use this code for Qalsody.
AHA: 1Q,24

J1305 **Injection, evinacumab-dgnb, 5 mg** G K2
Use this code for Evkeeza.
AHA: 4Q,21

J1306 **Injection, inclisiran, 1 mg** G K2
Use this code for Leqvio.
AHA: 3Q,22

● **J1307** **Injection, crovalimab-akkz, 10 mg**
Use this code for Piasky.

J1320 **Injection, amitriptyline HCl, up to 20 mg** N N1 ☑
Use this code for Elavil.

J1322 **Injection, elosulfase alfa, 1 mg** K K2 ☑
Use this code for Vimizim.

● **J1323** **Injection, elranatamab-bcmm, 1 mg**
Use this code for Elrexfio.
AHA: 2Q,24

J1324 **Injection, enfuvirtide, 1 mg**
Use this code for Fuzeon.
CMS: 100-02,15,50.5

J1325 **Injection, epoprostenol, 0.5 mg**
Use this code for Flolan and Veletri.
CMS: 100-04,20,180; 100-04,32,411.3

J1327 **Injection, eptifibatide, 5 mg**
Use this code for Integrilin.

J1330 **Injection, ergonovine maleate, up to 0.2 mg**
Medicare jurisdiction: local contractor. Use this code for Ergotrate Maleate.

J1335 **Injection, ertapenem sodium, 500 mg**
Use this code for Invanz.

J1364 **Injection, erythromycin lactobionate, per 500 mg**

J1380 **Injection, estradiol valerate, up to 10 mg**
Use this code for Delestrogen, Dioval, Dioval XX, Dioval 40, Duragen-10, Duragen-20, Duragen-40, Estradiol L.A., Estradiol L.A. 20, Estradiol L.A. 40, Gynogen L.A. 10, Gynogen L.A. 20, Gynogen L.A. 40, Valergen 10, Valergen 20, Valergen 40, Estra-L 20, Estra-L 40, L.A.E. 20.

J1410 **Injection, estrogen conjugated, per 25 mg**
Use this code for Natural Estrogenic Substance, Premarin Intravenous, Primestrin Aqueous.

J1411 **Injection, etranacogene dezaparvovec-drlb, per therapeutic dose**
Use this code for Hemgenix.
AHA: 2Q,23

J1412 **Injection, valoctocogene roxaparvovec-rvox, per ml, containing nominal 2 x 10^{13} vector genomes**
Use this code for Roctavian.
AHA: 1Q,24

J1413 **Injection, delandistrogene moxeparvovec-rokl, per therapeutic dose**
Use this code for Elevidys.
AHA: 1Q,24

● **J1414** **Injection, fidanacogene elaparvovec-dzkt, per therapeutic dose**
Use this code for Beqvez.

J1426 **Injection, casimersen, 10 mg**
Use this code for Amondys 45.
AHA: 4Q,21

J1427 **Injection, viltolarsen, 10 mg**
Use this code for Viltepso.
AHA: 1Q,21

J1428 **Injection, eteplirsen, 10 mg**
Use this code for Exondys 51.

J1429 **Injection, golodirsen, 10 mg**
Use this code for Vyondys 53.
AHA: 2Q,20

J1430 **Injection, ethanolamine oleate, 100 mg**
Use this code for Ethamolin.

● **J1434** **Injection, fosaprepitant (Focinvez), 1 mg**
AHA: 2Q,24

J1435 **Injection, estrone, per 1 mg**
Use this code for Estrone Aqueous, Estragyn, Estro-A, Estrone, Estronol, Theelin Aqueous, Estrone 5, Kestrone 5.

J1436 **Injection, etidronate disodium, per 300 mg**
Use this code for Didronel.

J1437 **Injection, ferric derisomaltose, 10 mg**
Use this code for Monoferric.
AHA: 4Q,20

J1438 **Injection, etanercept, 25 mg (code may be used for Medicare when drug administered under the direct supervision of a physician, not for use when drug is self-administered)**
Use this code for Enbrel.
CMS: 100-02,15,50.5

J1439 **Injection, ferric carboxymaltose, 1 mg**
Use this code for Injectafer.

J1440 **Fecal microbiota, live - jslm, 1 ml**
Use this code for Rebyota.
AHA: 3Q,23

J1442 **Injection, filgrastim (G-CSF), excludes biosimilars, 1 mcg**
Use this code for Neupogen.

J1443 **Injection, ferric pyrophosphate citrate solution (Triferic), 0.1 mg of iron**
Use this code for Triferic solution.

J1444 **Injection, ferric pyrophosphate citrate powder, 0.1 mg of iron**
Use this code for Triferic powder.
AHA: 3Q,19

J1445 **Injection, ferric pyrophosphate citrate solution (Triferic AVNU), 0.1 mg of iron**
AHA: 4Q,21

J1447 **Injection, tbo-filgrastim, 1 mcg**
Use this code for Granix.

J1448 **Injection, trilaciclib, 1 mg**
Use this code for Cosela.
AHA: 4Q,21

J1449 **Injection, eflapegrastim-xnst, 0.1 mg**
Use this code for Rolvedon.
AHA: 2Q,23

J1450 **Injection, fluconazole, 200 mg**
Use this code for Diflucan.
CMS: 100-02,15,50.6

J1451 **Injection, fomepizole, 15 mg**
Use this code for Antizol.
CMS: 100-02,15,50.6

J1452 **Injection, fomivirsen sodium, intraocular, 1.65 mg**
Use this code for Vitravene.
CMS: 100-02,15,50.4.2; 100-02,15,50.6

J1453 **Injection, fosaprepitant, 1 mg**
Use this code for Emend.
CMS: 100-02,15,50.6

J1454 **Injection, fosnetupitant 235 mg and palonosetron 0.25 mg**
Use this code for Akynzeo.
CMS: 100-02,15,50.6
AHA: 1Q,19; 4Q,18

J1455 **Injection, foscarnet sodium, per 1,000 mg**
Use this code for Foscavir.
CMS: 100-02,15,50.6; 100-04,20,180; 100-04,32,411.3

J1456 **Injection, fosaprepitant (Teva), not therapeutically equivalent to J1453, 1 mg**
Use this code for fosaprepitant manufactured by Teva.
CMS: 100-02,15,50.6
AHA: 1Q,23

J1457 Injection, gallium nitrate, 1 mg E1 ☑
Use this code for Ganite.
CMS: 100-02,15,50.6; 100-04,20,180; 100-04,32,411.3

J1458 Injection, galsulfase, 1 mg K K2 ☑
Use this code for Naglazyme.
CMS: 100-02,15,50.6

J1459 Injection, immune globulin (Privigen), intravenous, nonlyophilized (e.g., liquid), 500 mg K K2 ☑
CMS: 100-02,15,50.6; 100-04,20,213

J1460 Injection, gamma globulin, intramuscular, 1 cc K K2 ☑
Use this code for GamaSTAN SD.
CMS: 100-02,15,50.6; 100-04,17,80.6

J1551 Injection, immune globulin (Cutaquig), 100 mg K K2
CMS: 100-02,15,50.6; 100-04,32,411.3
AHA: 3Q,22

● **J1552** Injection, immune globulin (Alyglo), 500 mg
CMS: 100-02,15,50.6

J1554 Injection, immune globulin (Asceniv), 500 mg K K2
CMS: 100-02,15,50.6; 100-04,20,213
AHA: 1Q,21

J1555 Injection, immune globulin (Cuvitru), 100 mg K K2
CMS: 100-02,15,50.6; 100-04,20,180; 100-04,32,411.3

J1556 Injection, immune globulin (Bivigam), 500 mg K K2 ☑
CMS: 100-02,15,50.6; 100-04,20,213

J1557 Injection, immune globulin, (Gammaplex), intravenous, nonlyophilized (e.g., liquid), 500 mg K K2 ☑
CMS: 100-02,15,50.6; 100-04,20,213

J1558 Injection, immune globulin (xembify), 100 mg K K2
CMS: 100-02,15,50.6; 100-04,32,411.3
AHA: 2Q,20

J1559 Injection, immune globulin (Hizentra), 100 mg K K2 ☑
CMS: 100-02,15,50.6; 100-04,20,180; 100-04,32,411.3

J1560 Injection, gamma globulin, intramuscular, over 10 cc K K2 ☑
Use this code for GamaSTAN SD.
CMS: 100-02,15,50.6; 100-04,17,80.6

J1561 Injection, immune globulin, (Gamunex/Gamunex-C/Gammaked), nonlyophilized (e.g., liquid), 500 mg K K2 ☑
CMS: 100-02,15,50.6; 100-04,20,180; 100-04,20,213; 100-04,32,411.3

J1562 Injection, immune globulin (Vivaglobin), 100 mg E1 ☑
CMS: 100-02,15,50.6; 100-04,20,180; 100-04,32,411.3

J1566 Injection, immune globulin, intravenous, lyophilized (e.g., powder), not otherwise specified, 500 mg K K2 ☑
Use this code for Carimune, Gammagard S/D, Iveegam, Polygam, Polygam S/D.
CMS: 100-02,15,50.6; 100-04,20,213

J1568 Injection, immune globulin, (Octagam), intravenous, nonlyophilized (e.g., liquid), 500 mg K K2 ☑
CMS: 100-02,15,50.6; 100-04,20,213

J1569 Injection, immune globulin, (Gammagard liquid), nonlyophilized, (e.g., liquid), 500 mg K K2 ☑
CMS: 100-02,15,50.6; 100-04,20,180; 100-04,20,213; 100-04,32,411.3

J1570 Injection, ganciclovir sodium, 500 mg N N1 ☑
Use this code for Cytovene.
CMS: 100-04,20,180; 100-04,32,411.3

J1571 Injection, hepatitis B immune globulin (Hepagam B), intramuscular, 0.5 ml K K2 ☑

J1572 Injection, immune globulin, (Flebogamma/Flebogamma Dif), intravenous, nonlyophilized (e.g., liquid), 500 mg K K2 ☑
CMS: 100-04,20,213

J1573 Injection, hepatitis B immune globulin (Hepagam B), intravenous, 0.5 ml K K2 ☑

▲ **J1574** Injection, ganciclovir sodium (Exela), not therapeutically equivalent to J1570, 500 mg E1
Use this code for ganciclovir manufactured by Exela.
AHA: 1Q,23

J1575 Injection, immune globulin/hyaluronidase, 100 mg immuneglobulin K K2 ☑
Use this code for HyQvia.
CMS: 100-04,20,180; 100-04,32,411.3

J1576 Injection, immune globulin (Panzyga), intravenous, non-lyophilized (e.g., liquid), 500 mg K K2
CMS: 100-04,20,213
AHA: 3Q,23

J1580 Injection, garamycin, gentamicin, up to 80 mg N N1 ☑
Use this code for Gentamicin Sulfate, Jenamicin.

J1595 Injection, glatiramer acetate, 20 mg K K2 ☑
Use this code for Copaxone.
CMS: 100-02,15,50.5

J1596 Injection, glycopyrrolate, 0.1 mg N N1
AHA: 1Q,24

● **J1597** Injection, glycopyrrolate (Glyrx-PF), 0.1 mg N1
AHA: 3Q,24

● **J1598** Injection, glycopyrrolate (Fresenius Kabi), not therapeutically equivalent to J1596, 0.1 mg N1
AHA: 3Q,24

J1599 Injection, immune globulin, intravenous, nonlyophilized (e.g., liquid), not otherwise specified, 500 mg N N1 ☑
CMS: 100-04,20,213

J1600 Injection, gold sodium thiomalate, up to 50 mg E1 ☑
Use this code for Myochrysine.
CMS: 100-04,4,20.6.4

J1602 Injection, golimumab, 1 mg, for intravenous use K K2 ☑
Use this code for Simponi.

J1610 Injection, glucagon HCl, per 1 mg K K2 ☑
Use this code for Glucagen.

J1611 Injection, glucagon HCl (Fresenius Kabi), not therapeutically equivalent to J1610, per 1 mg K K2
Use this code for glucagon HCl manufactured by Fresenius Kabi.
AHA: 1Q,23

J1620 Injection, gonadorelin HCl, per 100 mcg E1 ☑
Use this code for Factrel, Lutrepulse.

J1626 Injection, granisetron HCl, 100 mcg N N1 ☑
Use this code for Kytril.
CMS: 100-04,4,20.6.4

J1627 Injection, granisetron, extended-release, 0.1 mg K K2
Use this code for Sustol.

J1628 Injection, guselkumab, 1 mg K K2
Use this code for Tremfya.
AHA: 1Q,19; 4Q,18

J1630 Injection, haloperidol, up to 5 mg N N1 ☑
Use this code for Haldol.
CMS: 100-04,4,20.6.4

J1631 Injection, haloperidol decanoate, per 50 mg N N1 ☑
Use this code for Haldol Decanoate-50.
CMS: 100-04,4,20.6.4

J1632 Injection, brexanolone, 1 mg K K2
Use this code for Zulresso.
AHA: 4Q,20

J1640 **Injection, hemin, 1 mg** K K2 ☑
Use this code for Panhematin.

J1642 **Injection, heparin sodium, (heparin lock flush), per 10 units** N N1 ☑
Use this code for Hep-Lock, Hep-Lock U/P, Hep-Pak, Lok-Pak.
CMS: 100-04,4,20.6.4

J1643 **Injection, heparin sodium (Pfizer), not therapeutically equivalent to J1644, per 1000 units** K K2
Use this code for heparin sodium manufactured by Pfizer.
AHA: 1Q,23

J1644 **Injection, Heparin sodium, per 1000 units** N N1 ☑
Use this code for Heparin Sodium, Liquaemin Sodium.
CMS: 100-04,4,20.6.4

J1645 **Injection, dalteparin sodium, per 2500 IU** N N1 ☑
Use this code for Fragmin.
CMS: 100-02,15,50.5; 100-04,4,20.6.4

J1650 **Injection, enoxaparin sodium, 10 mg** N N1 ☑
Use this code for Lovenox.
CMS: 100-02,15,50.5; 100-04,4,20.6.4

J1652 **Injection, fondaparinux sodium, 0.5 mg** N N1 ☑
Use this code for Atrixtra.
CMS: 100-02,15,50.5

J1655 **Injection, tinzaparin sodium, 1000 IU** E1 ☑
Use this code for Innohep.
CMS: 100-02,15,50.5; 100-04,4,20.6.4

J1670 **Injection, tetanus immune globulin, human, up to 250 units** K K2 ☑
Use this code for HyperTET SD.

J1675 **Injection, histrelin acetate, 10 mcg** B ☑
Use this code for Supprelin LA.

J1700 **Injection, hydrocortisone acetate, up to 25 mg** N N1 ☑
Use this code for Hydrocortone Acetate.
CMS: 100-04,4,20.6.4

J1710 **Injection, hydrocortisone sodium phosphate, up to 50 mg** N N1 ☑
Use this code for Hydrocortone Phosphate.
CMS: 100-04,4,20.6.4

J1720 **Injection, hydrocortisone sodium succinate, up to 100 mg** N N1 ☑
Use this code for Solu-Cortef, A-Hydrocort.
CMS: 100-04,4,20.6.4

J1726 **Injection, hydroxyprogesterone caproate, (Makena), 10 mg** K K2

J1729 **Injection, hydroxyprogesterone caproate, not otherwise specified, 10 mg** K K2

J1730 **Injection, diazoxide, up to 300 mg** E1 ☑

J1738 **Injection, meloxicam, 1 mg** N N1
Use this code for Anjeso.
AHA: 4Q,20

J1740 **Injection, ibandronate sodium, 1 mg** N N1 ☑
Use this code for Boniva.

J1741 **Injection, ibuprofen, 100 mg** N N1 ☑
Use this code for Caldolor.

J1742 **Injection, ibutilide fumarate, 1 mg** K K2 ☑
Use this code for Corvert.

J1743 **Injection, idursulfase, 1 mg** K K2 ☑
Use this code for Elaprase.

J1744 **Injection, icatibant, 1 mg** K K2 ☑
Use this code for Firazyr.
CMS: 100-02,15,50.5

J1745 **Injection, infliximab, excludes biosimilar, 10 mg** K K2 ☑
Use this code for Remicade.

J1746 **Injection, ibalizumab-uiyk, 10 mg** K K2
Use this code for Trogarzo.
CMS: 100-04,4,260.1; 100-04,4,260.1.1
AHA: 1Q,19; 4Q,18

J1747 **Injection, spesolimab-sbzo, 1 mg** G K2
Use this code for Spevigo.
AHA: 2Q,23

● **J1748** **Injection, infliximab-dyyb (Zymfentra), 10 mg**
AHA: 3Q,24

● **J1749** **Injection, iloprost, 0.1 mcg**
Use this code for Ventavis.

J1750 **Injection, iron dextran, 50 mg** K K2 ☑
Use this code for INFeD.

J1756 **Injection, iron sucrose, 1 mg** N N1 ☑
Use this code for Venofer.
CMS: 100-04,8,60.2.4; 100-04,8,60.2.4.2

J1786 **Injection, imiglucerase, 10 units** K K2 ☑
Use this code for Cerezyme.

J1790 **Injection, droperidol, up to 5 mg** N N1 ☑
Use this code for Inapsine.
CMS: 100-04,4,20.6.4

J1800 **Injection, propranolol HCl, up to 1 mg** N N1 ☑
Use this code for Inderal.
CMS: 100-04,4,20.6.4

J1805 **Injection, esmolol HCl, 10 mg** K K2
AHA: 3Q,23

▲ **J1806** **Injection, esmolol HCl (WG Critical Care), not therapeutically equivalent to J1805, 10 mg** K K2
Use this code for esmolol HCl manufactured by WG Critical Care.
AHA: 3Q,23

J1810 **Injection, droperidol and fentanyl citrate, up to 2 ml ampule** E1 ☑

J1811 **Insulin (Fiasp) for administration through DME (i.e., insulin pump) per 50 units** K K2
AHA: 3Q,23

J1812 **Insulin (Fiasp), per 5 units** N N1
AHA: 3Q,23

J1813 **Insulin (Lyumjev) for administration through DME (i.e., insulin pump) per 50 units** K K2
AHA: 3Q,23

J1814 **Insulin (Lyumjev), per 5 units** N N1
AHA: 3Q,23

J1815 **Injection, insulin, per 5 units** N N1 ☑
Use this code for Humalog, Humulin, Iletin, Insulin Lispro, Lantus, Levemir, NPH, Pork insulin, Regular insulin, Ultralente, Velosulin, Humulin R, Iletin II Regular Pork, Insulin Purified Pork, Relion, Lente Iletin I, Novolin R, Humulin R U-500.
CMS: 100-04,4,20.6.4

J1817 **Insulin for administration through DME (i.e., insulin pump) per 50 units** N N1 ☑
Use this code for Humalog, Humulin, Iletin II NPH Pork, Lispro-PFC, Novolin, Novolog, Novolog Flexpen, Novolog Mix, Relion Novolin.

J1823 **Injection, inebilizumab-cdon, 1 mg** G K2
Use this code for Uplinza.
AHA: 1Q,21

J1826 **Injection, interferon beta-1a, 30 mcg** K K2 ☑
Use this code for AVONEX, Rebif.

J1830 **Injection interferon beta-1b, 0.25 mg (code may be used for Medicare when drug administered under the direct supervision of a physician, not for use when drug is self-administered)** E ☑
Use this code for Betaseron.
CMS: 100-02,15,50.5

J1833 **Injection, isavuconazonium, 1 mg** K K2 ☑
Use this code for Cresemba.

J1835 **Injection, itraconazole, 50 mg** E ☑
Use this code for Sporonox IV.
CMS: 100-04,4,20.6.4

J1836 **Injection, metronidazole, 10 mg** K K2
AHA: 3Q,23

~~J1840~~ ~~**Injection, kanamycin sulfate, up to 500 mg**~~

~~J1850~~ ~~**Injection, kanamycin sulfate, up to 75 mg**~~

J1885 **Injection, ketorolac tromethamine, per 15 mg** N N1 ☑
Use this code for Toradol.
CMS: 100-04,4,20.6.4

J1890 **Injection, cephalothin sodium, up to 1 g** E ☑
CMS: 100-04,4,20.6.4

J1920 **Injection, labetalol HCl, 5 mg** K K2
AHA: 3Q,23

▲ **J1921** **Injection, labetalol HCl (Hikma), not therapeutically equivalent to J1920, 5 mg** K K2
Use this code for labetalol HCl manufactured by Hikma.
AHA: 4Q,23; 3Q,23

J1930 **Injection, lanreotide, 1 mg** K K2 ☑
Use this code for Somatuline.

J1931 **Injection, laronidase, 0.1 mg** K K2 ☑
Use this code for Aldurazyme.

J1932 **Injection, lanreotide, (Cipla), 1 mg** G K2
AHA: 4Q,22

J1939 **Injection, bumetanide, 0.5 mg** N N1
Use this code for Bumex.
AHA: 1Q,24

J1940 **Injection, furosemide, up to 20 mg** N N1 ☑
Use this code for Lasix.
CMS: 100-04,4,20.6.4

J1941 **Injection, furosemide (Furoscix), 20 mg** E
Use this code for Furoscix.
AHA: 3Q,23

J1943 **Injection, aripiprazole lauroxil, (Aristada Initio), 1 mg** K K2
AHA: 4Q,19

J1944 **Injection, aripiprazole lauroxil, (Aristada), 1 mg** K K2
AHA: 4Q,19

J1945 **Injection, lepirudin, 50 mg** E ☑
Use this code for Refludan.
This drug is used for patients with heparin-induced thrombocytopenia.

J1950 **Injection, leuprolide acetate (for depot suspension), per 3.75 mg** K K2 ☑
Use this code for Lupron Depot-Pedi.
AHA: 2Q,19; 4Q,18

J1951 **Injection, leuprolide acetate for depot suspension (Fensolvi), 0.25 mg** K K2
AHA: 3Q,21

J1952 **Leuprolide injectable, camcevi, 1 mg** G K2
Use this code for Camcevi.
AHA: 1Q,22

J1953 **Injection, levetiracetam, 10 mg** N N1 ☑
Use this code for Keppra.

J1954 **Injection, leuprolide acetate for depot suspension (Cipla), 7.5 mg** G K2
AHA: 2Q,23; 1Q,23

J1955 **Injection, levocarnitine, per 1 g** B ☑
Use this code for Carnitor.

J1956 **Injection, levofloxacin, 250 mg** N N1 ☑
Use this code for Levaquin.
CMS: 100-04,4,20.6.4

J1960 **Injection, levorphanol tartrate, up to 2 mg** N N1 ☑
Use this code for Levo-Dromoran.
CMS: 100-04,4,20.6.4

J1961 **Injection, lenacapavir, 1 mg** G K2
Use this code for Sunlenca.
AHA: 3Q,23

J1980 **Injection, hyoscyamine sulfate, up to 0.25 mg** N N1 ☑
Use this code for Levsin.
CMS: 100-04,4,20.6.4

J1990 **Injection, chlordiazepoxide HCl, up to 100 mg** E ☑
Use this code for Librium.
CMS: 100-04,4,20.6.4

~~J2001~~ ~~**Injection, lidocaine HCl for intravenous infusion, 10 mg**~~

● **J2002** **Injection, lidocaine HCl in 5% dextrose, 1 mg**

● **J2003** **Injection, lidocaine HCl , 1 mg**

● **J2004** **Injection, lidocaine HCl with epinephrine, 1 mg**

J2010 **Injection, lincomycin HCl, up to 300 mg** N N1 ☑
Use this code for Lincocin.
CMS: 100-04,4,20.6.4

J2020 **Injection, linezolid, 200 mg** N N1 ☑
Use this code for Zyvok.

▲ **J2021** **Injection, linezolid (Hospira), not therapeutically equivalent to J2020, 200 mg** K K2
Use this code for linezolid manufactured by Hospira.
AHA: 1Q,23

J2060 **Injection, lorazepam, 2 mg** N N1 ☑
Use this code for Ativan.
CMS: 100-04,4,20.6.4

J2062 **Loxapine for inhalation, 1 mg** E
Use this code for Adasuve.
AHA: 1Q,19

J2150 **Injection, mannitol, 25% in 50 ml** N N1 ☑
Use this code for Osmitrol.
CMS: 100-04,4,20.6.4

J2170 **Injection, mecasermin, 1 mg** N N1 ☑
Use this code for Iplex, Increlex.
CMS: 100-02,15,50.5; 100-04,4,20.6.4

J2175 **Injection, meperidine HCl, per 100 mg** N N1 ☑
Use this code for Demerol.
CMS: 100-04,20,180; 100-04,32,411.3; 100-04,4,20.6.4

J2180 Injection, meperidine and promethazine HCl, up to 50 mg N N1 ☑
Use this code for Mepergan Injection.
CMS: 100-04,4,20.6.4

J2182 Injection, mepolizumab, 1 mg K K2 ☑
Use this code for Nucala.

● **J2183** Injection, meropenem (WG Critical Care), not therapeutically equivalent to J2185, 100 mg N1
AHA: 3Q,24

▲ **J2184** Injection, meropenem (B. Braun), not therapeutically equivalent to J2185, 100 mg K N1
Use this code for meropenem manufactured by B. Braun.
AHA: 1Q,23

J2185 Injection, meropenem, 100 mg N N1 ☑
Use this code for Merrem.
CMS: 100-04,4,20.6.4

J2186 Injection, meropenem, vaborbactam, 10 mg/10 mg, (20 mg) K K2
Use this code for Vabomere.
CMS: 100-04,4,260.1; 100-04,4,260.1.1
AHA: 1Q,19; 4Q,18

J2210 Injection, methylergonovine maleate, up to 0.2 mg N N1 ☑
Use this code for Methergine.
CMS: 100-04,4,20.6.4

J2212 Injection, methylnaltrexone, 0.1 mg K K2 ☑
Use this code for Relistor.
CMS: 100-02,15,50.5

● **J2246** Injection, micafungin in sodium (Baxter), not therapeutically equivalent to J2248, 1 mg
AHA: 3Q,24

J2247 Injection, micafungin sodium (Par Pharm) not therapeutically equivalent to J2248, 1 mg K K2
Use this code for micafungin sodium manufactured by Par Pharm.
AHA: 1Q,23

J2248 Injection, micafungin sodium, 1 mg N N1 ☑
Use this code for Mycamine.

J2249 Injection, remimazolam, 1 mg N N1
Use this code for Byfavo.
AHA: 3Q,23

J2250 Injection, midazolam HCl, per 1 mg N N1 ☑
Use this code for Versed.
CMS: 100-04,4,20.6.4

▲ **J2251** Injection, midazolam in 0.9% sodium chloride, intravenous, not therapeutically equivalent to J2250, 1 mg K N1
AHA: 1Q,23

● **J2252** Injection, midazolam in 0.8% sodium chloride, intravenous, not therapeutically equivalent to J2250, 1 mg

● **J2253** Injection, midazolam (Seizalam), 1 mg

J2260 Injection, milrinone lactate, 5 mg N N1 ☑
Use this code for Primacor.
CMS: 100-04,20,180; 100-04,32,411.3; 100-04,4,20.6.4

J2265 Injection, minocycline HCl, 1 mg K K2 ☑
Use this code for MINOCIN.

● **J2267** Injection, mirikizumab-mrkz, 1 mg K2
Use this code for Omvoh.
AHA: 3Q,24

J2270 Injection, morphine sulfate, up to 10 mg N N1 ☑
Use this code for Depodur, Infumorph.
CMS: 100-04,20,180; 100-04,4,20.6.4

▲ **J2272** Injection, morphine sulfate (Fresenius Kabi), not therapeutically equivalent to J2270, up to 10 mg K N1
Use this code for morphine sulfate manufactured by Fresenius Kabi.
AHA: 1Q,23

J2274 Injection, morphine sulfate, preservative free for epidural or intrathecal use, 10 mg N N1 ☑
Use this code for DepoDur, Astromorph PF, Duramorph PF.
CMS: 100-04,20,180

● **J2277** Injection, motixafortide, 0.25 mg G K2
Use this code for Aphexda.
AHA: 2Q,24

J2278 Injection, ziconotide, 1 mcg K K2 ☑
Use this code for Prialt.
CMS: 100-04,20,180

J2280 Injection, moxifloxacin, 100 mg N N1 ☑
Use this code for Avelox.
CMS: 100-04,4,20.6.4

▲ **J2281** Injection, moxifloxacin (Fresenius Kabi), not therapeutically equivalent to J2280, 100 mg K K2
Use this code for moxifloxacin manufactured by Fresenius Kabi.
AHA: 1Q,23

○ **J2290** Injection, nafcillin sodium, 20 mg

J2300 Injection, nalbuphine HCl, per 10 mg N N1 ☑
Use this code for Nubain.
CMS: 100-04,4,20.6.4

J2305 Injection, nitroglycerin, 5 mg K K2
AHA: 3Q,23

J2310 Injection, naloxone HCl, per 1 mg N N1 ☑
Use this code for Narcan.

J2311 Injection, naloxone HCl (Zimhi), 1 mg K K2
Use this code for naloxone HCl (Zimhi) manufactured by Adamis.
AHA: 1Q,23

J2315 Injection, naltrexone, depot form, 1 mg K K2 ☑
Use this code for Vivitrol.

J2320 Injection, nandrolone decanoate, up to 50 mg N N1 ☑

J2323 Injection, natalizumab, 1 mg K K2 ☑
Use this code for Tysabri.

J2325 Injection, nesiritide, 0.1 mg E1 ☑
Use this code for Natrecor.
CMS: 100-03,200.1

J2326 Injection, nusinersen, 0.1 mg K K2
Use this code for Spinraza.
AHA: 1Q,21; 1Q,20; 4Q,18; 1Q,18

J2327 Injection, risankizumab-rzaa, intravenous, 1 mg G K2
AHA: 1Q,23

J2329 Injection, ublituximab-xiiy, 1mg G K2
Use this code for Briumvi.
AHA: 3Q,23

J2350 Injection, ocrelizumab, 1 mg K K2
Use this code for Ocrevus.

J2353 Injection, octreotide, depot form for intramuscular injection, 1 mg K K2 ☑
Use this code for Sandostatin LAR.

J2354 Injection, octreotide, nondepot form for subcutaneous or intravenous injection, 25 mcg N N1 ☑
Use this code for Sandostatin.
CMS: 100-02,15,50.5

J2355 **Injection, oprelvekin, 5 mg** E1 ☑
Use this code for Neumega.

J2356 **Injection, tezepelumab-ekko, 1 mg** G K2
Use this code for Tezspire.
AHA: 3Q,22

J2357 **Injection, omalizumab, 5 mg** K K2 ☑
Use this code for Xolair.

J2358 **Injection, olanzapine, long-acting, 1 mg** K K2 ☑
Use this code for ZYPREXA RELPREVV.

J2359 **Injection, olanzapine, 0.5 mg** K K2
AHA: 4Q,23

J2360 **Injection, orphenadrine citrate, up to 60 mg** N N1 ☑
Use this code for Norflex.

J2371 **Injection, phenylephrine HCl, 20 mcg** N N1
AHA: 3Q,23

J2372 **Injection, phenylephrine HCl (Biorphen), 20 mcg** K K2
AHA: 3Q,23

● **J2373** **Injection, phenylephrine HCl (Immphentiv), 20 mcg** N1
AHA: 3Q,24

J2401 **Injection, chloroprocaine HCl, per 1 mg** K K2
AHA: 1Q,23

J2402 **Injection, chloroprocaine HCl (Clorotekal), per 1 mg** E
Use this code for chloroprocaine HCl (Clorotekal) manufactured by B. Braun.
AHA: 1Q,23

J2403 **Chloroprocaine HCl ophthalmic, 3% gel, 1 mg** G K2
Use this code for Iheezo.
AHA: 2Q,23

J2404 **Injection, nicardipine, 0.1 mg** N N1
Use this code for Cardene IV.
AHA: 1Q,24

J2405 **Injection, ondansetron HCl, per 1 mg** N N1 ☑
Use this code for Zofran.

J2406 **Injection, oritavancin (Kimyrsa), 10 mg** G K2
AHA: 4Q,21

J2407 **Injection, oritavancin (Orbactiv), 10 mg** K K2 ☑
Use this code for Orbactiv.

J2410 **Injection, oxymorphone HCl, up to 1 mg** E1 ☑
Use this code for Numorphan, Oxymorphone HCl.

J2425 **Injection, palifermin, 50 mcg** K K2 ☑
Use this code for Kepivance.

J2426 **Injection, paliperidone palmitate extended release (Invega Sustenna), 1 mg** K K2 ☑
Use this code for INVEGA SUSTENNA.
AHA: 3Q,23; 4Q,18

J2427 **Injection, paliperidone palmitate extended release (Invega Hafyera or Invega Trinza), 1 mg** K K2
AHA: 3Q,23

J2430 **Injection, pamidronate disodium, per 30 mg** N N1 ☑
Use this code for Aredia.

J2440 **Injection, papaverine HCl, up to 60 mg** N N1 ☑

J2460 **Injection, oxytetracycline HCl, up to 50 mg** E1 ☑
Use this code for Terramycin IM.

▲ **J2468** **Injection, palonosetron HCl (Posfrea), 25 mcg**
AHA: 3Q,24

J2469 **Injection, palonosetron HCl, 25 mcg** N N1 ☑
Use this code for Aloxi.

● **J2470** **Injection, pantoprazole sodium, 40 mg** N1
AHA: 3Q,24

● **J2471** **Injection, pantoprazole (Hikma), not therapeutically equivalent to J2470, 40 mg** N1
AHA: 3Q,24

● **J2472** **Injection, pantoprazole sodium in sodium chloride (Baxter), 40 mg**

J2501 **Injection, paricalcitol, 1 mcg** N N1 ☑
Use this code For Zemplar.

J2502 **Injection, pasireotide long acting, 1 mg** K K2 ☑
Use this code for Signifor LAR.

J2503 **Injection, pegaptanib sodium, 0.3 mg** E1 ☑
Use this code for Macugen.

J2504 **Injection, pegademase bovine, 25 IU** E1 ☑
Use this code for Adagen.

J2506 **Injection, pegfilgrastim, excludes biosimilar, 0.5 mg** K K2
Use this code for Neulasta.
AHA: 1Q,22

J2507 **Injection, pegloticase, 1 mg** K K2 ☑
Use this code for KRYSTEXXA.

J2508 **Injection, pegunigalsidase alfa-iwxj, 1 mg** G K2
Use this code for Elfabrio.
AHA: 1Q,24

J2510 **Injection, penicillin G procaine, aqueous, up to 600,000 units** K K2 ☑
Use this code for Wycillin, Duracillin A.S., Pfizerpen A.S., Crysticillin 300 A.S., Crysticillin 600 A.S.

J2513 **Injection, pentastarch, 10% solution, 100 ml** E1 ☑

J2515 **Injection, pentobarbital sodium, per 50 mg** N N1 ☑
Use this code for Nembutal Sodium Solution.

J2540 **Injection, penicillin G potassium, up to 600,000 units** N N1 ☑
Use this code for Pfizerpen.

J2543 **Injection, piperacillin sodium/tazobactam sodium, 1 g/0.125 g (1.125 g)** N N1 ☑
Use this code for Zosyn.

J2545 **Pentamidine isethionate, inhalation solution, FDA-approved final product, noncompounded, administered through DME, unit dose form, per 300 mg** B ☑
Use this code for Nebupent, Pentam 300.

J2547 **Injection, peramivir, 1 mg** K K2 ☑
Use this code for Rapivab.

J2550 **Injection, promethazine HCl, up to 50 mg** N N1 ☑
Use this code for Phenergan.

J2560 **Injection, phenobarbital sodium, up to 120 mg** N N1 ☑

J2561 **Injection, phenobarbital sodium (Sezaby), 1 mg** N N1
AHA: 3Q,23

J2562 **Injection, plerixafor, 1 mg** K K2 ☑
Use this code for Mozobil.

J2590 **Injection, oxytocin, up to 10 units** N N1 ☑
Use this code for Pitocin, Syntocinon.

J2597 **Injection, desmopressin acetate, per 1 mcg** K K2 ☑
Use this code for DDAVP.

J2598 **Injection, vasopressin, 1 unit** K K2
AHA: 3Q,23

▲ **J2599** **Injection, vasopressin (American Regent), not therapeutically equivalent to J2598, 1 unit** K N1
Use this code for vasopressin manufactured by American Regent.
AHA: 3Q,23

● **J2601** **Injection, vasopressin (Baxter), 1 unit** K2
Use this code for vasopressin manufactured by Baxter.

J2650 **Injection, prednisolone acetate, up to 1 ml** E1 ☑

J2670 **Injection, tolazoline HCl, up to 25 mg** E1 ☑

J2675 **Injection, progesterone, per 50 mg** N N1 ☑
Use this code for Gesterone, Gestrin.

J2679 **Injection, fluphenazine HCl, 1.25 mg** N N1
AHA: 1Q,24

J2680 **Injection, fluphenazine decanoate, up to 25 mg** N N1 ☑

J2690 **Injection, procainamide HCl, up to 1 g** K K2 ☑
Use this code for Pronestyl.

J2700 **Injection, oxacillin sodium, up to 250 mg** N N1 ☑
Use this code for Bactocill

J2704 **Injection, propofol, 10 mg** N N1 ☑
Use this code for Diprivan.

J2710 **Injection, neostigmine methylsulfate, up to 0.5 mg** N N1 ☑
Use this code for Prostigmin.

J2720 **Injection, protamine sulfate, per 10 mg** N N1 ☑

J2724 **Injection, protein C concentrate, intravenous, human, 10 IU** K K2 ☑

J2725 **Injection, protirelin, per 250 mcg** E1 ☑
Use this code for Thyrel TRH.

J2730 **Injection, pralidoxime chloride, up to 1 g** N N1 ☑
Use this code for Protopam Chloride.

J2760 **Injection, phentolamine mesylate, up to 5 mg** K K2 ☑
Use this code for Regitine.

J2765 **Injection, metoclopramide HCl, up to 10 mg** N N1 ☑
Use this code for Reglan.

J2770 **Injection, quinupristin/dalfopristin, 500 mg (150/350)** K K2 ☑
Use this code for Synercid.

J2777 **Injection, faricimab-svoa, 0.1 mg** G K2
Use this code for Vabysmo.
AHA: 4Q,22

J2778 **Injection, ranibizumab, 0.1 mg** K K2 ☑
Use this code for Lucentis.

J2779 **Injection, ranibizumab, via intravitreal implant (Susvimo), 0.1 mg** G K2
AHA: 3Q,22

~~J2780 Injection, ranitidine hydrochloride, 25 mg~~

J2781 **Injection, pegcetacoplan, intravitreal, 1 mg** G K2
Use this code for Syfovre.
AHA: 4Q,23

● **J2782** **Injection, avacincaptad pegol, 0.1 mg** G K2
Use this code for Izervay.
AHA: 2Q,24

J2783 **Injection, rasburicase, 0.5 mg** K K2 ☑
Use this code for Elitek.

J2785 **Injection, regadenoson, 0.1 mg** N N1 ☑
Use this code for Lexiscan.

J2786 **Injection, reslizumab, 1 mg** K K2 ☑
Use this code for Cinqair.

J2787 **Riboflavin 5'-phosphate, ophthalmic solution, up to 3 ml** N N1
Use this code for Photrexa Viscous.
CMS: 100-04,4,260.1; 100-04,4,260.1.1
AHA: 1Q,19

J2788 **Injection, Rho D immune globulin, human, minidose, 50 mcg (250 IU)** N N1 ☑
Use this code for RhoGam, MiCRhoGAM.

J2790 **Injection, Rho D immune globulin, human, full dose, 300 mcg (1500 IU)** N N1 ☑
Use this code for RhoGam, HypRho SD.

J2791 **Injection, Rho D immune globulin (human), (Rhophylac), intramuscular or intravenous, 100 IU** N N1 ☑
Use this for Rhophylac.

J2792 **Injection, Rho D immune globulin, intravenous, human, solvent detergent, 100 IU** K K2 ☑
Use this code for WINRho SDF.

J2793 **Injection, rilonacept, 1 mg** E1 ☑
Use this code for Arcalyst.
CMS: 100-02,15,50.5

J2794 **Injection, risperidone (RISPERDAL CONSTA), 0.5 mg** K K2 ☑

J2795 **Injection, ropivacaine HCl, 1 mg** N N1 ☑
Use this code for Naropin.

~~J2796 Injection, romiplostim, 10 mcg~~

J2797 **Injection, rolapitant, 0.5 mg** E1
Use this code for Varubi.
AHA: 1Q,19; 4Q,18

J2798 **Injection, risperidone, (Perseris), 0.5 mg** K K2
AHA: 4Q,19

J2799 **Injection, risperidone (Uzedy), 1 mg** G K2
Use this code for Uzedy.
AHA: 1Q,24

J2800 **Injection, methocarbamol, up to 10 ml** N N1 ☑
Use this code for Robaxin.

● **J2801** **Injection, risperidone (Rykindo), 0.5 mg** K K2
AHA: 2Q,24

● **J2802** **Injection, romiplostim, 1 mcg**
Use this code for Nplate.

J2805 **Injection, sincalide, 5 mcg** N N1 ☑
Use this code for Kinevac.

~~J2806 Injection, sincalide (Maia), not therapeutically equivalent to J2805, 5 mcg~~

J2810 **Injection, theophylline, per 40 mg** E1 ☑

J2820 **Injection, sargramostim (GM-CSF), 50 mcg** K K2 ☑
Use this code for Leukine.

J2840 **Injection, sebelipase alfa, 1 mg** K K2 ☑
Use this code for Kanuma.

J2850 **Injection, secretin, synthetic, human, 1 mcg** K K2 ☑

J2860 **Injection, siltuximab, 10 mg** K K2 ☑
Use this code for Sylvant.

J2910 **Injection, aurothioglucose, up to 50 mg** E1 ☑
Use this code for Solganal.

J2916 **Injection, sodium ferric gluconate complex in sucrose injection, 12.5 mg** N N1 ☑
CMS: 100-03,110.10

● **J2919** **Injection, methylprednisolone sodium succinate, 5 mg** N
AHA: 2Q,24

~~J2920 Injection, methylprednisolone sodium succinate, up to 40 mg~~
To report, see ~J2919

~~J2930 Injection, methylprednisolone sodium succinate, up to 125 mg~~
To report, see ~J2919

J2940 Injection, somatrem, 1 mg E1 ☑
Use this code for Protropin.

J2941 Injection, somatropin, 1 mg K K2 ☑
Use this code for Humatrope, Genotropin Nutropin, Biotropin, Genotropin, Genotropin Miniquick, Norditropin, Nutropin, Nutropin AQ, Saizen, Saizen Somatropin RDNA Origin, Serostim, Serostim RDNA Origin, Zorbtive.
CMS: 100-02,15,50.5

J2950 Injection, promazine HCl, up to 25 mg N N1 ☑
Use this code for Sparine, Prozine-50.

J2993 Injection, reteplase, 18.1 mg K K2 ☑
Use this code for Retavase.
AHA: 3Q,21; 4Q,18

J2995 Injection, streptokinase, per 250,000 IU E1 ☑
Use this code for Streptase.
AHA: 3Q,21; 4Q,18

J2997 Injection, alteplase recombinant, 1 mg K K2 ☑
Use this code for Activase, Cathflo.
AHA: 3Q,21; 4Q,18

J2998 Injection, plasminogen, human-tvmh, 1 mg G K2
Use this code for Ryplazim.
AHA: 3Q,22

J3000 Injection, streptomycin, up to 1 g N N1 ☑
Use this code for Streptomycin Sulfate.

J3010 Injection, fentanyl citrate, 0.1 mg N N1 ☑
Use this code for Sublimaze.
CMS: 100-04,20,180; 100-04,32,411.3

J3030 Injection, sumatriptan succinate, 6 mg (code may be used for Medicare when drug administered under the direct supervision of a physician, not for use when drug is self-administered) N N1 ☑
Use this code for Imitrex.
CMS: 100-02,15,50.5

J3031 Injection, fremanezumab-vfrm, 1 mg (code may be used for Medicare when drug administered under the direct supervision of a physician, not for use when drug is self-administered) K K2
Use this code for Ajovy.
AHA: 4Q,19

J3032 Injection, eptinezumab-jjmr, 1 mg K K2
Use this code for Vyepti.
AHA: 4Q,20

● **J3055 Injection, talquetamab-tgvs, 0.25 mg** G K2
Use this code for Talvey.
AHA: 2Q,24

J3060 Injection, taliglucerase alfa, 10 units K K2 ☑
Use this code for Elelyso.

J3070 Injection, pentazocine, 30 mg N N1 ☑
Use this code for Talwin.

J3090 Injection, tedizolid phosphate, 1 mg K K2 ☑
Use this code for Sivextro.

J3095 Injection, telavancin, 10 mg K K2 ☑
Use this code for VIBATIV.

J3101 Injection, tenecteplase, 1 mg K K2 ☑
Use this code for TNKase.
AHA: 3Q,21; 3Q,20; 4Q,18

J3105 Injection, terbutaline sulfate, up to 1 mg N N1 ☑
For terbutaline in inhalation solution, see K0525 and K0526.

J3110 Injection, teriparatide, 10 mcg B ☑
Use this code for Forteo.
CMS: 100-02,15,50.5; 100-04,10,90.1

J3111 Injection, romosozumab-aqqg, 1 mg K K2
Use this code for Evenity.
CMS: 100-04,10,90.1

J3121 Injection, testosterone enanthate, 1 mg N N1 ☑
Use this code for Delatstryl.

J3145 Injection, testosterone undecanoate, 1 mg K K2 ☑
Use this code for Aveed.

J3230 Injection, chlorpromazine HCl, up to 50 mg N N1 ☑
Use this code for Thorazine.

J3240 Injection, thyrotropin alpha, 0.9 mg, provided in 1.1 mg vial K K2 ☑
Use this code for Thyrogen.

J3241 Injection, teprotumumab-trbw, 10 mg K K2
Use this code for Tepezza.
AHA: 4Q,20

J3243 Injection, tigecycline, 1 mg N N1 ☑
Use this code for Tygacil.

▲ **J3244 Injection, tigecycline (Accord), not therapeutically equivalent to J3243, 1 mg** K K2
Use this code for tigecycline manufactured by Accord.
AHA: 1Q,23

J3245 Injection, tildrakizumab, 1 mg K K2
Use this code for Ilumya.

J3246 Injection, tirofiban HCl, 0.25 mg K K2 ☑
Use this code for Aggrastat.

● **J3247 Injection, secukinumab, IV, 1 mg** K2
Use this code for Cosentyx.
AHA: 3Q,24

J3250 Injection, trimethobenzamide HCl, up to 200 mg N N1 ☑
Use this code for Tigan, Tiject-20, Arrestin.

J3260 Injection, tobramycin sulfate, up to 80 mg N N1 ☑
Use this code for Nebcin.

J3262 Injection, tocilizumab, 1 mg K K2 ☑
Use this code for ACTEMRA.

● **J3263 Injection, toripalimab-tpzi, 1 mg** K2
Use this code for Loqtorzi.
AHA: 3Q,24

J3265 Injection, torsemide, 10 mg/ml E1 ☑
Use this code for Demadex, Torsemide.

J3280 Injection, thiethylperazine maleate, up to 10 mg E1 ☑

J3285 Injection, treprostinil, 1 mg K K2 ☑
Use this code for Remodulin.
CMS: 100-04,20,180; 100-04,32,411.3

J3299 Injection, triamcinolone acetonide (Xipere), 1 mg G K2
AHA: 3Q,22

J3300 Injection, triamcinolone acetonide, preservative free, 1 mg N N1 ☑
Use this code for TRIVARIS, TRIESENCE.

J3301 **Injection, triamcinolone acetonide, not otherwise specified, 10 mg** N N1 ✓
Use this code for Kenalog-10, Kenalog-40, Tri-Kort, Kenaject-40, Cenacort A-40, Triam-A, Trilog.
AHA: 1Q,24; 4Q,18

J3302 **Injection, triamcinolone diacetate, per 5 mg** N N1 ✓
Use this code for Aristocort, Aristocort Intralesional, Aristocort Forte, Amcort, Trilone, Cenacort Forte.

J3303 **Injection, triamcinolone hexacetonide, per 5 mg** N N1 ✓
Use this code for Aristospan Intralesional, Aristospan Intra-articular.

J3304 **Injection, triamcinolone acetonide, preservative-free, extended-release, microsphere formulation, 1 mg** K K2
Use this code for Zilretta.
AHA: 1Q,19; 4Q,18

J3305 **Injection, trimetrexate glucuronate, per 25 mg** E1 ✓
Use this code for Neutrexin.

J3310 **Injection, perphenazine, up to 5 mg** N N1 ✓
Use this code for Trilafon.

J3315 **Injection, triptorelin pamoate, 3.75 mg** K K2 ✓
Use this code for Trelstar Depot, Trelstar Depot Plus Debioclip Kit, Trelstar LA.

J3316 **Injection, triptorelin, extended-release, 3.75 mg** K K2
Use this code for Triptodur.
AHA: 1Q,19; 4Q,18

J3320 **Injection, spectinomycin dihydrochloride, up to 2 g** E1 ✓
Use this code for Trobicin.

J3350 **Injection, urea, up to 40 g** E1 ✓

J3355 **Injection, urofollitropin, 75 IU** E1 ✓
Use this code for Metrodin, Bravelle, Fertinex.
CMS: 100-02,15,50.5

J3357 **Ustekinumab, for subcutaneous injection, 1 mg** K K2 ✓
Use this code for STELARA.
CMS: 100-02,15,50.5

J3358 **Ustekinumab, for intravenous injection, 1 mg** K K2
Use this code for Stelara.

J3360 **Injection, diazepam, up to 5 mg** N N1 ✓
Use this code for Diastat, Dizac, Valium.
CMS: 100-04,8,60.2.1

J3364 **Injection, urokinase, 5,000 IU vial** E1 ✓
Use this code for Kinlytic.
AHA: 3Q,21; 4Q,18

J3365 **Injection, IV, urokinase, 250,000 IU vial** E1 ✓
Use this code for Kinlytic.
AHA: 3Q,21; 4Q,18

J3370 **Injection, vancomycin HCl, 500 mg** N N1 ✓
Use this code for Vancocin.

▲ **J3371** **Injection, vancomycin HCl (Mylan), not therapeutically equivalent to J3370, 500 mg** K K2
Use this code for vancomycin HCl manufactured by Mylan.
AHA: 1Q,23

▲ **J3372** **Injection, vancomycin HCl (Xellia), not therapeutically equivalent to J3370, 500 mg** K K2
Use this code for vancomycin HCl manufactured by Xellia.
AHA: 1Q,23

▲ **J3380** **Injection, vedolizumab, IV, 1 mg** K K2 ✓
Use this code for Entyvio.
AHA: 2Q,24; 4Q,18

J3385 **Injection, velaglucerase alfa, 100 units** K K2 ✓
Use this code for VPRIV.

● **J3392** **Injection, exagamglogene autotemcel, per treatment**
Use this code for Casgevy.

● **J3393** **Injection, betibeglogene autotemcel, per treatment**
Use this code for Zynteglo.
AHA: 3Q,24

● **J3394** **Injection, lovotibeglogene autotemcel, per treatment**
Use this code for Lyfgenia.
AHA: 3Q,24

J3396 **Injection, verteporfin, 0.1 mg** K K2 ✓
Use this code for Visudyne.
CMS: 100-03,80.2; 100-03,80.2.1; 100-03,80.3; 100-03,80.3.1; 100-04,32,300; 100-04,32,300.1; 100-04,32,300.2
AHA: 1Q,20; 4Q,18

J3397 **Injection, vestronidase alfa-vjbk, 1 mg** E1
Use this code for Mepsevii.
CMS: 100-04,4,260.1; 100-04,4,260.1.1
AHA: 1Q,19; 4Q,18

J3398 **Injection, voretigene neparvovec-rzyl, 1 billion vector genomes** K K2
Use this code for Luxturna.
AHA: 1Q,19; 4Q,18

J3399 **Injection, onasemnogene abeparvovec-xioi, per treatment, up to $5x10^{15}$ vector genomes** K
Use this code for Zolgensma.
AHA: 2Q,20

J3400 **Injection, triflupromazine HCl, up to 20 mg** E1 ✓

J3401 **Beremagene geperpavec-svdt for topical administration, containing nominal 5×10^9 PFU/ml vector genomes, per 0.1 ml** G K2
Use this code for Vyjuvek.
AHA: 1Q,24

J3410 **Injection, hydroxyzine HCl, up to 25 mg** N N1 ✓
Use this code for Vistaril, Vistaject-25, Hyzine, Hyzine-50.

J3411 **Injection, thiamine HCl, 100 mg** N N1 ✓

J3415 **Injection, pyridoxine HCl, 100 mg** N N1 ✓

J3420 **Injection, vitamin B-12 cyanocobalamin, up to 1,000 mcg** N N1 ✓
Use this code for Sytobex, Redisol, Rubramin PC, Betalin 12, Berubigen, Cobex, Cobal, Crystal B12, Cyano, Cyanocobalamin, Hydroxocobalamin, Hydroxycobal, Nutri-Twelve.

● **J3424** **Injection, hydroxocobalamin, IV, 25 mg** K K2
Use this code for Cyanokit.
AHA: 2Q,24

▲ **J3425** **Injection, hydroxocobalamin, IM, 10 mcg** N N1
AHA: 2Q,24; 1Q,24

J3430 **Injection, phytonadione (vitamin K), per 1 mg** N N1 ✓
Use this code for AquaMephyton, Konakion, Menadione, Phytonadione.

J3465 **Injection, voriconazole, 10 mg** N N1 ✓

J3470 **Injection, hyaluronidase, up to 150 units** N N1 ✓

J3471 **Injection, hyaluronidase, ovine, preservative free, per 1 USP unit (up to 999 USP units)** N N1 ✓

J3472 **Injection, hyaluronidase, ovine, preservative free, per 1,000 USP units** N N1 ✓

J3473 **Injection, hyaluronidase, recombinant, 1 USP unit** N N1 ✓

J3475 **Injection, magnesium sulfate, per 500 mg** N N1 ✓
Use this code for Mag Sul, Sulfa Mag.

J3480 **Injection, potassium chloride, per 2 mEq** N N1 ✓

J3485 **Injection, zidovudine, 10 mg** N N1 ☑
Use this code for Retrovir, Zidovudine.

J3486 **Injection, ziprasidone mesylate, 10 mg** N N1 ☑
Use this code for Geodon.

J3489 **Injection, zoledronic acid, 1 mg** N N1 ☑
Use this code for Reclast and Zometa.

J3490 **Unclassified drugs** N N1 ☑
CMS: 100-02,15,50.5; 100-03,1,110.22; 100-03,110.22; 100-04,10,90.1; 100-04,32,280.1; 100-04,32,280.2; 100-04,32,400; 100-04,32,400.1; 100-04,32,400.2; 100-04,32,400.2.1; 100-04,32,400.2.2; 100-04,32,400.2.3; 100-04,32,400.2.3.1; 100-04,32,400.2.4; 100-04,32,400.2.5; 100-04,32,400.3; 100-04,32,400.4; 100-04,32,412.1; 100-04,4,260.1; 100-04,4,260.1.1; 100-04,8,60.2.1.1; 100-04,8,60.2.3
AHA: 3Q,23; 3Q,21

J3520 **Edetate disodium, per 150 mg** E1 ☑
Use this code for Endrate, Disotate, Meritate, Chealamide, E.D.T.A. This drug is used in chelation therapy, a treatment for atherosclerosis that is not covered by Medicare.

J3530 **Nasal vaccine inhalation** N N1 ☑

J3535 **Drug administered through a metered dose inhaler** E1 ☑

J3570 **Laetrile, amygdalin, vitamin B-17** E1 ☑
The FDA has found Laetrile to have no safe or effective therapeutic purpose.

J3590 **Unclassified biologics** N N1 ☑
CMS: 100-02,15,50.5; 100-03,1,110.22; 100-03,110.22; 100-04,10,90.1; 100-04,32,280.1; 100-04,32,280.2; 100-04,32,400; 100-04,32,400.1; 100-04,32,400.2; 100-04,32,400.2.1; 100-04,32,400.2.2; 100-04,32,400.2.3; 100-04,32,400.2.3.1; 100-04,32,400.2.4; 100-04,32,400.2.5; 100-04,32,400.3; 100-04,32,400.4; 100-04,32,412.1
AHA: 3Q,23

J3591 **Unclassified drug or biological used for ESRD on dialysis** B
CMS: 100-04,4,260.1; 100-04,4,260.1.1; 100-04,8,20
AHA: 1Q,19

J7030 **Infusion, normal saline solution, 1,000 cc** N N1 ☑

J7040 **Infusion, normal saline solution, sterile (500 ml=1 unit)** N N1 ☑

J7042 **5% dextrose/normal saline (500 ml = 1 unit)** N N1 ☑

J7050 **Infusion, normal saline solution, 250 cc** N N1 ☑

J7060 **5% dextrose/water (500 ml = 1 unit)** N N1 ☑

J7070 **Infusion, D-5-W, 1,000 cc** N N1 ☑

J7100 **Infusion, dextran 40, 500 ml** N N1 ☑
Use this code for Gentran, 10% LMD, Rheomacrodex.

J7110 **Infusion, dextran 75, 500 ml** N N1 ☑
Use this code for Gentran 75.

J7120 **Ringers lactate infusion, up to 1,000 cc** N N1 ☑

J7121 **5% dextrose in lactated ringers infusion, up to 1000 cc** N N1 ☑

J7131 **Hypertonic saline solution, 1 ml** N N1 ☑

● **J7165** **Injection, prothrombin complex concentrate, human-lans, per IU of Factor IX activity** G K2
Use this code for Balfaxar.
AHA: 2Q,24

J7168 **Prothrombin complex concentrate (human), Kcentra, per IU of Factor IX activity** K K2
AHA: 3Q,21

J7169 **Injection, coagulation Factor Xa (recombinant), inactivated-zhzo (Andexxa), 10 mg** K K2
AHA: 2Q,20

J7170 **Injection, emicizumab-kxwh, 0.5 mg** K K2
Use this code for Hemlibra.
AHA: 1Q,19; 4Q,18

● **J7171** **Injection, ADAMTS13, recombinant-krhn, 10 IU** K2
Use this code for Adzynma.
AHA: 3Q,24

J7175 **Injection, Factor X, (human), 1 IU** K K2 ☑
Use this code for Coagadex.

J7177 **Injection, human fibrinogen concentrate (Fibryga), 1 mg** K K2
CMS: 100-04,4,260.1; 100-04,4,260.1.1
AHA: 1Q,19; 4Q,18

J7178 **Injection, human fibrinogen concentrate, not otherwise specified, 1 mg** K K2 ☑
Use this code for RiaSTAP.

J7179 **Injection, von Willebrand factor (recombinant), (Vonvendi), 1 IU VWF:RCo** K K2 ☑

J7180 **Injection, Factor XIII (antihemophilic factor, human), 1 IU** K K2 ☑
Use this code for Corifact.

J7181 **Injection, Factor XIII A-subunit, (recombinant), per IU** K K2 ☑

J7182 **Injection, Factor VIII, (antihemophilic factor, recombinant), (NovoEight), per IU** K K2 ☑

J7183 **Injection, von Willebrand factor complex (human), Wilate, 1 IU VWF:RCO** K K2 ☑

J7185 **Injection, Factor VIII (antihemophilic factor, recombinant) (Xyntha), per IU** K K2 ☑

J7186 **Injection, antihemophilic Factor VIII/von Willebrand factor complex (human), per Factor VIII IU** K K2 ☑
Use this code for Alphanate.
CMS: 100-04,17,80.4.1

J7187 **Injection, von Willebrand factor complex (Humate-P), per IU VWF:RCO** K K2 ☑
CMS: 100-04,17,80.4.1

J7188 **Injection, Factor VIII (antihemophilic factor, recombinant) (Obizur), per IU** K K2 ☑

J7189 **Factor VIIa (antihemophilic factor, recombinant), (NovoSeven RT), 1 mcg** K K2 ☑
CMS: 100-04,17,80.4.1

J7190 **Factor VIII (antihemophilic factor, human) per IU** K K2 ☑
Use this code for Koate-DVI, Monarc-M, Monoclate-P.
CMS: 100-04,17,80.4; 100-04,17,80.4.1

J7191 **Factor VIII (antihemophilic factor (porcine)), per IU** E1 ☑
CMS: 100-04,17,80.4; 100-04,17,80.4.1

J7192 **Factor VIII (antihemophilic factor, recombinant) per IU, not otherwise specified** K K2 ☑
Use this code for Advate rAHF-PFM, Antihemophilic Factor Human Method M Monoclonal Purified, Bioclate, Kogenate FS, Recombinate, Refacto.
CMS: 100-04,17,80.4; 100-04,17,80.4.1

J7193 **Factor IX (antihemophilic factor, purified, nonrecombinant) per IU** K K2 ☑
Use this code for AlphaNine SD, Mononine.
CMS: 100-04,17,80.4; 100-04,17,80.4.1

J7194 **Factor IX complex, per IU** K K2 ☑
Use this code for Konyne-80, Profilnine SD, Proplex T, Proplex T, Bebulin VH, factor IX+ complex, Profilnine SD.
CMS: 100-04,17,80.4; 100-04,17,80.4.1

J7195 **Injection, Factor IX (antihemophilic factor, recombinant) per IU, not otherwise specified** K K2 ☑
Use this code for Antithrombin III, Benefix, Thrombate III.
CMS: 100-04,17,80.4; 100-04,17,80.4.1

J7196 **Injection, antithrombin recombinant, 50 IU** E1 ☑
Use this code for ATryn.

J7197 **Antithrombin III (human), per IU** K K2 ☑
Use this code for Thrombate III, ATnativ.
CMS: 100-04,17,80.4.1

J7198 **Antiinhibitor, per IU** K K2 ☑
Medicare jurisdiction: local contractor. Use this code for Autoplex T, Feiba VH AICC.
CMS: 100-03,110.3; 100-04,17,80.4; 100-04,17,80.4.1

J7199 **Hemophilia clotting factor, not otherwise classified** B ☑
Medicare jurisdiction: local contractor.
CMS: 100-04,17,80.4; 100-04,17,80.4.1

J7200 **Injection, Factor IX, (antihemophilic factor, recombinant), Rixubis, per IU** K K2 ☑

J7201 **Injection, Factor IX, Fc fusion protein, (recombinant), Alprolix, 1 IU** K K2 ☑

J7202 **Injection, Factor IX, albumin fusion protein, (recombinant), Idelvion, 1 IU** K K2 ☑

J7203 **Injection Factor IX, (antihemophilic factor, recombinant), glycoPEGylated, (Rebinyn), 1 IU** K K2
AHA: 1Q,19; 4Q,18

J7204 **Injection, Factor VIII, antihemophilic factor (recombinant), (Esperoct), glycopegylated-exei, per IU** K K2
AHA: 2Q,20

J7205 **Injection, Factor VIII Fc fusion protein (recombinant), per IU** K K2 ☑
Use this code for Eloctate.

J7207 **Injection, Factor VIII, (antihemophilic factor, recombinant), PEGylated, 1 IU** K K2 ☑
Use this code for Adynovate.

J7208 **Injection, Factor VIII, (antihemophilic factor, recombinant), PEGylated-aucl, (Jivi), 1 IU** K K2
AHA: 3Q,19

J7209 **Injection, Factor VIII, (antihemophilic factor, recombinant), (Nuwiq), 1 IU** K K2 ☑

J7210 **Injection, Factor VIII, (antihemophilic factor, recombinant), (Afstyla), 1 IU** K K2

J7211 **Injection, Factor VIII, (antihemophilic factor, recombinant), (Kovaltry), 1 IU** K K2

J7212 **Factor VIIa (antihemophilic factor, recombinant)-jncw (Sevenfact), 1 mcg** K K2
AHA: 1Q,21

J7213 **Injection, coagulation factor IX (recombinant), Ixinity, 1 IU** K K2
AHA: 3Q,23

J7214 **Injection, Factor VIII/von Willebrand factor complex, recombinant (Altuviiio), per Factor VIII IU** G K2
AHA: 4Q,23

J7294 **Segesterone acetate and ethinyl estradiol 0.15 mg, 0.013 mg per 24 hours; yearly vaginal system, ea** E1
Use this code for Annovera vaginal ring.
AHA: 4Q,21

J7295 **Ethinyl estradiol and etonogestrel 0.015 mg, 0.12 mg per 24 hours; monthly vaginal ring, ea** E1
Use this code for NuvaRing vaginal ring.
AHA: 4Q,21

J7296 **Levonorgestrel-releasing intrauterine contraceptive system, (Kyleena), 19.5 mg** E1

J7297 **Levonorgestrel-releasing intrauterine contraceptive system (Liletta), 52 mg** M E1 ☑

J7298 **Levonorgestrel-releasing intrauterine contraceptive system (Mirena), 52 mg** M E1 ☑
AHA: 1Q,23

J7300 **Intrauterine copper contraceptive** E1 ☑
Use this code for Paragard T380A.

J7301 **Levonorgestrel-releasing intrauterine contraceptive system (Skyla), 13.5 mg** M E1 ☑

J7304 **Contraceptive supply, hormone containing patch, each** E1 ☑

J7306 **Levonorgestrel (contraceptive) implant system, including implants and supplies** E1 ☑

J7307 **Etonogestrel (contraceptive) implant system, including implant and supplies** E1 ☑
Use this code for Implanon and Nexplanon.

J7308 **Aminolevulinic acid HCl for topical administration, 20%, single unit dosage form (354 mg)** K K2 ☑
Use this code for Levulan Kerastick.
AHA: 1Q,20

J7309 **Methyl aminolevulinate (MAL) for topical administration, 16.8%, 1 g** E1 ☑
Use this code for Metvixia.
AHA: 1Q,20

J7310 **Ganciclovir, 4.5 mg, long-acting implant** E1 ☑
Use this code for Vitrasert.

J7311 **Injection, fluocinolone acetonide, intravitreal implant (Retisert), 0.01 mg** K K2 ☑

J7312 **Injection, dexamethasone, intravitreal implant, 0.1 mg** K K2 ☑
Use this code for OZURDEX.

J7313 **Injection, fluocinolone acetonide, intravitreal implant (Iluvien), 0.01 mg** K K2 ☑

J7314 **Injection, fluocinolone acetonide, intravitreal implant (Yutiq), 0.01 mg** K K2
AHA: 4Q,19

J7315 **Mitomycin, opthalmic, 0.2 mg** N N1 ☑
Use this code for Mitosol.

J7316 **Injection, ocriplasmin, 0.125 mg** N N1 ☑
Use this code for Jetrea.

J7318 **Hyaluronan or derivative, Durolane, for intra-articular injection, 1 mg** K K2
AHA: 1Q,19; 4Q,18

J7320 **Hyaluronan or derivative, GenVisc 850, for intra-articular injection, 1 mg** K K2 ☑

J7321 **Hyaluronan or derivative, Hyalgan, Supartz or Visco-3, for intra-articular injection, per dose** N N1 ☑
AHA: 1Q,21; 2Q,20; 4Q,18

J7322 **Hyaluronan or derivative, Hymovis, for intra-articular injection, 1 mg** K K2 ☑

J7323 **Hyaluronan or derivative, Euflexxa, for intra-articular injection, per dose** K K2 ☑

J7324 **Hyaluronan or derivative, Orthovisc, for intra-articular injection, per dose** K K2 ☑

J7325 **Hyaluronan or derivative, Synvisc or Synvisc-One, for intra-articular injection, 1 mg** K K2 ☑

J7326 **Hyaluronan or derivative, Gel-One, for intra-articular injection, per dose** K K2 ☑

J7327 **Hyaluronan or derivative, Monovisc, for intra-articular injection, per dose** K K2 ☑

J7328 **Hyaluronan or derivative, GELSYN-3, for intra-articular injection, 0.1 mg** K K2 ☑

J7329 **Hyaluronan or derivative, Trivisc, for intra-articular injection, 1 mg** K K2
CMS: 100-04,4,260.1; 100-04,4,260.1.1
AHA: 1Q,19; 4Q,18

J7330 **Autologous cultured chondrocytes, implant** B ☑
Medicare jurisdiction: local contractor. Use this code for Carticel.

J7331 **Hyaluronan or derivative, SYNOJOYNT, for intra-articular injection, 1 mg** K K2
AHA: 4Q,19

J7332 **Hyaluronan or derivative, Triluron, for intra-articular injection, 1 mg** K K2
AHA: 4Q,19

J7336 **Capsaicin 8% patch, per sq cm** K K2 ☑
Use this code for Qutenza.

J7340 **Carbidopa 5 mg/levodopa 20 mg enteral suspension, 100 ml** K K2 ☑
Use this code for Duopa.

J7342 **Instillation, ciprofloxacin otic suspension, 6 mg** K K2 ☑
Use this code for Otiprio.

J7345 **Aminolevulinic acid HCl for topical administration, 10% gel, 10 mg** K K2
Use this code for Ameluz.
AHA: 1Q,20; 1Q,18

J7351 **Injection, bimatoprost, intracameral implant, 1 mcg** K K2
Use this code for Durysta.
AHA: 4Q,20

J7352 **Afamelanotide implant, 1 mg** K K2
Use this code for Scenesse.
AHA: 1Q,21

J7353 **Anacaulase-bcdb, 8.8% gel, 1 gm** N K2
Use this code for Nexobrid.
AHA: 4Q,23

● **J7354** **Cantharidin for topical administration, 0.7%, single unit dose applicator (3.2 mg)** G K2
Use this code for Ycanth.
AHA: 2Q,24

● **J7355** **Injection, travoprost, intracameral implant, 1 mcg** K2
Use this code for iDose TR.
AHA: 3Q,24

J7402 **Mometasone furoate sinus implant, (Sinuva), 10 mcg** K K2
AHA: 1Q,21

J7500 **Azathioprine, oral, 50 mg** N N1 ☑
Use this code for Azasan, Imuran.
CMS: 100-04,17,80.3

J7501 **Azathioprine, parenteral, 100 mg** K K2 ☑
CMS: 100-04,17,80.3

J7502 **Cyclosporine, oral, 100 mg** N N1 ☑
Use this code for Neoral, Sandimmune, Gengraf, Sangcya.
CMS: 100-04,17,80.3

J7503 **Tacrolimus, extended release, (Envarsus XR), oral, 0.25 mg** N N1 ☑

J7504 **Lymphocyte immune globulin, antithymocyte globulin, equine, parenteral, 250 mg** K K2 ☑
Use this code for Atgam.
CMS: 100-03,260.7; 100-04,17,80.3

J7505 **Muromonab-CD3, parenteral, 5 mg** E1 ☑
Use this code for Orthoclone OKT3.
CMS: 100-04,17,80.3

J7507 **Tacrolimus, immediate release, oral, 1 mg** N N1 ☑
Use this code for Prograf.
CMS: 100-04,17,80.3

J7508 **Tacrolimus, extended release, (Astagraf XL), oral, 0.1 mg** N N1 ☑

J7509 **Methylprednisolone, oral, per 4 mg** N N1 ☑
Use this code for Medrol, Methylpred.
CMS: 100-04,17,80.3

J7510 **Prednisolone, oral, per 5 mg** N N1 ☑
Use this code for Delta-Cortef, Cotolone, Pediapred, Prednoral, Prelone.
CMS: 100-04,17,80.3

J7511 **Lymphocyte immune globulin, antithymocyte globulin, rabbit, parenteral, 25 mg** K K2 ☑
Use this code for Thymoglobulin.
CMS: 100-04,17,80.3

J7512 **Prednisone, immediate release or delayed release, oral, 1 mg** N N1 ☑

J7513 **Daclizumab, parenteral, 25 mg** E1 ☑
Use this code for Zenapax.
CMS: 100-04,17,80.3

● **J7514** **Mycophenolate mofetil (Myhibbin), oral suspension, 100 mg**

J7515 **Cyclosporine, oral, 25 mg** N N1 ☑
Use this code for Neoral, Sandimmune, Gengraf, Sangcya.
CMS: 100-04,17,80.3

▲ **J7516** **Injection, cyclosporine, 250 mg** N N1 ☑
Use this code for Neoral, Sandimmune, Gengraf, Sangcya.
CMS: 100-04,17,80.3
AHA: 2Q,24

J7517 **Mycophenolate mofetil, oral, 250 mg** N N1 ☑
Use this code for CellCept.
CMS: 100-04,17,80.3

J7518 **Mycophenolic acid, oral, 180 mg** N N1 ☑
Use this code for Myfortic Delayed Release.
CMS: 100-04,17,80.3.1

J7519 **Injection, mycophenolate mofetil, 10 mg** K K2
Use this code for CellCept.
AHA: 4Q,23

J7520 **Sirolimus, oral, 1 mg** N N1 ☑
Use this code for Rapamune.
CMS: 100-04,17,80.3

J7525 **Tacrolimus, parenteral, 5 mg** K K2 ☑
Use this code for Prograf.
CMS: 100-04,17,80.3

J7527 **Everolimus, oral, 0.25 mg** N N1 ☑
Use this code for Zortress, Afinitor.

J7599 **Immunosuppressive drug, not otherwise classified** N N1 ☑
Determine if an alternative HCPCS Level II or a CPT code better describes the service being reported. This code should be used only if a more specific code is unavailable.
CMS: 100-04,17,80.3

Inhalation Drugs

● **J7601** **Ensifentrine, inhalation suspension, FDA-approved final product, noncompounded, administered through DME, unit dose form, 3 mg**
Use this code for Ohtuvayre.

J7604 **Acetylcysteine, inhalation solution, compounded product, administered through DME, unit dose form, per g** M ☑

J7605 **Arformoterol, inhalation solution, FDA-approved final product, noncompounded, administered through DME, unit dose form, 15 mcg** M ☑
CMS: 100-02,15,50.5

J7606 **Formoterol fumarate, inhalation solution, FDA-approved final product, noncompounded, administered through DME, unit dose form, 20 mcg** M ☑
Use this code for PERFOROMIST.
CMS: 100-02,15,50.5

J7607 **Levalbuterol, inhalation solution, compounded product, administered through DME, concentrated form, 0.5 mg** M ☑
CMS: 100-03,200.2

J7608 **Acetylcysteine, inhalation solution, FDA-approved final product, noncompounded, administered through DME, unit dose form, per g** M ☑
Use this code for Acetadote, Mucomyst, Mucosil.

J7609 **Albuterol, inhalation solution, compounded product, administered through DME, unit dose, 1 mg** M ☑

J7610 **Albuterol, inhalation solution, compounded product, administered through DME, concentrated form, 1 mg** M ☑

J7611 **Albuterol, inhalation solution, FDA-approved final product, noncompounded, administered through DME, concentrated form, 1 mg** M ☑
Use this code for Accuneb, Proventil, Respirol, Ventolin.

J7612 **Levalbuterol, inhalation solution, FDA-approved final product, noncompounded, administered through DME, concentrated form, 0.5 mg** M ☑
Use this code for Xopenex HFA.
CMS: 100-03,200.2

J7613 **Albuterol, inhalation solution, FDA-approved final product, noncompounded, administered through DME, unit dose, 1 mg** M ☑
Use this code for Accuneb, Proventil, Respirol, Ventolin.

J7614 **Levalbuterol, inhalation solution, FDA-approved final product, noncompounded, administered through DME, unit dose, 0.5 mg** M ☑
Use this code for Xopenex.
CMS: 100-03,200.2

J7615 **Levalbuterol, inhalation solution, compounded product, administered through DME, unit dose, 0.5 mg** M ☑
CMS: 100-03,200.2

J7620 **Albuterol, up to 2.5 mg and ipratropium bromide, up to 0.5 mg, FDA-approved final product, noncompounded, administered through DME** M ☑

J7622 **Beclomethasone, inhalation solution, compounded product, administered through DME, unit dose form, per mg** M ☑
Use this code for Beclovent, Beconase.

J7624 **Betamethasone, inhalation solution, compounded product, administered through DME, unit dose form, per mg** M ☑

J7626 **Budesonide, inhalation solution, FDA-approved final product, noncompounded, administered through DME, unit dose form, up to 0.5 mg** M ☑
Use this code for Pulmicort, Pulmicort Flexhaler, Pulmicort Respules, Vanceril.

J7627 **Budesonide, inhalation solution, compounded product, administered through DME, unit dose form, up to 0.5 mg** M ☑

J7628 **Bitolterol mesylate, inhalation solution, compounded product, administered through DME, concentrated form, per mg** M ☑

J7629 **Bitolterol mesylate, inhalation solution, compounded product, administered through DME, unit dose form, per mg** M ☑

J7631 **Cromolyn sodium, inhalation solution, FDA-approved final product, noncompounded, administered through DME, unit dose form, per 10 mg** M ☑
Use this code for Intal, Nasalcrom.

J7632 **Cromolyn sodium, inhalation solution, compounded product, administered through DME, unit dose form, per 10 mg** M ☑

J7633 **Budesonide, inhalation solution, FDA-approved final product, noncompounded, administered through DME, concentrated form, per 0.25 mg** M ☑
Use this code for Pulmicort, Pulmicort Flexhaler, Pulmicort Respules, Vanceril.

J7634 **Budesonide, inhalation solution, compounded product, administered through DME, concentrated form, per 0.25 mg** M ☑

J7635 **Atropine, inhalation solution, compounded product, administered through DME, concentrated form, per mg** M ☑

J7636 **Atropine, inhalation solution, compounded product, administered through DME, unit dose form, per mg** M ☑

J7637 **Dexamethasone, inhalation solution, compounded product, administered through DME, concentrated form, per mg** M ☑

J7638 **Dexamethasone, inhalation solution, compounded product, administered through DME, unit dose form, per mg** M ☑

J7639 **Dornase alfa, inhalation solution, FDA-approved final product, noncompounded, administered through DME, unit dose form, per mg** M ☑
Use this code for Pulmozyme.
CMS: 100-02,15,50.5

J7640 **Formoterol, inhalation solution, compounded product, administered through DME, unit dose form, 12 mcg** E1 ☑

J7641 **Flunisolide, inhalation solution, compounded product, administered through DME, unit dose, per mg** M ☑
Use this code for Aerobid, Flunisolide.

J7642 **Glycopyrrolate, inhalation solution, compounded product, administered through DME, concentrated form, per mg** M ☑

J7643 **Glycopyrrolate, inhalation solution, compounded product, administered through DME, unit dose form, per mg** M ☑

J7644 **Ipratropium bromide, inhalation solution, FDA-approved final product, noncompounded, administered through DME, unit dose form, per mg** M ☑
Use this code for Atrovent.

J7645 **Ipratropium bromide, inhalation solution, compounded product, administered through DME, unit dose form, per mg** M ☑

J7647 **Isoetharine HCl, inhalation solution, compounded product, administered through DME, concentrated form, per mg** M ☑

J7648 **Isoetharine HCl, inhalation solution, FDA-approved final product, noncompounded, administered through DME, concentrated form, per mg** M ☑
Use this code for Beta-2.

J7649 Isoetharine HCl, inhalation solution, FDA-approved final product, noncompounded, administered through DME, unit dose form, per mg M ☑

J7650 Isoetharine HCl, inhalation solution, compounded product, administered through DME, unit dose form, per mg M ☑

J7657 Isoproterenol HCl, inhalation solution, compounded product, administered through DME, concentrated form, per mg M ☑

J7658 Isoproterenol HCl, inhalation solution, FDA-approved final product, noncompounded, administered through DME, concentrated form, per mg M ☑
Use this code for Isuprel HCl.

J7659 Isoproterenol HCl, inhalation solution, FDA-approved final product, noncompounded, administered through DME, unit dose form, per mg M ☑
Use this code for Isuprel HCl.

J7660 Isoproterenol HCl, inhalation solution, compounded product, administered through DME, unit dose form, per mg M ☑

J7665 Mannitol, administered through an inhaler, 5 mg N N1 ☑
Use this code for ARIDOL.

J7667 Metaproterenol sulfate, inhalation solution, compounded product, concentrated form, per 10 mg M ☑

J7668 Metaproterenol sulfate, inhalation solution, FDA-approved final product, noncompounded, administered through DME, concentrated form, per 10 mg M ☑
Use this code for Alupent.

J7669 Metaproterenol sulfate, inhalation solution, FDA-approved final product, noncompounded, administered through DME, unit dose form, per 10 mg M ☑
Use this code for Alupent.

J7670 Metaproterenol sulfate, inhalation solution, compounded product, administered through DME, unit dose form, per 10 mg M ☑

J7674 Methacholine chloride administered as inhalation solution through a nebulizer, per 1 mg N N1 ☑

J7676 Pentamidine isethionate, inhalation solution, compounded product, administered through DME, unit dose form, per 300 mg M ☑

J7677 Revefenacin inhalation solution, FDA-approved final product, noncompounded, administered through DME, 1 mcg M
Use this code for Yupelri.

J7680 Terbutaline sulfate, inhalation solution, compounded product, administered through DME, concentrated form, per mg M ☑
Use this code for Brethine.

J7681 Terbutaline sulfate, inhalation solution, compounded product, administered through DME, unit dose form, per mg M ☑
Use this code for Brethine.

J7682 Tobramycin, inhalation solution, FDA-approved final product, noncompounded, unit dose form, administered through DME, per 300 mg M ☑
Use this code for Tobi.
CMS: 100-02,15,50.5

J7683 Triamcinolone, inhalation solution, compounded product, administered through DME, concentrated form, per mg M ☑
Use this code for Azmacort.

J7684 Triamcinolone, inhalation solution, compounded product, administered through DME, unit dose form, per mg M ☑
Use this code for Azmacort.

J7685 Tobramycin, inhalation solution, compounded product, administered through DME, unit dose form, per 300 mg M ☑

J7686 Treprostinil, inhalation solution, FDA-approved final product, noncompounded, administered through DME, unit dose form, 1.74 mg M ☑
Use this code for Tyvaso.
CMS: 100-02,15,50.5

J7699 NOC drugs, inhalation solution administered through DME M ☑
CMS: 100-02,15,50.5

J7799 NOC drugs, other than inhalation drugs, administered through DME N N1 ☑
CMS: 100-04,20,180; 100-04,32,411.4; 100-04,32,411.5; 100-04,32,411.6

J7999 Compounded drug, not otherwise classified N N1 ☑
CMS: 100-04,20,180; 100-04,32,411.4; 100-04,32,411.5; 100-04,32,411.6

J8498 Antiemetic drug, rectal/suppository, not otherwise specified B ☑

J8499 Prescription drug, oral, nonchemotherapeutic, NOS E ☑
CMS: 100-02,15,50.5

J Codes Chemotherapy Drugs J8501-J9999

Oral Chemotherapy Drugs

J8501 Aprepitant, oral, 5 mg N N1 ☑
Use this code for Emend.
CMS: 100-02,15,50.5.4; 100-03,110.18; 100-04,17,80.2.1; 100-04,17,80.2.4

J8510 Busulfan, oral, 2 mg N N1 ☑
Use this code for Busulfex, Myleran.
CMS: 100-04,17,80.1.1

J8515 Cabergoline, oral, 0.25 mg E ☑
Use this code for Dostinex.

~~**J8520** Capecitabine, oral, 150 mg~~

~~**J8521** Capecitabine, oral, 500 mg~~

● **J8522** Capecitabine, oral, 50 mg
Use this code for Xeloda.

J8530 Cyclophosphamide, oral, 25 mg N N1 ☑
Use this code for Cytoxan.
CMS: 100-04,17,80.1.1

J8540 Dexamethasone, oral, 0.25 mg N N1 ☑
Use this code for Decadron.

● **J8541** Dexamethasone (Hemady), oral, 0.25 mg

J8560 Etoposide, oral, 50 mg K K2 ☑
Use this code for VePesid.
CMS: 100-04,17,80.1.1

J8562 Fludarabine phosphate, oral, 10 mg E ☑
Use this code for Oforta.

J8565 Gefitinib, oral, 250 mg E ☑
Use this code for Iressa.
CMS: 100-04,17,80.1.1

J8597 Antiemetic drug, oral, not otherwise specified N N1 ☑

J8600 Melphalan, oral, 2 mg E ☑
Use this code for Alkeran.
CMS: 100-04,17,80.1.1

J8610 Methotrexate, oral, 2.5 mg N N1 ☑
Use this code for Trexall, RHEUMATREX.
CMS: 100-04,17,80.1.1

● **J8611** Methotrexate (Jylamvo), oral, 2.5 mg K2
AHA: 3Q,24

● **J8612** Methotrexate (Xatmep), oral, 2.5 mg K2
AHA: 3Q,24

J8650 **Nabilone, oral, 1 mg** E ☑
Use this code for Cesamet.

J8655 **Netupitant 300 mg and palonosetron 0.5 mg, oral** K K2 ☑
Use this code for Akynzeo.

J8670 **Rolapitant, oral, 1 mg** K K2 ☑
Use this code for Varubi.

J8700 **Temozolomide, oral, 5 mg** N N1 ☑
Use this code for Temodar.

J8705 **Topotecan, oral, 0.25 mg** K K2 ☑
Use this code for Hycamtin.

J8999 **Prescription drug, oral, chemotherapeutic, NOS** B ☑
Determine if an alternative HCPCS Level II or a CPT code better describes the service being reported. This code should be used only if a more specific code is unavailable.
CMS: 100-04,17,80.1.1; 100-04,17,80.1.2

Injectable Chemotherapy Drugs

These codes cover the cost of the chemotherapy drug only, not the administration.

J9000 **Injection, doxorubicin HCl, 10 mg** N N1 ☑ ⊘
Use this code for Adriamycin PFS, Adriamycin RDF, Rubex.
CMS: 100-04,20,180; 100-04,32,411.3

J9015 **Injection, aldesleukin, per single use vial** K K2 ☑ ⊘
Use this code for Proleukin, IL-2, Interleukin.

J9017 **Injection, arsenic trioxide, 1 mg** K K2 ☑ ⊘
Use this code for Trisenox.

J9019 **Injection, asparaginase (Erwinaze), 1,000 IU** E ☑

J9020 **Injection, asparaginase, not otherwise specified, 10,000 units** E ☑ ⊘
Use this code for Elspar.

J9021 **Injection, asparaginase, recombinant, (Rylaze), 0.1 mg** G K2
Use this code for Rylaze.
AHA: 1Q,22

J9022 **Injection, atezolizumab, 10 mg** K K2
Use this code for Tecentriq.

J9023 **Injection, avelumab, 10 mg** K K2
Use this code for Bavencio.

J9025 **Injection, azacitidine, 1 mg** N N1 ☑ ⊘
Use this code for Vidaza.

● **J9026** **Injection, tarlatamab-dlle, 1 mg**
Use this code for Imdelltra.

J9027 **Injection, clofarabine, 1 mg** K K2 ☑ ⊘
Use this code for Clolar.

● **J9028** **Injection, nogapendekin alfa inbakicept-pmln, for intravesical use, 1 mcg**
Use this code for Anktiva.

▲ **J9029** **Intravesical instillation, nadofaragene firadenovec-vncg, per therapeutic dose** G K2
Use this code for Adstiladrin.
AHA: 2Q,24; 3Q,23

J9030 **BCG live intravesical instillation, 1 mg** N N1
Use this code for Pacis, TICE BCG.
AHA: 3Q,19

J9032 **Injection, belinostat, 10 mg** K K2 ☑
Use this code for Beleodaq.

▲ **J9033** **Injection, bendamustine HCl, 1 mg** K K2 ☑ ⊘
Use this code for Treanda.

J9034 **Injection, bendamustine HCl (Bendeka), 1 mg** K K2 ☑

J9035 **Injection, bevacizumab, 10 mg** K K2 ☑ ⊘
Use this code for Avastin.
CMS: 100-03,110.17

J9036 **Injection, bendamustine HCl, (Belrapzo/bendamustine), 1 mg** K K2
AHA: 3Q,19

J9037 **Injection, belantamab mafodotin-blmf, 0.5 mg** K K2
Use this code for Blenrep.
AHA: 1Q,21

J9039 **Injection, blinatumomab, 1 mcg** K K2 ☑
Use this code for Blincyto.
CMS: 100-04,20,180; 100-04,32,411.3

J9040 **Injection, bleomycin sulfate, 15 units** N N1 ☑ ⊘
Use this code for Blenoxane.
CMS: 100-04,20,180; 100-04,32,411.3

J9041 **Injection, bortezomib, 0.1 mg** K K2 ☑ ⊘
AHA: 1Q,23; 4Q,18

J9042 **Injection, brentuximab vedotin, 1 mg** K K2 ☑
Use this code for Adcentris.

J9043 **Injection, cabazitaxel, 1 mg** K K2 ☑
Use this code for Jevtana.

J9045 **Injection, carboplatin, 50 mg** N N1 ☑ ⊘
Use this code for Paraplatin.

▲ **J9046** **Injection, bortezomib (Dr. Reddy's), not therapeutically equivalent to J9041, 0.1 mg** K K2
Use this code for bortezomib manufactured by Dr. Reddy's.
AHA: 1Q,23

J9047 **Injection, carfilzomib, 1 mg** K K2 ☑
Use this code for Kyprolis.

J9048 **Injection, bortezomib (Fresenius Kabi), not therapeutically equivalent to J9041, 0.1 mg** K K2
Use this code for bortezomib manufactured by Fresenius Kabi.
AHA: 1Q,23

J9049 **Injection, bortezomib (Hospira), not therapeutically equivalent to J9041, 0.1 mg** K K2
Use this code for bortezomib manufactured by Hospira.
AHA: 1Q,23

J9050 **Injection, carmustine, 100 mg** K K2 ☑ ⊘
Use this code for BiCNU.

J9051 **Injection, bortezomib (MAIA), not therapeutically equivalent to J9041, 0.1 mg** E1
AHA: 4Q,23

J9052 **Injection, carmustine (Accord), not therapeutically equivalent to J9050, 100 mg** K K2
AHA: 1Q,24

J9055 **Injection, cetuximab, 10 mg** K K2 ☑ ⊘
Use this code for Erbitux.
CMS: 100-03,110.17

J9056 **Injection, bendamustine HCl (Vivimusta), 1 mg** G K2
AHA: 3Q,23

J9057 **Injection, copanlisib, 1 mg** K K2
Use this code for Aliqopa.
AHA: 1Q,19; 4Q,18

J9058 ~~**Injection, bendamustine HCl (Apotex), 1 mg**~~

J9059 ~~**Injection, bendamustine HCl (Baxter), 1 mg**~~

J9060 **Injection, cisplatin, powder or solution, 10 mg** N N1 ☑ ⊘
Use this code for Plantinol AQ.

J9061 Injection, amivantamab-vmjw, 2 mg G K2
Use this code for Rybrevant.
AHA: 1Q,22

J9063 Injection, mirvetuximab soravtansine-gynx, 1 mg G K2
Use this code for Elahere.
AHA: 3Q,23

J9064 Injection, cabazitaxel (Sandoz), not therapeutically equivalent to J9043, 1 mg E
AHA: 4Q,23

J9065 Injection, cladribine, per 1 mg K K2 ☑ ⊘
Use this code for Leustatin.
CMS: 100-04,20,180; 100-04,32,411.3

J9070 ~~Cyclophosphamide, 100 mg~~
To report, see ~J9075

▲ **J9071** Injection, cyclophosphamide (AuroMedics), 5 mg G K2
AHA: 2Q,22

▲ **J9072** Injection, cyclophosphamide (Avyxa), 5 mg G
AHA: 1Q,24

● **J9073** Injection, cyclophosphamide (Ingenus), 5 mg K K2
Use this code for cyclophosphamide manufactured by Ingenus.
AHA: 2Q,24

● **J9074** Injection, cyclophosphamide (Sandoz), 5 mg E K2
Use this code for cyclophosphamide manufactured by Sandoz.
AHA: 2Q,24

● **J9075** Injection, cyclophosphamide, not otherwise specified, 5 mg K K2
AHA: 2Q,24

● **J9076** Injection, cyclophosphamide (Baxter), 5 mg

J9098 Injection, cytarabine liposome, 10 mg E ☑ ⊘
Use this code for Depocyt.

J9100 Injection, cytarabine, 100 mg N N1 ☑ ⊘
Use this code for Cytosar-U, Ara-C, Tarabin CFS.
CMS: 100-04,20,180; 100-04,32,411.3

J9118 Injection, calaspargase pegol-mknl, 10 units E
Use this code for Asparlas.
AHA: 4Q,19

J9119 Injection, cemiplimab-rwlc, 1 mg K K2
Use this code for Libtayo.
AHA: 4Q,19

J9120 Injection, dactinomycin, 0.5 mg K K2 ☑ ⊘
Use this code for Cosmegen.

J9130 Dacarbazine, 100 mg N N1 ☑ ⊘
Use this code for DTIC-Dome.

J9144 Injection, daratumumab, 10 mg and hyaluronidase-fihj K K2
Use this code for Darzalex Faspro.
AHA: 1Q,21

J9145 Injection, daratumumab, 10 mg K K2 ☑
Use this code for Darzalex.

J9150 Injection, daunorubicin, 10 mg K K2 ☑ ⊘
Use this code for Cerubidine.

J9151 Injection, daunorubicin citrate, liposomal formulation, 10 mg E ☑ ⊘
Use this code for Daunoxome.

J9153 Injection, liposomal, 1 mg daunorubicin and 2.27 mg cytarabine K K2
Use this code for Vyxeos.
AHA: 1Q,19; 4Q,18

J9155 Injection, degarelix, 1 mg K K2 ☑
CMS: 100-02,15,50.5

J9165 Injection, diethylstilbestrol diphosphate, 250 mg E ☑

J9171 Injection, docetaxel, 1 mg N N1 ☑ ⊘
Use this code for Taxotere.

▲ **J9172** Injection, docetaxel (Docivyx), 1 mg E K2
AHA: 1Q,24

J9173 Injection, durvalumab, 10 mg K K2
Use this code for Imfinzi.
AHA: 1Q,19; 4Q,18

J9175 Injection, Elliotts' B solution, 1 ml N N1 ☑

J9176 Injection, elotuzumab, 1 mg K K2 ☑
Use this code for Empliciti.

J9177 Injection, enfortumab vedotin-ejfv, 0.25 mg K K2
Use this code for PADCEV.
AHA: 2Q,20

J9178 Injection, epirubicin HCl, 2 mg N N1 ☑ ⊘
Use this code for Ellence.

J9179 Injection, eribulin mesylate, 0.1 mg K K2 ☑
Use this code for Halaven.

J9181 Injection, etoposide, 10 mg N N1 ☑ ⊘
Use this code for VePesid, Toposar.

J9185 Injection, fludarabine phosphate, 50 mg K K2 ☑ ⊘
Use this code for Fludara.

J9190 Injection, fluorouracil, 500 mg N N1 ☑
Use this code for Adrucil.
CMS: 100-04,20,180; 100-04,32,411.3

J9196 Injection, gemcitabine HCl (Accord), not therapeutically equivalent to J9201, 200 mg K K2
Use this code for gemcitabine HCl manufactured by Accord.
AHA: 2Q,23

J9198 Injection, gemcitabine HCl, (Infugem), 100 mg K K2
AHA: 2Q,20

J9200 Injection, floxuridine, 500 mg K K2 ☑ ⊘
Use this code for FUDR.
CMS: 100-04,20,180

J9201 Injection, gemcitabine HCl, not otherwise specified, 200 mg N N1 ☑ ⊘
Use this code for Gemzar.

J9202 Goserelin acetate implant, per 3.6 mg K K2 ☑
Use this code for Zoladex.

J9203 Injection, gemtuzumab ozogamicin, 0.1 mg K K2
Use this code for Mylotarg.

J9204 Injection, mogamulizumab-kpkc, 1 mg K K2
Use this code for Poteligeo.
AHA: 4Q,19

J9205 Injection, irinotecan liposome, 1 mg K K2 ☑
Use this code for Onivyde.

J9206 Injection, irinotecan, 20 mg N N1 ☑ ⊘
Use this code for Camptosar.
CMS: 100-03,110.17

J9207 Injection, ixabepilone, 1 mg K K2 ☑ ⊘
Use this code for IXEMPRA.

J9208 Injection, ifosfamide, 1 g N N1 ☑ ⊘
Use this code for IFEX, Mitoxana.

J9209 **Injection, mesna, 200 mg** N N1 ☑
Use this code for Mesnex.

J9210 **Injection, emapalumab-lzsg, 1 mg** K K2
Use this code for Gamifant.
AHA: 4Q,19

J9211 **Injection, idarubicin HCl, 5 mg** N N1 ☑ ⃠
Use this code for Idamycin.

J9212 **Injection, interferon alfacon-1, recombinant, 1 mcg** E1 ☑
Use this code for Infergen.

J9213 **Injection, interferon, alfa-2a, recombinant, 3 million units** E1 ☑
Use this code for Roferon-A.

J9214 **Injection, interferon, alfa-2b, recombinant, 1 million units** K K2 ☑
Use this code for Intron A, Rebetron Kit.
CMS: 100-02,15,50.5

J9215 **Injection, interferon, alfa-N3, (human leukocyte derived), 250,000 IU** E1 ☑
Use this code for Alferon N.

J9216 **Injection, interferon, gamma 1-b, 3 million units** E1 ☑
Use this code for Actimmune.
CMS: 100-02,15,50.5

J9217 **Leuprolide acetate (for depot suspension), 7.5 mg** K K2 ☑
Use this code for Lupron Depot, Eligard.
AHA: 2Q,19; 4Q,18

J9218 **Leuprolide acetate, per 1 mg** K K2 ☑
Use this code for Lupron.
CMS: 100-02,15,50.5
AHA: 2Q,19; 4Q,18

J9219 **Leuprolide acetate implant, 65 mg** E1 ☑
Use this code for Lupron Implant, Viadur.

J9223 **Injection, lurbinectedin, 0.1 mg** K K2
Use this code for Zepzelca.
AHA: 1Q,21

J9225 **Histrelin implant (Vantas), 50 mg** K K2 ☑ ⃠

J9226 **Histrelin implant (Supprelin LA), 50 mg** K K2 ☑

J9227 **Injection, isatuximab-irfc, 10 mg** K K2
Use this code for Sarclisa.
AHA: 4Q,20

J9228 **Injection, ipilimumab, 1 mg** K K2 ☑
Use this code for YERVOY.

J9229 **Injection, inotuzumab ozogamicin, 0.1 mg** K K2
Use this code for Besponsa.
AHA: 1Q,19; 4Q,18

J9230 **Injection, mechlorethamine HCl, (nitrogen mustard), 10 mg** N N1 ☑ ⃠
Use this code for Mustargen.

J9245 **Injection, melphalan HCl, not otherwise specified, 50 mg** K K2 ☑ ⃠
AHA: 2Q,20; 4Q,18

J9246 **Injection, melphalan (Evomela), 1 mg** K K2
AHA: 2Q,20

J9247 **Injection, melphalan flufenamide, 1 mg** G
Use this code for Pepaxto.
AHA: 4Q,21

● **J9248** **Injection, melphalan (Hepzato), 1 mg** G K2
AHA: 2Q,24

● **J9249** **Injection, melphalan (Apotex), 1 mg** E1
Use this code for melphalan manufactured by Apotex.
AHA: 2Q,24

J9250 ~~**Methotrexate sodium, 5 mg**~~
To report, see ~J9260

▲ **J9255** **Injection, methotrexate (Accord), not therapeutically equivalent to J9260, 50 mg** E1
AHA: 2Q,24; 1Q,24

J9258 ~~**Injection, paclitaxel protein-bound particles (Teva), not therapeutically equivalent to J9264, 1 mg**~~

J9259 ~~**Injection, paclitaxel protein-bound particles (American Regent), not therapeutically equivalent to J9264, 1 mg**~~

▲ **J9260** **Injection, methotrexate sodium, 50 mg** N N1 ☑
Use this code for Folex, Folex PFS, Methotrexate LPF.
AHA: 2Q,24; 4Q,18

J9261 **Injection, nelarabine, 50 mg** K K2 ☑ ⃠
Use this code for Arranon.

J9262 **Injection, omacetaxine mepesuccinate, 0.01 mg** K K2 ☑
Use this code for Synribo.
CMS: 100-02,15,50.5

J9263 **Injection, oxaliplatin, 0.5 mg** N N1 ☑ ⃠
Use this code for Eloxatin.

J9264 **Injection, paclitaxel protein-bound particles, 1 mg** K K2 ☑ ⃠
Use this code for Abraxane.

J9266 **Injection, pegaspargase, per single dose vial** K K2 ☑ ⃠
Use this code for Oncaspar.

J9267 **Injection, paclitaxel, 1 mg** N N1 ☑
Use this code for Taxol.

J9268 **Injection, pentostatin, 10 mg** K K2 ☑ ⃠
Use this code for Nipent.

J9269 **Injection, tagraxofusp-erzs, 10 mcg** K K2
Use this code for Elzonris.
AHA: 4Q,19

J9270 **Injection, plicamycin, 2.5 mg** E1 ☑ ⃠
Use this code for Mithracin.

J9271 **Injection, pembrolizumab, 1 mg** K K2 ☑
Use this code for Keytruda.

J9272 **Injection, dostarlimab-gxly, 10 mg** G K2
Use this code for Jemperli.
AHA: 1Q,22

J9273 **Injection, tisotumab vedotin-tftv, 1 mg** G K2
Use this code for Tivdak.
AHA: 2Q,22

J9274 **Injection, tebentafusp-tebn, 1 mcg** G K2
Use this code for Kimmtrak.
AHA: 4Q,22

J9280 **Injection, mitomycin, 5 mg** K K2 ☑ ⃠
Use this code for Mutamycin.

J9281 **Mitomycin pyelocalyceal instillation, 1 mg** K K2
Use this code for Jelmyto.
AHA: 1Q,21

J9285 **Injection, olaratumab, 10 mg** E1
Use this code for Lartruvo.

J9286 **Injection, glofitamab-gxbm, 2.5 mg** G K2
Use this code for Columvi.
AHA: 1Q,24

● **J9292** **Injection, pemetrexed (Avyxa), not therapeutically equivalent to J9305, 10 mg**

J9293 **Injection, mitoxantrone HCl, per 5 mg** K K2 ☑ ⊘
Use this code for Novantrone.

▲ **J9294** **Injection, pemetrexed (Hospira), not therapeutically equivalent to J9305, 10 mg** K K2
Use this code for pemetrexed manufactured by Hospira.
AHA: 2Q,23

J9295 **Injection, necitumumab, 1 mg** K K2 ☑
Use this code for Portrazza.

▲ **J9296** **Injection, pemetrexed (Accord), not therapeutically equivalent to J9305, 10 mg** K K2
Use this code for pemetrexed manufactured by Accord.
AHA: 2Q,23

J9297 **Injection, pemetrexed (Sandoz), not therapeutically equivalent to J9305, 10 mg** K K2
Use this code for pemetrexed manufactured by Sandoz.
AHA: 2Q,23

J9298 **Injection, nivolumab and relatlimab-rmbw, 3 mg/1 mg** G K2
Use this code for Opdualag.
AHA: 4Q,22

J9299 **Injection, nivolumab, 1 mg** K K2 ☑
Use this code for Opdivo.

J9301 **Injection, obinutuzumab, 10 mg** K K2 ☑
Use this code for Gazyva.

J9302 **Injection, ofatumumab, 10 mg** K K2 ☑
Use this code for Arzerra.

J9303 **Injection, panitumumab, 10 mg** K K2 ☑ ⊘
Use this code for Vectibix.

J9304 **Injection, pemetrexed (Pemfexy), 10 mg** G K2
AHA: 4Q,20

J9305 **Injection, pemetrexed, NOS, 10 mg** K K2 ☑ ⊘
AHA: 4Q,20; 4Q,18

J9306 **Injection, pertuzumab, 1 mg** K K2 ☑
Use this code for Perjeta.

J9307 **Injection, pralatrexate, 1 mg** K K2 ☑
Use this code for FOLOTYN.

J9308 **Injection, ramucirumab, 5 mg** K K2 ☑
Use this code for Cyramza.

J9309 **Injection, polatuzumab vedotin-piiq, 1 mg** K K2
Use this code for Polivy.

J9311 **Injection, rituximab 10 mg and hyaluronidase** K K2
Use this code for Rituxan Hycela.
AHA: 1Q,19; 4Q,18

J9312 **Injection, rituximab, 10 mg** K K2
Use this code for Rituxan.
AHA: 1Q,19; 4Q,18

J9313 **Injection, moxetumomab pasudotox-tdfk, 0.01 mg** K K2
Use this code for Lumoxiti.
AHA: 4Q,19

▲ **J9314** **Injection, pemetrexed (Teva), not therapeutically equivalent to J9305, 10 mg** K K2
Use this code for pemetrexed manufactured by Teva.
AHA: 2Q,23; 1Q,23

J9316 **Injection, pertuzumab, trastuzumab, and hyaluronidase-zzxf, per 10 mg** K K2
Use this code for PHESGO.
AHA: 1Q,21

J9317 **Injection, sacituzumab govitecan-hziy, 2.5 mg** K K2
Use this code for Trodelvy.
AHA: 1Q,21

J9318 **Injection, romidepsin, nonlyophilized, 0.1 mg** K K2
AHA: 4Q,21

J9319 **Injection, romidepsin, lyophilized, 0.1 mg** K K2
Use this code for Istodax.
AHA: 4Q,21

J9320 **Injection, streptozocin, 1 g** K K2 ☑ ⊘
Use this code for Zanosar.

J9321 **Injection, epcoritamab-bysp, 0.16 mg** G K2
Use this code for Epkinly.
AHA: 1Q,24

▲ **J9322** **Injection, pemetrexed (BluePoint), not therapeutically equivalent to J9305, 10 mg** E1
Use this code for pemetrexed manufactured by BluePoint.
AHA: 3Q,23

J9323 **Injection, pemetrexed ditromethamine, 10 mg** K K2
Use this code for pemetrexed manufactured by Hospira.
AHA: 3Q,23

J9324 **Injection, pemetrexed (Pemrydi RTU), 10 mg** E1 K2
AHA: 1Q,24

J9325 **Injection, talimogene laherparepvec, per 1 million plaque forming units** K K2 ☑
Use this code for Imlygic.
AHA: 2Q,19; 4Q,18

J9328 **Injection, temozolomide, 1 mg** K K2 ☑ ⊘
Use this code for Temodar.

● **J9329** **Injection, tislelizumab-jsgr, 1mg**
Use this code for Tevimbra.

J9330 **Injection, temsirolimus, 1 mg** K K2 ☑ ⊘
Use this code for TORISEL.

J9331 **Injection, sirolimus protein-bound particles, 1 mg** G K2
AHA: 3Q,22

J9332 **Injection, efgartigimod alfa-fcab, 2 mg** G K2
Use this code for Vyvgart.
AHA: 3Q,22

J9333 **Injection, rozanolixizumab-noli, 1 mg** G K2
Use this code for Rystiggo.
AHA: 1Q,24

J9334 **Injection, efgartigimod alfa, 2 mg and hyaluronidase-qvfc** K K2
Use this code for Vyvgart.
AHA: 1Q,24

J9340 **Injection, thiotepa, 15 mg** K K2 ☑ ⊘
Use this code for Thioplex.

J9345 **Injection, retifanlimab-dlwr, 1 mg** K K2
Use this code for Zynyz.
AHA: 4Q,23

J9347 **Injection, tremelimumab-actl, 1 mg** G K2
Use this code for Imjudo.
AHA: 3Q,23

J9348 **Injection, naxitamab-gqgk, 1 mg** G K2
AHA: 3Q,21

J9349 **Injection, tafasitamab-cxix, 2 mg** K K2
Use this code for Monjuvi.
AHA: 1Q,21

J9350 **Injection, mosunetuzumab-axgb, 1 mg** G K2
Use this code for Lunsumio.
AHA: 3Q,23

J9351 **Injection, topotecan, 0.1 mg** N N1 ☑
Use this code for Hycamtin.

J9352 **Injection, trabectedin, 0.1 mg** K K2 ☑
Use this code for Yondelis.

J9353 **Injection, margetuximab-cmkb, 5 mg** G K2
AHA: 3Q,21

J9354 **Injection, ado-trastuzumab emtansine, 1 mg** K K2 ☑
Use this code for Kadcyla.

J9355 **Injection, trastuzumab, excludes biosimilar, 10 mg** K K2 ☑ ⊘
Use this code for Herceptin.
AHA: 3Q,19; 4Q,18

J9356 **Injection, trastuzumab, 10 mg and hyaluronidase-oysk** K K2
Use this code for Herceptin Hylecta.
AHA: 3Q,19

J9357 **Injection, valrubicin, intravesical, 200 mg** K K2 ☑ ⊘
Use this code for Valstar.

J9358 **Injection, fam-trastuzumab deruxtecan-nxki, 1 mg** K K2
Use this code for Enhertu.
AHA: 2Q,20

J9359 **Injection, loncastuximab tesirine-lpyl, 0.075 mg** G K2
Use this code for Zylonta.
AHA: 2Q,22

J9360 **Injection, vinblastine sulfate, 1 mg** N N1 ☑ ⊘
Use this code for Velban.
CMS: 100-04,20,180; 100-04,32,411.3

● **J9361** **Injection, efbemalenograstim alfa-vuxw, 0.5 mg**
Use this code for Ryzneuta.
AHA: 3Q,24

J9370 **Vincristine sulfate, 1 mg** N N1 ☑ ⊘
Use this code for Oncovin, Vincasar PFS.
CMS: 100-04,20,180; 100-04,32,411.3

~~J9371~~ ~~**Injection, vincristine sulfate liposome, 1 mg**~~

● **J9376** **Injection, pozelimab-bbfg, 1 mg** E1
Use this code for Veopoz.
AHA: 2Q,24

J9380 **Injection, teclistamab-cqyv, 0.5 mg** G K2
Use this code for Tecvayli.
AHA: 3Q,23

J9381 **Injection, teplizumab-mzwv, 5 mcg** G K2
Use this code for Tzield.
AHA: 3Q,23

J9390 **Injection, vinorelbine tartrate, 10 mg** N N1 ☑ ⊘
Use this code for Navelbine.

▲ **J9393** **Injection, fulvestrant (Teva), not therapeutically equivalent to J9395, 25 mg** K K2
Use this code for fulvestrant manufactured by Teva.
AHA: 1Q,23

J9394 **Injection, fulvestrant (Fresenius Kabi) not therapeutically equivalent to J9395, 25 mg** K K2
Use this code for fulvestrant manufactured by Fresenius Kabi.
AHA: 1Q,23

J9395 **Injection, fulvestrant, 25 mg** K K2 ☑ ⊘
Use this code for Faslodex.

J9400 **Injection, ziv-aflibercept, 1 mg** K K2 ☑
Use this code for Zaltrap.

J9600 **Injection, porfimer sodium, 75 mg** K K2 ☑ ⊘
Use this code for Photofrin.
AHA: 1Q,20; 4Q,18

J9999 **Not otherwise classified, antineoplastic drugs** N N1 ☑
Determine if an alternative HCPCS Level II or a CPT code better describes the service being reported. This code should be used only if a more specific code is unavailable.
CMS: 100-02,15,50.5; 100-04,32,400; 100-04,32,400.1; 100-04,32,400.2; 100-04,32,400.2.1; 100-04,32,400.2.2; 100-04,32,400.2.3; 100-04,32,400.2.3.1; 100-04,32,400.2.4; 100-04,32,400.2.5; 100-04,32,400.3; 100-04,32,400.4; 100-04,32,411.3; 100-04,4,260.1; 100-04,4,260.1.1

Temporary Codes K0001-K1037

The K codes were established for use by the DME Medicare Administrative Contractors (DME MACs). The K codes are developed when the currently existing permanent national codes for supplies and certain product categories do not include the codes needed to implement a DME MAC medical review policy.

Wheelchairs and Accessories

K0001 Standard wheelchair Y (RR)

K0002 Standard hemi (low seat) wheelchair Y (RR)

K0003 Lightweight wheelchair Y (RR)

K0004 High strength, lightweight wheelchair Y (RR)

K0007 Extra heavy-duty wheelchair Y (RR)

K0008 Custom manual wheelchair/base Y

K0010 Standard-weight frame motorized/power wheelchair Y (RR)

K0011 Standard-weight frame motorized/power wheelchair with programmable control parameters for speed adjustment, tremor dampening, acceleration control and braking Y (RR)
CMS: 100-04,20,30.9

K0012 Lightweight portable motorized/power wheelchair Y (RR)

K0037 High mount flip-up footrest, each Y ☑ (NU, RR, UE)

K0038 Leg strap, each Y ☑ (NU, RR, UE)

K0039 Leg strap, H style, each Y ☑ (NU, RR, UE)

K0040 Adjustable angle footplate, each Y ☑ (NU, RR, UE)

K0041 Large size footplate, each Y ☑ (NU, RR, UE)

K0042 Standard size footplate, replacement only, each Y ☑ (NU, RR, UE)

K0043 Footrest, lower extension tube, replacement only, each Y ☑ (NU, RR, UE)

K0044 Footrest, upper hanger bracket, replacement only, each Y ☑ (NU, RR, UE)

K0045 Footrest, complete assembly, replacement only, each Y (NU, RR, UE)

K0046 Elevating legrest, lower extension tube, replacement only, each Y ☑ (NU, RR, UE)

K0047 Elevating legrest, upper hanger bracket, replacement only, each Y ☑ (NU, RR, UE)

K0050 Ratchet assembly, replacement only Y (NU, RR, UE)

K0051 Cam release assembly, footrest or legrest, replacement only, each Y ☑ (NU, RR, UE)

K0052 Swingaway, detachable footrests, replacement only, each Y ☑ (NU, RR, UE)

K0053 Elevating footrests, articulating (telescoping), each Y ☑ (NU, RR, UE)

K0056 Seat height less than 17 in or equal to or greater than 21 in for a high-strength, lightweight, or ultralightweight wheelchair Y ☑ (NU, RR, UE)

K0065 Spoke protectors, each Y ☑ (NU, RR, UE)

K0069 Rear wheel assembly, complete, with solid tire, spokes or molded, replacement only, each Y ☑ (NU, RR, UE)

K0070 Rear wheel assembly, complete, with pneumatic tire, spokes or molded, replacement only, each Y ☑ (RR)

K0071 Front caster assembly, complete, with pneumatic tire, replacement only, each Y ☑ (NU, RR, UE)

K0072 Front caster assembly, complete, with semi-pneumatic tire, replacement only, each Y ☑ (NU, RR, UE)

K0073 Caster pin lock, each Y ☑ (NU, RR, UE)

K0077 Front caster assembly, complete, with solid tire, replacement only, each Y ☑ (NU, RR, UE)

K0098 Drive belt for power wheelchair, replacement only Y (NU, RR, UE)

K0105 IV hanger, each Y ☑ (NU, RR, UE)

K0108 Wheelchair component or accessory, not otherwise specified Y

K0195 Elevating legrests, pair (for use with capped rental wheelchair base) Y (RR)

Equipment, Replacement, Repair, Rental

K0455 Infusion pump used for uninterrupted parenteral administration of medication, (e.g., epoprostenol or treprostinol) Y (RR)

K0462 Temporary replacement for patient-owned equipment being repaired, any type Y
CMS: 100-04,20,40.1

K0552 Supplies for external noninsulin drug infusion pump, syringe type cartridge, sterile, each Y ☑

K0601 Replacement battery for external infusion pump owned by patient, silver oxide, 1.5 volt, each Y ☑ (NU)

K0602 Replacement battery for external infusion pump owned by patient, silver oxide, 3 volt, each Y ☑ (NU)

K0603 Replacement battery for external infusion pump owned by patient, alkaline, 1.5 volt, each Y ☑ (NU)

K0604 Replacement battery for external infusion pump owned by patient, lithium, 3.6 volt, each Y ☑ (NU)

K0605 Replacement battery for external infusion pump owned by patient, lithium, 4.5 volt, each Y ☑ (NU)

K0606 Automatic external defibrillator, with integrated electrocardiogram analysis, garment type Y (RR)

K0607 Replacement battery for automated external defibrillator, garment type only, each Y ☑ (RR)

K0608 Replacement garment for use with automated external defibrillator, each Y ☑ (NU, RR, UE)

K0609 Replacement electrodes for use with automated external defibrillator, garment type only, each Y ☑ (KF)

K0669 Wheelchair accessory, wheelchair seat or back cushion, does not meet specific code criteria or no written coding verification from DME PDAC Y

K0672 Addition to lower extremity orthotic, removable soft interface, all components, replacement only, each A ☑

K0730 Controlled dose inhalation drug delivery system Y (RR)

K0733 Power wheelchair accessory, 12 to 24 amp hour sealed lead acid battery, each (e.g., gel cell, absorbed glassmat) Y (NU, RR, UE)

K0738 Portable gaseous oxygen system, rental; home compressor used to fill portable oxygen cylinders; includes portable containers, regulator, flowmeter, humidifier, cannula or mask, and tubing Y (RR)
CMS: 100-04,20,130.6

K0739 Repair or nonroutine service for durable medical equipment other than oxygen equipment requiring the skill of a technician, labor component, per 15 minutes Y ☑
CMS: 100-04,23,60.3

K0740 Repair or nonroutine service for oxygen equipment requiring the skill of a technician, labor component, per 15 minutes E1 ☑

K0743 Suction pump, home model, portable, for use on wounds Y

K0744 Absorptive wound dressing for use with suction pump, home model, portable, pad size 16 sq in or less A ☑

K0745 Absorptive wound dressing for use with suction pump, home model, portable, pad size more than 16 sq in but less than or equal to 48 sq in A ☑

K0746 Absorptive wound dressing for use with suction pump, home model, portable, pad size greater than 48 sq in A

Power Operated Vehicle and Accessories

K0800 Power operated vehicle, group 1 standard, patient weight capacity up to and including 300 pounds Y ♿ (NU, RR, UE)
CMS: 100-04,12,30.6.15.4

K0801 Power operated vehicle, group 1 heavy-duty, patient weight capacity 301 to 450 pounds Y ♿ (NU, RR, UE)
CMS: 100-04,12,30.6.15.4

K0802 Power operated vehicle, group 1 very heavy-duty, patient weight capacity 451 to 600 pounds Y ♿ (NU, RR, UE)
CMS: 100-04,12,30.6.15.4

K0806 Power operated vehicle, group 2 standard, patient weight capacity up to and including 300 pounds Y ♿ (NU, RR, UE)
CMS: 100-04,12,30.6.15.4

K0807 Power operated vehicle, group 2 heavy-duty, patient weight capacity 301 to 450 pounds Y ♿ (NU, RR, UE)
CMS: 100-04,12,30.6.15.4

K0808 Power operated vehicle, group 2 very heavy-duty, patient weight capacity 451 to 600 pounds Y ♿ (NU, RR, UE)
CMS: 100-04,12,30.6.15.4

K0812 Power operated vehicle, not otherwise classified Y
CMS: 100-04,12,30.6.15.4

Power Wheelchairs

K0813 Power wheelchair, group 1 standard, portable, sling/solid seat and back, patient weight capacity up to and including 300 pounds Y ♿ (RR)

K0814 Power wheelchair, group 1 standard, portable, captain's chair, patient weight capacity up to and including 300 pounds Y ♿ (RR)

K0815 Power wheelchair, group 1 standard, sling/solid seat and back, patient weight capacity up to and including 300 pounds Y ♿ (RR)

K0816 Power wheelchair, group 1 standard, captain's chair, patient weight capacity up to and including 300 pounds Y ♿ (RR)

K0820 Power wheelchair, group 2 standard, portable, sling/solid seat/back, patient weight capacity up to and including 300 pounds Y ♿ (RR)

K0821 Power wheelchair, group 2 standard, portable, captain's chair, patient weight capacity up to and including 300 pounds Y ♿ (RR)

K0822 Power wheelchair, group 2 standard, sling/solid seat/back, patient weight capacity up to and including 300 pounds Y ♿ (RR)

K0823 Power wheelchair, group 2 standard, captain's chair, patient weight capacity up to and including 300 pounds Y ♿ (RR)

K0824 Power wheelchair, group 2 heavy-duty, sling/solid seat/back, patient weight capacity 301 to 450 pounds Y ♿ (RR)

K0825 Power wheelchair, group 2 heavy-duty, captain's chair, patient weight capacity 301 to 450 pounds Y ♿ (RR)

K0826 Power wheelchair, group 2 very heavy-duty, sling/solid seat/back, patient weight capacity 451 to 600 pounds Y ♿ (RR)

K0827 Power wheelchair, group 2 very heavy-duty, captain's chair, patient weight capacity 451 to 600 pounds Y ♿ (RR)

K0828 Power wheelchair, group 2 extra heavy-duty, sling/solid seat/back, patient weight capacity 601 pounds or more Y ♿ (RR)

K0829 Power wheelchair, group 2 extra heavy-duty, captain's chair, patient weight 601 pounds or more Y ♿ (RR)

K0830 Power wheelchair, group 2 standard, seat elevator, sling/solid seat/back, patient weight capacity up to and including 300 pounds Y

K0831 Power wheelchair, group 2 standard, seat elevator, captain's chair, patient weight capacity up to and including 300 pounds Y

K0835 Power wheelchair, group 2 standard, single power option, sling/solid seat/back, patient weight capacity up to and including 300 pounds Y ♿ (RR)

K0836 Power wheelchair, group 2 standard, single power option, captain's chair, patient weight capacity up to and including 300 pounds Y ♿ (RR)

K0837 Power wheelchair, group 2 heavy-duty, single power option, sling/solid seat/back, patient weight capacity 301 to 450 pounds Y ♿ (RR)

K0838 Power wheelchair, group 2 heavy-duty, single power option, captain's chair, patient weight capacity 301 to 450 pounds Y ♿ (RR)

K0839 Power wheelchair, group 2 very heavy-duty, single power option sling/solid seat/back, patient weight capacity 451 to 600 pounds Y ♿ (RR)

K0840 Power wheelchair, group 2 extra heavy-duty, single power option, sling/solid seat/back, patient weight capacity 601 pounds or more Y ♿ (RR)

K0841 Power wheelchair, group 2 standard, multiple power option, sling/solid seat/back, patient weight capacity up to and including 300 pounds Y ♿ (RR)

K0842 Power wheelchair, group 2 standard, multiple power option, captain's chair, patient weight capacity up to and including 300 pounds Y ♿ (RR)

K0843 Power wheelchair, group 2 heavy-duty, multiple power option, sling/solid seat/back, patient weight capacity 301 to 450 pounds Y ♿ (RR)

K0848 Power wheelchair, group 3 standard, sling/solid seat/back, patient weight capacity up to and including 300 pounds Y ♿ (RR)
CMS: 100-04,20,30.9

K0849 Power wheelchair, group 3 standard, captain's chair, patient weight capacity up to and including 300 pounds Y ♿ (RR)
CMS: 100-04,20,30.9

K0850 Power wheelchair, group 3 heavy-duty, sling/solid seat/back, patient weight capacity 301 to 450 pounds Y ♿ (RR)
CMS: 100-04,20,30.9

K0851 Power wheelchair, group 3 heavy-duty, captain's chair, patient weight capacity 301 to 450 pounds Y ♿ (RR)
CMS: 100-04,20,30.9

K0852 Power wheelchair, group 3 very heavy-duty, sling/solid seat/back, patient weight capacity 451 to 600 pounds Y ♿ (RR)
CMS: 100-04,20,30.9

K0853 Power wheelchair, group 3 very heavy-duty, captain's chair, patient weight capacity 451 to 600 pounds Y ♿ (RR)
CMS: 100-04,20,30.9

K0854 Power wheelchair, group 3 extra heavy-duty, sling/solid seat/back, patient weight capacity 601 pounds or more Y ♿ (RR)
CMS: 100-04,20,30.9

K0855 Power wheelchair, group 3 extra heavy-duty, captain's chair, patient weight capacity 601 pounds or more Y ♿ (RR)
CMS: 100-04,20,30.9

K0856 Power wheelchair, group 3 standard, single power option, sling/solid seat/back, patient weight capacity up to and including 300 pounds Y ♿ (RR)
CMS: 100-04,20,30.9

K0857 Power wheelchair, group 3 standard, single power option, captain's chair, patient weight capacity up to and including 300 pounds Y ♿ (RR)
CMS: 100-04,20,30.9

K0858 Power wheelchair, group 3 heavy-duty, single power option, sling/solid seat/back, patient weight 301 to 450 pounds Y ♿ (RR)
CMS: 100-04,20,30.9

K0859 Power wheelchair, group 3 heavy-duty, single power option, captain's chair, patient weight capacity 301 to 450 pounds Y ♿ (RR)
CMS: 100-04,20,30.9

K0860 Power wheelchair, group 3 very heavy-duty, single power option, sling/solid seat/back, patient weight capacity 451 to 600 pounds Y ♿ (RR)
CMS: 100-04,20,30.9

K0861 Power wheelchair, group 3 standard, multiple power option, sling/solid seat/back, patient weight capacity up to and including 300 pounds Y ♿ (RR)
CMS: 100-04,20,30.9

K0862 Power wheelchair, group 3 heavy-duty, multiple power option, sling/solid seat/back, patient weight capacity 301 to 450 pounds Y ♿ (RR)
CMS: 100-04,20,30.9

K0863 Power wheelchair, group 3 very heavy-duty, multiple power option, sling/solid seat/back, patient weight capacity 451 to 600 pounds Y ♿ (RR)
CMS: 100-04,20,30.9

K0864 Power wheelchair, group 3 extra heavy-duty, multiple power option, sling/solid seat/back, patient weight capacity 601 pounds or more Y ♿ (RR)
CMS: 100-04,20,30.9

K0868 Power wheelchair, group 4 standard, sling/solid seat/back, patient weight capacity up to and including 300 pounds Y

K0869 Power wheelchair, group 4 standard, captain's chair, patient weight capacity up to and including 300 pounds Y

K0870 Power wheelchair, group 4 heavy-duty, sling/solid seat/back, patient weight capacity 301 to 450 pounds Y

K0871 Power wheelchair, group 4 very heavy-duty, sling/solid seat/back, patient weight capacity 451 to 600 pounds Y

K0877 Power wheelchair, group 4 standard, single power option, sling/solid seat/back, patient weight capacity up to and including 300 pounds Y

K0878 Power wheelchair, group 4 standard, single power option, captain's chair, patient weight capacity up to and including 300 pounds Y

K0879 Power wheelchair, group 4 heavy-duty, single power option, sling/solid seat/back, patient weight capacity 301 to 450 pounds Y

K0880 Power wheelchair, group 4 very heavy-duty, single power option, sling/solid seat/back, patient weight 451 to 600 pounds Y

K0884 Power wheelchair, group 4 standard, multiple power option, sling/solid seat/back, patient weight capacity up to and including 300 pounds Y

K0885 Power wheelchair, group 4 standard, multiple power option, captain's chair, patient weight capacity up to and including 300 pounds Y

K0886 Power wheelchair, group 4 heavy-duty, multiple power option, sling/solid seat/back, patient weight capacity 301 to 450 pounds Y

K0890 Power wheelchair, group 5 pediatric, single power option, sling/solid seat/back, patient weight capacity up to and including 125 pounds Y

K0891 Power wheelchair, group 5 pediatric, multiple power option, sling/solid seat/back, patient weight capacity up to and including 125 pounds Y

K0898 Power wheelchair, not otherwise classified Y

K0899 Power mobility device, not coded by DME PDAC or does not meet criteria Y
CMS: 100-04,12,30.6.15.4

Other DME

K0900 Customized durable medical equipment, other than wheelchair Y

K1004 Low frequency ultrasonic diathermy treatment device for home use Y
AHA: 4Q,23

K1007 Bilateral hip, knee, ankle, foot (HKAFO) device, powered, includes pelvic component, single or double upright(s), knee joints any type, with or without ankle joints any type, includes all components and accessories, motors, microprocessors, sensors Y

K1027 Oral device/appliance used to reduce upper airway collapsibility, without fixed mechanical hinge, custom fabricated, includes fitting and adjustment Y

K1030 External recharging system for battery (internal) for use with implanted cardiac contractility modulation generator, replacement only Y

K1034 Provision of COVID-19 test, nonprescription self-administered and self-collected use, FDA approved, authorized or cleared, one test count E1
AHA: 3Q,22

K1035 Molecular diagnostic test reader, nonprescription self-administered and self-collected use, FDA approved, authorized or cleared E1
AHA: 2Q,23

K1036 Supplies and accessories (e.g., transducer) for low frequency ultrasonic diathermy treatment device, per month E1
AHA: 4Q,23

● **K1037** Docking station for use with oral device/appliance used to reduce upper airway collapsibility E1

Orthotic Procedures and Devices L0112-L4631

L codes include orthotic and prosthetic procedures and devices, as well as scoliosis equipment, orthopedic shoes, and prosthetic implants.

Cervical

L0112 **Cranial cervical orthosis, congenital torticollis type, with or without soft interface material, adjustable range of motion joint, custom fabricated** A ♿

L0113 **Cranial cervical orthosis, torticollis type, with or without joint, with or without soft interface material, prefabricated, includes fitting and adjustment** A ♿

L0120 **Cervical, flexible, nonadjustable, prefabricated, off-the-shelf (foam collar)** A ♿

L0130 **Cervical, flexible, thermoplastic collar, molded to patient** A ♿

L0140 **Cervical, semi-rigid, adjustable (plastic collar)** A ♿

L0150 **Cervical, semi-rigid, adjustable molded chin cup (plastic collar with mandibular/occipital piece)** A ♿

L0160 **Cervical, semi-rigid, wire frame occipital/mandibular support, prefabricated, off-the-shelf** A ♿

L0170 **Cervical, collar, molded to patient model** A ♿

L0172 **Cervical, collar, semi-rigid thermoplastic foam, two piece, prefabricated, off-the-shelf** A ♿

L0174 **Cervical, collar, semi-rigid, thermoplastic foam, two piece with thoracic extension, prefabricated, off-the-shelf** A ♿

Multiple Post Collar

L0180 **Cervical, multiple post collar, occipital/mandibular supports, adjustable** A ♿

L0190 **Cervical, multiple post collar, occipital/mandibular supports, adjustable cervical bars (SOMI, Guilford, Taylor types)** A ♿

L0200 **Cervical, multiple post collar, occipital/mandibular supports, adjustable cervical bars, and thoracic extension** A ♿

Thoracic

L0220 **Thoracic, rib belt, custom fabricated** A ♿

L0450 **Thoracic-lumbar-sacral orthosis (TLSO), flexible, provides trunk support, upper thoracic region, produces intracavitary pressure to reduce load on the intervertebral disks with rigid stays or panel(s), includes shoulder straps and closures, prefabricated, off-the-shelf** A ♿

TLSO brace with adjustable straps and pads (L0450). The model at right and similar devices such as the Boston brace are molded polymer over foam and may be bivalve (front and back components)

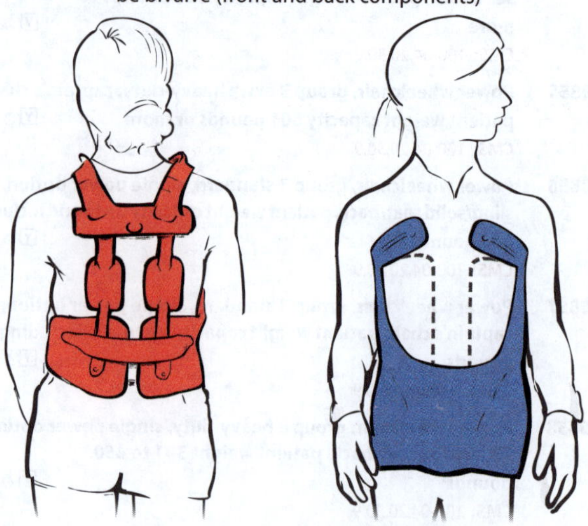

Thoracic lumbar sacral othosis (TLSO)

L0452 **Thoracic-lumbar-sacral orthosis (TLSO), flexible, provides trunk support, upper thoracic region, produces intracavitary pressure to reduce load on the intervertebral disks with rigid stays or panel(s), includes shoulder straps and closures, custom fabricated** A ♿

L0454 **Thoracic-lumbar-sacral orthosis (TLSO), flexible, provides trunk support, extends from sacrococcygeal junction to above T-9 vertebra, restricts gross trunk motion in the sagittal plane, produces intracavitary pressure to reduce load on the intervertebral disks with rigid stays or panel(s), includes shoulder straps and closures, prefabricated item that has been trimmed, bent, molded, assembled, or otherwise customized to fit a specific patient by an individual with expertise** A ♿

L0455 **Thoracic-lumbar-sacral orthosis (TLSO), flexible, provides trunk support, extends from sacrococcygeal junction to above T-9 vertebra, restricts gross trunk motion in the sagittal plane, produces intracavitary pressure to reduce load on the intervertebral disks with rigid stays or panel(s), includes shoulder straps and closures, prefabricated, off-the-shelf** A ♿

L0456 **Thoracic-lumbar-sacral orthosis (TLSO), flexible, provides trunk support, thoracic region, rigid posterior panel and soft anterior apron, extends from the sacrococcygeal junction and terminates just inferior to the scapular spine, restricts gross trunk motion in the sagittal plane, produces intracavitary pressure to reduce load on the intervertebral disks, includes straps and closures, prefabricated item that has been trimmed, bent, molded, assembled, or otherwise customized to fit a specific patient by an individual with expertise** A ♿

L0457 **Thoracic-lumbar-sacral orthosis (TLSO), flexible, provides trunk support, thoracic region, rigid posterior panel and soft anterior apron, extends from the sacrococcygeal junction and terminates just inferior to the scapular spine, restricts gross trunk motion in the sagittal plane, produces intracavitary pressure to reduce load on the intervertebral disks, includes straps and closures, prefabricated, off-the-shelf** A ♿

L0458 Thoracic-lumbar-sacral orthosis (TLSO), triplanar control, modular segmented spinal system, two rigid plastic shells, posterior extends from the sacrococcygeal junction and terminates just inferior to the scapular spine, anterior extends from the symphysis pubis to the xiphoid, soft liner, restricts gross trunk motion in the sagittal, coronal, and transverse planes, lateral strength is provided by overlapping plastic and stabilizing closures, includes straps and closures, prefabricated, includes fitting and adjustment A ♿

L0460 Thoracic-lumbar-sacral orthosis (TLSO), triplanar control, modular segmented spinal system, two rigid plastic shells, posterior extends from the sacrococcygeal junction and terminates just inferior to the scapular spine, anterior extends from the symphysis pubis to the sternal notch, soft liner, restricts gross trunk motion in the sagittal, coronal, and transverse planes, lateral strength is provided by overlapping plastic and stabilizing closures, includes straps and closures, prefabricated item that has been trimmed, bent, molded, assembled, or otherwise customized to fit a specific patient by an individual with expertise A ♿

L0462 Thoracic-lumbar-sacral orthosis (TLSO), triplanar control, modular segmented spinal system, three rigid plastic shells, posterior extends from the sacrococcygeal junction and terminates just inferior to the scapular spine, anterior extends from the symphysis pubis to the sternal notch, soft liner, restricts gross trunk motion in the sagittal, coronal, and transverse planes, lateral strength is provided by overlapping plastic and stabilizing closures, includes straps and closures, prefabricated, includes fitting and adjustment A ♿

L0464 Thoracic-lumbar-sacral orthosis (TLSO), triplanar control, modular segmented spinal system, four rigid plastic shells, posterior extends from sacrococcygeal junction and terminates just inferior to scapular spine, anterior extends from symphysis pubis to the sternal notch, soft liner, restricts gross trunk motion in sagittal, coronal, and transverse planes, lateral strength is provided by overlapping plastic and stabilizing closures, includes straps and closures, prefabricated, includes fitting and adjustment A ♿

L0466 Thoracic-lumbar-sacral orthosis (TLSO), sagittal control, rigid posterior frame and flexible soft anterior apron with straps, closures and padding, restricts gross trunk motion in sagittal plane, produces intracavitary pressure to reduce load on intervertebral disks, prefabricated item that has been trimmed, bent, molded, assembled, or otherwise customized to fit a specific patient by an individual with expertise A ♿

L0467 Thoracic-lumbar-sacral orthosis (TLSO), sagittal control, rigid posterior frame and flexible soft anterior apron with straps, closures and padding, restricts gross trunk motion in sagittal plane, produces intracavitary pressure to reduce load on intervertebral disks, prefabricated, off-the-shelf A ♿

L0468 Thoracic-lumbar-sacral orthosis (TLSO), sagittal-coronal control, rigid posterior frame and flexible soft anterior apron with straps, closures and padding, extends from sacrococcygeal junction over scapulae, lateral strength provided by pelvic, thoracic, and lateral frame pieces, restricts gross trunk motion in sagittal, and coronal planes, produces intracavitary pressure to reduce load on intervertebral disks, prefabricated item that has been trimmed, bent, molded, assembled, or otherwise customized to fit a specific patient by an individual with expertise A ♿

L0469 Thoracic-lumbar-sacral orthosis (TLSO), sagittal-coronal control, rigid posterior frame and flexible soft anterior apron with straps, closures and padding, extends from sacrococcygeal junction over scapulae, lateral strength provided by pelvic, thoracic, and lateral frame pieces, restricts gross trunk motion in sagittal and coronal planes, produces intracavitary pressure to reduce load on intervertebral disks, prefabricated, off-the-shelf A ♿

L0470 Thoracic-lumbar-sacral orthosis (TLSO), triplanar control, rigid posterior frame and flexible soft anterior apron with straps, closures and padding extends from sacrococcygeal junction to scapula, lateral strength provided by pelvic, thoracic, and lateral frame pieces, rotational strength provided by subclavicular extensions, restricts gross trunk motion in sagittal, coronal, and transverse planes, provides intracavitary pressure to reduce load on the intervertebral disks, includes fitting and shaping the frame, prefabricated, includes fitting and adjustment A ♿

L0472 Thoracic-lumbar-sacral orthosis (TLSO), triplanar control, hyperextension, rigid anterior and lateral frame extends from symphysis pubis to sternal notch with two anterior components (one pubic and one sternal), posterior and lateral pads with straps and closures, limits spinal flexion, restricts gross trunk motion in sagittal, coronal, and transverse planes, includes fitting and shaping the frame, prefabricated, includes fitting and adjustment A ♿

L0480 Thoracic-lumbar-sacral orthosis (TLSO), triplanar control, one-piece rigid plastic shell without interface liner, with multiple straps and closures, posterior extends from sacrococcygeal junction and terminates just inferior to scapular spine, anterior extends from symphysis pubis to sternal notch, anterior or posterior opening, restricts gross trunk motion in sagittal, coronal, and transverse planes, includes a carved plaster or CAD-CAM model, custom fabricated A ♿

L0482 Thoracic-lumbar-sacral orthosis (TLSO), triplanar control, one-piece rigid plastic shell with interface liner, multiple straps and closures, posterior extends from sacrococcygeal junction and terminates just inferior to scapular spine, anterior extends from symphysis pubis to sternal notch, anterior or posterior opening, restricts gross trunk motion in sagittal, coronal, and transverse planes, includes a carved plaster or CAD-CAM model, custom fabricated A ♿

L0484 Thoracic-lumbar-sacral orthosis (TLSO), triplanar control, two-piece rigid plastic shell without interface liner, with multiple straps and closures, posterior extends from sacrococcygeal junction and terminates just inferior to scapular spine, anterior extends from symphysis pubis to sternal notch, lateral strength is enhanced by overlapping plastic, restricts gross trunk motion in the sagittal, coronal, and transverse planes, includes a carved plaster or CAD-CAM model, custom fabricated A ♿

L0486 Thoracic-lumbar-sacral orthosis (TLSO), triplanar control, two-piece rigid plastic shell with interface liner, multiple straps and closures, posterior extends from sacrococcygeal junction and terminates just inferior to scapular spine, anterior extends from symphysis pubis to sternal notch, lateral strength is enhanced by overlapping plastic, restricts gross trunk motion in the sagittal, coronal, and transverse planes, includes a carved plaster or CAD-CAM model, custom fabricated A ♿

L0488 Thoracic-lumbar-sacral orthosis (TLSO), triplanar control, one-piece rigid plastic shell with interface liner, multiple straps and closures, posterior extends from sacrococcygeal junction and terminates just inferior to scapular spine, anterior extends from symphysis pubis to sternal notch, anterior or posterior opening, restricts gross trunk motion in sagittal, coronal, and transverse planes, prefabricated, includes fitting and adjustment A ♿

L0490 Thoracic-lumbar-sacral orthosis (TLSO), sagittal-coronal control, one-piece rigid plastic shell, with overlapping reinforced anterior, with multiple straps and closures, posterior extends from sacrococcygeal junction and terminates at or before the T-9 vertebra, anterior extends from symphysis pubis to xiphoid, anterior opening, restricts gross trunk motion in sagittal and coronal planes, prefabricated, includes fitting and adjustment A ♿

L0491 Thoracic-lumbar-sacral orthosis (TLSO), sagittal-coronal control, modular segmented spinal system, two rigid plastic shells, posterior extends from the sacrococcygeal junction and terminates just inferior to the scapular spine, anterior extends from the symphysis pubis to the xiphoid, soft liner, restricts gross trunk motion in the sagittal and coronal planes, lateral strength is provided by overlapping plastic and stabilizing closures, includes straps and closures, prefabricated, includes fitting and adjustment A

L0492 Thoracic-lumbar-sacral orthosis (TLSO), sagittal-coronal control, modular segmented spinal system, three rigid plastic shells, posterior extends from the sacrococcygeal junction and terminates just inferior to the scapular spine, anterior extends from the symphysis pubis to the xiphoid, soft liner, restricts gross trunk motion in the sagittal and coronal planes, lateral strength is provided by overlapping plastic and stabilizing closures, includes straps and closures, prefabricated, includes fitting and adjustment A

Cervical-Thoracic-Lumbar-Sacral Orthoses

L0621 Sacroiliac orthosis (SO), flexible, provides pelvic-sacral support, reduces motion about the sacroiliac joint, includes straps, closures, may include pendulous abdomen design, prefabricated, off-the-shelf A

L0622 Sacroiliac orthosis (SO), flexible, provides pelvic-sacral support, reduces motion about the sacroiliac joint, includes straps, closures, may include pendulous abdomen design, custom fabricated A

L0623 Sacroiliac orthosis (SO), provides pelvic-sacral support, with rigid or semi-rigid panels over the sacrum and abdomen, reduces motion about the sacroiliac joint, includes straps, closures, may include pendulous abdomen design, prefabricated, off-the-shelf A

L0624 Sacroiliac orthosis (SO), provides pelvic-sacral support, with rigid or semi-rigid panels placed over the sacrum and abdomen, reduces motion about the sacroiliac joint, includes straps, closures, may include pendulous abdomen design, custom fabricated A

L0625 Lumbar orthosis (LO), flexible, provides lumbar support, posterior extends from L-1 to below L-5 vertebra, produces intracavitary pressure to reduce load on the intervertebral discs, includes straps, closures, may include pendulous abdomen design, shoulder straps, stays, prefabricated, off-the-shelf A

L0626 Lumbar orthosis (LO), sagittal control, with rigid posterior panel(s), posterior extends from L-1 to below L-5 vertebra, produces intracavitary pressure to reduce load on the intervertebral discs, includes straps, closures, may include padding, stays, shoulder straps, pendulous abdomen design, prefabricated item that has been trimmed, bent, molded, assembled, or otherwise customized to fit a specific patient by an individual with expertise A

L0627 Lumbar orthosis (LO), sagittal control, with rigid anterior and posterior panels, posterior extends from L-1 to below L-5 vertebra, produces intracavitary pressure to reduce load on the intervertebral discs, includes straps, closures, may include padding, shoulder straps, pendulous abdomen design, prefabricated item that has been trimmed, bent, molded, assembled, or otherwise customized to fit a specific patient by an individual with expertise A

L0628 Lumbar-sacral orthosis (LSO), flexible, provides lumbo-sacral support, posterior extends from sacrococcygeal junction to T-9 vertebra, produces intracavitary pressure to reduce load on the intervertebral discs, includes straps, closures, may include stays, shoulder straps, pendulous abdomen design, prefabricated, off-the-shelf A

L0629 Lumbar-sacral orthosis (LSO), flexible, provides lumbo-sacral support, posterior extends from sacrococcygeal junction to T-9 vertebra, produces intracavitary pressure to reduce load on the intervertebral discs, includes straps, closures, may include stays, shoulder straps, pendulous abdomen design, custom fabricated A

L0630 Lumbar-sacral orthosis (LSO), sagittal control, with rigid posterior panel(s), posterior extends from sacrococcygeal junction to T-9 vertebra, produces intracavitary pressure to reduce load on the intervertebral discs, includes straps, closures, may include padding, stays, shoulder straps, pendulous abdomen design, prefabricated item that has been trimmed, bent, molded, assembled, or otherwise customized to fit a specific patient by an individual with expertise A

L0631 Lumbar-sacral orthosis (LSO), sagittal control, with rigid anterior and posterior panels, posterior extends from sacrococcygeal junction to T-9 vertebra, produces intracavitary pressure to reduce load on the intervertebral discs, includes straps, closures, may include padding, shoulder straps, pendulous abdomen design, prefabricated item that has been trimmed, bent, molded, assembled, or otherwise customized to fit a specific patient by an individual with expertise A

L0632 Lumbar-sacral orthosis (LSO), sagittal control, with rigid anterior and posterior panels, posterior extends from sacrococcygeal junction to T-9 vertebra, produces intracavitary pressure to reduce load on the intervertebral discs, includes straps, closures, may include padding, shoulder straps, pendulous abdomen design, custom fabricated A

L0633 Lumbar-sacral orthosis (LSO), sagittal-coronal control, with rigid posterior frame/panel(s), posterior extends from sacrococcygeal junction to T-9 vertebra, lateral strength provided by rigid lateral frame/panels, produces intracavitary pressure to reduce load on intervertebral discs, includes straps, closures, may include padding, stays, shoulder straps, pendulous abdomen design, prefabricated item that has been trimmed, bent, molded, assembled, or otherwise customized to fit a specific patient by an individual with expertise A

L0634 Lumbar-sacral orthosis (LSO), sagittal-coronal control, with rigid posterior frame/panel(s), posterior extends from sacrococcygeal junction to T-9 vertebra, lateral strength provided by rigid lateral frame/panel(s), produces intracavitary pressure to reduce load on intervertebral discs, includes straps, closures, may include padding, stays, shoulder straps, pendulous abdomen design, custom fabricated A

L0635 Lumbar-sacral orthosis (LSO), sagittal-coronal control, lumbar flexion, rigid posterior frame/panel(s), lateral articulating design to flex the lumbar spine, posterior extends from sacrococcygeal junction to T-9 vertebra, lateral strength provided by rigid lateral frame/panel(s), produces intracavitary pressure to reduce load on intervertebral discs, includes straps, closures, may include padding, anterior panel, pendulous abdomen design, prefabricated, includes fitting and adjustment A

L0636 Lumbar-sacral orthosis (LSO), sagittal-coronal control, lumbar flexion, rigid posterior frame/panels, lateral articulating design to flex the lumbar spine, posterior extends from sacrococcygeal junction to T-9 vertebra, lateral strength provided by rigid lateral frame/panels, produces intracavitary pressure to reduce load on intervertebral discs, includes straps, closures, may include padding, anterior panel, pendulous abdomen design, custom fabricated A

L0637 Lumbar-sacral orthosis (LSO), sagittal-coronal control, with rigid anterior and posterior frame/panels, posterior extends from sacrococcygeal junction to T-9 vertebra, lateral strength provided by rigid lateral frame/panels, produces intracavitary pressure to reduce load on intervertebral discs, includes straps, closures, may include padding, shoulder straps, pendulous abdomen design, prefabricated item that has been trimmed, bent, molded, assembled, or otherwise customized to fit a specific patient by an individual with expertise

L0638 Lumbar-sacral orthosis (LSO), sagittal-coronal control, with rigid anterior and posterior frame/panels, posterior extends from sacrococcygeal junction to T-9 vertebra, lateral strength provided by rigid lateral frame/panels, produces intracavitary pressure to reduce load on intervertebral discs, includes straps, closures, may include padding, shoulder straps, pendulous abdomen design, custom fabricated

L0639 Lumbar-sacral orthosis (LSO), sagittal-coronal control, rigid shell(s)/panel(s), posterior extends from sacrococcygeal junction to T-9 vertebra, anterior extends from symphysis pubis to xyphoid, produces intracavitary pressure to reduce load on the intervertebral discs, overall strength is provided by overlapping rigid material and stabilizing closures, includes straps, closures, may include soft interface, pendulous abdomen design, prefabricated item that has been trimmed, bent, molded, assembled, or otherwise customized to fit a specific patient by an individual with expertise

L0640 Lumbar-sacral orthosis (LSO), sagittal-coronal control, rigid shell(s)/panel(s), posterior extends from sacrococcygeal junction to T-9 vertebra, anterior extends from symphysis pubis to xyphoid, produces intracavitary pressure to reduce load on the intervertebral discs, overall strength is provided by overlapping rigid material and stabilizing closures, includes straps, closures, may include soft interface, pendulous abdomen design, custom fabricated

L0641 Lumbar orthosis (LO), sagittal control, with rigid posterior panel(s), posterior extends from L-1 to below L-5 vertebra, produces intracavitary pressure to reduce load on the intervertebral discs, includes straps, closures, may include padding, stays, shoulder straps, pendulous abdomen design, prefabricated, off-the-shelf

L0642 Lumbar orthosis (LO), sagittal control, with rigid anterior and posterior panels, posterior extends from L-1 to below L-5 vertebra, produces intracavitary pressure to reduce load on the intervertebral discs, includes straps, closures, may include padding, shoulder straps, pendulous abdomen design, prefabricated, off-the-shelf

L0643 Lumbar-sacral orthosis (LSO), sagittal control, with rigid posterior panel(s), posterior extends from sacrococcygeal junction to T-9 vertebra, produces intracavitary pressure to reduce load on the intervertebral discs, includes straps, closures, may include padding, stays, shoulder straps, pendulous abdomen design, prefabricated, off-the-shelf

L0648 Lumbar-sacral orthosis (LSO), sagittal control, with rigid anterior and posterior panels, posterior extends from sacrococcygeal junction to T-9 vertebra, produces intracavitary pressure to reduce load on the intervertebral discs, includes straps, closures, may include padding, shoulder straps, pendulous abdomen design, prefabricated, off-the-shelf

L0649 Lumbar-sacral orthosis (LSO), sagittal-coronal control, with rigid posterior frame/panel(s), posterior extends from sacrococcygeal junction to T-9 vertebra, lateral strength provided by rigid lateral frame/panels, produces intracavitary pressure to reduce load on intervertebral discs, includes straps, closures, may include padding, stays, shoulder straps, pendulous abdomen design, prefabricated, off-the-shelf

L0650 Lumbar-sacral orthosis (LSO), sagittal-coronal control, with rigid anterior and posterior frame/panel(s), posterior extends from sacrococcygeal junction to T-9 vertebra, lateral strength provided by rigid lateral frame/panel(s), produces intracavitary pressure to reduce load on intervertebral discs, includes straps, closures, may include padding, shoulder straps, pendulous abdomen design, prefabricated, off-the-shelf

L0651 Lumbar-sacral orthosis (LSO), sagittal-coronal control, rigid shell(s)/panel(s), posterior extends from sacrococcygeal junction to T-9 vertebra, anterior extends from symphysis pubis to xyphoid, produces intracavitary pressure to reduce load on the intervertebral discs, overall strength is provided by overlapping rigid material and stabilizing closures, includes straps, closures, may include soft interface, pendulous abdomen design, prefabricated, off-the-shelf

L0700 Cervical-thoracic-lumbar-sacral orthosis (CTLSO), anterior-posterior-lateral control, molded to patient model, (Minerva type)

L0710 Cervical-thoracic-lumbar-sacral orthosis (CTLSO), anterior-posterior-lateral control, molded to patient model, with interface material, (Minerva type)

Halo Procedure

L0810 Halo procedure, cervical halo incorporated into jacket vest

L0820 Halo procedure, cervical halo incorporated into plaster body jacket

L0830 Halo procedure, cervical halo incorporated into Milwaukee type orthotic

L0859 Addition to halo procedure, magnetic resonance image compatible systems, rings and pins, any material

L0861 Addition to halo procedure, replacement liner/interface material

Additions to Spinal Orthoses

L0970 Thoracic-lumbar-sacral orthosis (TLSO), corset front

L0972 Lumbar-sacral orthosis (LSO), corset front

L0974 Thoracic-lumbar-sacral orthosis (TLSO), full corset

L0976 Lumbar-sacral orthosis (LSO), full corset

L0978 Axillary crutch extension

L0980 Peroneal straps, prefabricated, off-the-shelf, pair

L0982 Stocking supporter grips, prefabricated, off-the-shelf, set of four (4)

L0984 Protective body sock, prefabricated, off-the-shelf, each

L0999 Addition to spinal orthosis, not otherwise specified

Determine if an alternative HCPCS Level II or a CPT code better describes the service being reported. This code should be used only if a more specific code is unavailable.

Orthotic Devices - Scoliosis Procedures

The orthotic care of scoliosis differs from other orthotic care in that the treatment is more dynamic in nature and uses continual modification of the orthosis to the patient's changing condition. This coding structure uses the proper names - or eponyms - of the procedures because they have historic and universal acceptance in the profession. It should be recognized that variations to the basic procedures described by the founders/developers are accepted in various medical and orthotic practices throughout the country. All procedures include model of patient when indicated.

L1000 Cervical-thoracic-lumbar-sacral orthosis (CTLSO) (Milwaukee), inclusive of furnishing initial orthotic, including model A ♿

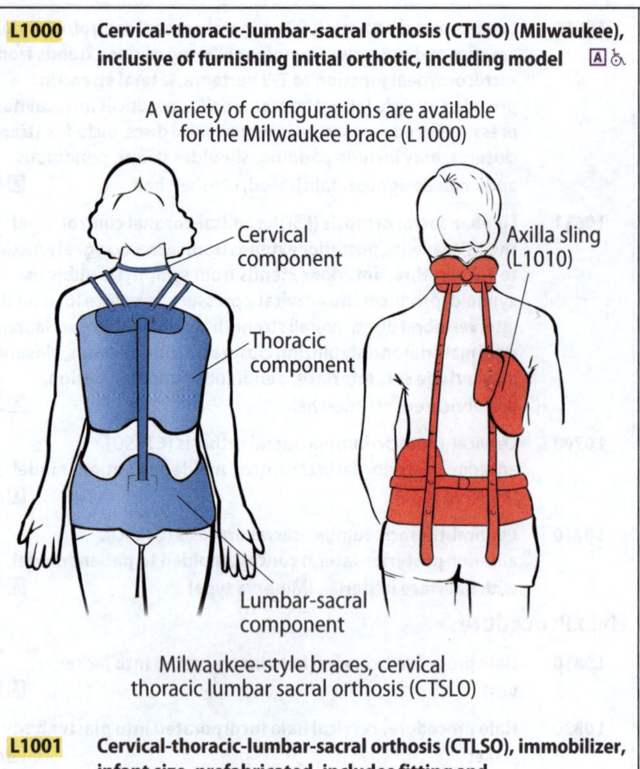

Milwaukee-style braces, cervical thoracic lumbar sacral orthosis (CTSLO)

L1001 Cervical-thoracic-lumbar-sacral orthosis (CTLSO), immobilizer, infant size, prefabricated, includes fitting and adjustment A A ♿

L1005 Tension based scoliosis orthosis and accessory pads, includes fitting and adjustment A ♿

● **L1006** Scoliosis orthosis (SO), sagittal-coronal control provided by a rigid lateral frame, extends from axilla to trochanter, includes all accessory pads, straps and interface, prefabricated item that has been trimmed, bent, molded, assembled, or otherwise customized to fit a specific patient by an individual with expertise

L1010 Addition to cervical-thoracic-lumbar-sacral orthosis (CTLSO) or scoliosis orthosis, axilla sling A ♿

L1020 Addition to cervical-thoracic-lumbar-sacral orthosis (CTLSO) or scoliosis orthosis, kyphosis pad A ♿

L1025 Addition to cervical-thoracic-lumbar-sacral orthosis (CTLSO) or scoliosis orthosis, kyphosis pad, floating A ♿

L1030 Addition to cervical-thoracic-lumbar-sacral orthosis (CTLSO) or scoliosis orthosis, lumbar bolster pad A ♿

L1040 Addition to cervical-thoracic-lumbar-sacral orthosis (CTLSO) or scoliosis orthosis, lumbar or lumbar rib pad A ♿

L1050 Addition to cervical-thoracic-lumbar-sacral orthosis (CTLSO) or scoliosis orthosis, sternal pad A ♿

L1060 Addition to cervical-thoracic-lumbar-sacral orthosis (CTLSO) or scoliosis orthosis, thoracic pad A ♿

L1070 Addition to cervical-thoracic-lumbar-sacral orthosis (CTLSO) or scoliosis orthosis, trapezius sling A ♿

L1080 Addition to cervical-thoracic-lumbar-sacral orthosis (CTLSO) or scoliosis orthosis, outrigger A ♿

L1085 Addition to cervical-thoracic-lumbar-sacral orthosis (CTLSO) or scoliosis orthosis, outrigger, bilateral with vertical extensions A ♿

L1090 Addition to cervical-thoracic-lumbar-sacral orthosis (CTLSO) or scoliosis orthosis, lumbar sling A ♿

L1100 Addition to cervical-thoracic-lumbar-sacral orthosis (CTLSO) or scoliosis orthosis, ring flange, plastic or leather A ♿

L1110 Addition to cervical-thoracic-lumbar-sacral orthosis (CTLSO) or scoliosis orthosis, ring flange, plastic or leather, molded to patient model A ♿

L1120 Addition to cervical-thoracic-lumbar-sacral orthosis (CTLSO), scoliosis orthosis, cover for upright, each A ☑ ♿

Thoracic-Lumbar-Sacral Orthosis (TLSO) (Low Profile)

L1200 Thoracic-lumbar-sacral orthosis (TLSO), inclusive of furnishing initial orthosis only A ♿

L1210 Addition to thoracic-lumbar-sacral orthosis (TLSO), (low profile), lateral thoracic extension A ♿

L1220 Addition to thoracic-lumbar-sacral orthosis (TLSO), (low profile), anterior thoracic extension A ♿

L1230 Addition to thoracic-lumbar-sacral orthosis (TLSO), (low profile), Milwaukee type superstructure A ♿

L1240 Addition to thoracic-lumbar-sacral orthosis (TLSO), (low profile), lumbar derotation pad A ♿

L1250 Addition to thoracic-lumbar-sacral orthosis (TLSO), (low profile), anterior ASIS pad A ♿

L1260 Addition to thoracic-lumbar-sacral orthosis (TLSO), (low profile), anterior thoracic derotation pad A ♿

L1270 Addition to thoracic-lumbar-sacral orthosis (TLSO), (low profile), abdominal pad A ♿
AHA: 2Q,19

L1280 Addition to thoracic-lumbar-sacral orthosis (TLSO), (low profile), rib gusset (elastic), each A ☑ ♿

L1290 Addition to thoracic-lumbar-sacral orthosis (TLSO), (low profile), lateral trochanteric pad A ♿

Other Scoliosis Procedures

L1300 Other scoliosis procedure, body jacket molded to patient model A ♿

L1310 Other scoliosis procedure, postoperative body jacket A ♿

● **L1320** Thoracic, pectus carinatum orthosis, sternal compression, rigid circumferential frame with anterior and posterior rigid pads, custom fabricated A

L1499 Spinal orthosis, not otherwise specified A
Determine if an alternative HCPCS Level II or a CPT code better describes the service being reported. This code should be used only if a more specific code is unavailable.

Hip Orthoses (HO) - Flexible

L1600 Hip orthosis (HO), abduction control of hip joints, flexible, Frejka type with cover, prefabricated item that has been trimmed, bent, molded, assembled, or otherwise customized to fit a specific patient by an individual with expertise A ♿

L1610 Hip orthosis (HO), abduction control of hip joints, flexible, (Frejka cover only), prefabricated item that has been trimmed, bent, molded, assembled, or otherwise customized to fit a specific patient by an individual with expertise A ♿

L1620 Hip orthosis (HO), abduction control of hip joints, flexible, (Pavlik harness), prefabricated item that has been trimmed, bent, molded, assembled, or otherwise customized to fit a specific patient by an individual with expertise A ♿

L1630 Hip orthosis (HO), abduction control of hip joints, semi-flexible (Von Rosen type), custom fabricated A ♿

L1640 Hip orthosis (HO), abduction control of hip joints, static, pelvic band or spreader bar, thigh cuffs, custom fabricated A ♿

L1650 Hip orthosis (HO), abduction control of hip joints, static, adjustable, (Ilfled type), prefabricated, includes fitting and adjustment A ♿

▲**L1652** Hip orthosis (HO), bilateral thigh cuffs with adjustable abductor spreader bar, adult size, prefabricated, includes fitting and adjustment, prefabricated item that has been trimmed, bent, molded, assembled, or otherwise customized to fit a specific patient by an individual with expertise A ♿

●**L1653** Hip orthosis (HO), bilateral thigh cuffs with adjustable abductor spreader bar, adult size, prefabricated, off the shelf

L1660 Hip orthosis (HO), abduction control of hip joints, static, plastic, prefabricated, includes fitting and adjustment A ♿

L1680 Hip orthosis (HO), abduction control of hip joints, dynamic, pelvic control, adjustable hip motion control, thigh cuffs (Rancho hip action type), custom fabricated A ♿

L1681 Hip orthosis (HO), bilateral hip joints and thigh cuffs, adjustable flexion, extension, abduction control of hip joint, postoperative hip abduction type, prefabricated item that has been trimmed, bent, molded, assembled, or otherwise customized to fit a specific patient by an individual with expertise A
AHA: 4Q,23

L1685 Hip orthosis (HO), abduction control of hip joint, postoperative hip abduction type, custom fabricated A ♿

L1686 Hip orthosis (HO), abduction control of hip joint, postoperative hip abduction type, prefabricated, includes fitting and adjustment A ♿

L1690 Combination, bilateral, lumbo-sacral, hip, femur orthosis providing adduction and internal rotation control, prefabricated, includes fitting and adjustment A ♿

Legg Perthes

L1700 Legg Perthes orthosis, (Toronto type), custom fabricated A ♿

L1710 Legg Perthes orthosis, (Newington type), custom fabricated A ♿

L1720 Legg Perthes orthosis, trilateral, (Tachdijan type), custom fabricated A ♿

L1730 Legg Perthes orthosis, (Scottish Rite type), custom fabricated A ♿

L1755 Legg Perthes orthosis, (Patten bottom type), custom fabricated A ♿

Knee Orthosis

L1810 Knee orthosis (KO), elastic with joints, prefabricated item that has been trimmed, bent, molded, assembled, or otherwise customized to fit a specific patient by an individual with expertise A ♿

L1812 Knee orthosis (KO), elastic with joints, prefabricated, off-the-shelf A ♿

▲**L1820** Knee orthosis (KO), elastic with condylar pads and joints, with or without patellar control, prefabricated item that has been trimmed, bent, molded, assembled, or otherwise customized to fit a specific patient by an individual with expertise A ♿

●**L1821** Knee orthosis (KO), elastic with condylar pads and joints, with or without patellar control, prefabricated, off the shelf

L1830 Knee orthosis (KO), immobilizer, canvas longitudinal, prefabricated, off-the-shelf A ♿

L1831 Knee orthosis (KO), locking knee joint(s), positional orthosis, prefabricated, includes fitting and adjustment A ♿

L1832 Knee orthosis (KO), adjustable knee joints (unicentric or polycentric), positional orthosis, rigid support, prefabricated item that has been trimmed, bent, molded, assembled, or otherwise customized to fit a specific patient by an individual with expertise A ♿

L1833 Knee orthosis (KO), adjustable knee joints (unicentric or polycentric), positional orthosis, rigid support, prefabricated, off-the shelf A ♿

L1834 Knee orthosis (KO), without knee joint, rigid, custom fabricated A ♿

L1836 Knee orthosis (KO), rigid, without joint(s), includes soft interface material, prefabricated, off-the-shelf A ♿

L1840 Knee orthosis (KO), derotation, medial-lateral, anterior cruciate ligament, custom fabricated A ♿

L1843 Knee orthosis (KO), single upright, thigh and calf, with adjustable flexion and extension joint (unicentric or polycentric), medial-lateral and rotation control, with or without varus/valgus adjustment, prefabricated item that has been trimmed, bent, molded, assembled, or otherwise customized to fit a specific patient by an individual with expertise A ♿

L1844 Knee orthosis (KO), single upright, thigh and calf, with adjustable flexion and extension joint (unicentric or polycentric), medial-lateral and rotation control, with or without varus/valgus adjustment, custom fabricated A ♿

L1845 Knee orthosis (KO), double upright, thigh and calf, with adjustable flexion and extension joint (unicentric or polycentric), medial-lateral and rotation control, with or without varus/valgus adjustment, prefabricated item that has been trimmed, bent, molded, assembled, or otherwise customized to fit a specific patient by an individual with expertise A ♿

L1846 Knee orthosis (KO), double upright, thigh and calf, with adjustable flexion and extension joint (unicentric or polycentric), medial-lateral and rotation control, with or without varus/valgus adjustment, custom fabricated A ♿

L1847 Knee orthosis (KO), double upright with adjustable joint, with inflatable air support chamber(s), prefabricated item that has been trimmed, bent, molded, assembled, or otherwise customized to fit a specific patient by an individual with expertise A ♿

L1848 Knee orthosis (KO), double upright with adjustable joint, with inflatable air support chamber(s), prefabricated, off-the-shelf A ♿

L1850 Knee orthosis (KO), Swedish type, prefabricated, off-the-shelf A ♿

L1851 Knee orthosis (KO), single upright, thigh and calf, with adjustable flexion and extension joint (unicentric or polycentric), medial-lateral and rotation control, with or without varus/valgus adjustment, prefabricated, off-the-shelf A ♿

L1852 Knee orthosis (KO), double upright, thigh and calf, with adjustable flexion and extension joint (unicentric or polycentric), medial-lateral and rotation control, with or without varus/valgus adjustment, prefabricated, off-the-shelf A ♿

L1860 Knee orthosis (KO), modification of supracondylar prosthetic socket, custom fabricated (SK) A ♿

Ankle-Foot Orthosis (AFO)

L1900 Ankle-foot orthosis (AFO), spring wire, dorsiflexion assist calf band, custom fabricated A ♿

L1902 Ankle orthosis (AO), ankle gauntlet or similar, with or without joints, prefabricated, off-the-shelf A ♿

L1904 Ankle orthosis (AO), ankle gauntlet or similar, with or without joints, custom fabricated A ♿

L1906 Ankle foot orthosis (AFO), multiligamentous ankle support, prefabricated, off-the-shelf A ♿

L1907 Ankle orthosis (AO), supramalleolar with straps, with or without interface/pads, custom fabricated A ♿

L1910 Ankle-foot orthosis (AFO), posterior, single bar, clasp attachment to shoe counter, prefabricated, includes fitting and adjustment A ♿

L1920 Ankle-foot orthosis (AFO), single upright with static or adjustable stop (Phelps or Perlstein type), custom fabricated A ♿

L1930 Ankle-foot orthosis (AFO), plastic or other material, prefabricated, includes fitting and adjustment A ♿

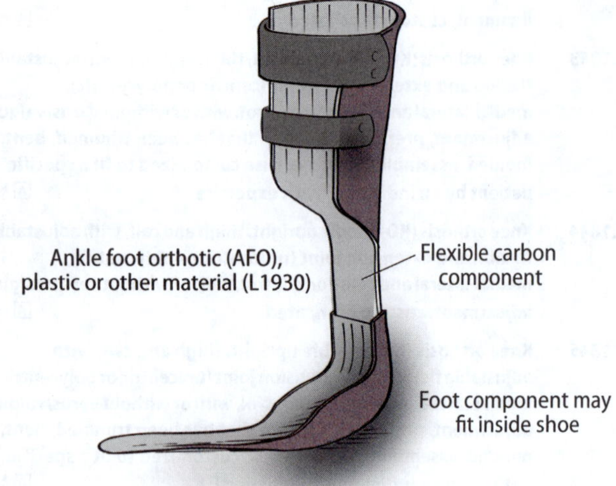

L1932 Ankle-foot orthosis (AFO), rigid anterior tibial section, total carbon fiber or equal material, prefabricated, includes fitting and adjustment A ♿

L1940 Ankle-foot orthosis (AFO), plastic or other material, custom fabricated A ♿

L1945 Ankle-foot orthosis (AFO), plastic, rigid anterior tibial section (floor reaction), custom fabricated A ♿

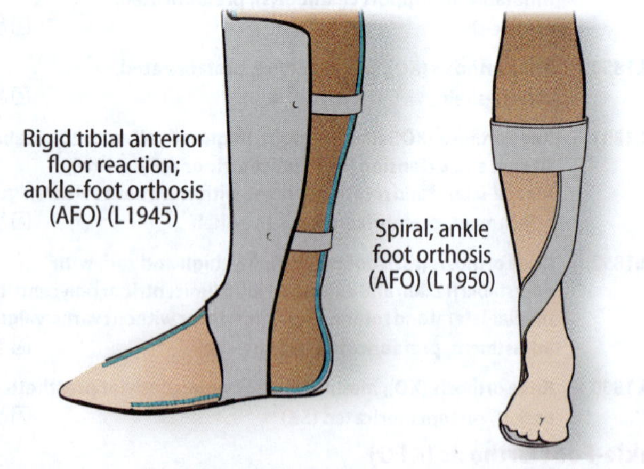

L1950 Ankle-foot orthosis (AFO), spiral, (Institute of Rehabilitative Medicine type), plastic, custom fabricated A ♿

L1951 Ankle-foot orthosis (AFO), spiral, (Institute of rehabilitative Medicine type), plastic or other material, prefabricated, includes fitting and adjustment A ♿

L1960 Ankle-foot orthosis (AFO), posterior solid ankle, plastic, custom fabricated A ♿

L1970 Ankle-foot orthosis (AFO), plastic with ankle joint, custom fabricated A ♿

L1971 Ankle-foot orthosis (AFO), plastic or other material with ankle joint, prefabricated, includes fitting and adjustment A ♿

L1980 Ankle-foot orthosis (AFO), single upright free plantar dorsiflexion, solid stirrup, calf band/cuff (single bar 'BK' orthosis), custom fabricated A ♿

L1990 Ankle-foot orthosis (AFO), double upright free plantar dorsiflexion, solid stirrup, calf band/cuff (double bar 'BK' orthosis), custom fabricated A ♿

Knee-Ankle-Foot Orthosis (KAFO) - Or Any Combination

L2000 Knee-ankle-foot orthosis (KAFO), single upright, free knee, free ankle, solid stirrup, thigh and calf bands/cuffs (single bar 'AK' orthosis), custom fabricated A ♿

L2005 Knee-ankle-foot orthosis (KAFO), any material, single or double upright, stance control, automatic lock and swing phase release, any type activation, includes ankle joint, any type, custom fabricated A ♿

L2006 Knee ankle foot device, any material, single or double upright, swing and stance phase microprocessor control with adjustability, includes all components (e.g., sensors, batteries, charger), any type activation, with or without ankle joint(s), custom fabricated A

L2010 Knee-ankle-foot orthosis (KAFO), single upright, free ankle, solid stirrup, thigh and calf bands/cuffs (single bar 'AK' orthosis), without knee joint, custom fabricated A ♿

L2020 Knee-ankle-foot orthosis (KAFO), double upright, free ankle, solid stirrup, thigh and calf bands/cuffs (double bar 'AK' orthosis), custom fabricated A ♿

L2030 Knee-ankle-foot orthosis (KAFO), double upright, free ankle, solid stirrup, thigh and calf bands/cuffs, (double bar 'AK' orthosis), without knee joint, custom fabricated A ♿

L2034 Knee-ankle-foot orthosis (KAFO), full plastic, single upright, with or without free motion knee, medial-lateral rotation control, with or without free motion ankle, custom fabricated A ♿

L2035 Knee-ankle-foot orthosis (KAFO), full plastic, static (pediatric size), without free motion ankle, prefabricated, includes fitting and adjustment A ♿

L2036 Knee-ankle-foot orthosis (KAFO), full plastic, double upright, with or without free motion knee, with or without free motion ankle, custom fabricated A ♿

L2037 Knee-ankle-foot orthosis (KAFO), full plastic, single upright, with or without free motion knee, with or without free motion ankle, custom fabricated A ♿

L2038 Knee-ankle-foot orthosis (KAFO), full plastic, with or without free motion knee, multi-axis ankle, custom fabricated A ♿

Torsion Control: Hip-Knee-Ankle-Foot Orthosis (HKAFO)

L2040 Hip-knee-ankle-foot orthosis (HKAFO), torsion control, bilateral rotation straps, pelvic band/belt, custom fabricated A ♿

L2050 Hip-knee-ankle-foot orthosis (HKAFO), torsion control, bilateral torsion cables, hip joint, pelvic band/belt, custom fabricated A ♿

L2060 Hip-knee-ankle-foot orthosis (HKAFO), torsion control, bilateral torsion cables, ball bearing hip joint, pelvic band/ belt, custom fabricated A ♿

L2070 Hip-knee-ankle-foot orthosis (HKAFO), torsion control, unilateral rotation straps, pelvic band/belt, custom fabricated A ♿

L2080 Hip-knee-ankle-foot orthosis (HKAFO), torsion control, unilateral torsion cable, hip joint, pelvic band/belt, custom fabricated

L2090 Hip-knee-ankle-foot orthosis (HKAFO), torsion control, unilateral torsion cable, ball bearing hip joint, pelvic band/ belt, custom fabricated

L2106 Ankle-foot orthosis (AFO), fracture orthosis, tibial fracture cast orthosis, thermoplastic type casting material, custom fabricated

L2108 Ankle-foot orthosis (AFO), fracture orthosis, tibial fracture cast orthosis, custom fabricated

L2112 Ankle-foot orthosis (AFO), fracture orthosis, tibial fracture orthosis, soft, prefabricated, includes fitting and adjustment

L2114 Ankle-foot orthosis (AFO), fracture orthosis, tibial fracture orthosis, semi-rigid, prefabricated, includes fitting and adjustment

L2116 Ankle-foot orthosis (AFO), fracture orthosis, tibial fracture orthosis, rigid, prefabricated, includes fitting and adjustment

L2126 Knee-ankle-foot orthosis (KAFO), fracture orthosis, femoral fracture cast orthosis, thermoplastic type casting material, custom fabricated

L2128 Knee-ankle-foot orthosis (KAFO), fracture orthosis, femoral fracture cast orthosis, custom fabricated

L2132 Knee-ankle-foot orthosis (KAFO), fracture orthosis, femoral fracture cast orthosis, soft, prefabricated, includes fitting and adjustment

L2134 Knee-ankle-foot orthosis (KAFO), fracture orthosis, femoral fracture cast orthosis, semi-rigid, prefabricated, includes fitting and adjustment

L2136 Knee-ankle-foot orthosis (KAFO), fracture orthosis, femoral fracture cast orthosis, rigid, prefabricated, includes fitting and adjustment

Additions to Fracture Orthosis

L2180 Addition to lower extremity fracture orthosis, plastic shoe insert with ankle joints

L2182 Addition to lower extremity fracture orthosis, drop lock knee joint

L2184 Addition to lower extremity fracture orthosis, limited motion knee joint

L2186 Addition to lower extremity fracture orthosis, adjustable motion knee joint, Lerman type

L2188 Addition to lower extremity fracture orthosis, quadrilateral brim

L2190 Addition to lower extremity fracture orthosis, waist belt

L2192 Addition to lower extremity fracture orthosis, hip joint, pelvic band, thigh flange, and pelvic belt

Additions to Lower Extremity Orthosis: Shoe-Ankle-Shin-Knee

L2200 Addition to lower extremity, limited ankle motion, each joint

L2210 Addition to lower extremity, dorsiflexion assist (plantar flexion resist), each joint

L2220 Addition to lower extremity, dorsiflexion and plantar flexion assist/resist, each joint

L2230 Addition to lower extremity, split flat caliper stirrups and plate attachment

L2232 Addition to lower extremity orthosis, rocker bottom for total contact ankle-foot orthosis (AFO), for custom fabricated orthosis only

L2240 Addition to lower extremity, round caliper and plate attachment

L2250 Addition to lower extremity, foot plate, molded to patient model, stirrup attachment

L2260 Addition to lower extremity, reinforced solid stirrup (Scott-Craig type)

L2265 Addition to lower extremity, long tongue stirrup

L2270 Addition to lower extremity, varus/valgus correction (T) strap, padded/lined or malleolus pad

L2275 Addition to lower extremity, varus/valgus correction, plastic modification, padded/lined

L2280 Addition to lower extremity, molded inner boot

L2300 Addition to lower extremity, abduction bar (bilateral hip involvement), jointed, adjustable

L2310 Addition to lower extremity, abduction bar, straight

L2320 Addition to lower extremity, nonmolded lacer, for custom fabricated orthosis only

L2330 Addition to lower extremity, lacer molded to patient model, for custom fabricated orthosis only

L2335 Addition to lower extremity, anterior swing band

L2340 Addition to lower extremity, pretibial shell, molded to patient model

L2350 Addition to lower extremity, prosthetic type, (BK) socket, molded to patient model, (used for PTB, AFO orthoses)

L2360 Addition to lower extremity, extended steel shank

L2370 Addition to lower extremity, Patten bottom

L2375 Addition to lower extremity, torsion control, ankle joint and half solid stirrup

L2380 Addition to lower extremity, torsion control, straight knee joint, each joint

L2385 Addition to lower extremity, straight knee joint, heavy-duty, each joint

L2387 Addition to lower extremity, polycentric knee joint, for custom fabricated knee-ankle-foot orthosis (KAFO), each joint

L2390 Addition to lower extremity, offset knee joint, each joint

L2395 Addition to lower extremity, offset knee joint, heavy-duty, each joint

L2397 Addition to lower extremity orthosis, suspension sleeve

Additions to Straight Knee or Offset Knee Joints

L2405 Addition to knee joint, drop lock, each

L2415 Addition to knee lock with integrated release mechanism (bail, cable, or equal), any material, each joint

L2425 Addition to knee joint, disc or dial lock for adjustable knee flexion, each joint

L2430 Addition to knee joint, ratchet lock for active and progressive knee extension, each joint

L2492 Addition to knee joint, lift loop for drop lock ring

Additions: Thigh/Weight Bearing - Gluteal/Ischial Weight Bearing

L2500 Addition to lower extremity, thigh/weight bearing, gluteal/ischial weight bearing, ring

L2510 Addition to lower extremity, thigh/weight bearing, quadri-lateral brim, molded to patient model

L2520 Addition to lower extremity, thigh/weight bearing, quadri-lateral brim, custom fitted

L2525 Addition to lower extremity, thigh/weight bearing, ischial containment/narrow M-L brim molded to patient model

L2526 Addition to lower extremity, thigh/weight bearing, ischial containment/narrow M-L brim, custom fitted

L2530 Addition to lower extremity, thigh/weight bearing, lacer, nonmolded

L2540 Addition to lower extremity, thigh/weight bearing, lacer, molded to patient model

L2550 Addition to lower extremity, thigh/weight bearing, high roll cuff

Additions: Pelvic and Thoracic Control

L2570 Addition to lower extremity, pelvic control, hip joint, Clevis type two-position joint, each

L2580 Addition to lower extremity, pelvic control, pelvic sling

L2600 Addition to lower extremity, pelvic control, hip joint, Clevis type, or thrust bearing, free, each

L2610 Addition to lower extremity, pelvic control, hip joint, Clevis or thrust bearing, lock, each

L2620 Addition to lower extremity, pelvic control, hip joint, heavy-duty, each

L2622 Addition to lower extremity, pelvic control, hip joint, adjustable flexion, each

L2624 Addition to lower extremity, pelvic control, hip joint, adjustable flexion, extension, abduction control, each

L2627 Addition to lower extremity, pelvic control, plastic, molded to patient model, reciprocating hip joint and cables

L2628 Addition to lower extremity, pelvic control, metal frame, reciprocating hip joint and cables

L2630 Addition to lower extremity, pelvic control, band and belt, unilateral

L2640 Addition to lower extremity, pelvic control, band and belt, bilateral

L2650 Addition to lower extremity, pelvic and thoracic control, gluteal pad, each

L2660 Addition to lower extremity, thoracic control, thoracic band

L2670 Addition to lower extremity, thoracic control, paraspinal uprights

L2680 Addition to lower extremity, thoracic control, lateral support uprights

Additions: General

L2750 Addition to lower extremity orthosis, plating chrome or nickel, per bar

L2755 Addition to lower extremity orthosis, high strength, lightweight material, all hybrid lamination/prepreg composite, per segment, for custom fabricated orthosis only

L2760 Addition to lower extremity orthosis, extension, per extension, per bar (for lineal adjustment for growth)

L2768 Orthotic side bar disconnect device, per bar

L2780 Addition to lower extremity orthosis, noncorrosive finish, per bar

L2785 Addition to lower extremity orthosis, drop lock retainer, each

L2795 Addition to lower extremity orthosis, knee control, full kneecap

L2800 Addition to lower extremity orthosis, knee control, knee cap, medial or lateral pull, for use with custom fabricated orthosis only

L2810 Addition to lower extremity orthosis, knee control, condylar pad

L2820 Addition to lower extremity orthosis, soft interface for molded plastic, below knee section

L2830 Addition to lower extremity orthosis, soft interface for molded plastic, above knee section

L2840 Addition to lower extremity orthosis, tibial length sock, fracture or equal, each

L2850 Addition to lower extremity orthosis, femoral length sock, fracture or equal, each

L2861 Addition to lower extremity joint, knee or ankle, concentric adjustable torsion style mechanism for custom fabricated orthotics only, each

L2999 Lower extremity orthoses, not otherwise specified

Determine if an alternative HCPCS Level II or a CPT code better describes the service being reported. This code should be used only if a more specific code is unavailable.

Orthopedic Footwear

Inserts

L3000 Foot insert, removable, molded to patient model, UCB type, Berkeley shell, each

L3001 Foot, insert, removable, molded to patient model, Spenco, each

L3002 Foot insert, removable, molded to patient model, Plastazote or equal, each

L3003 Foot insert, removable, molded to patient model, silicone gel, each

L3010 Foot insert, removable, molded to patient model, longitudinal arch support, each

L3020 Foot insert, removable, molded to patient model, longitudinal/metatarsal support, each

L3030 Foot insert, removable, formed to patient foot, each

L3031 Foot, insert/plate, removable, addition to lower extremity orthosis, high strength, lightweight material, all hybrid lamination/prepreg composite, each

Arch Support, Removable, Premolded

L3040 Foot, arch support, removable, premolded, longitudinal, each

L3050 Foot, arch support, removable, premolded, metatarsal, each

L3060 Foot, arch support, removable, premolded, longitudinal/metatarsal, each

Arch Support, Nonremovable, Attached to Shoe

L3070 Foot, arch support, nonremovable, attached to shoe, longitudinal, each

L3080 Foot, arch support, nonremovable, attached to shoe, metatarsal, each

L3090 Foot, arch support, nonremovable, attached to shoe, longitudinal/metatarsal, each

L3100 Hallus-valgus night dynamic splint, prefabricated, off-the-shelf

Abduction and Rotation Bars

L3140 Foot, abduction rotation bar, including shoes

A Denis-Browne style splint is a bar that can be applied by a strap or mounted on a shoe. This type of splint generally corrects congenital conditions such as genu varus

The angle may be adjusted on a plate on the sole of the shoe

Denis-Browne splint

L3150 Foot, abduction rotation bar, without shoes

L3160 Foot, adjustable shoe-styled positioning device

L3161 Foot, adductus positioning device, adjustable

L3170 Foot, plastic, silicone or equal, heel stabilizer, prefabricated, off-the-shelf, each

Orthopedic Shoes and Boots

L3201 Orthopedic shoe, Oxford with supinator or pronator, infant

L3202 Orthopedic shoe, Oxford with supinator or pronator, child

L3203 Orthopedic shoe, Oxford with supinator or pronator, junior

L3204 Orthopedic shoe, hightop with supinator or pronator, infant

L3206 Orthopedic shoe, hightop with supinator or pronator, child

L3207 Orthopedic shoe, hightop with supinator or pronator, junior

L3208 Surgical boot, each, infant

L3209 Surgical boot, each, child

L3211 Surgical boot, each, junior

L3212 Benesch boot, pair, infant

L3213 Benesch boot, pair, child

L3214 Benesch boot, pair, junior

L3215 Orthopedic footwear, ladies shoe, Oxford, each

L3216 Orthopedic footwear, ladies shoe, depth inlay, each

L3217 Orthopedic footwear, ladies shoe, hightop, depth inlay, each

L3219 Orthopedic footwear, mens shoe, Oxford, each

L3221 Orthopedic footwear, mens shoe, depth inlay, each

L3222 Orthopedic footwear, mens shoe, hightop, depth inlay, each

L3224 Orthopedic footwear, woman's shoe, Oxford, used as an integral part of a brace (orthosis)

L3225 Orthopedic footwear, man's shoe, Oxford, used as an integral part of a brace (orthosis)

L3230 Orthopedic footwear, custom shoe, depth inlay, each

L3250 Orthopedic footwear, custom molded shoe, removable inner mold, prosthetic shoe, each

L3251 Foot, shoe molded to patient model, silicone shoe, each

L3252 Foot, shoe molded to patient model, Plastazote (or similar), custom fabricated, each

L3253 Foot, molded shoe, Plastazote (or similar), custom fitted, each

L3254 Nonstandard size or width

L3255 Nonstandard size or length

L3257 Orthopedic footwear, additional charge for split size

L3260 Surgical boot/shoe, each

L3265 Plastazote sandal, each

Shoe Modification - Lifts

L3300 Lift, elevation, heel, tapered to metatarsals, per in

L3310 Lift, elevation, heel and sole, neoprene, per in

L3320 Lift, elevation, heel and sole, cork, per in

L3330 Lift, elevation, metal extension (skate)

L3332 Lift, elevation, inside shoe, tapered, up to one-half in

L3334 Lift, elevation, heel, per in

Shoe Modification - Wedges

L3340 Heel wedge, SACH

L3350 Heel wedge

L3360 Sole wedge, outside sole

L3370 Sole wedge, between sole

L3380 Clubfoot wedge

L3390 Outflare wedge

L3400 Metatarsal bar wedge, rocker

L3410 Metatarsal bar wedge, between sole

L3420 Full sole and heel wedge, between sole

Shoe Modifications - Heels

L3430 Heel, counter, plastic reinforced

L3440 Heel, counter, leather reinforced

L3450 Heel, SACH cushion type

L3455 Heel, new leather, standard

L3460 Heel, new rubber, standard

L3465 Heel, Thomas with wedge

L3470 Heel, Thomas extended to ball

L3480 Heel, pad and depression for spur

L3485 Heel, pad, removable for spur

Miscellaneous Shoe Additions

L3500 Orthopedic shoe addition, insole, leather

L3510 Orthopedic shoe addition, insole, rubber

L3520 Orthopedic shoe addition, insole, felt covered with leather

L3530 Orthopedic shoe addition, sole, half

L3540 Orthopedic shoe addition, sole, full

L3550 Orthopedic shoe addition, toe tap, standard

L3560 Orthopedic shoe addition, toe tap, horseshoe

L3570 Orthopedic shoe addition, special extension to instep (leather with eyelets)

L3580 Orthopedic shoe addition, convert instep to Velcro closure

L3590 Orthopedic shoe addition, convert firm shoe counter to soft counter

L3595 Orthopedic shoe addition, March bar

Transfer or Replacement

L3600 Transfer of an orthosis from one shoe to another, caliper plate, existing

L3610 Transfer of an orthosis from one shoe to another, caliper plate, new

L3620 Transfer of an orthosis from one shoe to another, solid stirrup, existing

L3630 Transfer of an orthosis from one shoe to another, solid stirrup, new

L3640 Transfer of an orthosis from one shoe to another, Dennis Browne splint (Riveton), both shoes

L3649 Orthopedic shoe, modification, addition or transfer, not otherwise specified

Determine if an alternative HCPCS Level II or a CPT code better describes the service being reported. This code should be used only if a more specific code is unavailable.

Shoulder Orthosis (SO)

L3650 Shoulder orthosis (SO), figure of eight design abduction restrainer, prefabricated, off-the-shelf

L3660 Shoulder orthosis (SO), figure of eight design abduction restrainer, canvas and webbing, prefabricated, off-the-shelf

L3670 Shoulder orthosis (SO), acromio/clavicular (canvas and webbing type), prefabricated, off-the-shelf

L3671 Shoulder orthosis (SO), shoulder joint design, without joints, may include soft interface, straps, custom fabricated, includes fitting and adjustment

L3674 Shoulder orthosis (SO), abduction positioning (airplane design), thoracic component and support bar, with or without nontorsion joint/turnbuckle, may include soft interface, straps, custom fabricated, includes fitting and adjustment

L3675 Shoulder orthosis (SO), vest type abduction restrainer, canvas webbing type or equal, prefabricated, off-the-shelf

L3677 Shoulder orthosis (SO), shoulder joint design, without joints, may include soft interface, straps, prefabricated item that has been trimmed, bent, molded, assembled, or otherwise customized to fit a specific patient by an individual with expertise

L3678 Shoulder orthosis (SO), shoulder joint design, without joints, may include soft interface, straps, prefabricated, off-the-shelf

Elbow Orthosis (EO)

L3702 Elbow orthosis (EO), without joints, may include soft interface, straps, custom fabricated, includes fitting and adjustment

L3710 Elbow orthosis (EO), elastic with metal joints, prefabricated, off-the-shelf

L3720 Elbow orthosis (EO), double upright with forearm/arm cuffs, free motion, custom fabricated

L3730 Elbow orthosis (EO), double upright with forearm/arm cuffs, extension/ flexion assist, custom fabricated

L3740 Elbow orthosis (EO), double upright with forearm/arm cuffs, adjustable position lock with active control, custom fabricated

L3760 Elbow orthosis (EO), with adjustable position locking joint(s), prefabricated, item that has been trimmed, bent, molded, assembled, or otherwise customized to fit a specific patient by an individual with expertise

L3761 Elbow orthosis (EO), with adjustable position locking joint(s), prefabricated, off-the-shelf

L3762 Elbow orthosis (EO), rigid, without joints, includes soft interface material, prefabricated, off-the-shelf

L3763 Elbow-wrist-hand orthosis (EWHO), rigid, without joints, may include soft interface, straps, custom fabricated, includes fitting and adjustment

L3764 Elbow-wrist-hand orthosis (EWHO), includes one or more nontorsion joints, elastic bands, turnbuckles, may include soft interface, straps, custom fabricated, includes fitting and adjustment

L3765 Elbow-wrist-hand-finger orthosis (EWHFO), rigid, without joints, may include soft interface, straps, custom fabricated, includes fitting and adjustment

L3766 Elbow-wrist-hand-finger orthosis (EWHFO), includes one or more nontorsion joints, elastic bands, turnbuckles, may include soft interface, straps, custom fabricated, includes fitting and adjustment

Wrist-Hand-Finger Orthosis (WHFO)

L3806 Wrist-hand-finger orthosis (WHFO), includes one or more nontorsion joint(s), turnbuckles, elastic bands/springs, may include soft interface material, straps, custom fabricated, includes fitting and adjustment

L3807 Wrist-hand-finger orthosis (WHFO), without joint(s), prefabricated item that has been trimmed, bent, molded, assembled, or otherwise customized to fit a specific patient by an individual with expertise

L3808 Wrist-hand-finger orthosis (WHFO), rigid without joints, may include soft interface material; straps, custom fabricated, includes fitting and adjustment

L3809 Wrist-hand-finger orthosis (WHFO), without joint(s), prefabricated, off-the-shelf, any type

Additions to Upper Extremity Orthosis

L3891 Addition to upper extremity joint, wrist or elbow, concentric adjustable torsion style mechanism for custom fabricated orthotics only, each

Dynamic Flexor Hinge, Reciprocal Wrist Extension/Flexion, Finger Flexion/Extension

L3900 Wrist-hand-finger orthosis (WHFO), dynamic flexor hinge, reciprocal wrist extension/ flexion, finger flexion/extension, wrist or finger driven, custom fabricated

L3901 Wrist-hand-finger orthosis (WHFO), dynamic flexor hinge, reciprocal wrist extension/ flexion, finger flexion/extension, cable driven, custom fabricated

External Power

L3904 Wrist-hand-finger orthosis (WHFO), external powered, electric, custom fabricated

Other Upper Extremity Orthoses

L3905 Wrist-hand orthosis (WHO), includes one or more nontorsion joints, elastic bands, turnbuckles, may include soft interface, straps, custom fabricated, includes fitting and adjustment

L3906 Wrist-hand orthosis (WHO), without joints, may include soft interface, straps, custom fabricated, includes fitting and adjustment

L3908 Wrist-hand orthosis (WHO), wrist extension control cock-up, nonmolded, prefabricated, off-the-shelf

L3912 Hand-finger orthosis (HFO), flexion glove with elastic finger control, prefabricated, off-the-shelf

L3913 Hand-finger orthosis (HFO), without joints, may include soft interface, straps, custom fabricated, includes fitting and adjustment

L3915 Wrist-hand orthosis (WHO), includes one or more nontorsion joint(s), elastic bands, turnbuckles, may include soft interface, straps, prefabricated item that has been trimmed, bent, molded, assembled, or otherwise customized to fit a specific patient by an individual with expertise

L3916 Wrist-hand orthosis (WHO), includes one or more nontorsion joint(s), elastic bands, turnbuckles, may include soft interface, straps, prefabricated, off-the-shelf

L3917 Hand orthosis (HO), metacarpal fracture orthosis, prefabricated item that has been trimmed, bent, molded, assembled, or otherwise customized to fit a specific patient by an individual with expertise

L3918 Hand orthosis (HO), metacarpal fracture orthosis, prefabricated, off-the-shelf

L3919 Hand orthosis (HO), without joints, may include soft interface, straps, custom fabricated, includes fitting and adjustment

L3921 Hand-finger orthosis (HFO), includes one or more nontorsion joints, elastic bands, turnbuckles, may include soft interface, straps, custom fabricated, includes fitting and adjustment

L3923 Hand-finger orthosis (HFO), without joints, may include soft interface, straps, prefabricated item that has been trimmed, bent, molded, assembled, or otherwise customized to fit a specific patient by an individual with expertise

L3924 Hand-finger orthosis (HFO), without joints, may include soft interface, straps, prefabricated, off-the-shelf

L3925 Finger orthosis (FO), proximal interphalangeal (PIP)/distal interphalangeal (DIP), nontorsion joint/spring, extension/flexion, may include soft interface material, prefabricated, off-the-shelf

L3927 Finger orthosis (FO), proximal interphalangeal (PIP)/distal interphalangeal (DIP), without joint/spring, extension/flexion (e.g., static or ring type), may include soft interface material, prefabricated, off-the-shelf

L3929 Hand-finger orthosis (HFO), includes one or more nontorsion joint(s), turnbuckles, elastic bands/springs, may include soft interface material, straps, prefabricated item that has been trimmed, bent, molded, assembled, or otherwise customized to fit a specific patient by an individual with expertise

L3930 Hand-finger orthosis (HFO), includes one or more nontorsion joint(s), turnbuckles, elastic bands/springs, may include soft interface material, straps, prefabricated, off-the-shelf

L3931 Wrist-hand-finger orthosis (WHFO), includes one or more nontorsion joint(s), turnbuckles, elastic bands/springs, may include soft interface material, straps, prefabricated, includes fitting and adjustment

L3933 Finger orthosis (FO); without joints, may include soft interface, custom fabricated, includes fitting and adjustment

L3935 Finger orthosis (FO), nontorsion joint, may include soft interface, custom fabricated, includes fitting and adjustment

L3956 Addition of joint to upper extremity orthosis, any material; per joint

Shoulder, Elbow, Wrist, Hand Orthosis

L3960 Shoulder-elbow-wrist-hand orthosis (SEWHO), abduction positioning, airplane design, prefabricated, includes fitting and adjustment

L3961 Shoulder-elbow-wrist-hand orthosis (SEWHO), shoulder cap design, without joints, may include soft interface, straps, custom fabricated, includes fitting and adjustment

L3962 Shoulder-elbow-wrist-hand orthosis (SEWHO), abduction positioning, Erb's palsy design, prefabricated, includes fitting and adjustment

L3967 Shoulder-elbow-wrist-hand orthosis (SEWHO), abduction positioning (airplane design), thoracic component and support bar, without joints, may include soft interface, straps, custom fabricated, includes fitting and adjustment

Additions to Mobile Arm Supports

L3971 Shoulder-elbow-wrist-hand orthotic (SEWHO), shoulder cap design, includes one or more nontorsion joints, elastic bands, turnbuckles, may include soft interface, straps, custom fabricated, includes fitting and adjustment

L3973 Shoulder-elbow-wrist-hand orthosis (SEWHO), abduction positioning (airplane design), thoracic component and support bar, includes one or more nontorsion joints, elastic bands, turnbuckles, may include soft interface, straps, custom fabricated, includes fitting and adjustment

L3975 Shoulder-elbow-wrist-hand-finger orthosis (SEWHO), shoulder cap design, without joints, may include soft interface, straps, custom fabricated, includes fitting and adjustment

L3976 Shoulder-elbow-wrist-hand-finger orthosis (SEWHO), abduction positioning (airplane design), thoracic component and support bar, without joints, may include soft interface, straps, custom fabricated, includes fitting and adjustment

L3977 Shoulder-elbow-wrist-hand-finger orthosis (SEWHO), shoulder cap design, includes one or more nontorsion joints, elastic bands, turnbuckles, may include soft interface, straps, custom fabricated, includes fitting and adjustment

L3978 Shoulder-elbow-wrist-hand-finger orthosis (SEWHO), abduction positioning (airplane design), thoracic component and support bar, includes one or more nontorsion joints, elastic bands, turnbuckles, may include soft interface, straps, custom fabricated, includes fitting and adjustment

Fracture Orthotic

L3980 Upper extremity fracture orthosis, humeral, prefabricated, includes fitting and adjustment

L3981 Upper extremity fracture orthosis, humeral, prefabricated, includes shoulder cap design, with or without joints, forearm section, may include soft interface, straps, includes fitting and adjustments

L3982 Upper extremity fracture orthosis, radius/ulnar, prefabricated, includes fitting and adjustment

L3984 Upper extremity fracture orthosis, wrist, prefabricated, includes fitting and adjustment

L3995 Addition to upper extremity orthosis, sock, fracture or equal, each

L3999 Upper limb orthosis, not otherwise specified

Repairs

L4000 Replace girdle for spinal orthosis (cervical-thoracic-lumbar-sacral orthosis (CTLSO) or spinal orthosis SO)

L4002 Replacement strap, any orthosis, includes all components, any length, any type

L4010 Replace trilateral socket brim

L4020 Replace quadrilateral socket brim, molded to patient model

L4030 Replace quadrilateral socket brim, custom fitted

L4040 Replace molded thigh lacer, for custom fabricated orthosis only

L4045 Replace nonmolded thigh lacer, for custom fabricated orthosis only

L4050 Replace molded calf lacer, for custom fabricated orthosis only

L4055 Replace nonmolded calf lacer, for custom fabricated orthosis only

L4060 Replace high roll cuff

L4070 Replace proximal and distal upright for KAFO

L4080 Replace metal bands KAFO, proximal thigh

L4090 Replace metal bands KAFO-AFO, calf or distal thigh

L4100 Replace leather cuff KAFO, proximal thigh

L4110 Replace leather cuff KAFO-AFO, calf or distal thigh

L4130 Replace pretibial shell

L4205 Repair of orthotic device, labor component, per 15 minutes

CMS: 100-04,23,60.3

L4210 Repair of orthotic device, repair or replace minor parts

Miscellaneous Lower Limb Supports

L4350 Ankle control orthosis, stirrup style, rigid, includes any type interface (e.g., pneumatic, gel), prefabricated, off-the-shelf

L4360 Walking boot, pneumatic and/or vacuum, with or without joints, with or without interface material, prefabricated item that has been trimmed, bent, molded, assembled, or otherwise customized to fit a specific patient by an individual with expertise

L4361 Walking boot, pneumatic and/or vacuum, with or without joints, with or without interface material, prefabricated, off-the-shelf

L4370 Pneumatic full leg splint, prefabricated, off-the-shelf

L4386 Walking boot, nonpneumatic, with or without joints, with or without interface material, prefabricated item that has been trimmed, bent, molded, assembled, or otherwise customized to fit a specific patient by an individual with expertise

L4387 Walking boot, nonpneumatic, with or without joints, with or without interface material, prefabricated, off-the-shelf

L4392 Replacement, soft interface material, static AFO

L4394 Replace soft interface material, foot drop splint

L4396 Static or dynamic ankle foot orthosis, including soft interface material, adjustable for fit, for positioning, may be used for minimal ambulation, prefabricated item that has been trimmed, bent, molded, assembled, or otherwise customized to fit a specific patient by an individual with expertise

L4397 Static or dynamic ankle foot orthosis, including soft interface material, adjustable for fit, for positioning, may be used for minimal ambulation, prefabricated, off-the-shelf

L4398 Foot drop splint, recumbent positioning device, prefabricated, off-the-shelf

L4631 Ankle-foot orthosis (AFO), walking boot type, varus/valgus correction, rocker bottom, anterior tibial shell, soft interface, custom arch support, plastic or other material, includes straps and closures, custom fabricated

Prosthetic Procedures L5000-L9900

The codes in this section are considered as "base" or "basic procedures or prosthetics" and may be modified by listing items/procedures or special materials from the "additions" sections and adding them to the base procedure.

Partial Foot

L5000 Partial foot, shoe insert with longitudinal arch, toe filler

L5010 Partial foot, molded socket, ankle height, with toe filler

L5020 Partial foot, molded socket, tibial tubercle height, with toe filler

Ankle

L5050 Ankle, Symes, molded socket, SACH foot

L5060 Ankle, Symes, metal frame, molded leather socket, articulated ankle/foot (SACH)

Below Knee

L5100 Below knee (BK), molded socket, shin, SACH foot

L5105 Below knee (BK), plastic socket, joints and thigh lacer, SACH foot

Knee Disarticulation

L5150 Knee disarticulation (or through knee), molded socket, external knee joints, shin, SACH foot

L5160 Knee disarticulation (or through knee), molded socket, bent knee configuration, external knee joints, shin, SACH foot

Above Knee

L5200 Above knee (AK), molded socket, single axis constant friction knee, shin, SACH foot

L5210 Above knee (AK), short prosthesis, no knee joint (stubbies), with foot blocks, no ankle joints, each

L5220 Above knee (AK), short prosthesis, no knee joint (stubbies), with articulated ankle/foot, dynamically aligned, each

L5230 Above knee (AK), for proximal femoral focal deficiency, constant friction knee, shin, SACH foot

Hip Disarticulation

L5250 Hip disarticulation, Canadian type; molded socket, hip joint, single axis constant friction knee, shin, SACH foot

L5270 Hip disarticulation, tilt table type; molded socket, locking hip joint, single axis constant friction knee, shin, SACH foot

Hemipelvectomy

L5280 Hemipelvectomy, Canadian type; molded socket, hip joint, single axis constant friction knee, shin, SACH foot

L5301 Below knee (BK), molded socket, shin, SACH foot, endoskeletal system

L5312 Knee disarticulation (or through knee), molded socket, single axis knee, pylon, SACH foot, endoskeletal system

L5321 Above knee (AK), molded socket, open end, SACH foot, endoskeletal system, single axis knee

L5331 Hip disarticulation, Canadian type, molded socket, endoskeletal system, hip joint, single axis knee, SACH foot

L5341 Hemipelvectomy, Canadian type, molded socket, endoskeletal system, hip joint, single axis knee, SACH foot

Immediate Postsurgical or Early Fitting Procedures

L5400 Immediate postsurgical or early fitting, application of initial rigid dressing, including fitting, alignment, suspension, and one cast change, below knee (BK)

Above-the-knee test socket

Below-the-knee early fitting rigid dressing (L5400)

Test sockets are often made of clear plastic so the prosthetist can visualize the fit against the residual limb

L5410 Immediate postsurgical or early fitting, application of initial rigid dressing, including fitting, alignment and suspension, below knee (BK), each additional cast change and realignment

L5420 Immediate postsurgical or early fitting, application of initial rigid dressing, including fitting, alignment and suspension and one cast change above knee (AK) or knee disarticulation

L5430 Immediate postsurgical or early fitting, application of initial rigid dressing, including fitting, alignment and suspension, above knee (AK) or knee disarticulation, each additional cast change and realignment

L5450 Immediate postsurgical or early fitting, application of nonweight bearing rigid dressing, below knee (BK)

L5460 Immediate postsurgical or early fitting, application of nonweight bearing rigid dressing, above knee (AK)

Initial Prosthesis

L5500 Initial, below knee (BK) PTB type socket, nonalignable system, pylon, no cover, SACH foot, plaster socket, direct formed

L5505 Initial, above knee (AK), knee disarticulation, ischial level socket, nonalignable system, pylon, no cover, SACH foot, plaster socket, direct formed

Preparatory Prosthesis

L5510 Preparatory, below knee (BK) PTB type socket, nonalignable system, pylon, no cover, SACH foot, plaster socket, molded to model

L5520 Preparatory, below knee (BK) PTB type socket, nonalignable system, pylon, no cover, SACH foot, thermoplastic or equal, direct formed

L5530 Preparatory, below knee (BK) PTB type socket, nonalignable system, pylon, no cover, SACH foot, thermoplastic or equal, molded to model

L5535 Preparatory, below knee (BK) PTB type socket, nonalignable system, no cover, SACH foot, prefabricated, adjustable open end socket

L5540 Preparatory, below knee (BK) PTB type socket, nonalignable system, pylon, no cover, SACH foot, laminated socket, molded to model

L5560 Preparatory, above knee (AK), knee disarticulation, ischial level socket, nonalignable system, pylon, no cover, SACH foot, plaster socket, molded to model

L5570 Preparatory, above knee (AK), knee disarticulation, ischial level socket, nonalignable system, pylon, no cover, SACH foot, thermoplastic or equal, direct formed

L5580 Preparatory, above knee (AK), knee disarticulation, ischial level socket, nonalignable system, pylon, no cover, SACH foot, thermoplastic or equal, molded to model

L5585 Preparatory, above knee (AK), knee disarticulation, ischial level socket, nonalignable system, pylon, no cover, SACH foot, prefabricated adjustable open end socket

L5590 Preparatory, above knee (AK), knee disarticulation, ischial level socket, nonalignable system, pylon, no cover, SACH foot, laminated socket, molded to model

L5595 Preparatory, hip disarticulation/hemipelvectomy, pylon, no cover, SACH foot, thermoplastic or equal, molded to patient model

L5600 Preparatory, hip disarticulation/hemipelvectomy, pylon, no cover, SACH foot, laminated socket, molded to patient model

Additions

Additions: Lower Extremity

L5610 Addition to lower extremity, endoskeletal system, above knee (AK), hydracadence system

L5611 Addition to lower extremity, endoskeletal system, above knee (AK), knee disarticulation, four-bar linkage, with friction swing phase control

L5613 Addition to lower extremity, endoskeletal system, above knee (AK), knee disarticulation, four-bar linkage, with hydraulic swing phase control

L5614 Addition to lower extremity, exoskeletal system, above knee (AK), knee disarticulation, four-bar linkage, with pneumatic swing phase control

L5615 Addition, endoskeletal knee-shin system, 4 bar linkage or multiaxial, fluid swing and stance phase control

L5616 Addition to lower extremity, endoskeletal system, above knee (AK), universal multiplex system, friction swing phase control

L5617 Addition to lower extremity, quick change self-aligning unit, above knee (AK) or below knee (BK), each

Additions: Test Sockets

L5618 Addition to lower extremity, test socket, Symes

L5620 Addition to lower extremity, test socket, below knee (BK)

L5622 Addition to lower extremity, test socket, knee disarticulation

L5624 Addition to lower extremity, test socket, above knee (AK)

L5626 Addition to lower extremity, test socket, hip disarticulation

L5628 Addition to lower extremity, test socket, hemipelvectomy

L5629 Addition to lower extremity, below knee, acrylic socket

Additions: Socket Variations

L5630 Addition to lower extremity, Symes type, expandable wall socket

L5631 Addition to lower extremity, above knee (AK) or knee disarticulation, acrylic socket

L5632 Addition to lower extremity, Symes type, PTB brim design socket

L5634 Addition to lower extremity, Symes type, posterior opening (Canadian) socket

L5636 Addition to lower extremity, Symes type, medial opening socket

L5637 Addition to lower extremity, below knee (BK), total contact

L5638 Addition to lower extremity, below knee (BK), leather socket

L5639 Addition to lower extremity, below knee (BK), wood socket

L5640 Addition to lower extremity, knee disarticulation, leather socket

L5642 Addition to lower extremity, above knee (AK), leather socket

L5643 Addition to lower extremity, hip disarticulation, flexible inner socket, external frame

L5644 Addition to lower extremity, above knee (AK), wood socket

L5645 Addition to lower extremity, below knee (BK), flexible inner socket, external frame

L5646 Addition to lower extremity, below knee (BK), air, fluid, gel or equal, cushion socket

L5647 Addition to lower extremity, below knee (BK), suction socket

L5648 Addition to lower extremity, above knee (AK), air, fluid, gel or equal, cushion socket

L5649 Addition to lower extremity, ischial containment/narrow M-L socket

L5650 Additions to lower extremity, total contact, above knee (AK) or knee disarticulation socket

L5651 Addition to lower extremity, above knee (AK), flexible inner socket, external frame

L5652 Addition to lower extremity, suction suspension, above knee (AK) or knee disarticulation socket

L5653 Addition to lower extremity, knee disarticulation, expandable wall socket

Additions: Socket Insert and Suspension

L5654 Addition to lower extremity, socket insert, Symes, (Kemblo, Pelite, Aliplast, Plastazote or equal)

L5655 Addition to lower extremity, socket insert, below knee (BK) (Kemblo, Pelite, Aliplast, Plastazote or equal)

L5656 Addition to lower extremity, socket insert, knee disarticulation (Kemblo, Pelite, Aliplast, Plastazote or equal)

L5658 Addition to lower extremity, socket insert, above knee (AK) (Kemblo, Pelite, Aliplast, Plastazote or equal)

L5661 Addition to lower extremity, socket insert, multidurometer Symes

L5665 Addition to lower extremity, socket insert, multidurometer, below knee (BK)

L5666 Addition to lower extremity, below knee (BK), cuff suspension

L5668 Addition to lower extremity, below knee (BK), molded distal cushion

L5670 Addition to lower extremity, below knee (BK), molded supracondylar suspension (PTS or similar)

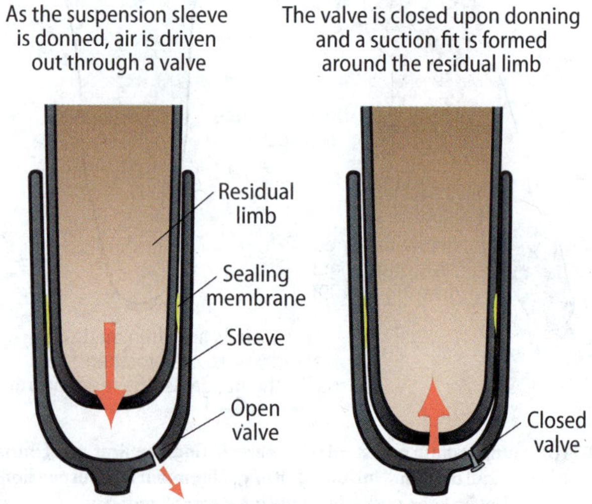

L5671 Addition to lower extremity, below knee (BK)/above knee (AK) suspension locking mechanism (shuttle, lanyard, or equal), excludes socket insert

L5672 Addition to lower extremity, below knee (BK), removable medial brim suspension

L5673 Addition to lower extremity, below knee (BK)/above knee (AK), custom fabricated from existing mold or prefabricated, socket insert, silicone gel, elastomeric or equal, for use with locking mechanism

L5676 Additions to lower extremity, below knee (BK), knee joints, single axis, pair

L5677 Additions to lower extremity, below knee (BK), knee joints, polycentric, pair

L5678 Additions to lower extremity, below knee (BK), joint covers, pair

L5679 Addition to lower extremity, below knee (BK)/above knee (AK), custom fabricated from existing mold or prefabricated, socket insert, silicone gel, elastomeric or equal, not for use with locking mechanism

L5680 Addition to lower extremity, below knee (BK), thigh lacer, nonmolded

L5681 Addition to lower extremity, below knee (BK)/above knee (AK), custom fabricated socket insert for congenital or atypical traumatic amputee, silicone gel, elastomeric or equal, for use with or without locking mechanism, initial only (for other than initial, use code L5673 or L5679)

L5682 Addition to lower extremity, below knee (BK), thigh lacer, gluteal/ischial, molded

L5683 Addition to lower extremity, below knee (BK)/above knee (AK), custom fabricated socket insert for other than congenital or atypical traumatic amputee, silicone gel, elastomeric or equal, for use with or without locking mechanism, initial only (for other than initial, use code L5673 or L5679)

L5684 Addition to lower extremity, below knee, fork strap

L5685 Addition to lower extremity prosthesis, below knee, suspension/sealing sleeve, with or without valve, any material, each

L5686 Addition to lower extremity, below knee (BK), back check (extension control)

L5688 Addition to lower extremity, below knee (BK), waist belt, webbing

L5690 Addition to lower extremity, below knee (BK), waist belt, padded and lined

L5692 Addition to lower extremity, above knee (AK), pelvic control belt, light

L5694 Addition to lower extremity, above knee (AK), pelvic control belt, padded and lined

L5695 Addition to lower extremity, above knee (AK), pelvic control, sleeve suspension, neoprene or equal, each

L5696 Addition to lower extremity, above knee (AK) or knee disarticulation, pelvic joint

L5697 Addition to lower extremity, above knee (AK) or knee disarticulation, pelvic band

L5698 Addition to lower extremity, above knee (AK) or knee disarticulation, Silesian bandage

L5699 All lower extremity prostheses, shoulder harness

Replacements

L5700 Replacement, socket, below knee (BK), molded to patient model

L5701 Replacement, socket, above knee (AK)/knee disarticulation, including attachment plate, molded to patient model

L5702 Replacement, socket, hip disarticulation, including hip joint, molded to patient model

L5703 Ankle, Symes, molded to patient model, socket without solid ankle cushion heel (SACH) foot, replacement only

L5704 Custom shaped protective cover, below knee (BK)

L5705 Custom shaped protective cover, above knee (AK)

L5706 Custom shaped protective cover, knee disarticulation

L5707 Custom shaped protective cover, hip disarticulation

Additions: Exoskeletal Knee-Shin System

L5710 Addition, exoskeletal knee-shin system, single axis, manual lock

L5711 Additions exoskeletal knee-shin system, single axis, manual lock, ultra-light material

L5712 Addition, exoskeletal knee-shin system, single axis, friction swing and stance phase control (safety knee)

L5714 Addition, exoskeletal knee-shin system, single axis, variable friction swing phase control

L5716 Addition, exoskeletal knee-shin system, polycentric, mechanical stance phase lock

L5718 Addition, exoskeletal knee-shin system, polycentric, friction swing and stance phase control

L5722 Addition, exoskeletal knee-shin system, single axis, pneumatic swing, friction stance phase control

L5724 Addition, exoskeletal knee-shin system, single axis, fluid swing phase control

L5726 Addition, exoskeletal knee-shin system, single axis, external joints, fluid swing phase control

L5728 Addition, exoskeletal knee-shin system, single axis, fluid swing and stance phase control

L5780 Addition, exoskeletal knee-shin system, single axis, pneumatic/hydra pneumatic swing phase control

L5781 Addition to lower limb prosthesis, vacuum pump, residual limb volume management and moisture evacuation system

L5782 Addition to lower limb prosthesis, vacuum pump, residual limb volume management and moisture evacuation system, heavy-duty

● **L5783** Addition to lower extremity, user adjustable, mechanical, residual limb volume management system

Component Modification

L5785 Addition, exoskeletal system, below knee (BK), ultra-light material (titanium, carbon fiber or equal)

L5790 Addition, exoskeletal system, above knee (AK), ultra-light material (titanium, carbon fiber or equal)

L5795 Addition, exoskeletal system, hip disarticulation, ultra-light material (titanium, carbon fiber or equal)

Additions: Endoskeletal Knee-Shin System

L5810 Addition, endoskeletal knee-shin system, single axis, manual lock

L5811 Addition, endoskeletal knee-shin system, single axis, manual lock, ultra-light material

L5812 Addition, endoskeletal knee-shin system, single axis, friction swing and stance phase control (safety knee)

L5814 Addition, endoskeletal knee-shin system, polycentric, hydraulic swing phase control, mechanical stance phase lock

L5816 Addition, endoskeletal knee-shin system, polycentric, mechanical stance phase lock

L5818 Addition, endoskeletal knee-shin system, polycentric, friction swing and stance phase control

L5822 Addition, endoskeletal knee-shin system, single axis, pneumatic swing, friction stance phase control

L5824 Addition, endoskeletal knee-shin system, single axis, fluid swing phase control

L5826 Addition, endoskeletal knee-shin system, single axis, hydraulic swing phase control, with miniature high activity frame

L5828 Addition, endoskeletal knee-shin system, single axis, fluid swing and stance phase control

L5830 Addition, endoskeletal knee-shin system, single axis, pneumatic/swing phase control

L5840 Addition, endoskeletal knee-shin system, four-bar linkage or multiaxial, pneumatic swing phase control

● **L5841** Addition, endoskeletal knee-shin system, polycentric, pneumatic swing, and stance phase control

L5845 Addition, endoskeletal knee-shin system, stance flexion feature, adjustable

L5848 Addition to endoskeletal knee-shin system, fluid stance extension, dampening feature, with or without adjustability

L5850 Addition, endoskeletal system, above knee (AK) or hip disarticulation, knee extension assist

L5855 Addition, endoskeletal system, hip disarticulation, mechanical hip extension assist

L5856 Addition to lower extremity prosthesis, endoskeletal knee-shin system, microprocessor control feature, swing and stance phase, includes electronic sensor(s), any type

L5857 Addition to lower extremity prosthesis, endoskeletal knee-shin system, microprocessor control feature, swing phase only, includes electronic sensor(s), any type

L5858 Addition to lower extremity prosthesis, endoskeletal knee-shin system, microprocessor control feature, stance phase only, includes electronic sensor(s), any type

L5859 Addition to lower extremity prosthesis, endoskeletal knee-shin system, powered and programmable flexion/extension assist control, includes any type motor(s)

L5910 Addition, endoskeletal system, below knee (BK), alignable system

L5920 Addition, endoskeletal system, above knee (AK) or hip disarticulation, alignable system

L5925 Addition, endoskeletal system, above knee (AK), knee disarticulation or hip disarticulation, manual lock

L5926 Addition to lower extremity prosthesis, endoskeletal, knee disarticulation, above knee, hip disarticulation, positional rotation unit, any type

L5930 Addition, endoskeletal system, high activity knee control frame

L5940 Addition, endoskeletal system, below knee (BK), ultra-light material (titanium, carbon fiber or equal)

L5950 Addition, endoskeletal system, above knee (AK), ultra-light material (titanium, carbon fiber or equal)

L5960 Addition, endoskeletal system, hip disarticulation, ultra-light material (titanium, carbon fiber or equal)

L5961 Addition, endoskeletal system, polycentric hip joint, pneumatic or hydraulic control, rotation control, with or without flexion and/or extension control

L5962 Addition, endoskeletal system, below knee (BK), flexible protective outer surface covering system

L5964 Addition, endoskeletal system, above knee (AK), flexible protective outer surface covering system

L5966 Addition, endoskeletal system, hip disarticulation, flexible protective outer surface covering system

L5968 Addition to lower limb prosthesis, multiaxial ankle with swing phase active dorsiflexion feature

L5969 Addition, endoskeletal ankle-foot or ankle system, power assist, includes any type motor(s)

L5970 All lower extremity prostheses, foot, external keel, SACH foot

L5971 All lower extremity prostheses, solid ankle cushion heel (SACH) foot, replacement only

L5972 All lower extremity prostheses, foot, flexible keel

L5973 Endoskeletal ankle foot system, microprocessor controlled feature, dorsiflexion and/or plantar flexion control, includes power source

L5974 All lower extremity prostheses, foot, single axis ankle/foot

Foot prosthesis (L5974)
Energy storing foot (L5976)
Carbon

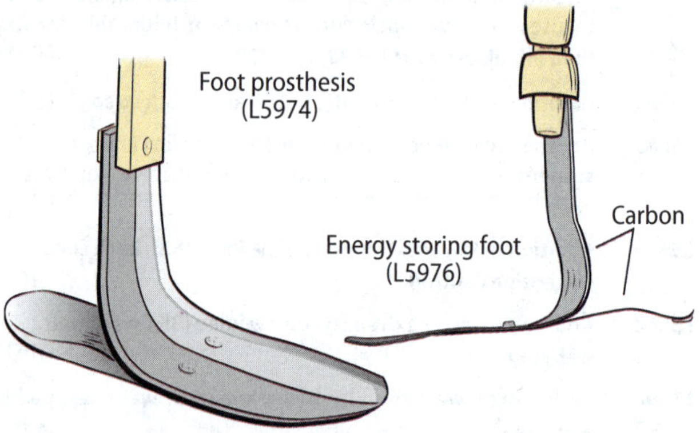

L5975 All lower extremity prostheses, combination single axis ankle and flexible keel foot

L5976 All lower extremity prostheses, energy storing foot (Seattle Carbon Copy II or equal)

L5978 All lower extremity prostheses, foot, multiaxial ankle/foot

Foot prosthesis, multi-axial ankle (L5978)

L5979 All lower extremity prostheses, multiaxial ankle, dynamic response foot, one-piece system

L5980 All lower extremity prostheses, flex-foot system

L5981 All lower extremity prostheses, flex-walk system or equal

L5982 All exoskeletal lower extremity prostheses, axial rotation unit

L5984 All endoskeletal lower extremity prostheses, axial rotation unit, with or without adjustability

L5985 All endoskeletal lower extremity prostheses, dynamic prosthetic pylon

L5986 All lower extremity prostheses, multiaxial rotation unit (MCP or equal)

L5987 All lower extremity prostheses, shank foot system with vertical loading pylon

L5988 Addition to lower limb prosthesis, vertical shock reducing pylon feature

L5990 Addition to lower extremity prosthesis, user adjustable heel height

L5991 Addition to lower extremity prostheses, osseointegrated external prosthetic connector
AHA: 4Q,23

L5999 Lower extremity prosthesis, not otherwise specified
Determine if an alternative HCPCS Level II or a CPT code better describes the service being reported. This code should be used only if a more specific code is unavailable.

Partial Hand

L6000 Partial hand, thumb remaining

L6010 Partial hand, little and/or ring finger remaining

L6020 Partial hand, no finger remaining

L6026 Transcarpal/metacarpal or partial hand disarticulation prosthesis, external power, self-suspended, inner socket with removable forearm section, electrodes and cables, two batteries, charger, myoelectric control of terminal device, excludes terminal device(s)

Wrist Disarticulation

L6050 Wrist disarticulation, molded socket, flexible elbow hinges, triceps pad

L6055 Wrist disarticulation, molded socket with expandable interface, flexible elbow hinges, triceps pad

Below Elbow

L6100 Below elbow, molded socket, flexible elbow hinge, triceps pad

L6110 Below elbow, molded socket (Muenster or Northwestern suspension types)

L6120 Below elbow, molded double wall split socket, step-up hinges, half cuff

L6130 Below elbow, molded double wall split socket, stump activated locking hinge, half cuff

Elbow Disarticulation

L6200 Elbow disarticulation, molded socket, outside locking hinge, forearm

L6205 Elbow disarticulation, molded socket with expandable interface, outside locking hinges, forearm

Above Elbow

L6250 Above elbow, molded double wall socket, internal locking elbow, forearm

Shoulder Disarticulation

L6300 Shoulder disarticulation, molded socket, shoulder bulkhead, humeral section, internal locking elbow, forearm

L6310 Shoulder disarticulation, passive restoration (complete prosthesis)

L6320 Shoulder disarticulation, passive restoration (shoulder cap only)

Interscapular Thoracic

L6350 Interscapular thoracic, molded socket, shoulder bulkhead, humeral section, internal locking elbow, forearm

L6360 Interscapular thoracic, passive restoration (complete prosthesis)

L6370 Interscapular thoracic, passive restoration (shoulder cap only)

Immediate and Early Postsurgical Procedures

L6380 Immediate postsurgical or early fitting, application of initial rigid dressing, including fitting alignment and suspension of components, and one cast change, wrist disarticulation or below elbow

L6382 Immediate postsurgical or early fitting, application of initial rigid dressing including fitting alignment and suspension of components, and one cast change, elbow disarticulation or above elbow

L6384 Immediate postsurgical or early fitting, application of initial rigid dressing including fitting alignment and suspension of components, and one cast change, shoulder disarticulation or interscapular thoracic

L6386 Immediate postsurgical or early fitting, each additional cast change and realignment

L6388 Immediate postsurgical or early fitting, application of rigid dressing only

Molded Socket

L6400 Below elbow, molded socket, endoskeletal system, including soft prosthetic tissue shaping

L6450 Elbow disarticulation, molded socket, endoskeletal system, including soft prosthetic tissue shaping

L6500 Above elbow, molded socket, endoskeletal system, including soft prosthetic tissue shaping

L6550 Shoulder disarticulation, molded socket, endoskeletal system, including soft prosthetic tissue shaping

L6570 Interscapular thoracic, molded socket, endoskeletal system, including soft prosthetic tissue shaping

Preparatory Socket

L6580 Preparatory, wrist disarticulation or below elbow, single wall plastic socket, friction wrist, flexible elbow hinges, figure of eight harness, humeral cuff, Bowden cable control, USMC or equal pylon, no cover, molded to patient model

L6582 Preparatory, wrist disarticulation or below elbow, single wall socket, friction wrist, flexible elbow hinges, figure of eight harness, humeral cuff, Bowden cable control, USMC or equal pylon, no cover, direct formed

L6584 Preparatory, elbow disarticulation or above elbow, single wall plastic socket, friction wrist, locking elbow, figure of eight harness, fair lead cable control, USMC or equal pylon, no cover, molded to patient model

L6586 Preparatory, elbow disarticulation or above elbow, single wall socket, friction wrist, locking elbow, figure of eight harness, fair lead cable control, USMC or equal pylon, no cover, direct formed

L6588 Preparatory, shoulder disarticulation or interscapular thoracic, single wall plastic socket, shoulder joint, locking elbow, friction wrist, chest strap, fair lead cable control, USMC or equal pylon, no cover, molded to patient model

L6590 Preparatory, shoulder disarticulation or interscapular thoracic, single wall socket, shoulder joint, locking elbow, friction wrist, chest strap, fair lead cable control, USMC or equal pylon, no cover, direct formed

Additions: Upper Limb

The following procedures/modifications/components may be added to other base procedures. The items in this section should reflect the additional complexity of each modification procedure, in addition to the base procedure, at the time of the original order.

L6600 Upper extremity additions, polycentric hinge, pair

L6605 Upper extremity additions, single pivot hinge, pair

L6610 Upper extremity additions, flexible metal hinge, pair

L6611 Addition to upper extremity prosthesis, external powered, additional switch, any type

L6615 Upper extremity addition, disconnect locking wrist unit

L6616 Upper extremity addition, additional disconnect insert for locking wrist unit, each

L6620 Upper extremity addition, flexion/extension wrist unit, with or without friction

L6621 Upper extremity prosthesis addition, flexion/extension wrist with or without friction, for use with external powered terminal device

L6623 Upper extremity addition, spring assisted rotational wrist unit with latch release

L6624 Upper extremity addition, flexion/extension and rotation wrist unit

L6625 Upper extremity addition, rotation wrist unit with cable lock

L6628 Upper extremity addition, quick disconnect hook adapter, Otto Bock or equal

L6629 Upper extremity addition, quick disconnect lamination collar with coupling piece, Otto Bock or equal

L6630 Upper extremity addition, stainless steel, any wrist

L6632 Upper extremity addition, latex suspension sleeve, each

L6635 Upper extremity addition, lift assist for elbow

L6637 Upper extremity addition, nudge control elbow lock

L6638 Upper extremity addition to prosthesis, electric locking feature, only for use with manually powered elbow

L6640 Upper extremity additions, shoulder abduction joint, pair

L6641 Upper extremity addition, excursion amplifier, pulley type

L6642 Upper extremity addition, excursion amplifier, lever type

L6645 Upper extremity addition, shoulder flexion-abduction joint, each

L6646 Upper extremity addition, shoulder joint, multipositional locking, flexion, adjustable abduction friction control, for use with body powered or external powered system

L6647 Upper extremity addition, shoulder lock mechanism, body powered actuator

L6648 Upper extremity addition, shoulder lock mechanism, external powered actuator

L6650 Upper extremity addition, shoulder universal joint, each

L6655 Upper extremity addition, standard control cable, extra

L6660 Upper extremity addition, heavy-duty control cable

L6665 Upper extremity addition, Teflon, or equal, cable lining

L6670 Upper extremity addition, hook to hand, cable adapter

L6672 Upper extremity addition, harness, chest or shoulder, saddle type

L6675 Upper extremity addition, harness, (e.g., figure of eight type), single cable design

L6676 Upper extremity addition, harness, (e.g., figure of eight type), dual cable design

L6677 Upper extremity addition, harness, triple control, simultaneous operation of terminal device and elbow

L6680 Upper extremity addition, test socket, wrist disarticulation or below elbow

L6682 Upper extremity addition, test socket, elbow disarticulation or above elbow

L6684 Upper extremity addition, test socket, shoulder disarticulation or interscapular thoracic

L6686 Upper extremity addition, suction socket

L6687 Upper extremity addition, frame type socket, below elbow or wrist disarticulation

L6688 Upper extremity addition, frame type socket, above elbow or elbow disarticulation

L6689 Upper extremity addition, frame type socket, shoulder disarticulation

L6690 Upper extremity addition, frame type socket, interscapular-thoracic

L6691 Upper extremity addition, removable insert, each

L6692 Upper extremity addition, silicone gel insert or equal, each

L6693 Upper extremity addition, locking elbow, forearm counterbalance

L6694 Addition to upper extremity prosthesis, below elbow/above elbow, custom fabricated from existing mold or prefabricated, socket insert, silicone gel, elastomeric or equal, for use with locking mechanism

L6695 Addition to upper extremity prosthesis, below elbow/above elbow, custom fabricated from existing mold or prefabricated, socket insert, silicone gel, elastomeric or equal, not for use with locking mechanism

L6696 Addition to upper extremity prosthesis, below elbow/above elbow, custom fabricated socket insert for congenital or atypical traumatic amputee, silicone gel, elastomeric or equal, for use with or without locking mechanism, initial only (for other than initial, use code L6694 or L6695)

L6697 Addition to upper extremity prosthesis, below elbow/above elbow, custom fabricated socket insert for other than congenital or atypical traumatic amputee, silicone gel, elastomeric or equal, for use with or without locking mechanism, initial only (for other than initial, use code L6694 or L6695)

L6698 Addition to upper extremity prosthesis, below elbow/above elbow, lock mechanism, excludes socket insert

Terminal Device

L6703 Terminal device, passive hand/mitt, any material, any size

L6704 Terminal device, sport/recreational/work attachment, any material, any size

L6706 Terminal device, hook, mechanical, voluntary opening, any material, any size, lined or unlined

L6707 Terminal device, hook, mechanical, voluntary closing, any material, any size, lined or unlined

L6708 Terminal device, hand, mechanical, voluntary opening, any material, any size

L6709 Terminal device, hand, mechanical, voluntary closing, any material, any size

L6711 Terminal device, hook, mechanical, voluntary opening, any material, any size, lined or unlined, pediatric

L6712 Terminal device, hook, mechanical, voluntary closing, any material, any size, lined or unlined, pediatric

L6713 Terminal device, hand, mechanical, voluntary opening, any material, any size, pediatric

L6714 Terminal device, hand, mechanical, voluntary closing, any material, any size, pediatric

L6715 Terminal device, multiple articulating digit, includes motor(s), initial issue or replacement

L6721 Terminal device, hook or hand, heavy-duty, mechanical, voluntary opening, any material, any size, lined or unlined

L6722 Terminal device, hook or hand, heavy-duty, mechanical, voluntary closing, any material, any size, lined or unlined

Addition to Terminal Device

L6805 Addition to terminal device, modifier wrist unit

L6810 Addition to terminal device, precision pinch device

L6880 Electric hand, switch or myoelectric controlled, independently articulating digits, any grasp pattern or combination of grasp patterns, includes motor(s)

L6881 Automatic grasp feature, addition to upper limb electric prosthetic terminal device

L6882 Microprocessor control feature, addition to upper limb prosthetic terminal device

Replacement Socket

L6883 Replacement socket, below elbow/wrist disarticulation, molded to patient model, for use with or without external power

L6884 Replacement socket, above elbow/elbow disarticulation, molded to patient model, for use with or without external power

L6885 Replacement socket, shoulder disarticulation/interscapular thoracic, molded to patient model, for use with or without external power

Hand Restoration

L6890 Addition to upper extremity prosthesis, glove for terminal device, any material, prefabricated, includes fitting and adjustment

L6895 Addition to upper extremity prosthesis, glove for terminal device, any material, custom fabricated

L6900 Hand restoration (casts, shading and measurements included), partial hand, with glove, thumb or one finger remaining

L6905 Hand restoration (casts, shading and measurements included), partial hand, with glove, multiple fingers remaining

L6910 Hand restoration (casts, shading and measurements included), partial hand, with glove, no fingers remaining

L6915 Hand restoration (shading and measurements included), replacement glove for above

External Power

L6920 Wrist disarticulation, external power, self-suspended inner socket, removable forearm shell, Otto Bock or equal switch, cables, two batteries and one charger, switch control of terminal device

L6925 Wrist disarticulation, external power, self-suspended inner socket, removable forearm shell, Otto Bock or equal electrodes, cables, two batteries and one charger, myoelectronic control of terminal device

L6930 Below elbow, external power, self-suspended inner socket, removable forearm shell, Otto Bock or equal switch, cables, two batteries and one charger, switch control of terminal device

L6935 Below elbow, external power, self-suspended inner socket, removable forearm shell, Otto Bock or equal electrodes, cables, two batteries and one charger, myoelectronic control of terminal device

L6940 Elbow disarticulation, external power, molded inner socket, removable humeral shell, outside locking hinges, forearm, Otto Bock or equal switch, cables, two batteries and one charger, switch control of terminal device

L6945 Elbow disarticulation, external power, molded inner socket, removable humeral shell, outside locking hinges, forearm, Otto Bock or equal electrodes, cables, two batteries and one charger, myoelectronic control of terminal device

L6950 Above elbow, external power, molded inner socket, removable humeral shell, internal locking elbow, forearm, Otto Bock or equal switch, cables, two batteries and one charger, switch control of terminal device

L6955 Above elbow, external power, molded inner socket, removable humeral shell, internal locking elbow, forearm, Otto Bock or equal electrodes, cables, two batteries and one charger, myoelectronic control of terminal device

L6960 Shoulder disarticulation, external power, molded inner socket, removable shoulder shell, shoulder bulkhead, humeral section, mechanical elbow, forearm, Otto Bock or equal switch, cables, two batteries and one charger, switch control of terminal device

L6965 Shoulder disarticulation, external power, molded inner socket, removable shoulder shell, shoulder bulkhead, humeral section, mechanical elbow, forearm, Otto Bock or equal electrodes, cables, two batteries and one charger, myoelectronic control of terminal device

L6970 Interscapular-thoracic, external power, molded inner socket, removable shoulder shell, shoulder bulkhead, humeral section, mechanical elbow, forearm, Otto Bock or equal switch, cables, two batteries and one charger, switch control of terminal device

L6975 Interscapular-thoracic, external power, molded inner socket, removable shoulder shell, shoulder bulkhead, humeral section, mechanical elbow, forearm, Otto Bock or equal electrodes, cables, two batteries and one charger, myoelectronic control of terminal device

Electric Hand and Accessories

L7007 Electric hand, switch or myoelectric controlled, adult

L7008 Electric hand, switch or myoelectric, controlled, pediatric

L7009 Electric hook, switch or myoelectric controlled, adult

L7040 Prehensile actuator, switch controlled

L7045 Electric hook, switch or myoelectric controlled, pediatric

Electronic Elbow and Accessories

L7170 Electronic elbow, Hosmer or equal, switch controlled

L7180 Electronic elbow, microprocessor sequential control of elbow and terminal device

L7181 Electronic elbow, microprocessor simultaneous control of elbow and terminal device

L7185 Electronic elbow, adolescent, Variety Village or equal, switch controlled

L7186 Electronic elbow, child, Variety Village or equal, switch controlled

L7190 Electronic elbow, adolescent, Variety Village or equal, myoelectronically controlled

L7191 Electronic elbow, child, Variety Village or equal, myoelectronically controlled

Electronic Wrist and Accessories

L7259 Electronic wrist rotator, any type

Battery Components

L7360 Six volt battery, each

L7362 Battery charger, six volt, each

L7364 Twelve volt battery, each

L7366 Battery charger, 12 volt, each

L7367 Lithium ion battery, rechargeable, replacement

L7368 Lithium ion battery charger, replacement only

Additions to Upper Extremity Prosthesis

L7400 Addition to upper extremity prosthesis, below elbow/wrist disarticulation, ultra-light material (titanium, carbon fiber or equal)

L7401 Addition to upper extremity prosthesis, above elbow disarticulation, ultra-light material (titanium, carbon fiber or equal)

L7402 Addition to upper extremity prosthesis, shoulder disarticulation/interscapular thoracic, ultra-light material (titanium, carbon fiber or equal)

L7403 Addition to upper extremity prosthesis, below elbow/wrist disarticulation, acrylic material

L7404 Addition to upper extremity prosthesis, above elbow disarticulation, acrylic material

L7405 Addition to upper extremity prosthesis, shoulder disarticulation/interscapular thoracic, acrylic material

L7499 Upper extremity prosthesis, not otherwise specified

Repairs

L7510 Repair of prosthetic device, repair or replace minor parts

Medicare jurisdiction: local contractor if repair of implanted prosthetic device.

L7520 Repair prosthetic device, labor component, per 15 minutes

Medicare jurisdiction: local contractor if repair of implanted prosthetic device.

CMS: 100-04,23,60.3

Prosthesis Supplies

L7600 Prosthetic donning sleeve, any material, each

L7700 Gasket or seal, for use with prosthetic socket insert, any type, each

Male Prosthetic

L7900 Male vacuum erection system

L7902 Tension ring, for vacuum erection device, any type, replacement only, each

Breast Prosthesis

L8000 Breast prosthesis, mastectomy bra, without integrated breast prosthesis form, any size, any type

L8001 Breast prosthesis, mastectomy bra, with integrated breast prosthesis form, unilateral, any size, any type

L8002 Breast prosthesis, mastectomy bra, with integrated breast prosthesis form, bilateral, any size, any type

L8010 Breast prosthesis, mastectomy sleeve

L8015 External breast prosthesis garment, with mastectomy form, post mastectomy

L8020 Breast prosthesis, mastectomy form

L8030 Breast prosthesis, silicone or equal, without integral adhesive

L8031 Breast prosthesis, silicone or equal, with integral adhesive

L8032 Nipple prosthesis, prefabricated, reusable, any type, each

L8033 Nipple prosthesis, custom fabricated, reusable, any material, any type, each A

L8035 Custom breast prosthesis, post mastectomy, molded to patient model A

L8039 Breast prosthesis, not otherwise specified A

Face and Ear Prosthesis

L8040 Nasal prosthesis, provided by a nonphysician A (KM, KN)
CMS: 100-04,20,30.9

Nasal prosthesis (L8040)

Orbital and midfacial prosthesis (L8041-L8042)

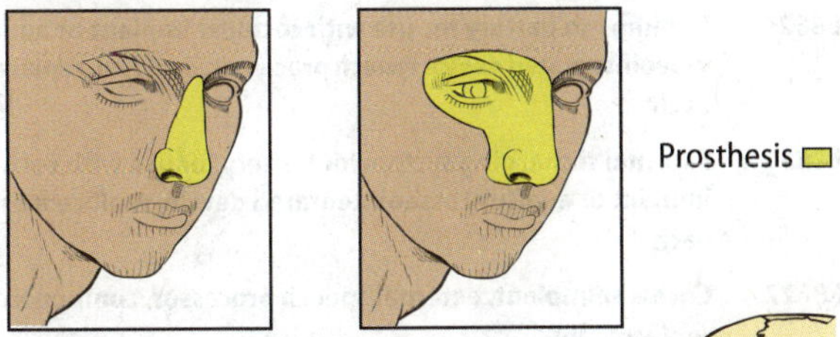

Prosthesis

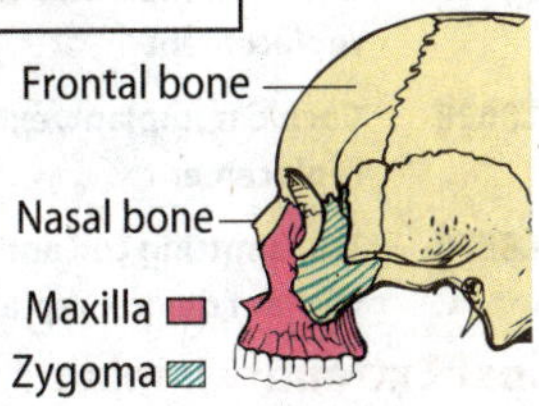

Facial prosthetics are typically custom manufactured from polymers and carefully matched to the original features. The maxilla, zygoma, frontal, and nasal bones are often involved, either singly or in combination (L8040-L8044)

Frontal bone

Nasal bone

Maxilla

Zygoma

(L8043–L8044)

L8041 Midfacial prosthesis, provided by a nonphysician A (KM, KN)
CMS: 100-04,20,30.9

L8042 Orbital prosthesis, provided by a nonphysician A (KM, KN)
CMS: 100-04,20,30.9

L8043 Upper facial prosthesis, provided by a nonphysician A (KM, KN)
CMS: 100-04,20,30.9

L8044 Hemi-facial prosthesis, provided by a nonphysician A (KM, KN)
CMS: 100-04,20,30.9

L8045 Auricular prosthesis, provided by a nonphysician A (KM, KN)
CMS: 100-04,20,30.9

L8046 Partial facial prosthesis, provided by a nonphysician A (KM, KN)
CMS: 100-04,20,30.9

L8047 Nasal septal prosthesis, provided by a nonphysician A (KM, KN)
CMS: 100-04,20,30.9

L8048 Unspecified maxillofacial prosthesis, by report, provided by a nonphysician A

L8049 Repair or modification of maxillofacial prosthesis, labor component, 15 minute increments, provided by a nonphysician A

Trusses

L8300 Truss, single with standard pad A

L8310 Truss, double with standard pads A

L8320 Truss, addition to standard pad, water pad A

L8330 Truss, addition to standard pad, scrotal pad A

Prosthetic Socks

L8400 Prosthetic sheath, below knee, each A ☑

L8410 Prosthetic sheath, above knee, each A ☑

L8415 Prosthetic sheath, upper limb, each A ☑

L8417 Prosthetic sheath/sock, including a gel cushion layer, below knee (BK) or above knee (AK), each A ☑

L8420 Prosthetic sock, multiple ply, below knee (BK), each A ☑

L8430 Prosthetic sock, multiple ply, above knee (AK), each A ☑

L8435 Prosthetic sock, multiple ply, upper limb, each A ☑

L8440 Prosthetic shrinker, below knee (BK), each A ☑

L8460 Prosthetic shrinker, above knee (AK), each A ☑

L8465 Prosthetic shrinker, upper limb, each A ☑

L8470 Prosthetic sock, single ply, fitting, below knee (BK), each A ☑

L8480 Prosthetic sock, single ply, fitting, above knee (AK), each A ☑

L8485 Prosthetic sock, single ply, fitting, upper limb, each A ☑

L8499 Unlisted procedure for miscellaneous prosthetic services A
Determine if an alternative HCPCS Level II or a CPT code better describes the service being reported. This code should be used only if a more specific code is unavailable.

Larynx and Trachea Prothetics and Accessories

L8500 Artificial larynx, any type A

L8501 Tracheostomy speaking valve A

L8505 Artificial larynx replacement battery/accessory, any type A

L8507 Tracheo-esophageal voice prosthesis, patient inserted, any type, each A ☑

L8509 Tracheo-esophageal voice prosthesis, inserted by a licensed health care provider, any type A

L8510 Voice amplifier A

L8511 Insert for indwelling tracheo-esophageal prosthesis, with or without valve, replacement only, each A ☑

L8512 Gelatin capsules or equivalent, for use with tracheo-esophageal voice prosthesis, replacement only, per 10 A ☑

L8513 Cleaning device used with tracheoesophageal voice prosthesis, pipet, brush, or equal, replacement only, each A ☑

L8514 Tracheo-esophageal puncture dilator, replacement only, each A ☑

L8515 Gelatin capsule, application device for use with tracheo-esophageal voice prosthesis, each A ☑

Breast Implant

L8600 **Implantable breast prosthesis, silicone or equal** N N1 ♿

Medicare covers implants inserted in post-mastectomy reconstruction in a breast cancer patient. Always report concurrent to the implant procedure.

CMS: 100-04,4,190

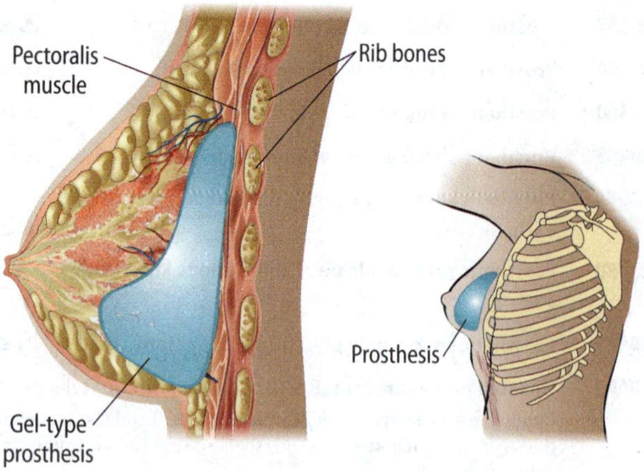

Pectoralis muscle

Rib bones

Prosthesis

Gel-type prosthesis

Bulking Agents

L8603 **Injectable bulking agent, collagen implant, urinary tract, 2.5 ml syringe, includes shipping and necessary supplies** N N1 ☑ ♿

CMS: 100-04,23,60.1; 100-04,4,190

L8604 **Injectable bulking agent, dextranomer/hyaluronic acid copolymer implant, urinary tract, 1 ml, includes shipping and necessary supplies** N N1 ☑

L8605 **Injectable bulking agent, dextranomer/hyaluronic acid copolymer implant, anal canal, 1 ml, includes shipping and necessary supplies** N N1 ♿

L8606 **Injectable bulking agent, synthetic implant, urinary tract, 1 ml syringe, includes shipping and necessary supplies** N N1 ☑ ♿

L8607 **Injectable bulking agent for vocal cord medialization, 0.1 ml, includes shipping and necessary supplies** N N1 ♿

Eye and Ear Implants and Accessories

L8608 **Miscellaneous external component, supply or accessory for use with the Argus II Retinal Prosthesis System** N N1

L8609 **Artificial cornea** N N1 ♿

L8610 **Ocular implant** N N1 ♿

CMS: 100-04,4,190

L8612 **Aqueous shunt** N N1 ♿

CMS: 100-04,4,190

L8613 **Ossicula implant** N N1 ♿

CMS: 100-04,4,190

L8614 **Cochlear device, includes all internal and external components** N N1 ♿

A cochlear implant is covered by Medicare when the patient has bilateral sensorineural deafness.

CMS: 100-04,14,40.8; 100-04,4,190; 100-04,4,60.4.2

L8615 **Headset/headpiece for use with cochlear implant device, replacement** A ♿

L8616 **Microphone for use with cochlear implant device, replacement** A ♿

L8617 **Transmitting coil for use with cochlear implant device, replacement** A ♿

L8618 **Transmitter cable for use with cochlear implant device or auditory osseointegrated device, replacement** A ♿

L8619 **Cochlear implant, external speech processor and controller, integrated system, replacement** A ♿

Medicare jurisdiction: local contractor.

L8621 **Zinc air battery for use with cochlear implant device and auditory osseointegrated sound processors, replacement, each** A ☑ ♿

L8622 **Alkaline battery for use with cochlear implant device, any size, replacement, each** A ☑ ♿

L8623 **Lithium ion battery for use with cochlear implant device speech processor, other than ear level, replacement, each** A ☑ ♿

L8624 **Lithium ion battery for use with cochlear implant or auditory osseointegrated device speech processor, ear level, replacement, each** A ☑ ♿

L8625 **External recharging system for battery for use with cochlear implant or auditory osseointegrated device, replacement only, each** A ♿

L8627 **Cochlear implant, external speech processor, component, replacement** A ♿

L8628 **Cochlear implant, external controller component, replacement** A ♿

L8629 **Transmitting coil and cable, integrated, for use with cochlear implant device, replacement** A ♿

Upper Extremity Implants

L8630 **Metacarpophalangeal joint implant** N N1 ♿

CMS: 100-04,4,190

Bone is cut at the MP joint (arthroplasty)

Bone may be hollowed out in both metacarpal and phalangeal sides in preparation for a prosthesis

Prosthetic joint implant

Prosthesis in place

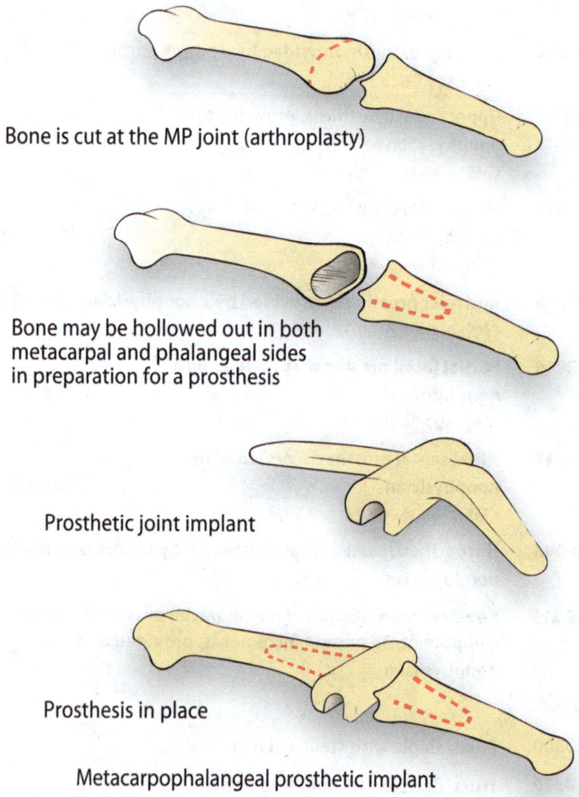

Metacarpophalangeal prosthetic implant

L8631 **Metacarpal phalangeal joint replacement, two or more pieces, metal (e.g., stainless steel or cobalt chrome), ceramic-like material (e.g., pyrocarbon), for surgical implantation (all sizes, includes entire system)** N N1 ♿

Lower Extremity Implants

L8641 Metatarsal joint implant N N1 ♿
CMS: 100-04,4,190

L8642 Hallux implant N N1 ♿
CMS: 100-04,4,190

Interphalangeal Implants

L8658 Interphalangeal joint spacer, silicone or equal, each N N1 ☑ ♿
CMS: 100-04,4,190

L8659 Interphalangeal finger joint replacement, two or more pieces, metal (e.g., stainless steel or cobalt chrome), ceramic-like material (e.g., pyrocarbon) for surgical implantation, any size N N1 ♿

Cardiovascular Implant

L8670 Vascular graft material, synthetic, implant N N1 ♿
CMS: 100-04,4,190

Neurostimulator and Accessories

L8678 Electrical stimulator supplies (external) for use with implantable neurostimulator, per month N N1
AHA: 2Q,23

L8679 Implantable neurostimulator, pulse generator, any type N N1 ♿

L8680 Implantable neurostimulator electrode, each E1 ☑

L8681 Patient programmer (external) for use with implantable programmable neurostimulator pulse generator, replacement only A ♿

L8682 Implantable neurostimulator radiofrequency receiver N N1 ♿

L8683 Radiofrequency transmitter (external) for use with implantable neurostimulator radiofrequency receiver A ♿

L8684 Radiofrequency transmitter (external) for use with implantable sacral root neurostimulator receiver for bowel and bladder management, replacement A ♿

L8685 Implantable neurostimulator pulse generator, single array, rechargeable, includes extension E1

L8686 Implantable neurostimulator pulse generator, single array, nonrechargeable, includes extension E1

L8687 Implantable neurostimulator pulse generator, dual array, rechargeable, includes extension E1

L8688 Implantable neurostimulator pulse generator, dual array, nonrechargeable, includes extension E1

L8689 External recharging system for battery (internal) for use with implantable neurostimulator, replacement only A ♿

Miscellaneous Prosthetics and Accessories

L8690 Auditory osseointegrated device, includes all internal and external components N N1 ♿
CMS: 100-04,14,40.8; 100-04,4,60.4.2

L8691 Auditory osseointegrated device, external sound processor, excludes transducer/actuator, replacement only, each A ♿

L8692 Auditory osseointegrated device, external sound processor, used without osseointegration, body worn, includes headband or other means of external attachment E1

L8693 Auditory osseointegrated device abutment, any length, replacement only A ♿

L8694 Auditory osseointegrated device, transducer/actuator, replacement only, each A ♿

L8695 External recharging system for battery (external) for use with implantable neurostimulator, replacement only A ♿

L8696 Antenna (external) for use with implantable diaphragmatic/phrenic nerve stimulation device, replacement, each A ♿

L8698 Miscellaneous component, supply or accessory for use with total artificial heart system A

L8699 Prosthetic implant, not otherwise specified N N1
Determine if an alternative HCPCS Level II or a CPT code better describes the service being reported. This code should be used only if a more specific code is unavailable.
CMS: 100-04,4,190

L8701 Powered upper extremity range of motion assist device, elbow, wrist, hand with single or double upright(s), includes microprocessor, sensors, all components and accessories, custom fabricated A

L8702 Powered upper extremity range of motion assist device, elbow, wrist, hand, finger, single or double upright(s), includes microprocessor, sensors, all components and accessories, custom fabricated A

● **L8720** External lower extremity sensory prosthetic, cutaneous stimulation of mechanoreceptors proximal to the ankle, per leg

● **L8721** Receptor sole for use with L8720, replacement, each

L9900 Orthotic and prosthetic supply, accessory, and/or service component of another HCPCS L code N N1

MIPS Value Pathways M0001-M0010

M0001 Advancing Cancer Care MIPS Value Pathways M

M0002 Optimal Care for Kidney Health MIPS Value Pathways M

M0003 ~~Optimal Care for Patients with Episodic Neurological Conditions MIPS Value Pathways~~

▲**M0004** Quality care for patients with neurological conditions MIPS value pathway M

M0005 Value in primary care MIPS value pathway M

M0010 Enhancing oncology model (EOM) monthly enhanced oncology services (MEOS) payment for EOM enhanced services M
AHA: 2Q,23

Medical Services M0075-M0301

Other Medical Services

M codes include office services, cellular therapy, prolotherapy, intragastric hypothermia, IV chelation therapy, and fabric wrapping of an abdominal aneurysm.

M0075 Cellular therapy E1
The therapeutic efficacy of injecting foreign proteins has not been established.

M0076 Prolotherapy E1
The therapeutic efficacy of prolotherapy and joint sclerotherapy has not been established.

M0100 Intragastric hypothermia using gastric freezing E1
Code with caution: This procedure is considered obsolete.

M0201 Administration of pneumococcal, influenza, hepatitis B, and/or COVID-19 vaccine inside a patient's home; reported only once per individual home per date of service when such vaccine administration(s) are performed at the patient's home S
AHA: 3Q,21

M0220 Injection, tixagevimab and cilgavimab, for the pre-exposure prophylaxis only, for certain adults and pediatric individuals (12 years of age and older weighing at least 40kg) with no known SARS-CoV-2 exposure, who either have moderate to severely compromised immune systems or for whom vaccination with any available COVID-19 vaccine is not recommended due to a history of severe adverse reaction to a COVID-19 vaccine(s) and/or COVID-19 vaccine component(s), includes injection and post administration monitoring S
AHA: 2Q,22

M0221 Injection, tixagevimab and cilgavimab, for the pre-exposure prophylaxis only, for certain adults and pediatric individuals (12 years of age and older weighing at least 40kg) with no known SARS-CoV-2 exposure, who either have moderate to severely compromised immune systems or for whom vaccination with any available COVID-19 vaccine is not recommended due to a history of severe adverse reaction to a COVID-19 vaccine(s) and/or COVID-19 vaccine component(s), includes injection and post administration monitoring in the home or residence; this includes a beneficiary's home that has been made provider-based to the hospital during the COVID-19 public health emergency S
AHA: 2Q,22

M0222 Intravenous injection, bebtelovimab, includes injection and post administration monitoring S
AHA: 2Q,22

M0223 Intravenous injection, bebtelovimab, includes injection and post administration monitoring in the home or residence; this includes a beneficiary's home that has been made provider-based to the hospital during the COVID-19 public health emergency S
AHA: 2Q,22

●**M0224** Intravenous infusion, pemivibart, for the pre-exposure prophylaxis only, for certain adults and adolescents (12 years of age and older weighing at least 40 kg) with no known SARS-CoV-2 exposure, who either have moderate-to-severe immune compromise due to a medical condition or receipt of immunosuppressive medications or treatments, includes infusion and post administration monitoring
AHA: 3Q,24

M0240 Intravenous infusion or subcutaneous injection, casirivimab and imdevimab, includes infusion or injection and post administration monitoring, subsequent repeat doses S
Use this code for casirivimab and imdevimab 600 mg administered as post exposure prophylaxis. Report also Q0240 for drug.
AHA: 4Q,21; 3Q,21

M0241 Intravenous infusion or subcutaneous injection, casirivimab and imdevimab, includes infusion or injection, and post administration monitoring in the home or residence. This includes a beneficiary's home that has been made provider-based to the hospital during the covid-19 public health emergency, subsequent repeat doses S
Use this code for casirivimab and imdevimab 600 mg administered as post exposure prophylaxis. Report also Q0240 for drug.
AHA: 4Q,21; 3Q,21

M0243 Intravenous infusion or subcutaneous injection, casirivimab and imdevimab, includes infusion or injection, and post administration monitoring S
Use this code for administration of Casirivimab and Imdevimab (REGN-COV2), Regeneron. Report also Q0243 for drug.
AHA: 2Q,22; 1Q,21; 4Q,20

M0244 Intravenous infusion or subcutaneous injection, casirivimab and imdevimab, includes infusion or injection and post administration monitoring in the home or residence; this includes a beneficiary's home that has been made provider-based to the hospital during the COVID-19 public health emergency S
Use this code for administration of casirivimab and imdevimab in the home setting. Report also Q0243 for drug.
AHA: 3Q,21

M0245 Intravenous infusion, bamlanivimab and etesevimab, includes infusion and post administration monitoring S
Use this code for administration of bamlanivimab (LY-CoV555) and etesevimab (LY-CoV016). Report also Q0245 for drug.
AHA: 1Q,21

M0246 Intravenous infusion, bamlanivimab and etesevimab, includes infusion and post administration monitoring in the home or residence; this includes a beneficiary's home that has been made provider-based to the hospital during the COVID-19 public health emergency S
Use this code for administration of bamlanivimab and etesevimab in the home setting. Report also Q0245 for drug.
AHA: 3Q,21

M0247 Intravenous infusion, sotrovimab, includes infusion and post administration monitoring S
AHA: 3Q,21

M0248 Intravenous infusion, sotrovimab, includes infusion and post administration monitoring in the home or residence; this includes a beneficiary's home that has been made provider-based to the hospital during the COVID-19 public health emergency S
AHA: 3Q,21

M0249 Intravenous infusion, tocilizumab, for hospitalized adults and pediatric patients (2 years of age and older) with COVID-19 who are receiving systemic corticosteroids and require supplemental oxygen, non-invasive or invasive mechanical ventilation, or extracorporeal membrane oxygenation (ECMO) only, includes infusion and post administration monitoring, first dose S
AHA: 4Q,21

M0250 Intravenous infusion, tocilizumab, for hospitalized adults and pediatric patients (2 years of age and older) with COVID-19 who are receiving systemic corticosteroids and require supplemental oxygen, non-invasive or invasive mechanical ventilation, or extracorporeal membrane oxygenation (ECMO) only, includes infusion and post administration monitoring, second dose S
AHA: 4Q,21

Cardiovascular Services

M0300 IV chelation therapy (chemical endarterectomy) E
Chelation therapy is considered experimental in the United States.
CMS: 100-03*; 100-03,20.22

M0301 Fabric wrapping of abdominal aneurysm E
Code with caution: This procedure has largely been replaced with more effective treatment modalities. Submit documentation.

Quality Measures M1003-M1425

Quality Measures

M1003 TB screening performed and results interpreted within 12 months prior to initiation of first-time biologic and/or immune response modifier therapy

M1004 Documentation of medical reason for not screening for TB or interpreting results (i.e., patient positive for TB and documentation of past treatment; patient who has recently completed a course of anti-TB therapy)

M1005 TB screening not performed or results not interpreted, reason not given

M1006 Disease activity not assessed, reason not given

M1007 >=50% of total number of a patient's outpatient RA encounters assessed

M1008 <50% of total number of a patient's outpatient RA encounters assessed

M1009 Discharge/discontinuation of the episode of care documented in the medical record

M1010 Discharge/discontinuation of the episode of care documented in the medical record

M1011 Discharge/discontinuation of the episode of care documented in the medical record

M1012 Discharge/discontinuation of the episode of care documented in the medical record

M1013 Discharge/discontinuation of the episode of care documented in the medical record

M1014 Discharge/discontinuation of the episode of care documented in the medical record

M1016 Female patients unable to bear children

M1018 Patients with an active diagnosis or history of cancer (except basal cell and squamous cell skin carcinoma), patients who are heavy tobacco smokers, lung cancer screening patients

M1019 Adolescent patients 12 to 17 years of age with major depression or dysthymia who reached remission at 12 months as demonstrated by a 12 month (+/-60 days) PHQ-9 or PHQ-9M score of less than 5

M1020 Adolescent patients 12 to 17 years of age with major depression or dysthymia who did not reach remission at 12 months as demonstrated by a 12 month (+/-60 days) PHQ-9 or PHQ-9M score of less than 5. Either PHQ-9 or PHQ-9M score was not assessed or is greater than or equal to 5

M1021 Patient had only urgent care visits during the performance period

M1027 Imaging of the head (CT or MRI) was obtained

M1028 Documentation of patients with primary headache diagnosis and imaging other than CT or MRI obtained

M1029 Imaging of the head (CT or MRI) was not obtained, reason not given

M1032 Adults currently taking pharmacotherapy for OUD

M1034 Adults who have at least 180 days of continuous pharmacotherapy with a medication prescribed for OUD without a gap of more than seven days

M1035 Adults who are deliberately phased out of medication assisted treatment (MAT) prior to 180 days of continuous treatment

M1036 Adults who have not had at least 180 days of continuous pharmacotherapy with a medication prescribed for OUD without a gap of more than seven days

M1037 Patients with a diagnosis of lumbar spine region cancer at the time of the procedure

M1038 Patients with a diagnosis of lumbar spine region fracture at the time of the procedure

M1039 Patients with a diagnosis of lumbar spine region infection at the time of the procedure

M1040 Patients with a diagnosis of lumbar idiopathic or congenital scoliosis

M1041 Patient had cancer, acute fracture or infection related to the lumbar spine or patient had neuromuscular, idiopathic or congenital lumbar scoliosis

M1043 Functional status was not measured by the Oswestry Disability Index (ODI version 2.1a) at 1 year (9 to 15 months) postoperatively

M1045 Functional status measured by the Oxford Knee Score (OKS) at one year (9 to 15 months) postoperatively was greater than or equal to 37 or knee injury and osteoarthritis outcome score joint replacement (KOOS, JR.) was greater than or equal to 71

M1046 Functional status measured by the Oxford Knee Score (OKS) at one year (9 to 15 months) postoperatively was less than 37 or the knee injury and osteoarthritis outcome score joint replacement (KOOS, JR.) was less than 71 postoperatively

M1049 Functional status was not measured by the Oswestry Disability Index (ODI version 2.1a) at 3 months (6 to 20 weeks) postoperatively

M1051 Patient had cancer, acute fracture or infection related to the lumbar spine or patient had neuromuscular, idiopathic or congenital lumbar scoliosis

M1052 Leg pain was not measured by the visual analog scale (VAS) or numeric pain scale at one year (9 to 15 months) postoperatively

M1054 Patient had only urgent care visits during the performance period

M1055 Aspirin or another antiplatelet therapy used

M1056 Prescribed anticoagulant medication during the performance period, history of GI bleeding, history of intracranial bleeding, bleeding disorder and specific provider documented reasons: allergy to aspirin or antiplatelets, use of nonsteroidal antiinflammatory agents, drug-drug interaction, uncontrolled hypertension > 180/110 mm Hg or gastroesophageal reflux disease

M1057 Aspirin or another antiplatelet therapy not used, reason not given

M1058 Patient was a permanent nursing home resident at any time during the performance period

M1059 Patient was in hospice or receiving palliative care at any time during the performance period

M1060 Patient died prior to the end of the performance period

M1067 Hospice services for patient provided any time during the measurement period

M1068 Adults who are not ambulatory

M1069 Patient screened for future fall risk

M1070 Patient not screened for future fall risk, reason not given

M1106 The start of an episode of care documented in the medical record M

M1107 Documentation stating patient has a diagnosis of a degenerative neurological condition such as ALS, MS, or Parkinson's diagnosed at any time before or during the episode of care M

M1108 Ongoing care not clinically indicated because the patient needed a home program only, referral to another provider or facility, or consultation only, as documented in the medical record M

M1109 Ongoing care not medically possible because the patient was discharged early due to specific medical events, documented in the medical record, such as the patient became hospitalized or scheduled for surgery M

M1110 Ongoing care not possible because the patient self-discharged early (e.g., financial or insurance reasons, transportation problems, or reason unknown) M

M1111 The start of an episode of care documented in the medical record M

M1112 Documentation stating patient has a diagnosis of a degenerative neurological condition such as ALS, MS, or Parkinson's diagnosed at any time before or during the episode of care M

M1113 Ongoing care not clinically indicated because the patient needed a home program only, referral to another provider or facility, or consultation only, as documented in the medical record M

M1114 Ongoing care not medically possible because the patient was discharged early due to specific medical events, documented in the medical record, such as the patient became hospitalized or scheduled for surgery M

M1115 Ongoing care not possible because the patient self-discharged early (e.g., financial or insurance reasons, transportation problems, or reason unknown) M

M1116 The start of an episode of care documented in the medical record M

M1117 Documentation stating patient has a diagnosis of a degenerative neurological condition such as ALS, MS, or Parkinson's diagnosed at any time before or during the episode of care M

M1118 Ongoing care not clinically indicated because the patient needed a home program only, referral to another provider or facility, or consultation only, as documented in the medical record M

M1119 Ongoing care not medically possible because the patient was discharged early due to specific medical events, documented in the medical record, such as the patient became hospitalized or scheduled for surgery M

M1120 Ongoing care not possible because the patient self-discharged early (e.g., financial or insurance reasons, transportation problems, or reason unknown) M

M1121 The start of an episode of care documented in the medical record M

M1122 Documentation stating patient has a diagnosis of a degenerative neurological condition such as ALS, MS, or Parkinson's diagnosed at any time before or during the episode of care M

M1123 Ongoing care not clinically indicated because the patient needed a home program only, referral to another provider or facility, or consultation only, as documented in the medical record M

M1124 Ongoing care not medically possible because the patient was discharged early due to specific medical events, documented in the medical record, such as the patient became hospitalized or scheduled for surgery M

M1125 Ongoing care not possible because the patient self-discharged early (e.g., financial or insurance reasons, transportation problems, or reason unknown) M

M1126 The start of an episode of care documented in the medical record M

M1127 Documentation stating patient has a diagnosis of a degenerative neurological condition such as ALS, MS, or Parkinson's diagnosed at any time before or during the episode of care M

M1128 Ongoing care not clinically indicated because the patient needed a home program only, referral to another provider or facility, or consultation only, as documented in the medical record M

M1129 Ongoing care not medically possible because the patient was discharged early due to specific medical events, documented in the medical record, such as the patient became hospitalized or scheduled for surgery M

M1130 Ongoing care not possible because the patient self-discharged early (e.g., financial or insurance reasons, transportation problems, or reason unknown) M

M1131 Documentation stating patient has a diagnosis of a degenerative neurological condition such as ALS, MS, or Parkinson's diagnosed at any time before or during the episode of care M

M1132 Ongoing care not clinically indicated because the patient needed a home program only, referral to another provider or facility, or consultation only, as documented in the medical record M

M1133 Ongoing care not medically possible because the patient was discharged early due to specific medical events, documented in the medical record, such as the patient became hospitalized or scheduled for surgery M

M1134 Ongoing care not possible because the patient self-discharged early (e.g., financial or insurance reasons, transportation problems, or reason unknown) M

M1135 The start of an episode of care documented in the medical record M

M1141 Functional status was not measured by the Oxford Knee Score (OKS) or the knee injury and osteoarthritis outcome score joint replacement (KOOS, JR.) at one year (9 to 15 months) postoperatively M

M1142 Emergent cases M

M1143 Initiated episode of rehabilitation therapy, medical, or chiropractic care for neck impairment M

M1146 Ongoing care not clinically indicated because the patient needed a home program only, referral to another provider or facility, or consultation only, as documented in the medical record M

M1147 Ongoing care not medically possible because the patient was discharged early due to specific medical events, documented in the medical record, such as the patient became hospitalized or scheduled for surgery M

M1148 Ongoing care not possible because the patient self-discharged early (e.g., financial or insurance reasons, transportation problems, or reason unknown) M

M1149 Patient unable to complete the neck FS PROM at initial evaluation and/or discharge due to blindness, illiteracy, severe mental incapacity or language incompatibility, and an adequate proxy is not available M

▲ M1150 Current or prior left ventricular ejection fraction (LVEF) less than or equal to 40% or documentation of moderately or severely depressed left ventricular systolic function M

M1151 Patients with a history of heart transplant or with a left ventricular assist device (LVAD) M

M1152 Patients with a history of heart transplant or with a left ventricular assist device (LVAD) M

M1153 Patient with diagnosis of osteoporosis on date of encounter M

M1154 ~~Hospice services provided to patient any time during the measurement period~~

M1155 ~~Patient had anaphylaxis due to the pneumococcal vaccine any time during or before the measurement period~~

M1159 Hospice services provided to patient any time during the measurement period M

M1160 Patient had anaphylaxis due to the meningococcal vaccine any time on or before the patient's 13th birthday M

M1161 Patient had anaphylaxis due to the tetanus, diphtheria or pertussis vaccine any time on or before the patient's 13th birthday M

M1162 Patient had encephalitis due to the tetanus, diphtheria or pertussis vaccine any time on or before the patient's 13th birthday M

M1163 Patient had anaphylaxis due to the HPV vaccine any time on or before the patient's 13th birthday M

M1164 Patients with dementia any time during the patient's history through the end of the measurement period M

M1165 Patients who use hospice services any time during the measurement period M

M1166 Pathology report for tissue specimens produced from wide local excisions or re-excisions M

M1167 In hospice or using hospice services during the measurement period M

M1168 Patient received an influenza vaccine on or between July 1 of the year prior to the measurement period and June 30 of the measurement period M

M1169 Documentation of medical reason(s) for not administering influenza vaccine (e.g., prior anaphylaxis due to the influenza vaccine) M

M1170 Patient did not receive an influenza vaccine on or between July 1 of the year prior to the measurement period and June 30 of the measurement period M

M1171 Patient received at least 1 TD vaccine or 1 TDaP vaccine between 9 years prior to the encounter and the end of the measurement period M

M1172 Documentation of medical reason(s) for not administering TD or TDaP vaccine (e.g., prior anaphylaxis due to the TD or TDaP vaccine or history of encephalopathy within 7 days after a previous dose of a TD-containing vaccine) M

M1173 Patient did not receive at least 1 TD vaccine or 1 TDaP vaccine between 9 years prior to the encounter and the end of the measurement oneperiod M

M1174 Patient received at least two doses of the herpes zoster recombinant vaccine (at least 28 days apart) anytime on or after the patient's 50th birthday before or during the measurement period M

M1175 Documentation of medical reason(s) for not administering zoster vaccine (e.g., prior anaphylaxis due to the zoster vaccine) M

▲ M1176 Patient did not receive two doses of the herpes zoster recombinant vaccine (at least 28 days apart) anytime on or after the patient's 50th birthday before or during the measurement period M

▲ M1177 Patient received any pneumococcal conjugate or polysaccharide vaccine on or after their 19th birthday and before the end of the measurement period M

M1178 Documentation of medical reason(s) for not administering pneumococcal vaccine (e.g., prior anaphylaxis due to the pneumococcal vaccine) M

▲ M1179 Patient did not receive any pneumococcal conjugate or polysaccharide vaccine, on or after their 19th birthday and before or during measurement period M

M1180 Patients on immune checkpoint inhibitor therapy M

M1181 Grade 2 or above diarrhea and/or Grade 2 or above colitis M

M1182 Patients not eligible due to pre-existing inflammatory bowel disease (IBD) (e.g., ulcerative colitis, Crohn's disease) M

M1183 Documentation of immune checkpoint inhibitor therapy held and corticosteroids or immunosuppressants prescribed or administered M

M1184 Documentation of medical reason(s) for not prescribing or administering corticosteroid or immunosuppressant treatment (e.g., allergy, intolerance, infectious etiology, pancreatic insufficiency, hyperthyroidism, prior bowel surgical interventions, celiac disease, receiving other medication, awaiting diagnostic workup results for alternative etiologies, other medical reasons/contraindication) M

M1185 Documentation of immune checkpoint inhibitor therapy not held and/or corticosteroids or immunosuppressants prescribed or administered was not performed, reason not given M

M1186 Patients who have an order for or are receiving hospice or palliative care M

M1187 Patients with a diagnosis of end stage renal disease (ESRD) M

M1188 Patients with a diagnosis of chronic kidney disease (CKD) Stage 5 M

M1189 Documentation of a kidney health evaluation defined by an estimated glomerular filtration rate (EGFR) and urine albumin-creatinine ratio (UACR) performed M

M1190 Documentation of a kidney health evaluation was not performed or defined by an estimated glomerular filtration rate (EGFR) and urine albumin-creatinine ratio (UACR) M

M1191 Hospice services provided to patient any time during the measurement period M

M1192 Patients with an existing diagnosis of squamous cell carcinoma of the esophagus M

M1193 Surgical pathology reports that contain impression or conclusion of or recommendation for testing of MMR by immunohistochemistry, MSI by DNA-based testing status, or both M

M1194 Documentation of medical reason(s) surgical pathology reports did not contain impression or conclusion of or recommendation for testing of MMR by immunohistochemistry, MSI by DNA-based testing status, or both tests were not included (e.g., patient will not be treated with checkpoint inhibitor therapy, no residual carcinoma is present in the sample [tissue exhausted or status post neoadjuvant treatment], insufficient tumor for testing) M

M1195 Surgical pathology reports that do not contain impression or conclusion of or recommendation for testing of MMR by immunohistochemistry, MSI by DNA-based testing status, or both, reason not given M

M1196 Initial (index visit) numeric rating scale (NRS), visual rating scale (VRS), or ItchyQuant assessment score of greater than or equal to 4 M

M1197 Itch severity assessment score is reduced by three or more points from the initial (index) assessment score to the follow-up visit score M

M1198 Itch severity assessment score was not reduced by at least three points from initial (index) score to the follow-up visit score or assessment was not completed during the follow-up encounter M

M1199 Patients receiving RRT M

M1200 Ace inhibitor (ACE-I) or ARB therapy prescribed during the measurement period M

M1201 Documentation of medical reason(s) for not prescribing ACE inhibitor (ACE-I) or ARB therapy during the measurement period (e.g., pregnancy, history of angioedema to ACE-I, other allergy to ACE-I and ARB, hyperkalemia or history of hyperkalemia while on ACE-I or ARB therapy, acute kidney injury due to ACE-I or ARB therapy), other medical reasons) M

M1202 Documentation of patient reason(s) for not prescribing ACE inhibitor or ARB therapy during the measurement period, (e.g., patient declined, other patient reasons) M

M1203 Ace inhibitor or ARB therapy not prescribed during the measurement period, reason not given M

M1204 Initial (index visit) numeric rating scale (NRS), visual rating scale (VRS), or ItchyQuant assessment score of greater than or equal to 4 M

M1205 Itch severity assessment score is reduced by three or more points from the initial (index) assessment score to the follow-up visit score M

M1206 Itch severity assessment score was not reduced by at least three points from initial (index) score to the follow-up visit score or assessment was not completed during the follow-up encounter M

M1207 Patient is screened for food insecurity, housing instability, transportation needs, utility difficulties, and interpersonal safety M

M1208 Patient is not screened for food insecurity, housing instability, transportation needs, utility difficulties, and interpersonal safety M

M1209 At least two orders for high-risk medications from the same drug class, (Table 4), without appropriate diagnoses M
AHA: 2Q,23

M1210 At least two orders for high-risk medications from the same drug class, (Table 4), not ordered M

▲ **M1211** Most recent glycemic status assessment (HbA1c or GMI) level > 9.0% M

▲ **M1212** Glycemic status assessment (HbA1c or GMI) level is missing, or was not performed during the measurement period M

M1213 No history of spirometry results with confirmed airflow obstruction (FEV1/FVC < 70%) and present spirometry is >= 70% M

M1214 Spirometry results with confirmed airflow obstruction (FEV1/FVC < 70%) documented and reviewed M

M1215 Documentation of medical reason(s) for not documenting and reviewing spirometry results (e.g., patients with dementia or tracheostomy) M

M1216 No spirometry results with confirmed airflow obstruction FEV1/FVC < 70%) documented and/or no spirometry performed with results documented during the encounter M

M1217 Documentation of system reason(s) for not documenting and reviewing spirometry results (e.g., spirometry equipment not available at the time of the encounter) M

M1218 Patient has COPD symptoms (e.g., dyspnea, cough/sputum, wheezing) M

~~M1219 Anaphylaxis due to the vaccine on or before the date of the encounter~~

M1220 Dilated retinal eye exam with interpretation by an ophthalmologist or optometrist or artificial intelligence (AI) interpretation documented and reviewed; with evidence of retinopathy M

M1221 Dilated retinal eye exam with interpretation by an ophthalmologist or optometrist or artificial intelligence (AI) interpretation documented and reviewed; without evidence of retinopathy M

M1222 Glaucoma plan of care not documented, reason not otherwise specified M

M1223 Glaucoma plan of care documented M

M1224 Intraocular pressure (IOP) reduced by a value less than 20% from the pre-intervention level M

M1225 Intraocular pressure (IOP) reduced by a value of greater than or equal to 20% from the pre-intervention level M

M1226 IOP measurement not documented, reason not otherwise specified M

M1227 Evidence-based therapy was prescribed M

M1228 Patient, who has a reactive HCV antibody test, and has a follow up HCV viral test that detected HCV viremia, has HCV treatment initiated within 3 months of the reactive HCV antibody test M

M1229 Patient, who has a reactive HCV antibody test, and has a follow up HCV viral test that detected HCV viremia, is referred within 1 month of the reactive HCV antibody test to a clinician who treats HCV infection M

M1230 Patient has a reactive HCV antibody test and does not have a follow-up HCV viral test, or patient has a reactive HCV antibody test and has a follow-up HCV viral test that detects HCV viremia and is not referred to a clinician who treats HCV infection within 1 month and does not have HCV treatment initiated within 3 months of the reactive HCV antibody test, reason not given M

M1231 Patient receives HCV antibody test with nonreactive result M

M1232 Patient receives HCV antibody test with reactive result M

M1233 Patient does not receive HCV antibody test or patient does receive HCV antibody test but results not documented, reason not given M

M1234 Patient has a reactive HCV antibody test, and has a follow-up HCV viral test that does not detect HCV viremia M

M1235 Documentation or patient report of HCV antibody test or HCV RNA test which occurred prior to the performance period M

M1236 Baseline MRS > 2 M

M1237 Patient reason for not screening for food insecurity, housing instability, transportation needs, utility difficulties, and interpersonal safety (e.g., patient declined or other patient reasons) M

M1238 Documentation that administration of second recombinant zoster vaccine could not occur during the performance period due to the recommended 2 to 6 month interval between doses (i.e, first dose received after October 31) M

M1239 Patient did not respond to the question of "Patient felt heard and understood by this provider and team" M

M1240 Patient did not respond to the question of "Patient felt this provider and team put my best interests first when making recommendations about my care" M

M1241 Patient did not respond to the question of "Patient felt this provider and team saw me as a person, not just someone with a medical problem" M

M1242 Patient did not respond to the question of "Patient felt this provider and team understood what is important to me in my life" M

M1243 Patient provided a response other than "completely true" for the question of "Patient felt heard and understood by this provider and team" M

M1244 Patient provided a response other than "completely true" for the question of "Patient felt this provider and team put my best interests first when making recommendations about my care" M

M1245 Patient provided a response other than "completely true" for the question of "Patient felt this provider and team saw me as a person, not just someone with a medical problem" M

M1246 Patient provided a response other than "completely true" for the question of "Patient felt this provider and team understood what is important to me in my life" M

M1247 Patient responded "completely true" for the question of "Patient felt this provider and team put my best interests first when making recommendations about my care" M

M1248 Patient responded "completely true" for the question of "Patient felt this provider and team saw me as a person, not just someone with a medical problem" M

M1249 Patient responded "completely true" for the question of "Patient felt this provider and team understood what is important to me in my life" M

M1250 Patient responded as "completely true" for the question of "Patient felt heard and understood by this provider and team" M

M1251 Patients for whom a proxy completed the entire HU survey on their behalf for any reason (no patient involvement) M

M1252 Patients who did not complete at least one of the four patient experience HU survey items and return the HU survey within 60 days of the ambulatory palliative care visit M

M1253 Patients who respond on the patient experience HU survey that they did not receive care by the listed ambulatory palliative care provider in the last 60 days (disavowal) M

M1254 Patients who were deceased when the HU survey reached them M

M1255 Patients who have another reason for visiting the clinic [not prenatal or postpartum care] and have a positive pregnancy test but have not established the clinic as an OB provider (e.g., plan to terminate the pregnancy or seek prenatal services elsewhere) M

M1256 Prior history of known CVD M

M1257 CVD risk assessment not performed or incomplete (e.g., CVD risk assessment was not documented), reason not otherwise specified M

M1258 CVD risk assessment performed, have a documented calculated risk score M

▲ M1259 Patient status documented within the first year of initiating dialysis M

▲ M1260 Patient status not documented within the first year of initiating dialysis M

M1261 Patients who were on the kidney or kidney-pancreas waitlist prior to initiation of dialysis M

M1262 Patients who had a transplant prior to initiation of dialysis M

M1263 Patients in hospice on their initiation of dialysis date or during the month of evaluation M

M1264 ~~Patients age 75 or older on their initiation of dialysis date~~

M1265 CMS Medical Evidence Form 2728 for dialysis patients: initial form completed M

M1266 Patients admitted to a skilled nursing facility (SNF) M

▲ M1267 Patients not observed in active status on any kidney or kidney-pancreas transplant waitlist as of the last day of each month during the measurement period M

▲ M1268 Patients observed in active status on any kidney or kidney-pancreas transplant waitlist as of the last day of each month during the measurement period M

M1269 Receiving ESRD MCP dialysis services by the provider on the last day of the reporting month M

M1270 Patients not on any kidney or kidney-pancreas transplant waitlist as of the last day of each month during the measurement period M

M1271 Patients with dementia at any time prior to or during the month M

▲ M1272 Patients observed on any kidney or kidney-pancreas transplant waitlist as of the last day of each month during the measurement period M

M1273 Patients who were admitted to a skilled nursing facility (SNF) within 1 year of dialysis initiation according to the CMS-2728 Form M

M1274 Patients who were admitted to a skilled nursing facility (SNF) during the month of evaluation were excluded from that month M

M1275 Patients determined to be in hospice were excluded from month of evaluation and the remainder of reporting period M

M1276 BMI documented outside normal parameters, no follow-up plan documented, no reason given M

M1277 Colorectal cancer screening results documented and reviewed M

M1278 Elevated or hypertensive blood pressure reading documented, and the indicated follow-up is documented M

M1279 Elevated or hypertensive blood pressure reading documented, indicated follow-up not documented, reason not given M

M1280 Women who had a bilateral mastectomy or who have a history of a bilateral mastectomy or for whom there is evidence of a right and a left unilateral mastectomy M

M1281 Blood pressure reading not documented, reason not given M

M1282 Patient screened for tobacco use and identified as a tobacco non-user M

M1283 Patient screened for tobacco use and identified as a tobacco user M

M1284 Patients age 66 or older in institutional special needs plans (SNP) or residing in long-term care with POS code 32, 33, 34, 54, or 56 for more than 90 consecutive days during the measurement period M

M1285 Screening, diagnostic, film, digital or digital breast tomosynthesis (3D) mammography results were not documented and reviewed, reason not otherwise specified M

M1286 BMI is documented as being outside of normal parameters, follow-up plan is not completed for documented medical reason M

M1287 BMI is documented below normal parameters and a follow-up plan is documented M

M1288 Documented reason for not screening or recommending a follow-up for high blood pressure M

M1289 Patient identified as tobacco user did not receive tobacco cessation intervention during the measurement period or in the 6 months prior to the measurement period (counseling and/or pharmacotherapy) M

M1290 Patient not eligible due to active diagnosis of hypertension M

M1291 Patients 66 years of age and older with at least one claim/encounter for frailty during the measurement period and a dispensed medication for dementia during the measurement period or the year prior to the measurement period M

▲ **M1292** Patients 66 years of age and older with at least one claim/encounter for frailty during the measurement period and an advanced illness diagnosis during the measurement period or the year prior to the measurement period M

M1293 BMI is documented above normal parameters and a follow-up plan is documented M

M1294 Normal blood pressure reading documented, follow-up not required M

M1295 Patients with a diagnosis or past history of total colectomy or colorectal cancer M

M1296 BMI is documented within normal parameters and no follow-up plan is required M

M1297 BMI not documented due to medical reason or patient refusal of height or weight measurement M

M1298 Documentation of patient pregnancy anytime during the measurement period prior to and including the current encounter M

M1299 Influenza immunization administered or previously received M

M1300 Influenza immunization was not administered for reasons documented by clinician (e.g., patient allergy or other medical reasons, patient declined or other patient reasons, vaccine not available or other system reasons) M

M1301 Patient identified as a tobacco user received tobacco cessation intervention during the measurement period or in the 6 months prior to the measurement period (counseling and/or pharmacotherapy) M

M1302 Screening, diagnostic, film digital or digital breast tomosynthesis (3D) mammography results documented and reviewed M

M1303 Hospice services provided to patient any time during the measurement period M

M1304 Patient did not receive any pneumococcal conjugate or polysaccharide vaccine on or after their 19th birthday and before the end of the measurement period M

M1305 Patient received any pneumococcal conjugate or polysaccharide vaccine on or after their 19th birthday and before the end of the measurement period M

M1306 Patient had anaphylaxis due to the pneumococcal vaccine any time during or before the measurement period M

M1307 Documentation stating the patient has received or is currently receiving palliative or hospice care M

M1308 Influenza immunization was not administered, reason not given M

M1309 Palliative care services provided to patient any time during the measurement period M

M1310 Patient screened for tobacco use and received tobacco cessation intervention during the measurement period or in the 6 months prior to the measurement period (counseling, pharmacotherapy, or both), if identified as a tobacco user M

M1311 Anaphylaxis due to the vaccine on or before the date of the encounter M

M1312 Patient not screened for tobacco use M

M1313 Tobacco screening not performed or tobacco cessation intervention not provided during the measurement period or in the 6 months prior to the measurement period M

M1314 BMI not documented and no reason is given M

M1315 Colorectal cancer screening results were not documented and reviewed; reason not otherwise specified M

M1316 Current tobacco non-user M

M1317 Patients who are counseled on connection with a CSP and explicitly opt out M

M1318 Patients who did not have documented contact with a CSP for at least one of their screened positive HRSNS within 60 days after screening or documentation that there was no contact with a CSP M

M1319 Patients who had documented contact with a CSP for at least one of their screened positive HRSNS within 60 days after screening M

M1320 Patients who screened positive for at least 1 of the 5 HRSNS M

M1321 Patients who were not seen within 7 weeks following the date of injection for follow-up or who did not have a documented IOP or no plan of care documented if the IOP was >25 mm Hg M

M1322 Patients seen within 7 weeks following the date of injection and are screened for elevated intraocular pressure (IOP) with tonometry with documented IOP =<25 mm Hg for injected eye M

M1323 Patients seen within 7 weeks following the date of injection and are screened for elevated intraocular pressure (IOP) with tonometry with documented IOP >25 mm Hg and a plan of care was documented M

M1324 Patients who had an intravitreal or periocular corticosteroid injection (e.g., triamcinolone, preservative-free triamcinolone, dexamethasone, dexamethasone intravitreal implant, or fluocinolone intravitreal implant) M

M1325 Patients who were not seen for reasons documented by clinician for patient or medical reasons (e.g., inadequate time for follow-up, patients who received a prior intravitreal or periocular steroid injection within the last 6 months and had a subsequent IOP evaluation with IOP <25mm Hg within 7 weeks of treatment) M

M1326 Patients with a diagnosis of hypotony M

M1327 Patients who were not appropriately evaluated during the initial exam and/or who were not re-evaluated within 8 weeks M

M1328 Patients with a diagnosis of acute vitreous hemorrhage M

M1329 Patients with a post-operative encounter of the eye with the acute PVD within 2 weeks before the initial encounter or 8 weeks after initial acute PVD encounter M

M1330 Documentation of patient reason(s) for not having a follow-up exam (e.g., inadequate time for follow-up) M

M1331 Patients who were appropriately evaluated during the initial exam and were re-evaluated no later than 8 weeks from initial exam M

M1332 Patients who were not appropriately evaluated during the initial exam and/or who were not re-evaluated within 2 weeks M

M1333 Acute vitreous hemorrhage M

M1334 Patients with a post-operative encounter of the eye with the acute PVD within 2 weeks before the initial encounter or 2 weeks after initial acute PVD encounter M

M1335 Documentation of patient reason(s) for not having a follow-up exam (e.g., inadequate time for follow-up) M

M1336 Patients who were appropriately evaluated during the initial exam and were re-evaluated no later than 2 weeks M

M1337 Acute PVD M

M1338 Patients who had follow-up assessment 30 to 180 days after the index assessment who did not demonstrate positive improvement or maintenance of functioning scores during the performance period M

M1339 Patients who had follow-up assessment 30 to 180 days after the index assessment who demonstrated positive improvement or maintenance of functioning scores during the performance period M

M1340 Index assessment completed using the 12-item WHODAS 2.0 or SDS during the denominator identification period M

M1341 Patients who did not have a follow-up assessment or did not have an assessment within 30 to 180 days after the index assessment during the performance period M

M1342 Patients who died during the performance period M

▲ **M1343** Patients who are at PAM level 4 at baseline or patients who are flagged with extreme straight line response sets on the PAM or with excessive missing responses M

▲ **M1344** Patients who did not have a baseline PAM score and/or a second score within 4 to 12 months of baseline PAM score M

▲ **M1345** Patients who had a baseline PAM score and a second score within 4 to 12 months of baseline PAM score M

▲ **M1346** Patients who did not have a net increase in PAM score of at least 6 points within a 4 to 12 month period M

▲ **M1347** Patients who achieved a net increase in PAM score of at least 3 points in a 4 to 12 month period (passing) M

▲ **M1348** Patients who achieved a net increase in PAM score of at least 6 points in a 4 to 12 month period (excellent) M

▲ **M1349** Patients who did not have a net increase in PAM score of at least 3 points within a 4 to 12 month period M

M1350 Patients who had a completed suicide safety plan initiated, reviewed, or updated in collaboration with their clinician (concurrent or within 24 hours of the index clinical encounter) M

M1351 Patients who had a suicide safety plan initiated, reviewed, or updated and reviewed and updated in collaboration with the patient and their clinician (concurrent or within 24 hours of clinical encounter and within 120 days after initiation) M

M1352 Suicidal ideation and/or behavior symptoms based on the C-SSRS or equivalent assessment M

M1353 Patients who did not have a completed suicide safety plan initiated, reviewed, or updated in collaboration with their clinician (concurrent or within 24 hours of the index clinical encounter) M

M1354 Patients who did not have a suicide safety plan initiated, reviewed, or updated or reviewed and updated in collaboration with the patient and their clinician (concurrent or within 24 hours of clinical encounter and within 120 days after initiation) M

M1355 Suicide risk based on their clinician's evaluation or a clinician-rated tool M

M1356 Patients who died during the measurement period M

M1357 Patients who had a reduction in suicidal ideation and/or behavior upon follow-up assessment within 120 days of index assessment M

M1358 Patients who did not have a reduction in suicidal ideation and/or behavior upon follow-up assessment within 120 days of index assessment M

M1359 Index assessment during the denominator period when the suicidal ideation and/or behavior symptoms or increased suicide risk by clinician determination occurs and a non-zero C-SSRS score is obtained M

M1360 Suicidal ideation and/or behavior symptoms based on the C-SSRS M

M1361 Suicide risk based on their clinician's evaluation or a clinician-rated tool M

M1362 Patients who died during the measurement period M

M1363 Patients who did not have a follow-up assessment within 120 days of the index assessment M

M1364 Calculated 10-year ASCVD risk score of >=20 percent during the performance period M

M1365 Patient encounter during the performance period with hospice and palliative care specialty code 17 M

M1366 Focusing on women's health MIPS value pathway M

M1367 Quality care for the treatment of ear, nose, and throat disorders MIPS value pathway M

M1368 Prevention and treatment of infectious disorders including hepatitis C and HIV MIPS value pathway M

M1369 Quality care in mental health and substance use disorders MIPS value pathway M

M1370 Rehabilitative support for musculoskeletal care MIPS value pathway M

● **M1371** Most recent glycemic status assessment (HbA1c or GMI) level < 7.0%

● M1372 Most recent glycemic status assessment (HbA1c or GMI) level >= 7.0% and < 8.0%

● M1373 Most recent glycemic status assessment (HbA1c or GMI) level >= 8.0% and <= 9.0%

● M1374 An additional encounter with an RA diagnosis during the performance period or prior performance period that is at least 90 days before or after an encounter with an RA diagnosis during the performance period

● M1375 An additional encounter with an RA diagnosis during the performance period or prior performance period that is at least 90 days before or after an encounter with an RA diagnosis during the performance period

● M1376 An additional encounter with an RA diagnosis during the performance period or prior performance period that is at least 90 days before or after an encounter with an RA diagnosis during the performance period

● M1377 Recommended follow-up interval for repeat colonoscopy of 10 years documented in colonoscopy report and communicated with patient

● M1378 Documentation of medical reason(s) for not recommending a 10 year follow-up interval (e.g., inadequate prep, familial or personal history of colonic polyps, patient had no adenoma and age is >= 66 years old, or life expectancy < 10 years, other medical reasons)

● M1379 A 10 year follow-up interval for colonoscopy not recommended, reason not otherwise specified

● M1380 Filled at least two prescriptions during the performance period for any combination of the qualifying oral antipsychotic medications listed under "denominator note" or the long-acting injectable antipsychotic medications listed under "denominator note"

● M1381 Patients with secondary stroke (e.g., a subsequent stroke that may occur with vasospasm in the setting of subarachnoid hemorrhage) within 5 days of the initial procedure

● M1382 Patient encounter during the performance period with Place of Service code 11

● M1383 Acute PVD

● M1384 Patients who died during the performance period

● M1385 Documentation of patient reasons for patients who were not seen for the second PAM survey (e.g., less than 4 months between baseline PAM assessment and follow-up)

● M1386 Patients with an excisional surgery for melanoma or melanoma in situ in the past 5 years with an initial AJCC staging of 0, I, or II at the start of the performance period

● M1387 Patients who died during the performance period

● M1388 Patients with documentation of an exam performed for recurrence of melanoma

● M1389 Documentation of patient reasons for no examination, (i.e., refusal of examination or lost to follow-up) (documentation must include information that the clinician was unable to reach the patient by phone, mail, or secure electronic mail - at least one method must be documented)

● M1390 Patients who do not have a documented exam performed for recurrence of melanoma or no documentation within the performance period

● M1391 All patients who were diagnosed with recurrent melanoma during the current performance period

● M1392 Documentation of patient reasons for no examination, (i.e., refusal of examination or lost to follow-up) (documentation must include information that the clinician was unable to reach the patient by phone, mail, or secure electronic mail - at least one method must be documented)

● M1393 Patients who were not diagnosed with recurrent melanoma during the current performance period

● M1394 Stages I-III breast cancer

● M1395 Patients receiving an initial chemotherapy regimen with a defined duration with the eligible clinician or group

● M1396 Patients on a therapeutic clinical trial

● M1397 Patients with recurrence/disease progression

● M1398 Patients with baseline and follow-up PROMIS surveys documented in the medical record

● M1399 Patients who leave the practice during the follow-up period

● M1400 Patients who died during the follow-up period

● M1401 Stages I-III breast cancer

● M1402 Patients receiving an initial chemotherapy regimen with a defined duration with the eligible clinician or group

● M1403 Patients with baseline and follow-up PROMIS surveys documented in the medical record

● M1404 Patients on a therapeutic clinical trial

● M1405 Patients with recurrence/disease progression

● M1406 Patients who leave the practice during the follow-up period

● M1407 Patients who died during the follow-up period

● M1408 Patients who have germline BRCA testing completed before diagnosis of epithelial ovarian, fallopian tube, or primary peritoneal cancer

● M1409 Patients who received germline testing for BRCA1 and BRCA2 or genetic counseling completed within 6 months of diagnosis

● M1410 Patients who did not have germline testing for BRCA1 and BRCA2 or genetic counseling completed within 6 months of diagnosis

● M1411 Currently on first-line immune checkpoint inhibitors without chemotherapy

● M1412 Patients with metastatic NSCLC with epidermal growth factor receptor (EGFR) mutations, ALK genomic tumor aberrations, or other targetable genomic abnormalities with approved first-line targeted therapy, such as NSCLC with ROS1 rearrangement, BRAF V600E mutation, NTRK 1/2/3 gene fusion, METex14 skipping mutation, and RET rearrangement

● M1413 Patients who had a positive PD-L1 biomarker expression test result prior to the initiation of first-line immune checkpoint inhibitor therapy

● M1414 Documentation of medical reason(s) for not performing the PD-L1 biomarker expression test prior to initiation of first-line immune checkpoint inhibitor therapy (e.g., patient is in an urgent or emergent situation where delay of treatment would jeopardize the patient's health status; other medical reasons/contraindication)

● M1415 Patients who did not have a positive PD-L1 biomarker expression test result prior to the initiation of first-line immune checkpoint inhibitor therapy

● M1416 Patient received hospice services any time during the performance period

● M1417 Patients who are up to date on their COVID-19 vaccinations as defined by CDC recommendations on current vaccination

● M1418 Patients who are not up to date on their COVID-19 vaccinations as defined by CDC recommendations on current vaccination because of a medical contraindication documented by clinician

● **M1419** **Patients who are not up to date on their COVID-19 vaccinations as defined by CDC recommendations on current vaccination**

● **M1420** **Complete ophthalmologic care MIPS value pathway**

● **M1421** **Dermatological care MIPS value pathway**

● **M1422** **Gastroenterology care MIPS value pathway**

● **M1423** **Optimal care for patients with urologic conditions MIPS value pathway**

● **M1424** **Pulmonology care MIPS value pathway**

● **M1425** **Surgical care MIPS value pathway**

Pathology and Laboratory Services P2028-P9615

P codes include chemistry, toxicology, and microbiology tests, screening Papanicolaou procedures, and various blood products.

Chemistry and Toxicology Tests

P2028 Cephalin flocculation, blood A
Code with caution: This test is considered obsolete. Submit documentation.

P2029 Congo red, blood A
Code with caution: This test is considered obsolete. Submit documentation.

P2031 Hair analysis (excluding arsenic) E1

P2033 Thymol turbidity, blood A
Code with caution: This test is considered obsolete. Submit documentation.

P2038 Mucoprotein, blood (seromucoid) (medical necessity procedure) A
Code with caution: This test is considered obsolete. Submit documentation.

Pathology Screening Tests

P3000 Screening Papanicolaou smear, cervical or vaginal, up to three smears, by technician under physician supervision A A
One Pap test is covered by Medicare every two years, unless the physician suspects cervical abnormalities and shortens the interval. See also G0123-G0124.
CMS: 100-02,15,280.4; 100-03,210.2.1; 100-04,18,1.2; 100-04,18,30.2.1; 100-04,18,30.5; 100-04,18,30.6

P3001 Screening Papanicolaou smear, cervical or vaginal, up to three smears, requiring interpretation by physician A B ⃠
One Pap test is covered by Medicare every two years, unless the physician suspects cervical abnormalities and shortens the interval. See also G0123-G0124.
CMS: 100-02,15,280.4; 100-03,210.2.1; 100-04,18,1.2; 100-04,18,30.2.1; 100-04,18,30.5; 100-04,18,30.6

Microbiology Tests

P7001 Culture, bacterial, urine; quantitative, sensitivity study E1

Miscellaneous

P9010 Blood (whole), for transfusion, per unit R ☑
CMS: 100-01,3,20.5; 100-01,3,20.5.2; 100-01,3,20.5.3; 100-02,1,10; 100-04,3,40.2.2

P9011 Blood, split unit R ☑
CMS: 100-01,3,20.5; 100-01,3,20.5.2; 100-01,3,20.5.3; 100-02,1,10; 100-04,3,40.2.2; 100-04,4,231.4

P9012 Cryoprecipitate, each unit R ☑
CMS: 100-02,1,10; 100-04,3,40.2.2

P9016 Red blood cells, leukocytes reduced, each unit R ☑
CMS: 100-02,1,10; 100-04,3,40.2.2

P9017 Fresh frozen plasma (single donor), frozen within 8 hours of collection, each unit R ☑
CMS: 100-02,1,10; 100-04,3,40.2.2

P9019 Platelets, each unit R ☑
CMS: 100-02,1,10; 100-04,3,40.2.2

P9020 Platelet rich plasma, each unit R ☑
CMS: 100-04,3,40.2.2

P9021 Red blood cells, each unit R ☑
CMS: 100-01,3,20.5; 100-01,3,20.5.2; 100-01,3,20.5.3; 100-02,1,10; 100-04,3,40.2.2

P9022 Red blood cells, washed, each unit R ☑
CMS: 100-01,3,20.5; 100-01,3,20.5.2; 100-01,3,20.5.3; 100-02,1,10; 100-04,3,40.2.2

P9023 Plasma, pooled multiple donor, solvent/detergent treated, frozen, each unit R ☑
CMS: 100-02,1,10; 100-04,3,40.2.2

P9025 Plasma, cryoprecipitate reduced, pathogen reduced, each unit R
AHA: 4Q,21

P9026 Cryoprecipitated fibrinogen complex, pathogen reduced, each unit R
AHA: 4Q,21

● **P9027** Red blood cells, leukocytes reduced, oxygen/ carbon dioxide reduced, each unit

P9031 Platelets, leukocytes reduced, each unit R ☑
CMS: 100-02,1,10; 100-04,3,40.2.2

P9032 Platelets, irradiated, each unit R ☑
CMS: 100-02,1,10; 100-04,3,40.2.2

P9033 Platelets, leukocytes reduced, irradiated, each unit R ☑
CMS: 100-02,1,10; 100-04,3,40.2.2

P9034 Platelets, pheresis, each unit R ☑
CMS: 100-02,1,10; 100-04,3,40.2.2

P9035 Platelets, pheresis, leukocytes reduced, each unit R ☑
CMS: 100-02,1,10; 100-04,3,40.2.2

P9036 Platelets, pheresis, irradiated, each unit R ☑
CMS: 100-02,1,10; 100-04,3,40.2.2

P9037 Platelets, pheresis, leukocytes reduced, irradiated, each unit R ☑
CMS: 100-02,1,10; 100-04,3,40.2.2

P9038 Red blood cells, irradiated, each unit R ☑
CMS: 100-01,3,20.5; 100-01,3,20.5.2; 100-01,3,20.5.3; 100-02,1,10; 100-04,3,40.2.2

P9039 Red blood cells, deglycerolized, each unit R ☑
CMS: 100-02,1,10; 100-04,3,40.2.2

P9040 Red blood cells, leukocytes reduced, irradiated, each unit R ☑
CMS: 100-02,1,10; 100-04,3,40.2.2

P9041 Infusion, albumin (human), 5%, 50 ml K K2 ☑
CMS: 100-02,1,10; 100-04,3,40.2.2

P9043 Infusion, plasma protein fraction (human), 5%, 50 ml R ☑
CMS: 100-02,1,10; 100-04,3,40.2.2

P9044 Plasma, cryoprecipitate reduced, each unit R ☑
CMS: 100-02,1,10; 100-04,3,40.2.2

P9045 Infusion, albumin (human), 5%, 250 ml K K2 ☑
CMS: 100-02,1,10; 100-04,3,40.2.2

P9046 Infusion, albumin (human), 25%, 20 ml K K2 ☑
CMS: 100-02,1,10; 100-04,3,40.2.2

P9047 Infusion, albumin (human), 25%, 50 ml K K2 ☑
CMS: 100-02,1,10; 100-04,3,40.2.2

P9048 Infusion, plasma protein fraction (human), 5%, 250 ml R ☑
CMS: 100-02,1,10; 100-04,3,40.2.2

P9050 Granulocytes, pheresis, each unit E1 ☑
CMS: 100-02,1,10; 100-03,110.5; 100-04,3,40.2.2

P9051 Whole blood or red blood cells, leukocytes reduced, CMV-negative, each unit R ☑
CMS: 100-02,1,10; 100-04,3,40.2.2

P9052 Platelets, HLA-matched leukocytes reduced, apheresis/pheresis, each unit R ☑
CMS: 100-02,1,10; 100-04,3,40.2.2

P9053 Platelets, pheresis, leukocytes reduced, CMV-negative, irradiated, each unit R ☑
CMS: 100-02,1,10; 100-04,3,40.2.2

Pathology and Laboratory Services

P2028 — P9053

P9054 **Whole blood or red blood cells, leukocytes reduced, frozen, deglycerol, washed, each unit** R ☑
CMS: 100-02,1,10; 100-04,3,40.2.2

P9055 **Platelets, leukocytes reduced, CMV-negative, apheresis/pheresis, each unit** R ☑
CMS: 100-02,1,10; 100-04,3,40.2.2

P9056 **Whole blood, leukocytes reduced, irradiated, each unit** R ☑
CMS: 100-02,1,10; 100-04,3,40.2.2

P9057 **Red blood cells, frozen/deglycerolized/washed, leukocytes reduced, irradiated, each unit** R ☑
CMS: 100-02,1,10; 100-04,3,40.2.2

P9058 **Red blood cells, leukocytes reduced, CMV-negative, irradiated, each unit** R ☑
CMS: 100-02,1,10; 100-04,3,40.2.2

P9059 **Fresh frozen plasma between 8-24 hours of collection, each unit** R ☑
CMS: 100-02,1,10; 100-04,3,40.2.2

P9060 **Fresh frozen plasma, donor retested, each unit** R ☑
CMS: 100-02,1,10; 100-04,3,40.2.2

P9070 **Plasma, pooled multiple donor, pathogen reduced, frozen, each unit** R

P9071 **Plasma (single donor), pathogen reduced, frozen, each unit** R

P9073 **Platelets, pheresis, pathogen-reduced, each unit** R

P9099 **Blood component or product not otherwise classified** R

P9100 **Pathogen(s) test for platelets** S

P9603 **Travel allowance, one way in connection with medically necessary laboratory specimen collection drawn from homebound or nursing homebound patient; prorated miles actually travelled** A ☑
CMS: 100-04,16,60; 100-04,16,60.2

P9604 **Travel allowance, one way in connection with medically necessary laboratory specimen collection drawn from homebound or nursing homebound patient; prorated trip charge** A ☑
CMS: 100-04,16,60; 100-04,16,60.2

P9612 **Catheterization for collection of specimen, single patient, all places of service** A
CMS: 100-04,16,60; 100-04,16,60.1.2

P9615 **Catheterization for collection of specimen(s) (multiple patients)** N
CMS: 100-04,16,60; 100-04,16,60.1.2; 100-04,16,60.1.4

Q Codes (Temporary) Q0035-Q9998

Temporary Q codes are used to pay health care providers for supplies, drugs, and biologicals to which no permanent code has been assigned.

Q0035 **Cardiokymography** Q1 N1

Covered only in conjunction with electrocardiographic stress testing in male patients with atypical angina or nonischemic chest pain, or female patients with angina.

Q0081 **Infusion therapy, using other than chemotherapeutic drugs, per visit** B ☑

Q0083 **Chemotherapy administration by other than infusion technique only (e.g., subcutaneous, intramuscular, push), per visit** B ☑

Q0084 **Chemotherapy administration by infusion technique only, per visit** B ☑

Q0085 **Chemotherapy administration by both infusion technique and other technique(s) (e.g. subcutaneous, intramuscular, push), per visit** B ☑

Q0091 **Screening Papanicolaou smear; obtaining, preparing and conveyance of cervical or vaginal smear to laboratory** A S ⊘

One pap test is covered by Medicare every two years for low risk patients and every one year for high risk patients. Q0091 can be reported with an E/M code when a separately identifiable E/M service is provided.

CMS: 100-02,13,220; 100-02,13,220.1; 100-02,13,220.3; 100-02,15,280.4; 100-03,210.2.1; 100-04,18,1.2; 100-04,18,30.2.1; 100-04,18,30.5; 100-04,18,30.6; 1004-04,13,220.1

AHA: 2Q,24

Q0092 **Set-up portable x-ray equipment** N N1

CMS: 100-04,13,90.4

Q0111 **Wet mounts, including preparations of vaginal, cervical or skin specimens** A

Q0112 **All potassium hydroxide (KOH) preparations** A

Q0113 **Pinworm examinations** A

Q0114 **Fern test** A

Q0115 **Postcoital direct, qualitative examinations of vaginal or cervical mucous** A A

Q0138 **Injection, ferumoxytol, for treatment of iron deficiency anemia, 1 mg (non-ESRD use)** K K2 ☑

Use this code for Feraheme.

Q0139 **Injection, ferumoxytol, for treatment of iron deficiency anemia, 1 mg (for ESRD on dialysis)** K K2 ☑

Use this code for Feraheme.

Q0144 **Azithromycin dihydrate, oral, capsules/powder, 1 g** E1 ☑

Use this code for Zithromax, Zithromax Z-PAK.

● **Q0155** **Dronabinol (Syndros), 0.1 mg, oral, FDA-approved prescription anti-emetic, for use as a complete therapeutic substitute for an IV anti-emetic at the time of chemotherapy treatment, not to exceed a 48 hour dosage regimen**

Q0161 **Chlorpromazine HCl, 5 mg, oral, FDA-approved prescription antiemetic, for use as a complete therapeutic substitute for an IV antiemetic at the time of chemotherapy treatment, not to exceed a 48-hour dosage regimen** N N1 ☑

CMS: 100-02,15,50.5.4; 100-03,110.18; 100-04,17,80.2.1

Q0162 **Ondansetron 1 mg, oral, FDA-approved prescription antiemetic, for use as a complete therapeutic substitute for an IV antiemetic at the time of chemotherapy treatment, not to exceed a 48-hour dosage regimen** N N1 ☑

Use this code for Zofran, Zuplenz.

CMS: 100-02,15,50.5.4; 100-03,110.18; 100-04,17,80.2.1

Q0163 **Diphenhydramine HCl, 50 mg, oral, FDA-approved prescription antiemetic, for use as a complete therapeutic substitute for an IV antiemetic at time of chemotherapy treatment not to exceed a 48-hour dosage regimen** N N1 ☑

See also J1200. Medicare covers at the time of chemotherapy if regimen doesn't exceed 48 hours. Submit on the same claim as the chemotherapy. Use this code for Truxadryl.

CMS: 100-02,15,50.5.4; 100-03,110.18; 100-04,17,80.2.1

AHA: 1Q,24; 4Q,19

Q0164 **Prochlorperazine maleate, 5 mg, oral, FDA-approved prescription antiemetic, for use as a complete therapeutic substitute for an IV antiemetic at the time of chemotherapy treatment, not to exceed a 48-hour dosage regimen** N N1 ☑

Medicare covers at the time of chemotherapy if regimen doesn't exceed 48 hours. Submit on the same claim as the chemotherapy. Use this code for Compazine.

CMS: 100-02,15,50.5.4; 100-03,110.18; 100-04,17,80.2.1

Q0166 **Granisetron HCl, 1 mg, oral, FDA-approved prescription antiemetic, for use as a complete therapeutic substitute for an IV antiemetic at the time of chemotherapy treatment, not to exceed a 24-hour dosage regimen** N N1 ☑

Medicare covers at the time of chemotherapy if regimen doesn't exceed 48 hours. Submit on the same claim as the chemotherapy. Use this code for Kytril.

CMS: 100-02,15,50.5.4; 100-03,110.18; 100-04,17,80.2.1

Q0167 **Dronabinol, 2.5 mg, oral, FDA-approved prescription antiemetic, for use as a complete therapeutic substitute for an IV antiemetic at the time of chemotherapy treatment, not to exceed a 48-hour dosage regimen** N N1 ☑

Medicare covers at the time of chemotherapy if regimen doesn't exceed 48 hours. Submit on the same claim as the chemotherapy. Use this code for Marinol.

CMS: 100-02,15,50.5.4; 100-03,110.18; 100-04,17,80.2.1

Q0169 **Promethazine HCl, 12.5 mg, oral, FDA-approved prescription antiemetic, for use as a complete therapeutic substitute for an IV antiemetic at the time of chemotherapy treatment, not to exceed a 48-hour dosage regimen** N N1 ☑

Medicare covers at the time of chemotherapy if regimen doesn't exceed 48 hours. Submit on the same claim as the chemotherapy. Use this code for Phenergan.

CMS: 100-02,15,50.5.4; 100-03,110.18; 100-04,17,80.2.1

Q0173 **Trimethobenzamide HCl, 250 mg, oral, FDA-approved prescription antiemetic, for use as a complete therapeutic substitute for an IV antiemetic at the time of chemotherapy treatment, not to exceed a 48-hour dosage regimen** E1 ☑

Medicare covers at the time of chemotherapy if regimen doesn't exceed 48 hours. Submit on the same claim as the chemotherapy. Use this code for Tebamide, T-Gen, Ticon, Tigan, Triban, Trimazide.

CMS: 100-02,15,50.5.4; 100-03,110.18; 100-04,17,80.2.1

Q0174 **Thiethylperazine maleate, 10 mg, oral, FDA-approved prescription antiemetic, for use as a complete therapeutic substitute for an IV antiemetic at the time of chemotherapy treatment, not to exceed a 48-hour dosage regimen** E1 ☑

Medicare covers at the time of chemotherapy if regimen doesn't exceed 48 hours. Submit on the same claim as the chemotherapy.

CMS: 100-02,15,50.5.4; 100-03,110.18; 100-04,17,80.2.1

Q0175 **Perphenazine, 4 mg, oral, FDA-approved prescription antiemetic, for use as a complete therapeutic substitute for an IV antiemetic at the time of chemotherapy treatment, not to exceed a 48-hour dosage regimen** N N1 ☑

Medicare covers at the time of chemotherapy if regimen doesn't exceed 48 hours. Submit on the same claim as the chemotherapy. Use this code for Trilifon.

CMS: 100-02,15,50.5.4; 100-03,110.18; 100-04,17,80.2.1

Q0177 **Hydroxyzine pamoate, 25 mg, oral, FDA-approved prescription antiemetic, for use as a complete therapeutic substitute for an IV antiemetic at the time of chemotherapy treatment, not to exceed a 48-hour dosage regimen** N N1 ☑

Medicare covers at the time of chemotherapy if regimen doesn't exceed 48 hours. Submit on the same claim as the chemotherapy. Use this code for Vistaril.

CMS: 100-02,15,50.5.4; 100-03,110.18; 100-04,17,80.2.1

Q0180 **Dolasetron mesylate, 100 mg, oral, FDA-approved prescription antiemetic, for use as a complete therapeutic substitute for an IV antiemetic at the time of chemotherapy treatment, not to exceed a 24-hour dosage regimen** N N1 ☑

Medicare covers at the time of chemotherapy if regimen doesn't exceed 24 hours. Submit on the same claim as the chemotherapy. Use this code for Anzemet.

CMS: 100-02,15,50.5.4; 100-03,110.18; 100-04,17,80.2.1

Q0181 **Unspecified oral dosage form, FDA-approved prescription antiemetic, for use as a complete therapeutic substitute for an IV antiemetic at the time of chemotherapy treatment, not to exceed a 48-hour dosage regimen** N N1 ☑

Medicare covers at the time of chemotherapy if regimen doesn't exceed 48-hours. Submit on the same claim as the chemotherapy.

CMS: 100-02,15,50.5.4; 100-03,110.18; 100-04,17,80.2.1

AHA: 1Q,24; 4Q,19

Q0220 **Injection, tixagevimab and cilgavimab, for the pre-exposure prophylaxis only, for certain adults and pediatric individuals (12 years of age and older weighing at least 40kg) with no known SARS-CoV-2 exposure, who either have moderate to severely compromised immune systems or for whom vaccination with any available COVID-19 vaccine is not recommended due to a history of severe adverse reaction to a COVID-19 vaccine(s) and/or COVID-19 vaccine component(s), 300 mg** L L1

Use this code for tixagevimab and cilgavimab (Evusheld) 300 mg administered as pre-exposure prophylaxis. Report also M0220 or M0221 for administration.

Q0221 **Injection, tixagevimab and cilgavimab, for the pre-exposure prophylaxis only, for certain adults and pediatric individuals (12 years of age and older weighing at least 40kg) with no known SARS-CoV-2 exposure, who either have moderate to severely compromised immune systems or for whom vaccination with any available COVID-19 vaccine is not recommended due to a history of severe adverse reaction to a COVID-19 vaccine(s) and/or COVID-19 vaccine component(s), 600 mg** L L1

AHA: 2Q,22

Q0222 **Injection, bebtelovimab, 175 mg** K L1

AHA: 2Q,22

● **Q0224** **Injection, pemivibart, for the pre-exposure prophylaxis only, for certain adults and adolescents (12 years of age and older weighing at least 40 kg) with no known SARS-CoV-2 exposure, and who either have moderate-to-severe immune compromise due to a medical condition or receipt of immunosuppressive medications or treatments, and are unlikely to mount an adequate immune response to COVID-19 vaccination, 4500 mg** L1

AHA: 3Q,24

Q0240 **Injection, casirivimab and imdevimab, 600 mg** L L1

Use this code for casirivimab and imdevimab 600 mg administered as post exposure prophylaxis. Report also M0240 or M0241 for administration.

AHA: 4Q,21; 3Q,21

Q0243 **Injection, casirivimab and imdevimab, 2400 mg** L L1

Use this code for Casirivimab and Imdevimab (REGN-COV2), Regeneron.

AHA: 1Q,21; 4Q,20

Q0244 **Injection, casirivimab and imdevimab, 1200 mg** L L1

AHA: 4Q,21

Q0245 **Injection, bamlanivimab and etesevimab, 2100 mg** L L1

Use this code for Eli Lilly's bamlanivimab (LY-CoV555) 700 mg and etesevimab (LY-CoV016) 1400 mg, administered together.

AHA: 1Q,21

Q0247 **Injection, sotrovimab, 500 mg** L L1

AHA: 3Q,21

Q0249 **Injection, tocilizumab, for hospitalized adults and pediatric patients (2 years of age and older) with COVID-19 who are receiving systemic corticosteroids and require supplemental oxygen, non-invasive or invasive mechanical ventilation, or extracorporeal membrane oxygenation (ECMO) only, 1 mg** L L1

AHA: 4Q,21

Q0477 **Power module patient cable for use with electric or electric/pneumatic ventricular assist device, replacement only** A ♿

Q0478 **Power adapter for use with electric or electric/pneumatic ventricular assist device, vehicle type** A ♿

Q0479 **Power module for use with electric or electric/pneumatic ventricular assist device, replacement only** A ♿

Q0480 **Driver for use with pneumatic ventricular assist device, replacement only** A ♿

CMS: 100-04,32,320.3.4

Q0481 **Microprocessor control unit for use with electric ventricular assist device, replacement only** A ♿

CMS: 100-04,32,320.3.4

Q0482 **Microprocessor control unit for use with electric/pneumatic combination ventricular assist device, replacement only** A ♿

CMS: 100-04,32,320.3.4

Q0483 **Monitor/display module for use with electric ventricular assist device, replacement only** A ♿

CMS: 100-04,32,320.3.4

Q0484 **Monitor/display module for use with electric or electric/pneumatic ventricular assist device, replacement only** A ♿

CMS: 100-04,32,320.3.4

Q0485 **Monitor control cable for use with electric ventricular assist device, replacement only** A ♿

CMS: 100-04,32,320.3.4

Q0486 **Monitor control cable for use with electric/pneumatic ventricular assist device, replacement only** A ♿

CMS: 100-04,32,320.3.4

Q0487 **Leads (pneumatic/electrical) for use with any type electric/pneumatic ventricular assist device, replacement only** A ♿

CMS: 100-04,32,320.3.4

Q0488 **Power pack base for use with electric ventricular assist device, replacement only** A

CMS: 100-04,32,320.3.4

Q0489 **Power pack base for use with electric/pneumatic ventricular assist device, replacement only** A ♿

CMS: 100-04,32,320.3.4

Q0490 **Emergency power source for use with electric ventricular assist device, replacement only** A ♿

CMS: 100-04,32,320.3.4

Q0491 **Emergency power source for use with electric/pneumatic ventricular assist device, replacement only** A ♿

CMS: 100-04,32,320.3.4

Q0492 Emergency power supply cable for use with electric ventricular assist device, replacement only
CMS: 100-04,32,320.3.4

Q0493 Emergency power supply cable for use with electric/pneumatic ventricular assist device, replacement only
CMS: 100-04,32,320.3.4

Q0494 Emergency hand pump for use with electric or electric/pneumatic ventricular assist device, replacement only
CMS: 100-04,32,320.3.4

Q0495 Battery/power pack charger for use with electric or electric/pneumatic ventricular assist device, replacement only
CMS: 100-04,32,320.3.4

Q0496 Battery, other than lithium-ion, for use with electric or electric/pneumatic ventricular assist device, replacement only
CMS: 100-04,32,320.3.4

Q0497 Battery clips for use with electric or electric/pneumatic ventricular assist device, replacement only
CMS: 100-04,32,320.3.4

Q0498 Holster for use with electric or electric/pneumatic ventricular assist device, replacement only
CMS: 100-04,32,320.3.4

Q0499 Belt/vest/bag for use to carry external peripheral components of any type ventricular assist device, replacement only
CMS: 100-04,32,320.3.4

Q0500 Filters for use with electric or electric/pneumatic ventricular assist device, replacement only
The base unit for this code is for each filter.
CMS: 100-04,32,320.3.4

Q0501 Shower cover for use with electric or electric/pneumatic ventricular assist device, replacement only
CMS: 100-04,32,320.3.4

Q0502 Mobility cart for pneumatic ventricular assist device, replacement only
CMS: 100-04,32,320.3.4

Q0503 Battery for pneumatic ventricular assist device, replacement only, each
CMS: 100-04,32,320.3.4

Q0504 Power adapter for pneumatic ventricular assist device, replacement only, vehicle type
CMS: 100-04,32,320.3.4

Q0506 Battery, lithium-ion, for use with electric or electric/pneumatic ventricular assist device, replacement only
CMS: 100-04,32,320.3.4

Q0507 Miscellaneous supply or accessory for use with an external ventricular assist device
CMS: 100-04,32,320.3.4

Q0508 Miscellaneous supply or accessory for use with an implanted ventricular assist device
CMS: 100-04,32,320.3.4

Q0509 Miscellaneous supply or accessory for use with any implanted ventricular assist device for which payment was not made under Medicare Part A
CMS: 100-04,32,320.3.4

Q0510 Pharmacy supply fee for initial immunosuppressive drug(s), first month following transplant

Q0511 Pharmacy supply fee for oral anticancer, oral antiemetic, or immunosuppressive drug(s); for the first prescription in a 30-day period

Q0512 Pharmacy supply fee for oral anticancer, oral antiemetic, or immunosuppressive drug(s); for a subsequent prescription in a 30-day period

Q0513 Pharmacy dispensing fee for inhalation drug(s); per 30 days

Q0514 Pharmacy dispensing fee for inhalation drug(s); per 90 days

Q0515 Injection, sermorelin acetate, 1 mcg

Q0516 ~~Pharmacy supplying fee for HIV pre-exposure prophylaxis (PrEP) FDA-approved prescription oral drug, per 30-days~~

Q0517 ~~Pharmacy supplying fee for HIV pre-exposure prophylaxis (PrEP) FDA-approved prescription oral drug, per 60-days~~

Q0518 ~~Pharmacy supplying fee for HIV pre-exposure prophylaxis (PrEP) FDA-approved prescription oral drug, per 90-days~~

Q0519 ~~Pharmacy supplying fee for HIV pre-exposure prophylaxis (PrEP) FDA-approved prescription injectable drug, per 30-days~~

Q0520 ~~Pharmacy supplying fee for HIV pre-exposure prophylaxis (PrEP) FDA-approved prescription injectable drug, per 60-days~~

● **Q0521** Pharmacy supplying fee for HIV pre-exposure prophylaxis FDA-approved prescription

Q1004 New technology, intraocular lens, category 4 as defined in Federal Register notice

Q1005 New technology, intraocular lens, category 5 as defined in Federal Register notice

Q2004 Irrigation solution for treatment of bladder calculi, for example renacidin, per 500 ml

Q2009 Injection, fosphenytoin, 50 mg phenytoin equivalent
Use this code for Cerebyx.

Q2017 Injection, teniposide, 50 mg
Use this code for Vumon.

Q2026 Injection, Radiesse, 0.1 ml
CMS: 100-03,250.5; 100-04,32,260.1; 100-04,32,260.1.1; 100-04,32,260.2.1; 100-04,32,260.2.2

Q2028 Injection, sculptra, 0.5 mg
CMS: 100-04,32,260.1.1; 100-04,32,260.2.2

Q2034 Influenza virus vaccine, split virus, for intramuscular use (Agriflu)

Q2035 Influenza virus vaccine, split virus, when administered to individuals 3 years of age and older, for intramuscular use (AFLURIA)
CMS: 100-02,15,50.4.4.2

Q2036 Influenza virus vaccine, split virus, when administered to individuals 3 years of age and older, for intramuscular use (FLULAVAL)
CMS: 100-02,15,50.4.4.2

Q2037 Influenza virus vaccine, split virus, when administered to individuals 3 years of age and older, for intramuscular use (FLUVIRIN)
CMS: 100-02,15,50.4.4.2

Q2038 Influenza virus vaccine, split virus, when administered to individuals 3 years of age and older, for intramuscular use (Fluzone)
CMS: 100-02,15,50.4.4.2

Q2039 Influenza virus vaccine, not otherwise specified
CMS: 100-02,15,50.4.4.2

Q2041 **Axicabtagene ciloleucel, up to 200 million autologous anti-CD19 CAR positive T cells, including leukapheresis and dose preparation procedures, per therapeutic dose** K

Use this code for Yescarta.

CMS: 100-04,32,400; 100-04,32,400.1; 100-04,32,400.2; 100-04,32,400.2.1; 100-04,32,400.2.2; 100-04,32,400.2.3; 100-04,32,400.2.3.1; 100-04,32,400.2.4; 100-04,32,400.2.5; 100-04,32,400.3; 100-04,32,400.4; 100-04,32,66.2

AHA: 2Q,19; 2Q,18; 1Q,18

Q2042 **Tisagenlecleucel, up to 600 million CAR-positive viable T cells, including leukapheresis and dose preparation procedures, per therapeutic dose** K

Use this code for Kymriah.

CMS: 100-04,32,400; 100-04,32,400.1; 100-04,32,400.2; 100-04,32,400.2.1; 100-04,32,400.2.2; 100-04,32,400.2.3; 100-04,32,400.2.3.1; 100-04,32,400.2.4; 100-04,32,400.2.5; 100-04,32,400.3; 100-04,32,400.4; 100-04,32,66.2

AHA: 2Q,19; 1Q,19

Q2043 **Sipuleucel-T, minimum of 50 million autologous CD54+ cells activated with PAP-GM-CSF, including leukapheresis and all other preparatory procedures, per infusion** K K2 ☑

Use this code for PROVENGE.

CMS: 100-03,1,110.22; 100-03,110.22; 100-04,32,280.1; 100-04,32,280.2; 100-04,32,280.4; 100-04,32,280.5

Q2049 **Injection, doxorubicin HCl, liposomal, imported Lipodox, 10 mg** K K2 ☑

Q2050 **Injection, doxorubicin HCl, liposomal, not otherwise specified, 10 mg** K K2 ☑ ⃠

▲ **Q2052** **Services, supplies and accessories used in the home for the administration of intravenous immune globulin (IVIG)** A ☑

CMS: 100-04,20,213

AHA: 1Q,24

Q2053 **Brexucabtagene autoleucel, up to 200 million autologous anti-CD19 CAR positive viable T cells, including leukapheresis and dose preparation procedures, per therapeutic dose** K

Use this code for Tecartus.

CMS: 100-04,32,400; 100-04,32,400.1; 100-04,32,400.2; 100-04,32,400.2.1; 100-04,32,400.2.2; 100-04,32,400.2.3; 100-04,32,400.2.3.1; 100-04,32,400.2.4; 100-04,32,400.2.5; 100-04,32,400.3; 100-04,32,400.4

AHA: 1Q,21

Q2054 **Lisocabtagene maraleucel, up to 110 million autologous anti-CD19 CAR-positive viable T cells, including leukapheresis and dose preparation procedures, per therapeutic dose** G

Use this code for Breyanzi.

CMS: 100-04,32,400; 100-04,32,400.1; 100-04,32,400.2; 100-04,32,400.2.2; 100-04,32,400.2.3; 100-04,32,400.2.3.1; 100-04,32,400.2.4; 100-04,32,400.2.5; 100-04,32,400.3; 100-04,32,400.4

AHA: 4Q,21

▲ **Q2055** **Idecabtagene vicleucel, up to 510 million autologous B-cell maturation antigen (BCMA) directed CAR-positive T cells, including leukapheresis and dose preparation procedures, per therapeutic dose** G

Use this code for Abecma.

CMS: 100-04,32,400; 100-04,32,400.1; 100-04,32,400.2; 100-04,32,400.2.2; 100-04,32,400.2.3; 100-04,32,400.2.3.1; 100-04,32,400.2.4; 100-04,32,400.2.5; 100-04,32,400.3; 100-04,32,400.4

AHA: 3Q,24; 1Q,22

Q2056 **Ciltacabtagene autoleucel, up to 100 million autologous B-cell maturation antigen (BCMA) directed CAR-positive T cells, including leukapheresis and dose preparation procedures, per therapeutic dose** G

Use this code for Carvykti.

CMS: 100-04,32,400; 100-04,32,400.1; 100-04,32,400.2; 100-04,32,400.2.2; 100-04,32,400.2.3; 100-04,32,400.2.3.1; 100-04,32,400.2.4; 100-04,32,400.2.5; 100-04,32,400.3; 100-04,32,400.4

AHA: 4Q,22

Q3001 **Radioelements for brachytherapy, any type, each** B ☑ ⃠

Q3014 **Telehealth originating site facility fee** A ⃠

CMS: 100-04,12,190.5; 100-04,12,190.6; 100-04,39,30.5

Q3027 **Injection, interferon beta-1a, 1 mcg for intramuscular use** K K2 ☑

Use this code for Avonex.

CMS: 100-02,15,50.5

Q3028 **Injection, interferon beta-1a, 1 mcg for subcutaneous use** E1 ☑

Use this code for Rebif.

CMS: 100-02,15,50.5

Q3031 **Collagen skin test** N N1

Q4001 **Casting supplies, body cast adult, with or without head, plaster** A B ♿

CMS: 100-04,20,170

Q4002 **Cast supplies, body cast adult, with or without head, fiberglass** A B ♿

CMS: 100-04,20,170

Q4003 **Cast supplies, shoulder cast, adult (11 years +), plaster** A B ♿

CMS: 100-04,20,170

Q4004 **Cast supplies, shoulder cast, adult (11 years +), fiberglass** A B ♿

CMS: 100-04,20,170

Q4005 **Cast supplies, long arm cast, adult (11 years +), plaster** A B ♿

CMS: 100-04,20,170

Q4006 **Cast supplies, long arm cast, adult (11 years +), fiberglass** A B ♿

CMS: 100-04,20,170

Q4007 **Cast supplies, long arm cast, pediatric (0-10 years), plaster** A B ♿

CMS: 100-04,20,170

Q4008 **Cast supplies, long arm cast, pediatric (0-10 years), fiberglass** A B ♿

CMS: 100-04,20,170

Q4009 **Cast supplies, short arm cast, adult (11 years +), plaster** A B ♿

CMS: 100-04,20,170

Q4010 **Cast supplies, short arm cast, adult (11 years +), fiberglass** A B ♿

CMS: 100-04,20,170

Q4011 **Cast supplies, short arm cast, pediatric (0-10 years), plaster** A B ♿

CMS: 100-04,20,170

Q4012 **Cast supplies, short arm cast, pediatric (0-10 years), fiberglass** A B ♿

CMS: 100-04,20,170

Q4013 **Cast supplies, gauntlet cast (includes lower forearm and hand), adult (11 years +), plaster** A B ♿

CMS: 100-04,20,170

Q4014 **Cast supplies, gauntlet cast (includes lower forearm and hand), adult (11 years +), fiberglass** A B ♿

CMS: 100-04,20,170

Q4015 **Cast supplies, gauntlet cast (includes lower forearm and hand), pediatric (0-10 years), plaster** A B ♿

CMS: 100-04,20,170

Q4016 Cast supplies, gauntlet cast (includes lower forearm and hand), pediatric (0-10 years), fiberglass A B ♿
CMS: 100-04,20,170

Q4017 Cast supplies, long arm splint, adult (11 years +), plaster A B ♿
CMS: 100-04,20,170

Q4018 Cast supplies, long arm splint, adult (11 years +), fiberglass A B ♿
CMS: 100-04,20,170

Q4019 Cast supplies, long arm splint, pediatric (0-10 years), plaster A B ♿
CMS: 100-04,20,170

Q4020 Cast supplies, long arm splint, pediatric (0-10 years), fiberglass A B ♿
CMS: 100-04,20,170

Q4021 Cast supplies, short arm splint, adult (11 years +), plaster A B ♿
CMS: 100-04,20,170

Q4022 Cast supplies, short arm splint, adult (11 years +), fiberglass A B ♿
CMS: 100-04,20,170

Q4023 Cast supplies, short arm splint, pediatric (0-10 years), plaster A B ♿
CMS: 100-04,20,170

Q4024 Cast supplies, short arm splint, pediatric (0-10 years), fiberglass A B ♿
CMS: 100-04,20,170

Q4025 Cast supplies, hip spica (one or both legs), adult (11 years +), plaster A B ♿
CMS: 100-04,20,170

Q4026 Cast supplies, hip spica (one or both legs), adult (11 years +), fiberglass A B ♿
CMS: 100-04,20,170

Q4027 Cast supplies, hip spica (one or both legs), pediatric (0-10 years), plaster A B ♿
CMS: 100-04,20,170

Q4028 Cast supplies, hip spica (one or both legs), pediatric (0-10 years), fiberglass A B ♿
CMS: 100-04,20,170

Q4029 Cast supplies, long leg cast, adult (11 years +), plaster A B ♿
CMS: 100-04,20,170

Q4030 Cast supplies, long leg cast, adult (11 years +), fiberglass A B ♿
CMS: 100-04,20,170

Q4031 Cast supplies, long leg cast, pediatric (0-10 years), plaster A B ♿
CMS: 100-04,20,170

Q4032 Cast supplies, long leg cast, pediatric (0-10 years), fiberglass A B ♿
CMS: 100-04,20,170

Q4033 Cast supplies, long leg cylinder cast, adult (11 years +), plaster A B ♿
CMS: 100-04,20,170

Q4034 Cast supplies, long leg cylinder cast, adult (11 years +), fiberglass A B ♿
CMS: 100-04,20,170

Q4035 Cast supplies, long leg cylinder cast, pediatric (0-10 years), plaster A B ♿
CMS: 100-04,20,170

Q4036 Cast supplies, long leg cylinder cast, pediatric (0-10 years), fiberglass A B ♿
CMS: 100-04,20,170

Q4037 Cast supplies, short leg cast, adult (11 years +), plaster A B ♿
CMS: 100-04,20,170

Q4038 Cast supplies, short leg cast, adult (11 years +), fiberglass A B ♿
CMS: 100-04,20,170

Q4039 Cast supplies, short leg cast, pediatric (0-10 years), plaster A B ♿
CMS: 100-04,20,170

Q4040 Cast supplies, short leg cast, pediatric (0-10 years), fiberglass A B ♿
CMS: 100-04,20,170

Q4041 Cast supplies, long leg splint, adult (11 years +), plaster A B ♿
CMS: 100-04,20,170

Q4042 Cast supplies, long leg splint, adult (11 years +), fiberglass A B ♿
CMS: 100-04,20,170

Q4043 Cast supplies, long leg splint, pediatric (0-10 years), plaster A B ♿
CMS: 100-04,20,170

Q4044 Cast supplies, long leg splint, pediatric (0-10 years), fiberglass A B ♿
CMS: 100-04,20,170

Q4045 Cast supplies, short leg splint, adult (11 years +), plaster A B ♿
CMS: 100-04,20,170

Q4046 Cast supplies, short leg splint, adult (11 years +), fiberglass A B ♿
CMS: 100-04,20,170

Q4047 Cast supplies, short leg splint, pediatric (0-10 years), plaster A B ♿
CMS: 100-04,20,170

Q4048 Cast supplies, short leg splint, pediatric (0-10 years), fiberglass A B ♿
CMS: 100-04,20,170

Q4049 Finger splint, static B ♿
CMS: 100-04,20,170

Q4050 Cast supplies, for unlisted types and materials of casts B
CMS: 100-04,20,170

Q4051 Splint supplies, miscellaneous (includes thermoplastics, strapping, fasteners, padding and other supplies) B
CMS: 100-04,20,170

Q4074 Iloprost, inhalation solution, FDA-approved final product, noncompounded, administered through DME, unit dose form, up to 20 mcg Y ☑
CMS: 100-02,15,50.5

Q4081 Injection, epoetin alfa, 100 units (for ESRD on dialysis) N ☑
CMS: 100-04,8,60.4; 100-04,8,60.4.1; 100-04,8,60.4.2; 100-04,8,60.4.4; 100-04,8,60.4.4.1; 100-04,8,60.4.4.2; 100-04,8,60.4.5.1

Q4082 Drug or biological, not otherwise classified, Part B drug competitive acquisition program (CAP) B ☑

Q4100 Skin substitute, not otherwise specified N N1 ☑
CMS: 100-04,4,260.1; 100-04,4,260.1.1
AHA: 2Q,22; 2Q,18

Q4101 **Apligraf, per sq cm** N N1 ☑
CMS: 100-04,4,260.1; 100-04,4,260.1.1

Q4102 **Oasis wound matrix, per sq cm** N N1 ☑
CMS: 100-04,4,260.1; 100-04,4,260.1.1

Q4103 **Oasis burn matrix, per sq cm** N N1 ☑
CMS: 100-04,4,260.1; 100-04,4,260.1.1

Q4104 **Integra bilayer matrix wound dressing (BMWD), per sq cm** N N1 ☑
CMS: 100-04,4,260.1; 100-04,4,260.1.1

Q4105 **Integra dermal regeneration template (DRT) or Integra Omnigraft dermal regeneration matrix, per sq cm** N N1 ☑
CMS: 100-04,4,260.1; 100-04,4,260.1.1

Q4106 **Dermagraft, per sq cm** N N1 ☑
CMS: 100-04,4,260.1; 100-04,4,260.1.1

Q4107 **GRAFTJACKET, per sq cm** N N1 ☑
CMS: 100-04,4,260.1; 100-04,4,260.1.1

Q4108 **Integra matrix, per sq cm** N N1 ☑
CMS: 100-04,4,260.1; 100-04,4,260.1.1

Q4110 **PriMatrix, per sq cm** N N1 ☑
CMS: 100-04,4,260.1; 100-04,4,260.1.1

Q4111 **GammaGraft, per sq cm** N N1 ☑
CMS: 100-04,4,260.1; 100-04,4,260.1.1

Q4112 **Cymetra, injectable, 1 cc** N N1 ☑

Q4113 **GRAFTJACKET XPRESS, injectable, 1 cc** N N1 ☑

Q4114 **Integra flowable wound matrix, injectable, 1 cc** N N1 ☑

Q4115 **AlloSkin, per sq cm** N N1 ☑
CMS: 100-04,4,260.1; 100-04,4,260.1.1

Q4116 **AlloDerm, per sq cm** N N1 ☑
CMS: 100-04,4,260.1; 100-04,4,260.1.1

Q4117 **HYALOMATRIX, per sq cm** N N1 ☑
CMS: 100-04,4,260.1; 100-04,4,260.1.1

Q4118 **MatriStem micromatrix, 1 mg** N N1 ☑

Q4121 **TheraSkin, per sq cm** N N1 ☑
CMS: 100-04,4,260.1; 100-04,4,260.1.1

Q4122 **DermACELL, DermACELL AWM or DermACELL AWM Porous, per sq cm** N N1 ☑
CMS: 100-04,4,260.1; 100-04,4,260.1.1

Q4123 **AlloSkin RT, per sq cm** N N1 ☑
CMS: 100-04,4,260.1; 100-04,4,260.1.1

Q4124 **OASIS ultra tri-layer wound matrix, per sq cm** N N1 ☑
CMS: 100-04,4,260.1; 100-04,4,260.1.1

Q4125 **ArthroFlex, per sq cm** N N1 ☑

Q4126 **MemoDerm, DermaSpan, TranZgraft or InteguPly, per sq cm** N N1 ☑
CMS: 100-04,4,260.1; 100-04,4,260.1.1

Q4127 **Talymed, per sq cm** N N1 ☑
CMS: 100-04,4,260.1; 100-04,4,260.1.1

Q4128 **FlexHD, or AllopatchHD, per sq cm** N N1 ☑
CMS: 100-04,4,260.1; 100-04,4,260.1.1
AHA: 4Q,22

Q4130 **Strattice, per sq cm** N N1 ☑

Q4132 **Grafix Core and GrafixPL Core, per sq cm** N N1 ☑
CMS: 100-04,4,260.1; 100-04,4,260.1.1

Q4133 **Grafix PRIME, GrafixPL PRIME, Stravix and StravixPL, per sq cm** N N1 ☑
CMS: 100-04,4,260.1; 100-04,4,260.1.1

Q4134 **HMatrix, per sq cm** N N1 ☑
CMS: 100-04,4,260.1; 100-04,4,260.1.1

Q4135 **Mediskin, per sq cm** N N1 ☑
CMS: 100-04,4,260.1; 100-04,4,260.1.1

Q4136 **EZ Derm, per sq cm** N N1 ☑
CMS: 100-04,4,260.1; 100-04,4,260.1.1

Q4137 **AmnioExcel, AmnioExcel Plus or BioDExcel, per sq cm** N N1 ☑
CMS: 100-04,4,260.1; 100-04,4,260.1.1

Q4138 **BioDFence DryFlex, per sq cm** N N1 ☑
CMS: 100-04,4,260.1; 100-04,4,260.1.1

Q4139 **AmnioMatrix or BioDMatrix, injectable, 1 cc** N N1 ☑

Q4140 **BioDFence, per sq cm** N N1 ☑
CMS: 100-04,4,260.1; 100-04,4,260.1.1

Q4141 **AlloSkin AC, per sq cm** N N1 ☑
CMS: 100-04,4,260.1; 100-04,4,260.1.1

Q4142 **XCM biologic tissue matrix, per sq cm** N N1 ☑

Q4143 **Repriza, per sq cm** N N1 ☑
CMS: 100-04,4,260.1; 100-04,4,260.1.1

Q4145 **EpiFix, injectable, 1 mg** N N1 ☑

Q4146 **TENSIX, per sq cm** N N1 ☑
CMS: 100-04,4,260.1; 100-04,4,260.1.1

Q4147 **Architect, Architect PX, or Architect FX, extracellular matrix, per sq cm** N N1 ☑
CMS: 100-04,4,260.1; 100-04,4,260.1.1

Q4148 **Neox Cord 1K, Neox Cord RT, or Clarix Cord 1K, per sq cm** N N1 ☑
CMS: 100-04,4,260.1; 100-04,4,260.1.1

Q4149 **Excellagen, 0.1 cc** N N1 ☑

Q4150 **AlloWrap DS or dry, per sq cm** N N1 ☑
CMS: 100-04,4,260.1; 100-04,4,260.1.1

Q4151 **AmnioBand or Guardian, per sq cm** N N1 ☑
CMS: 100-04,4,260.1; 100-04,4,260.1.1

Q4152 **DermaPure, per sq cm** N N1 ☑
CMS: 100-04,4,260.1; 100-04,4,260.1.1

Q4153 **Dermavest and Plurivest, per sq cm** N N1 ☑
CMS: 100-04,4,260.1; 100-04,4,260.1.1

Q4154 **Biovance, per sq cm** N N1 ☑
CMS: 100-04,4,260.1; 100-04,4,260.1.1

Q4155 **Neox Flo or Clarix Flo 1 mg** N N1 ☑

Q4156 **Neox 100 or Clarix 100, per sq cm** N N1 ☑
CMS: 100-04,4,260.1; 100-04,4,260.1.1

Q4157 **Revitalon, per sq cm** N N1 ☑
CMS: 100-04,4,260.1; 100-04,4,260.1.1

Q4158 **Kerecis Omega3, per sq cm** N N1 ☑
CMS: 100-04,4,260.1; 100-04,4,260.1.1

Q4159 **Affinity, per sq cm** N N1 ☑
CMS: 100-04,4,260.1; 100-04,4,260.1.1

Q4160 **NuShield, per sq cm** N N1 ☑
CMS: 100-04,4,260.1; 100-04,4,260.1.1

Q4161 **bio-ConneKt wound matrix, per sq cm** N N1 ☑
CMS: 100-04,4,260.1; 100-04,4,260.1.1

Q4162 **WoundEx Flow, BioSkin Flow, 0.5 cc** N N1 ☑

Q4163 WoundEx, BioSkin, per sq cm
CMS: 100-04,4,260.1; 100-04,4,260.1.1

Q4164 Helicoll, per sq cm
CMS: 100-04,4,260.1; 100-04,4,260.1.1

Q4165 Keramatrix or Kerasorb, per sq cm
CMS: 100-04,4,260.1; 100-04,4,260.1.1

Q4166 Cytal, per sq cm
CMS: 100-04,4,260.1; 100-04,4,260.1.1

Q4167 Truskin, per sq cm
CMS: 100-04,4,260.1; 100-04,4,260.1.1

Q4168 AmnioBand, 1 mg

Q4169 Artacent wound, per sq cm
CMS: 100-04,4,260.1; 100-04,4,260.1.1

Q4170 Cygnus, per sq cm
CMS: 100-04,4,260.1; 100-04,4,260.1.1

Q4171 Interfyl, 1 mg

Q4173 PalinGen or PalinGen XPlus, per sq cm
CMS: 100-04,4,260.1; 100-04,4,260.1.1

Q4174 PalinGen or ProMatrX, 0.36 mg per 0.25 cc

Q4175 Miroderm, per sq cm
CMS: 100-04,4,260.1; 100-04,4,260.1.1

Q4176 NeoPatch or Therion, per sq cm
CMS: 100-04,4,260.1; 100-04,4,260.1.1
AHA: 2Q,20; 1Q,18

Q4177 FlowerAmnioFlo, 0.1 cc

Q4178 FlowerAmnioPatch, per sq cm
CMS: 100-04,4,260.1; 100-04,4,260.1.1

Q4179 FlowerDerm, per sq cm
CMS: 100-04,4,260.1; 100-04,4,260.1.1

Q4180 Revita, per sq cm
CMS: 100-04,4,260.1; 100-04,4,260.1.1

Q4181 Amnio Wound, per sq cm
CMS: 100-04,4,260.1; 100-04,4,260.1.1

Q4182 TransCyte, per sq cm
CMS: 100-04,4,260.1; 100-04,4,260.1.1

Q4183 surgiGRAFT, per sq cm
CMS: 100-04,4,260.1; 100-04,4,260.1.1
AHA: 1Q,19

Q4184 Cellesta or Cellesta Duo, per sq cm
CMS: 100-04,4,260.1; 100-04,4,260.1.1
AHA: 1Q,19

Q4185 Cellesta Flowable Amnion (25 mg per cc); per 0.5 cc
CMS: 100-04,4,260.1; 100-04,4,260.1.1
AHA: 1Q,19

Q4186 Epifix, per sq cm
CMS: 100-04,4,260.1; 100-04,4,260.1.1
AHA: 1Q,19

Q4187 Epicord, per sq cm
CMS: 100-04,4,260.1; 100-04,4,260.1.1
AHA: 1Q,19

Q4188 AmnioArmor, per sq cm
CMS: 100-04,4,260.1; 100-04,4,260.1.1
AHA: 1Q,19

Q4189 Artacent AC, 1 mg
CMS: 100-04,4,260.1; 100-04,4,260.1.1
AHA: 1Q,19

Q4190 Artacent AC, per sq cm
CMS: 100-04,4,260.1; 100-04,4,260.1.1
AHA: 1Q,19

Q4191 Restorigin, per sq cm
CMS: 100-04,4,260.1; 100-04,4,260.1.1
AHA: 1Q,19

Q4192 Restorigin, 1 cc
CMS: 100-04,4,260.1; 100-04,4,260.1.1
AHA: 1Q,19

Q4193 Coll-e-Derm, per sq cm
CMS: 100-04,4,260.1; 100-04,4,260.1.1
AHA: 1Q,19

Q4194 Novachor, per sq cm
CMS: 100-04,4,260.1; 100-04,4,260.1.1
AHA: 1Q,19

Q4195 PuraPly, per sq cm
CMS: 100-04,4,260.1; 100-04,4,260.1.1
AHA: 1Q,19

Q4196 PuraPly AM, per sq cm
CMS: 100-04,4,260.1; 100-04,4,260.1.1
AHA: 1Q,19

Q4197 PuraPly XT, per sq cm
CMS: 100-04,4,260.1; 100-04,4,260.1.1
AHA: 1Q,19

Q4198 Genesis Amniotic Membrane, per sq cm
CMS: 100-04,4,260.1; 100-04,4,260.1.1
AHA: 1Q,19

Q4199 Cygnus matrix, per sq cm
AHA: 1Q,22

Q4200 SkinTE, per sq cm
CMS: 100-04,4,260.1; 100-04,4,260.1.1
AHA: 1Q,19

Q4201 Matrion, per sq cm
CMS: 100-04,4,260.1; 100-04,4,260.1.1
AHA: 1Q,19

Q4202 Keroxx (2.5 g/cc), 1 cc
CMS: 100-04,4,260.1; 100-04,4,260.1.1
AHA: 1Q,19

Q4203 Derma-Gide, per sq cm
CMS: 100-04,4,260.1; 100-04,4,260.1.1
AHA: 1Q,19

Q4204 XWRAP, per sq cm
CMS: 100-04,4,260.1; 100-04,4,260.1.1
AHA: 1Q,19

Q4205 Membrane Graft or Membrane Wrap, per sq cm
AHA: 4Q,19

Q4206 Fluid Flow or Fluid GF, 1 cc
AHA: 4Q,19

Q4208 Novafix, per sq cm
AHA: 4Q,19

Q4209 SurGraft, per sq cm
AHA: 4Q,19

~~Q4210 Axolotl Graft or Axolotl DualGraft, per sq cm~~

Q4211 Amnion Bio or AxoBioMembrane, per sq cm
AHA: 4Q,19

Q4212 AlloGen, per cc
AHA: 4Q,19

Q4213 Ascent, 0.5 mg N N1
AHA: 4Q,19

Q4214 Cellesta Cord, per sq cm N N1
AHA: 4Q,19

Q4215 Axolotl Ambient or Axolotl Cryo, 0.1 mg N N1
AHA: 4Q,19

Q4216 Artacent Cord, per sq cm N N1
AHA: 4Q,19

Q4217 WoundFix, BioWound, WoundFix Plus, BioWound Plus, WoundFix Xplus or BioWound Xplus, per sq cm N N1
AHA: 4Q,19

Q4218 SurgiCORD, per sq cm N N1
AHA: 4Q,19

Q4219 SurgiGRAFT-DUAL, per sq cm N N1
AHA: 4Q,19

Q4220 BellaCell HD or SureDerm, per sq cm N N1
AHA: 4Q,19

Q4221 Amnio Wrap2, per sq cm N N1
AHA: 4Q,19

Q4222 ProgenaMatrix, per sq cm N N1
AHA: 4Q,19

Q4224 Human Health Factor 10 Amniotic Patch (HHF10-P), per sq cm N N1
AHA: 2Q,22

Q4225 AmnioBind or DermaBind TL, per sq cm N N1
AHA: 1Q,24; 2Q,22

Q4226 MyOwn Skin, includes harvesting and preparation procedures, per sq cm N N1
AHA: 4Q,19

Q4227 AmnioCore, per sq cm N N1
AHA: 2Q,20

Q4229 Cogenex Amniotic Membrane, per sq cm N N1
AHA: 2Q,20

Q4230 Cogenex Flowable Amnion, per 0.5 cc N N1
AHA: 2Q,20

Q4231 Corplex P, per cc N N1
AHA: 2Q,20

Q4232 Corplex, per sq cm N N1
AHA: 2Q,20

Q4233 SurFactor or NuDyn, per 0.5 cc N N1
AHA: 2Q,20

Q4234 XCellerate, per sq cm N N1
AHA: 2Q,20

Q4235 AMNIOREPAIR or AltiPly, per sq cm N N1
AHA: 2Q,20

Q4236 carePATCH, per sq cm N N1
AHA: 4Q,21; 2Q,20

Q4237 Cryo-Cord, per sq cm N N1
AHA: 2Q,20

Q4238 Derm-Maxx, per sq cm N N1
AHA: 2Q,20

Q4239 Amnio-Maxx or Amnio-Maxx Lite, per sq cm N N1
AHA: 2Q,20

Q4240 CoreCyte, for topical use only, per 0.5 cc N N1
AHA: 2Q,20

Q4241 PolyCyte, for topical use only, per 0.5 cc N N1
AHA: 2Q,20

Q4242 AmnioCyte Plus, per 0.5 cc N N1
AHA: 2Q,20

Q4244 ~~Procenta, per 200 mg~~
To report, see ~Q4310

Q4245 AmnioText, per cc N N1
AHA: 2Q,20

Q4246 CoreText or ProText, per cc N N1
AHA: 2Q,20

Q4247 AmnioText Patch, per sq cm N N1
AHA: 2Q,20

Q4248 Dermacyte Amniotic Membrane Allograft, per sq cm N N1
AHA: 2Q,20

Q4249 AMNIPLY, for topical use only, per sq cm N N1
AHA: 4Q,20

Q4250 AmnioAmp-MP, per sq cm N N1
AHA: 4Q,20

Q4251 Vim, per sq cm N N1
AHA: 4Q,21

Q4252 Vendaje, per sq cm N N1
AHA: 4Q,21

Q4253 Zenith Amniotic Membrane, per sq cm N N1
AHA: 4Q,21

Q4254 Novafix DL, per sq cm N N1
AHA: 4Q,20

Q4255 REGUaRD, for topical use only, per sq cm N N1
AHA: 4Q,20

Q4256 MLG-Complete, per sq cm N N1
AHA: 2Q,22

Q4257 Relese, per sq cm N N1
AHA: 2Q,22

Q4258 Enverse, per sq cm N N1
AHA: 2Q,22

Q4259 Celera Dual Layer or Celera Dual Membrane, per sq cm N N1
AHA: 3Q,22

Q4260 Signature APatch, per sq cm N N1
AHA: 3Q,22

Q4261 TAG, per sq cm N N1
AHA: 3Q,22

Q4262 Dual Layer Impax Membrane, per sq cm N N1
AHA: 1Q,23

Q4263 SurGraft TL, per sq cm N N1
AHA: 1Q,23

Q4264 Cocoon Membrane, per sq cm N N1
AHA: 1Q,23

Q4265 NeoStim TL, per sq cm N N1
AHA: 2Q,23

Q4266 NeoStim Membrane, per sq cm N N1
AHA: 2Q,23

Q4267 NeoStim DL, per sq cm N N1
AHA: 2Q,23

Q4268 SurGraft FT, per sq cm N N1
AHA: 2Q,23

Q4269 SurGraft XT, per sq cm N N1
AHA: 2Q,23

Q4270 Complete SL, per sq cm N N1
AHA: 2Q,23

Q4271 Complete FT, per sq cm N N1
AHA: 2Q,23

Q4272 Esano A, per sq cm N N1
AHA: 3Q,23

Q4273 Esano AAA, per sq cm N N1
AHA: 3Q,23

Q4274 Esano AC, per sq cm N N1
AHA: 3Q,23

Q4275 Esano ACA, per sq cm N N1
AHA: 3Q,23

Q4276 ORION, per sq cm N N1
AHA: 3Q,23

Q4277 ~~WoundPlus membrane or E-Graft, per sq cm~~

Q4278 EPIEFFECT, per sq cm N N1
AHA: 3Q,23

Q4279 Vendaje AC, per sq cm N N1
AHA: 1Q,24

Q4280 Xcell Amnio Matrix, per sq cm N N1
AHA: 3Q,23

Q4281 Barrera SL or Barrera DL, per sq cm N N1
AHA: 3Q,23

Q4282 Cygnus Dual, per sq cm N N1
AHA: 3Q,23

Q4283 Biovance Tri-Layer or Biovance 3L, per sq cm N N1
AHA: 3Q,23

Q4284 DermaBind SL, per sq cm N N1
AHA: 3Q,23

Q4285 NuDYN DL or NuDYN DL MESH, per sq cm N N1
AHA: 4Q,23

Q4286 NuDYN SL or NuDYN SLW, per sq cm N N1
AHA: 4Q,23

Q4287 DermaBind DL, per sq cm N N1
AHA: 1Q,24

Q4288 DermaBind CH, per sq cm N N1
AHA: 1Q,24

Q4289 RevoShield+ Amniotic Barrier, per sq cm N N1

Q4290 Membrane Wrap-Hydro, per sq cm N N1
AHA: 1Q,24

Q4291 Lamellas XT, per sq cm N N1
AHA: 1Q,24

Q4292 Lamellas, per sq cm N N1
AHA: 1Q,24

Q4293 Acesso DL, per sq cm N N1
AHA: 1Q,24

Q4294 Amnio Quad-Core, per sq cm N N1
AHA: 1Q,24

Q4295 Amnio Tri-Core Amniotic, per sq cm N N1
AHA: 1Q,24

Q4296 Rebound Matrix, per sq cm N N1
AHA: 1Q,24

Q4297 Emerge Matrix, per sq cm N N1
AHA: 1Q,24

Q4298 AmniCore Pro, per sq cm N N1
AHA: 1Q,24

Q4299 AmniCore Pro+, per sq cm N N1
AHA: 1Q,24

Q4300 Acesso TL, per sq cm N N1
AHA: 1Q,24

Q4301 Activate Matrix, per sq cm N N1
AHA: 1Q,24

Q4302 Complete ACA, per sq cm N N1
AHA: 1Q,24

Q4303 Complete AA, per sq cm N N1
AHA: 1Q,24

Q4304 GRAFIX PLUS, per sq cm N
AHA: 1Q,24

● Q4305 American Amnion AC Tri-Layer, per sq cm N N1
AHA: 2Q,24

● Q4306 American Amnion AC, per sq cm N N1
AHA: 2Q,24

● Q4307 American Amnion, per sq cm N N1
AHA: 2Q,24

● Q4308 Sanopellis, per sq cm N N1
AHA: 2Q,24

● Q4309 VIA Matrix, per sq cm N N1
AHA: 2Q,24

● Q4310 Procenta, per 100 mg N N1
AHA: 2Q,24

● Q4311 Acesso, per sq cm N1
AHA: 3Q,24

● Q4312 Acesso AC, per sq cm N1
AHA: 3Q,24

● Q4313 DermaBind FM, per sq cm N1
AHA: 3Q,24

● Q4314 Reeva FT, per sq cm N1
AHA: 3Q,24

● Q4315 RegeneLink Amniotic Membrane Allograft, per sq cm N1
AHA: 3Q,24

● Q4316 AmchoPlast, per sq cm N1
AHA: 3Q,24

● Q4317 VitoGraft, per sq cm N1
AHA: 3Q,24

● Q4318 E-Graft, per sq cm N1
AHA: 3Q,24

● Q4319 SanoGraft, per sq cm N1
AHA: 3Q,24

● Q4320 PelloGraft, per sq cm N1
AHA: 3Q,24

● Q4321 RenoGraft, per sq cm N1
AHA: 3Q,24

● Q4322 CaregraFT, per sq cm N1
AHA: 3Q,24

● Q4323 alloPLY, per sq cm N1
AHA: 3Q,24

● Q4324 AmnioTX, per sq cm N1
AHA: 3Q,24

● Q4325 ACApatch, per sq cm N1
AHA: 3Q,24

● Q4326 WoundPlus, per sq cm N1
AHA: 3Q,24

● Q4327 DuoAmnion, per sq cm N1
AHA: 3Q,24

● Q4328 MOST, per sq cm N1
AHA: 3Q,24

● Q4329 Singlay, per sq cm N1
AHA: 3Q,24

● Q4330 TOTAL, per sq cm N1
AHA: 3Q,24

● Q4331 Axolotl Graft, per sq cm N1
AHA: 3Q,24

● Q4332 Axolotl DualGraft, per sq cm N1
AHA: 3Q,24

● Q4333 ArdeoGraft, per sq cm N1
AHA: 3Q,24

● Q4334 AmnioPlast 1, per sq cm N1

● Q4335 AmnioPlast 2, per sq cm N1

● Q4336 Artacent C, per sq cm N1

● Q4337 Artacent Trident, per sq cm N1

● Q4338 Artacent Velos, per sq cm N1

● Q4339 Artacent Vericlen, per sq cm N1

● Q4340 SimpliGraft, per sq cm N1

● Q4341 SimpliMax, per sq cm N1

● Q4342 TheraMend, per sq cm N1

● Q4343 Dermacyte AC Matrix Amniotic Membrane Allograft, per sq cm N1

● Q4344 Tri-Membrane Wrap, per sq cm N1

● Q4345 Matrix HD Allograft Dermis, per sq cm N1

● Q4346 Shelter DM Matrix, per sq cm

● Q4347 Rampart DL Matrix, per sq cm

● Q4348 Sentry SL Matrix, per sq cm

● Q4349 Mantle DL Matrix, per sq cm

● Q4350 Palisade DM Matrix, per sq cm

● Q4351 Enclose TL Matrix, per sq cm

● Q4352 Overlay SL Matrix, per sq cm

● Q4353 Xceed TL Matrix, per sq cm

Q5001 Hospice or home health care provided in patient's home/residence B
CMS: 100-01,3,30.3; 100-04,10,40.2; 100-04,11,10; 100-04,11,130.1; 100-04,11,30.3

Q5002 Hospice or home health care provided in assisted living facility B
CMS: 100-01,3,30.3; 100-04,10,40.2; 100-04,11,10; 100-04,11,130.1; 100-04,11,30.3

Q5003 Hospice care provided in nursing long-term care facility (LTC) or nonskilled nursing facility (NF) B
CMS: 100-01,3,30.3; 100-04,11,10; 100-04,11,130.1; 100-04,11,30.3

Q5004 Hospice care provided in skilled nursing facility (SNF) B
CMS: 100-01,3,30.3; 100-04,11,10; 100-04,11,130.1; 100-04,11,30.3

Q5005 Hospice care provided in inpatient hospital B
CMS: 100-01,3,30.3; 100-04,11,10; 100-04,11,130.1; 100-04,11,30.3

Q5006 Hospice care provided in inpatient hospice facility B
CMS: 100-01,3,30.3; 100-04,11,10; 100-04,11,130.1; 100-04,11,30.3

Q5007 Hospice care provided in long-term care facility B
CMS: 100-01,3,30.3; 100-04,11,10; 100-04,11,130.1; 100-04,11,30.3

Q5008 Hospice care provided in inpatient psychiatric facility B
CMS: 100-01,3,30.3; 100-04,11,10; 100-04,11,130.1; 100-04,11,30.3

Q5009 Hospice or home health care provided in place not otherwise specified (NOS) B
CMS: 100-01,3,30.3; 100-04,10,40.2; 100-04,11,10; 100-04,11,130.1; 100-04,11,30.3

Q5010 Hospice home care provided in a hospice facility B
CMS: 100-01,3,30.3; 100-04,11,10; 100-04,11,130.1; 100-04,11,30.3

Q5101 Injection, filgrastim-sndz, biosimilar, (Zarxio), 1 mcg K K2

Q5103 Injection, infliximab-dyyb, biosimilar, (Inflectra), 10 mg K K2

Q5104 Injection, infliximab-abda, biosimilar, (Renflexis), 10 mg K K2

Q5105 Injection, epoetin alfa-epbx, biosimilar, (Retacrit) (for ESRD on dialysis), 100 units K K2
CMS: 100-04,8,60.4.2

Q5106 Injection, epoetin alfa-epbx, biosimilar, (Retacrit) (for non-ESRD use), 1000 units K K2

Q5107 Injection, bevacizumab-awwb, biosimilar, (Mvasi), 10 mg K K2
CMS: 100-04,4,260.1; 100-04,4,260.1.1
AHA: 4Q,19; 1Q,19; 4Q,18

Q5108 Injection, pegfilgrastim-jmdb (Fulphila), biosimilar, 0.5 mg K K2
CMS: 100-04,4,260.1; 100-04,4,260.1.1
AHA: 2Q,23; 1Q,19; 4Q,18; 3Q,18

Q5109 Injection, infliximab-qbtx, biosimilar, (Ixifi), 10 mg E1
CMS: 100-04,4,260.1; 100-04,4,260.1.1
AHA: 1Q,19; 4Q,18

Q5110 Injection, filgrastim-aafi, biosimilar, (Nivestym), 1 mcg K K2
CMS: 100-04,4,260.1; 100-04,4,260.1.1
AHA: 1Q,19; 4Q,18; 3Q,18

Q5111 Injection, pegfilgrastim-cbqv (Udenyca), biosimilar, 0.5 mg K K2
CMS: 100-04,4,260.1; 100-04,4,260.1.1
AHA: 2Q,23; 1Q,19; 4Q,18

Q5112 Injection, trastuzumab-dttb, biosimilar, (Ontruzant), 10 mg K K2
AHA: 3Q,19

Q5113 Injection, trastuzumab-pkrb, biosimilar, (Herzuma), 10 mg K K2
AHA: 3Q,19

Q5114 Injection, Trastuzumab-dkst, biosimilar, (Ogivri), 10 mg K K2
AHA: 3Q,19

Q5115 Injection, rituximab-abbs, biosimilar, (Truxima), 10 mg K K2
AHA: 3Q,19

Q5116 Injection, trastuzumab-qyyp, biosimilar, (Trazimera), 10 mg K K2
AHA: 4Q,19

Q5117 Injection, trastuzumab-anns, biosimilar, (Kanjinti), 10 mg K K2
AHA: 4Q,19

Q5118 Injection, bevacizumab-bvzr, biosimilar, (Zirabev), 10 mg K K2
AHA: 4Q,19

Q5119 Injection, rituximab-pvvr, biosimilar, (RUXIENCE), 10 mg K K2
AHA: 2Q,20

Q5120 Injection, pegfilgrastim-bmez (ZIEXTENZO), biosimilar, 0.5 mg K K2
AHA: 2Q,23; 2Q,20

Q5121 Injection, infliximab-axxq, biosimilar, (AVSOLA), 10 mg K K2
AHA: 2Q,20

Q5122 Injection, pegfilgrastim-apgf (Nyvepria), biosimilar, 0.5 mg K K2
AHA: 2Q,23; 1Q,21

Q5123 Injection, rituximab-arrx, biosimilar, (Riabni), 10 mg G K2
AHA: 3Q,21

Q5124 Injection, ranibizumab-nuna, biosimilar, (Byooviz), 0.1 mg G K2
AHA: 2Q,22

Q5125 Injection, filgrastim-ayow, biosimilar, (Releuko), 1 mcg G K2
AHA: 4Q,22

Q5126 Injection, bevacizumab-maly, biosimilar, (Alymsys), 10 mg G K2
AHA: 1Q,23

Q5127 Injection, pegfilgrastim-fpgk (Stimufend), biosimilar, 0.5 mg K K2
Use this code for Stimufend.
AHA: 2Q,23

Q5128 Injection, ranibizumab-eqrn (Cimerli), biosimilar, 0.1 mg G K2
Use this code for Cimerli.
AHA: 2Q,23

Q5129 Injection, bevacizumab-adcd (Vegzelma), biosimilar, 10 mg G K2
Use this code for Vegzelma.
AHA: 2Q,23

Q5130 Injection, pegfilgrastim-pbbk (Fylnetra), biosimilar, 0.5 mg G K2
Use this code for Fylnetra.
AHA: 2Q,23

~~Q5131 Injection, adalimumab-aacf (Idacio), biosimilar, 20 mg~~

~~Q5132 Injection, adalimumab-afzb (Abrilada), biosimilar, 10 mg~~

● **Q5133** Injection, tocilizumab-bavi (Tofidence), biosimilar, 1 mg E1 K2
AHA: 2Q,24

● **Q5134** Injection, natalizumab-sztn (Tyruko), biosimilar, 1 mg E1
AHA: 2Q,24

● **Q5135** Injection, tocilizumab-aazg (Tyenne), biosimilar, 1 mg K2

● **Q5136** Injection, denosumab-bbdz (Jubbonti/Wyost), biosimilar, 1 mg

● **Q5137** Injection, ustekinumab-auub (Wezlana), biosimilar, SC, 1 mg N1
Use this code for subcutaneous formulation only.
AHA: 3Q,24

● **Q5138** Injection, ustekinumab-auub (Wezlana), biosimilar, IV, 1 mg N1
Use this code for intravenous formulation only.
AHA: 3Q,24

● **Q5139** Injection, eculizumab-aeeb (bkemv), biosimilar, 10 mg
Use this code for Bkemv.

● **Q5140** Injection, adalimumab-fkjp, biosimilar, 1 mg
Use this code for Hulio.

● **Q5141** Injection, adalimumab-aaty, biosimilar, 1 mg
Use this code for Yuflyma.

● **Q5142** Injection, adalimumab-ryvk biosimilar, 1 mg
Use this code for Simlandi.

● **Q5143** Injection, adalimumab-adbm, biosimilar, 1 mg
Use this code for Cyltezo.

● **Q5144** Injection, adalimumab-aacf (Idacio), biosimilar, 1 mg

● **Q5145** Injection, adalimumab-afzb (Abrilada), biosimilar, 1 mg

● **Q5146** Injection, trastuzumab-strf (Hercessi), biosimilar, 10 mg

Q9001 Assessment by chaplain services B
AHA: 1Q,24; 4Q,22

Q9002 Counseling, individual, by chaplain services B
AHA: 1Q,24; 4Q,22

Q9003 Counseling, group, by chaplain services B
AHA: 1Q,24; 4Q,22

Q9004 Department of Veterans Affairs Whole Health Partner Services E1

Q9950 Injection, sulfur hexafluoride lipid microspheres, per ml N N1
Use this code for Lumason.
CMS: 100-03,1,220.2

Q9951 Low osmolar contrast material, 400 or greater mg/ml iodine concentration, per ml N N1 ☑
CMS: 100-03,1,220.2

Q9953 Injection, iron-based magnetic resonance contrast agent, per ml N N1 ☑
CMS: 100-03,1,220.2

Q9954 Oral magnetic resonance contrast agent, per 100 ml N N1 ☑
CMS: 100-03,1,220.2

Q9955 Injection, perflexane lipid microspheres, per ml N N1 ☑

Q9956 Injection, octafluoropropane microspheres, per ml N N1 ☑
Use this code for Optison.

Q9957 Injection, perflutren lipid microspheres, per ml N N1 ☑
Use this code for Definity.

Q9958 High osmolar contrast material, up to 149 mg/ml iodine concentration, per ml N N1 ☑
CMS: 100-03,1,220.2

Q9959 High osmolar contrast material, 150-199 mg/ml iodine concentration, per ml N N1 ☑
CMS: 100-03,1,220.2

Q9960 High osmolar contrast material, 200-249 mg/ml iodine concentration, per ml N N1 ☑
CMS: 100-03,1,220.2

Q9961 High osmolar contrast material, 250-299 mg/ml iodine concentration, per ml N N1 ☑
CMS: 100-03,1,220.2

Q9962 High osmolar contrast material, 300-349 mg/ml iodine concentration, per ml N N1 ☑
CMS: 100-03,1,220.2

Q9963 High osmolar contrast material, 350-399 mg/ml iodine concentration, per ml N N1 ☑
CMS: 100-03,1,220.2

Q9964 High osmolar contrast material, 400 or greater mg/ml iodine concentration, per ml N N1 ☑
CMS: 100-03,1,220.2

Q9965 **Low osmolar contrast material, 100-199 mg/ml iodine concentration, per ml** N N1 ☑

Use this code for Omnipaque 140, Omnipaque 180, Optiray 160, Optiray 140, ULTRAVIST 150.

CMS: 100-03,1,220.2

Q9966 **Low osmolar contrast material, 200-299 mg/ml iodine concentration, per ml** N N1 ☑

Use this code for Omnipaque 240, Optiray 240, ULTRAVIST 240.

CMS: 100-03,1,220.2

Q9967 **Low osmolar contrast material, 300-399 mg/ml iodine concentration, per ml** N N1 ☑

Use this code for Omnipaque 300, Omnipaque 350, Optiray, Optiray 300, Optiray 320, Oxilan 300, Oxilan 350, ULTRAVIST 300, ULTRAVIST 370.

CMS: 100-03,1,220.2

Q9968 **Injection, nonradioactive, noncontrast, visualization adjunct (e.g., methylene blue, isosulfan blue), 1 mg** K K2 ☑

Q9969 **Tc-99m from nonhighly enriched uranium source, full cost recovery add-on, per study dose** K ☑

Q9982 **Flutemetamol F18, diagnostic, per study dose, up to 5 mCi** N N1

Use this code for Vizamyl.

CMS: 100-04,13,60.12; 100-04,32,60.12

Q9983 **Florbetaben F18, diagnostic, per study dose, up to 8.1 mCi** N N1

Use this code for Neuraceq.

CMS: 100-04,13,60.12; 100-04,32,60.12

Q9991 **Injection, buprenorphine extended-release (Sublocade), less than or equal to 100 mg** K K2

Q9992 **Injection, buprenorphine extended-release (Sublocade), greater than 100 mg** K K2

● **Q9996** **Injection, ustekinumab-ttwe (Pyzchiva), subcutaneous, 1 mg**

● **Q9997** **Injection, ustekinumab-ttwe (Pyzchiva), intravenous, 1 mg**

● **Q9998** **Injection, ustekinumab-aekn (Selarsdi), 1 mg**

Diagnostic Radiology Services R0070-R0076

R codes are used for the transportation of portable x-ray and/or EKG equipment.

R0070 **Transportation of portable x-ray equipment and personnel to home or nursing home, per trip to facility or location, one patient seen** B ☑

Only a single, reasonable transportation charge is allowed for each trip the portable x-ray supplier makes to a location. When more than one patient is x-rayed at the same location, prorate the single allowable transport charge among all patients.

CMS: 100-04,13,90.3

R0075 **Transportation of portable x-ray equipment and personnel to home or nursing home, per trip to facility or location, more than one patient seen** B ☑

Only a single, reasonable transportation charge is allowed for each trip the portable x-ray supplier makes to a location. When more than one patient is x-rayed at the same location, prorate the single allowable transport charge among all patients.

CMS: 100-04,13,90.3

R0076 **Transportation of portable EKG to facility or location, per patient** B ☑

Only a single, reasonable transportation charge is allowed for each trip the portable EKG supplier makes to a location. When more than one patient is tested at the same location, prorate the single allowable transport charge among all patients.

CMS: 100-04,13,90.3; 100-04,6,20.3

Temporary National Codes (Non-Medicare) S0012-S9999

The S codes are used by the Blue Cross/Blue Shield Association (BCBSA) and the Health Insurance Association of America (HIAA) to report drugs, services, and supplies for which there are no national codes but for which codes are needed by the private sector to implement policies, programs, or claims processing. They are for the purpose of meeting the particular needs of the private sector. These codes are also used by the Medicaid program, but they are not payable by Medicare.

S0012 **Butorphanol tartrate, nasal spray, 25 mg** ☑
Use this code for Stadol NS.

S0013 **Esketamine, nasal spray, 1 mg**
Use this code for Spravato.

S0014 **Tacrine HCl, 10 mg** ☑
Use this code for Cognex.

S0017 **Injection, aminocaproic acid, 5 g** ☑
Use this code for Amicar.

S0021 **Injection, cefoperazone sodium, 1 g** ☑
Use this code for Cefobid.

S0023 **Injection, cimetidine HCl, 300 mg** ☑
Use this code for Tagamet HCl.

S0028 **Injection, famotidine, 20 mg** ☑
Use this code for Pepcid.

S0032 **Injection, nafcillin sodium, 2 g** ☑
Use this code for Nallpen, Unipen.

S0034 **Injection, ofloxacin, 400 mg** ☑
Use this code for Floxin IV.

S0039 **Injection, sulfamethoxazole and trimethoprim, 10 ml** ☑
Use this code for Bactrim IV, Septra IV, SMZ-TMP, Sulfatrim.

S0040 **Injection, ticarcillin disodium and clavulanate potassium, 3.1 g** ☑
Use this code for Timentin.

S0074 **Injection, cefotetan disodium, 500 mg** ☑
Use this code for Cefotan.

S0078 **Injection, fosphenytoin sodium, 750 mg** ☑
Use this code for Cerebryx.

S0080 **Injection, pentamidine isethionate, 300 mg** ☑
Use this code for NebuPent, Pentam 300, Pentacarinat. See also code J2545.

S0081 **Injection, piperacillin sodium, 500 mg** ☑
Use this code for Pipracil.

S0088 **Imatinib, 100 mg** ☑
Use this code for Gleevec.

S0090 **Sildenafil citrate, 25 mg** A ☑
Use this code for Viagra.

S0091 **Granisetron HCl, 1 mg (for circumstances falling under the Medicare statute, use Q0166)** ☑
Use this code for Kytril.

S0092 **Injection, hydromorphone HCl, 250 mg (loading dose for infusion pump)** ☑
Use this code for Dilaudid, Hydromophone. See also J1171.

S0093 **Injection, morphine sulfate, 500 mg (loading dose for infusion pump)** ☑
Use this code for Duramorph, MS Contin, Morphine Sulfate. See also J2270, J2272.

S0104 **Zidovudine, oral, 100 mg** ☑
See also J3485 for Retrovir.

S0106 **Bupropion HCl sustained release tablet, 150 mg, per bottle of 60 tablets** ☑
Use this code for Wellbutrin SR tablets.

S0108 **Mercaptopurine, oral, 50 mg** ☑
Use this code for Purinethol oral.

S0109 **Methadone, oral, 5 mg** ☑
Use this code for Dolophine.

S0117 **Tretinoin, topical, 5 g** ☑

S0119 **Ondansetron, oral, 4 mg (for circumstances falling under the Medicare statute, use HCPCS Q code)** ☑
Use this code for Zofran, Zuplenz.

S0122 **Injection, menotropins, 75 IU** ☑
Use this code for Humegon, Pergonal, Repronex.
CMS: 100-02,15,50.5

S0126 **Injection, follitropin alfa, 75 IU** ☑
Use this code for Gonal-F.
CMS: 100-02,15,50.5

S0128 **Injection, follitropin beta, 75 IU** ☑
Use this code for Follistim.
CMS: 100-02,15,50.5

S0132 **Injection, ganirelix acetate, 250 mcg** ☑
Use this code for Antagon.
CMS: 100-02,15,50.5

S0136 **Clozapine, 25 mg** ☑
Use this code for Clozaril.

S0137 **Didanosine (ddI), 25 mg** ☑
Use this code for Videx.

S0138 **Finasteride, 5 mg** ☑
Use this code for Propecia (oral), Proscar (oral).

S0139 **Minoxidil, 10 mg** ☑

S0140 **Saquinavir, 200 mg** ☑
Use this code for Fortovase (oral), Invirase (oral).

S0142 **Colistimethate sodium, inhalation solution administered through DME, concentrated form, per mg** ☑

S0145 **Injection, PEGylated interferon alfa-2A, 180 mcg per ml** ☑
Use this code for Pegasys.
CMS: 100-02,15,50.5

S0148 **Injection, PEGylated interferon alfa-2B, 10 mcg** ☑
CMS: 100-02,15,50.5

S0155 **Sterile dilutant for epoprostenol, 50 ml** ☑
Use this code for Flolan.

S0156 **Exemestane, 25 mg** ☑
Use this code for Aromasin.

S0157 **Becaplermin gel 0.01%, 0.5 gm** ☑
Use this code for Regranex Gel.

S0160 **Dextroamphetamine sulfate, 5 mg** ☑

S0164 ~~Injection, pantoprazole sodium, 40 mg~~
To report, see ~J2470-J2471

S0169 **Calcitriol, 0.25 mcg** ☑
Use this code for Calcijex.

S0170 **Anastrozole, oral, 1 mg** ☑
Use this code for Arimidex.

S0172 **Chlorambucil, oral, 2 mg** ☑
Use this code for Leukeran.

S0174 **Dolasetron mesylate, oral 50 mg (for circumstances falling under the Medicare statute, use Q0180)** ☑
Use this code for Anzemet.

S0175 **Flutamide, oral, 125 mg** ☑
Use this code for Eulexin.

S0176 Hydroxyurea, oral, 500 mg ☑
Use this code for Droxia, Hydrea, Mylocel.

S0177 Levamisole HCl, oral, 50 mg ☑
Use this code for Ergamisol.

S0178 Lomustine, oral, 10 mg ☑
Use this code for Ceenu.

S0179 Megestrol acetate, oral, 20 mg ☑
Use this code for Megace.

S0182 Procarbazine HCl, oral, 50 mg ☑
Use this code for Matulane.

S0183 Prochlorperazine maleate, oral, 5 mg (for circumstances falling under the Medicare statute, use Q0164) ☑
Use this code for Compazine.

S0187 Tamoxifen citrate, oral, 10 mg ☑
Use this code for Nolvadex.

S0189 Testosterone pellet, 75 mg ☑

S0190 Mifepristone, oral, 200 mg ☑
Use this code for Mifoprex 200 mg oral.

S0191 Misoprostol, oral, 200 mcg ☑

S0194 Dialysis/stress vitamin supplement, oral, 100 capsules ☑

S0197 Prenatal vitamins, 30-day supply ☑

S0199 Medically induced abortion by oral ingestion of medication including all associated services and supplies (e.g., patient counseling, office visits, confirmation of pregnancy by HCG, ultrasound to confirm duration of pregnancy, ultrasound to confirm completion of abortion) except drugs

S0201 Partial hospitalization services, less than 24 hours, per diem

S0207 Paramedic intercept, nonhospital-based ALS service (nonvoluntary), nontransport

S0208 Paramedic intercept, hospital-based ALS service (nonvoluntary), nontransport

S0209 Wheelchair van, mileage, per mile ☑

S0215 Nonemergency transportation; mileage, per mile ☑
See also codes A0021-A0999 for transportation.

S0220 Medical conference by a physician with interdisciplinary team of health professionals or representatives of community agencies to coordinate activities of patient care (patient is present); approximately 30 minutes ☑

S0221 Medical conference by a physician with interdisciplinary team of health professionals or representatives of community agencies to coordinate activities of patient care (patient is present); approximately 60 minutes ☑

S0250 Comprehensive geriatric assessment and treatment planning performed by assessment team A

S0255 Hospice referral visit (advising patient and family of care options) performed by nurse, social worker, or other designated staff
CMS: 100-04,11,10

S0257 Counseling and discussion regarding advance directives or end of life care planning and decisions, with patient and/or surrogate (list separately in addition to code for appropriate evaluation and management service)

S0260 History and physical (outpatient or office) related to surgical procedure (list separately in addition to code for appropriate evaluation and management service)

S0265 Genetic counseling, under physician supervision, each 15 minutes ☑

S0270 Physician management of patient home care, standard monthly case rate (per 30 days) ☑

S0271 Physician management of patient home care, hospice monthly case rate (per 30 days) ☑

S0272 Physician management of patient home care, episodic care monthly case rate (per 30 days) ☑

S0273 Physician visit at member's home, outside of a capitation arrangement

S0274 Nurse practitioner visit at member's home, outside of a capitation arrangement

S0280 Medical home program, comprehensive care coordination and planning, initial plan

S0281 Medical home program, comprehensive care coordination and planning, maintenance of plan

S0285 Colonoscopy consultation performed prior to a screening colonoscopy procedure

S0302 Completed early periodic screening diagnosis and treatment (EPSDT) service (list in addition to code for appropriate evaluation and management service)

S0310 Hospitalist services (list separately in addition to code for appropriate evaluation and management service)

S0311 Comprehensive management and care coordination for advanced illness, per calendar month

S0315 Disease management program; initial assessment and initiation of the program

S0316 Disease management program, follow-up/reassessment

S0317 Disease management program; per diem ☑

S0320 Telephone calls by a registered nurse to a disease management program member for monitoring purposes; per month

S0340 Lifestyle modification program for management of coronary artery disease, including all supportive services; first quarter/stage

S0341 Lifestyle modification program for management of coronary artery disease, including all supportive services; second or third quarter/stage

S0342 Lifestyle modification program for management of coronary artery disease, including all supportive services; fourth quarter/stage

S0353 Treatment planning and care coordination management for cancer initial treatment

S0354 Treatment planning and care coordination management for cancer established patient with a change of regimen

S0390 Routine foot care; removal and/or trimming of corns, calluses and/or nails and preventive maintenance in specific medical conditions (e.g., diabetes), per visit

S0395 Impression casting of a foot performed by a practitioner other than the manufacturer of the orthotic

S0400 Global fee for extracorporeal shock wave lithotripsy treatment of kidney stone(s)

S0500 Disposable contact lens, per lens ☑

S0504 Single vision prescription lens (safety, athletic, or sunglass), per lens ☑

S0506 Bifocal vision prescription lens (safety, athletic, or sunglass), per lens ☑

S0508 Trifocal vision prescription lens (safety, athletic, or sunglass), per lens ☑

S0510 Nonprescription lens (safety, athletic, or sunglass), per lens ☑

S0512 Daily wear specialty contact lens, per lens ☑

S0514 Color contact lens, per lens ☑

S0515 Scleral lens, liquid bandage device, per lens

S0516 Safety eyeglass frames

S0518 Sunglasses frames

S0580 Polycarbonate lens (list this code in addition to the basic code for the lens)

S0581 Nonstandard lens (list this code in addition to the basic code for the lens)

S0590 Integral lens service, miscellaneous services reported separately

S0592 Comprehensive contact lens evaluation

S0595 Dispensing new spectacle lenses for patient supplied frame

S0596 Phakic intraocular lens for correction of refractive error ☑

S0601 Screening proctoscopy

S0610 Annual gynecological examination, new patient A

S0612 Annual gynecological examination, established patient A

S0613 Annual gynecological examination; clinical breast examination without pelvic evaluation

S0618 Audiometry for hearing aid evaluation to determine the level and degree of hearing loss

S0620 Routine ophthalmological examination including refraction; new patient

S0621 Routine ophthalmological examination including refraction; established patient

S0622 Physical exam for college, new or established patient (list separately in addition to appropriate evaluation and management code)

S0630 Removal of sutures; by a physician other than the physician who originally closed the wound

S0800 Laser in situ keratomileusis (LASIK)

S0810 Photorefractive keratectomy (PRK)

S0812 Phototherapeutic keratectomy (PTK)

S1001 Deluxe item, patient aware (list in addition to code for basic item)
CMS: 100-02,15,110

S1002 Customized item (list in addition to code for basic item)

S1015 IV tubing extension set

S1016 Non-PVC (polyvinyl chloride) intravenous administration set, for use with drugs that are not stable in PVC, e.g., Paclitaxel

S1030 Continuous noninvasive glucose monitoring device, purchase (for physician interpretation of data, use CPT code)

S1031 Continuous noninvasive glucose monitoring device, rental, including sensor, sensor replacement, and download to monitor (for physician interpretation of data, use CPT code)

S1034 Artificial pancreas device system (e.g., low glucose suspend [LGS] feature) including continuous glucose monitor, blood glucose device, insulin pump and computer algorithm that communicates with all of the devices

S1035 Sensor; invasive (e.g., subcutaneous), disposable, for use with artificial pancreas device system

S1036 Transmitter; external, for use with artificial pancreas device system

S1037 Receiver (monitor); external, for use with artificial pancreas device system

S1040 Cranial remolding orthotic, pediatric, rigid, with soft interface material, custom fabricated, includes fitting and adjustment(s)

S1091 Stent, noncoronary, temporary, with delivery system (Propel)

S2053 Transplantation of small intestine and liver allografts

S2054 Transplantation of multivisceral organs

S2055 Harvesting of donor multivisceral organs, with preparation and maintenance of allografts; from cadaver donor

S2060 Lobar lung transplantation

S2061 Donor lobectomy (lung) for transplantation, living donor

S2065 Simultaneous pancreas kidney transplantation

S2066 Breast reconstruction with gluteal artery perforator (GAP) flap, including harvesting of the flap, microvascular transfer, closure of donor site and shaping the flap into a breast, unilateral

S2067 Breast reconstruction of a single breast with "stacked" deep inferior epigastric perforator (DIEP) flap(s) and/or gluteal artery perforator (GAP) flap(s), including harvesting of the flap(s), microvascular transfer, closure of donor site(s) and shaping the flap into a breast, unilateral

S2068 Breast reconstruction with deep inferior epigastric perforator (DIEP) flap or superficial inferior epigastric artery (SIEA) flap, including harvesting of the flap, microvascular transfer, closure of donor site and shaping the flap into a breast, unilateral

S2070 Cystourethroscopy, with ureteroscopy and/or pyeloscopy; with endoscopic laser treatment of ureteral calculi (includes ureteral catheterization)

S2079 Laparoscopic esophagomyotomy (Heller type)

S2080 Laser-assisted uvulopalatoplasty (LAUP)
AHA: 2Q,22

S2083 Adjustment of gastric band diameter via subcutaneous port by injection or aspiration of saline

S2095 Transcatheter occlusion or embolization for tumor destruction, percutaneous, any method, using yttrium-90 microspheres

S2102 Islet cell tissue transplant from pancreas; allogeneic

S2103 Adrenal tissue transplant to brain

S2107 Adoptive immunotherapy i.e. development of specific antitumor reactivity (e.g., tumor-infiltrating lymphocyte therapy) per course of treatment

S2112 Arthroscopy, knee, surgical for harvesting of cartilage (chondrocyte cells)

S2115 Osteotomy, periacetabular, with internal fixation

S2117 Arthroereisis, subtalar

S2118 Metal-on-metal total hip resurfacing, including acetabular and femoral components

S2120 Low density lipoprotein (LDL) apheresis using heparin-induced extracorporeal LDL precipitation

S2140 Cord blood harvesting for transplantation, allogeneic

S2142 Cord blood-derived stem-cell transplantation, allogeneic

S2150 Bone marrow or blood-derived stem cells (peripheral or umbilical), allogeneic or autologous, harvesting, transplantation, and related complications; including: pheresis and cell preparation/storage; marrow ablative therapy; drugs, supplies, hospitalization with outpatient follow-up; medical/surgical, diagnostic, emergency, and rehabilitative services; and the number of days of pre- and posttransplant care in the global definition

S2152 Solid organ(s), complete or segmental, single organ or combination of organs; deceased or living donor(s), procurement, transplantation, and related complications; including: drugs; supplies; hospitalization with outpatient follow-up; medical/surgical, diagnostic, emergency, and rehabilitative services, and the number of days of pre- and posttransplant care in the global definition

S2202 Echosclerotherapy

S2205 Minimally invasive direct coronary artery bypass surgery involving mini-thoracotomy or mini-sternotomy surgery, performed under direct vision; using arterial graft(s), single coronary arterial graft

S2206 Minimally invasive direct coronary artery bypass surgery involving mini-thoracotomy or mini-sternotomy surgery, performed under direct vision; using arterial graft(s), two coronary arterial grafts

S2207 Minimally invasive direct coronary artery bypass surgery involving mini-thoracotomy or mini-sternotomy surgery, performed under direct vision; using venous graft only, single coronary venous graft

S2208 Minimally invasive direct coronary artery bypass surgery involving mini-thoracotomy or mini-sternotomy surgery, performed under direct vision; using single arterial and venous graft(s), single venous graft

S2209 Minimally invasive direct coronary artery bypass surgery involving mini-thoracotomy or mini-sternotomy surgery, performed under direct vision; using two arterial grafts and single venous graft

S2225 Myringotomy, laser-assisted

S2230 Implantation of magnetic component of semi-implantable hearing device on ossicles in middle ear

S2235 Implantation of auditory brain stem implant

S2260 Induced abortion, 17 to 24 weeks M

S2265 Induced abortion, 25 to 28 weeks M

S2266 Induced abortion, 29 to 31 weeks M

S2267 Induced abortion, 32 weeks or greater M

S2300 Arthroscopy, shoulder, surgical; with thermally-induced capsulorrhaphy

S2325 Hip core decompression

S2340 Chemodenervation of abductor muscle(s) of vocal cord

S2341 Chemodenervation of adductor muscle(s) of vocal cord

S2342 Nasal endoscopy for postoperative debridement following functional endoscopic sinus surgery, nasal and/or sinus cavity(s), unilateral or bilateral

S2348 Decompression procedure, percutaneous, of nucleus pulposus of intervertebral disc, using radiofrequency energy, single or multiple levels, lumbar

S2350 Diskectomy, anterior, with decompression of spinal cord and/or nerve root(s), including osteophytectomy; lumbar, single interspace

S2351 Diskectomy, anterior, with decompression of spinal cord and/or nerve root(s), including osteophytectomy; lumbar, each additional interspace (list separately in addition to code for primary procedure)

S2400 Repair, congenital diaphragmatic hernia in the fetus using temporary tracheal occlusion, procedure performed in utero M

S2401 Repair, urinary tract obstruction in the fetus, procedure performed in utero M

S2402 Repair, congenital cystic adenomatoid malformation in the fetus, procedure performed in utero M

S2403 Repair, extralobar pulmonary sequestration in the fetus, procedure performed in utero M

S2404 Repair, myelomeningocele in the fetus, procedure performed in utero M

S2405 Repair of sacrococcygeal teratoma in the fetus, procedure performed in utero M

S2409 Repair, congenital malformation of fetus, procedure performed in utero, not otherwise classified M

S2411 Fetoscopic laser therapy for treatment of twin-to-twin transfusion syndrome M

S2900 Surgical techniques requiring use of robotic surgical system (list separately in addition to code for primary procedure)

S3000 Diabetic indicator; retinal eye exam, dilated, bilateral

S3005 Performance measurement, evaluation of patient self assessment, depression

S3600 STAT laboratory request (situations other than S3601)

S3601 Emergency STAT laboratory charge for patient who is homebound or residing in a nursing facility

S3620 Newborn metabolic screening panel, includes test kit, postage and the laboratory tests specified by the state for inclusion in this panel (e.g., galactose; hemoglobin, electrophoresis; hydroxyprogesterone, 17-d; phenylalanine (PKU); and thyroxine, total) A

S3630 Eosinophil count, blood, direct

S3645 HIV-1 antibody testing of oral mucosal transudate

S3650 Saliva test, hormone level; during menopause A

S3652 Saliva test, hormone level; to assess preterm labor risk M

S3655 Antisperm antibodies test (immunobead) M

S3708 Gastrointestinal fat absorption study

S3722 Dose optimization by area under the curve (AUC) analysis, for infusional 5-fluorouracil

S3800 Genetic testing for amyotrophic lateral sclerosis (ALS)

S3840 DNA analysis for germline mutations of the RET proto-oncogene for susceptibility to multiple endocrine neoplasia type 2

S3841 Genetic testing for retinoblastoma

S3842 Genetic testing for Von Hippel-Lindau disease

S3844 DNA analysis of the connexin 26 gene (GJB2) for susceptibility to congenital, profound deafness

S3845 Genetic testing for alpha-thalassemia

S3846 Genetic testing for hemoglobin E beta-thalassemia

S3849 Genetic testing for Niemann-Pick disease

S3850 Genetic testing for sickle cell anemia

S3852 DNA analysis for APOE epsilon 4 allele for susceptibility to Alzheimer's disease

S3853 Genetic testing for myotonic muscular dystrophy

S3854 Gene expression profiling panel for use in the management of breast cancer treatment

S3861 Genetic testing, sodium channel, voltage-gated, type V, alpha subunit (SCN5A) and variants for suspected Brugada Syndrome

S3865 Comprehensive gene sequence analysis for hypertrophic cardiomyopathy

S3866 Genetic analysis for a specific gene mutation for hypertrophic cardiomyopathy (HCM) in an individual with a known HCM mutation in the family

S3870 Comparative genomic hybridization (CGH) microarray testing for developmental delay, autism spectrum disorder and/or intellectual disability

S3900 Surface electromyography (EMG)

S3902 Ballistocardiogram

S3904 Masters two step

S4005 Interim labor facility global (labor occurring but not resulting in delivery) M

S4011 In vitro fertilization; including but not limited to identification and incubation of mature oocytes, fertilization with sperm, incubation of embryo(s), and subsequent visualization for determination of development M

S4013 Complete cycle, gamete intrafallopian transfer (GIFT), case rate M

S4014 Complete cycle, zygote intrafallopian transfer (ZIFT), case rate M

S4015 Complete in vitro fertilization cycle, not otherwise specified, case rate M

S4016 Frozen in vitro fertilization cycle, case rate M

S4017 Incomplete cycle, treatment cancelled prior to stimulation, case rate M

S4018 Frozen embryo transfer procedure cancelled before transfer, case rate M

S4020 In vitro fertilization procedure cancelled before aspiration, case rate M

S4021 In vitro fertilization procedure cancelled after aspiration, case rate M

S4022 Assisted oocyte fertilization, case rate M

S4023 Donor egg cycle, incomplete, case rate M

S4025 Donor services for in vitro fertilization (sperm or embryo), case rate A

S4026 Procurement of donor sperm from sperm bank

S4027 Storage of previously frozen embryos M

S4028 Microsurgical epididymal sperm aspiration (MESA) A

S4030 Sperm procurement and cryopreservation services; initial visit A

S4031 Sperm procurement and cryopreservation services; subsequent visit A

S4035 Stimulated intrauterine insemination (IUI), case rate M

S4037 Cryopreserved embryo transfer, case rate M

S4040 Monitoring and storage of cryopreserved embryos, per 30 days M

S4042 Management of ovulation induction (interpretation of diagnostic tests and studies, nonface-to-face medical management of the patient), per cycle

S4981 Insertion of levonorgestrel-releasing intrauterine system

● S4988 Penile contracture device, manual, greater than 3 lbs traction force E1

AHA: 2Q,24

S4989 Contraceptive intrauterine device (e.g., Progestasert IUD), including implants and supplies M

S4990 Nicotine patches, legend ☑

S4991 Nicotine patches, nonlegend ☑

S4993 Contraceptive pills for birth control M ☑

S4995 Smoking cessation gum ☑

S5000 Prescription drug, generic ☑

S5001 Prescription drug, brand name ☑

S5010 5% dextrose and 0.45% normal saline, 1000 ml ☑

S5012 5% dextrose with potassium chloride, 1000 ml ☑

S5013 5% dextrose/0.45% normal saline with potassium chloride and magnesium sulfate, 1000 ml ☑

S5014 5% dextrose/0.45% normal saline with potassium chloride and magnesium sulfate, 1500 ml ☑

S5035 Home infusion therapy, routine service of infusion device (e.g., pump maintenance)

S5036 Home infusion therapy, repair of infusion device (e.g., pump repair)

S5100 Day care services, adult; per 15 minutes A ☑

S5101 Day care services, adult; per half day A ☑

S5102 Day care services, adult; per diem A ☑

S5105 Day care services, center-based; services not included in program fee, per diem ☑

S5108 Home care training to home care client, per 15 minutes ☑

S5109 Home care training to home care client, per session ☑

S5110 Home care training, family; per 15 minutes ☑

S5111 Home care training, family; per session

S5115 Home care training, nonfamily; per 15 minutes ☑

S5116 Home care training, nonfamily; per session ☑

S5120 Chore services; per 15 minutes ☑

S5121 Chore services; per diem ☑

S5125 Attendant care services; per 15 minutes ☑

S5126 Attendant care services; per diem ☑

S5130 Homemaker service, NOS; per 15 minutes ☑

S5131 Homemaker service, NOS; per diem ☑

S5135 Companion care, adult (e.g., IADL/ADL); per 15 minutes A ☑

S5136 Companion care, adult (e.g., IADL/ADL); per diem A ☑

S5140 Foster care, adult; per diem A ☑

S5141 Foster care, adult; per month A ☑

S5145 Foster care, therapeutic, child; per diem A ☑

S5146 Foster care, therapeutic, child; per month A ☑

S5150 Unskilled respite care, not hospice; per 15 minutes ☑

S5151 Unskilled respite care, not hospice; per diem ☑

S5160 Emergency response system; installation and testing

S5161 Emergency response system; service fee, per month (excludes installation and testing) ☑

S5162 Emergency response system; purchase only

S5165 Home modifications; per service

S5170 Home delivered meals, including preparation; per meal

S5175 Laundry service, external, professional; per order

S5180 Home health respiratory therapy, initial evaluation

S5181 Home health respiratory therapy, NOS, per diem

Code	Description
S5185	Medication reminder service, nonface-to-face; per month ☑
S5190	Wellness assessment, performed by nonphysician
S5199	Personal care item, NOS, each
S5497	Home infusion therapy, catheter care/maintenance, not otherwise classified; includes administrative services, professional pharmacy services, care coordination, and all necessary supplies and equipment (drugs and nursing visits coded separately), per diem ☑
S5498	Home infusion therapy, catheter care/maintenance, simple (single lumen), includes administrative services, professional pharmacy services, care coordination and all necessary supplies and equipment, (drugs and nursing visits coded separately), per diem ☑
S5501	Home infusion therapy, catheter care/maintenance, complex (more than one lumen), includes administrative services, professional pharmacy services, care coordination, and all necessary supplies and equipment (drugs and nursing visits coded separately), per diem ☑
S5502	Home infusion therapy, catheter care/maintenance, implanted access device, includes administrative services, professional pharmacy services, care coordination and all necessary supplies and equipment (drugs and nursing visits coded separately), per diem (use this code for interim maintenance of vascular access not currently in use) ☑
S5517	Home infusion therapy, all supplies necessary for restoration of catheter patency or declotting
S5518	Home infusion therapy, all supplies necessary for catheter repair
S5520	Home infusion therapy, all supplies (including catheter) necessary for a peripherally inserted central venous catheter (PICC) line insertion
S5521	Home infusion therapy, all supplies (including catheter) necessary for a midline catheter insertion
S5522	Home infusion therapy, insertion of peripherally inserted central venous catheter (PICC), nursing services only (no supplies or catheter included)
S5523	Home infusion therapy, insertion of midline venous catheter, nursing services only (no supplies or catheter included)
S5550	Insulin, rapid onset, 5 units ☑
S5551	Insulin, most rapid onset (Lispro or Aspart); 5 units ☑
S5552	Insulin, intermediate acting (NPH or LENTE); 5 units ☑
S5553	Insulin, long acting; 5 units ☑ CMS: 100-02,15,50.5
S5560	Insulin delivery device, reusable pen; 1.5 ml size ☑
S5561	Insulin delivery device, reusable pen; 3 ml size ☑
S5565	Insulin cartridge for use in insulin delivery device other than pump; 150 units ☑
S5566	Insulin cartridge for use in insulin delivery device other than pump; 300 units ☑
S5570	Insulin delivery device, disposable pen (including insulin); 1.5 ml size ☑ CMS: 100-02,15,50.5
S5571	Insulin delivery device, disposable pen (including insulin); 3 ml size ☑ CMS: 100-02,15,50.5
S8030	Scleral application of tantalum ring(s) for localization of lesions for proton beam therapy
S8035	Magnetic source imaging
S8037	Magnetic resonance cholangiopancreatography (MRCP)
S8040	Topographic brain mapping
S8042	Magnetic resonance imaging (MRI), low-field
S8055	Ultrasound guidance for multifetal pregnancy reduction(s), technical component (only to be used when the physician doing the reduction procedure does not perform the ultrasound, guidance is included in the CPT code for multifetal pregnancy reduction (59866) M
S8080	Scintimammography (radioimmunoscintigraphy of the breast), unilateral, including supply of radiopharmaceutical
S8085	Fluorine-18 fluorodeoxyglucose (F-18 FDG) imaging using dual-head coincidence detection system (nondedicated PET scan)
S8092	Electron beam computed tomography (also known as ultrafast CT, cine CT)
S8096	Portable peak flow meter
S8097	Asthma kit (including but not limited to portable peak expiratory flow meter, instructional video, brochure, and/or spacer) ☑
S8100	Holding chamber or spacer for use with an inhaler or nebulizer; without mask
S8101	Holding chamber or spacer for use with an inhaler or nebulizer; with mask
S8110	Peak expiratory flow rate (physician services)
S8120	Oxygen contents, gaseous, 1 unit equals 1 cubic foot ☑
S8121	Oxygen contents, liquid, 1 unit equals 1 pound ☑
S8130	Interferential current stimulator, 2 channel
S8131	Interferential current stimulator, 4 channel
S8185	Flutter device
S8186	Swivel adaptor
S8189	Tracheostomy supply, not otherwise classified
S8210	Mucus trap
S8265	Haberman feeder for cleft lip/palate
S8270	Enuresis alarm, using auditory buzzer and/or vibration device
S8301	Infection control supplies, not otherwise specified
S8415	Supplies for home delivery of infant M
S8420	Gradient pressure aid (sleeve and glove combination), custom made
S8421	Gradient pressure aid (sleeve and glove combination), ready made
S8422	Gradient pressure aid (sleeve), custom made, medium weight
S8423	Gradient pressure aid (sleeve), custom made, heavy weight
S8424	Gradient pressure aid (sleeve), ready made
S8425	Gradient pressure aid (glove), custom made, medium weight
S8426	Gradient pressure aid (glove), custom made, heavy weight
S8427	Gradient pressure aid (glove), ready made
S8428	Gradient pressure aid (gauntlet), ready made
S8429	Gradient pressure exterior wrap
S8430	Padding for compression bandage, roll ☑
S8431	Compression bandage, roll ☑

Special Coverage Instructions Noncovered by Medicare Carrier Discretion ☑ Quantity Alert ● New Code ○ Recycled/Reinstated ▲ Revised Code

 A2-Z3 ASC A-Y OPPS CMS: IOM AHA: Coding Clinic ♿ DMEPOS Paid ⊘ SNF Excluded A Age M Maternity

S8450 Splint, prefabricated, digit (specify digit by use of modifier) ☑

Various types of digit splints (S8450)

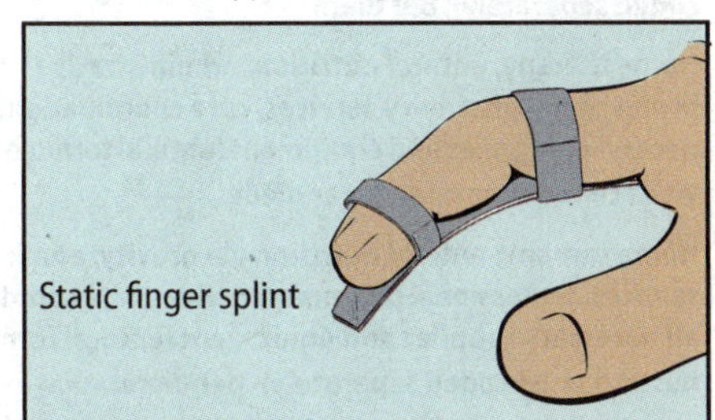

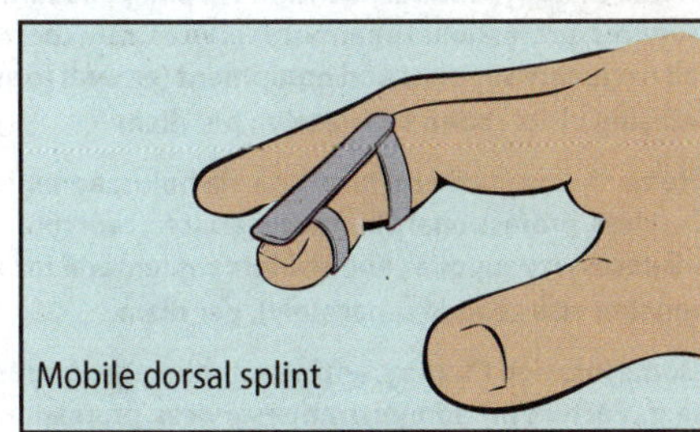

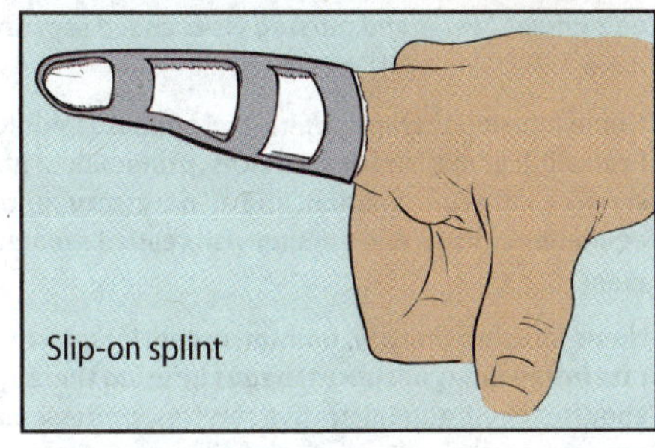

S8451 Splint, prefabricated, wrist or ankle ☑

S8452 Splint, prefabricated, elbow ☑

S8460 Camisole, postmastectomy

S8490 Insulin syringes (100 syringes, any size) ☑

S8930 Electrical stimulation of auricular acupuncture points; each 15 minutes of personal one-on-one contact with patient ☑

S8940 Equestrian/hippotherapy, per session

S8948 Application of a modality (requiring constant provider attendance) to one or more areas; low-level laser; each 15 minutes ☑

S8950 Complex lymphedema therapy, each 15 minutes ☑

S8990 Physical or manipulative therapy performed for maintenance rather than restoration

S8999 Resuscitation bag (for use by patient on artificial respiration during power failure or other catastrophic event)

S9001 Home uterine monitor with or without associated nursing services M

● **S9002** Intravaginal motion sensor system, provides biofeedback for pelvic floor muscle rehabilitation device E1

AHA: 2Q,24

S9007 Ultrafiltration monitor

S9024 Paranasal sinus ultrasound

S9025 Omnicardiogram/cardiointegram

S9034 Extracorporeal shockwave lithotripsy for gall stones (if performed with ERCP, use 43265)

S9055 Procuren or other growth factor preparation to promote wound healing

S9056 Coma stimulation per diem ☑

S9061 Home administration of aerosolized drug therapy (e.g., Pentamidine); administrative services, professional pharmacy services, care coordination, all necessary supplies and equipment (drugs and nursing visits coded separately), per diem ☑

S9083 Global fee urgent care centers

S9088 Services provided in an urgent care center (list in addition to code for service)

S9090 Vertebral axial decompression, per session ☑

S9097 Home visit for wound care

S9098 Home visit, phototherapy services (e.g., Bili-lite), including equipment rental, nursing services, blood draw, supplies, and other services, per diem ☑

S9110 Telemonitoring of patient in their home, including all necessary equipment; computer system, connections, and software; maintenance; patient education and support; per month

S9117 Back school, per visit ☑

S9122 Home health aide or certified nurse assistant, providing care in the home; per hour ☑

S9123 Nursing care, in the home; by registered nurse, per hour (use for general nursing care only, not to be used when CPT codes 99500-99602 can be used) ☑

S9124 Nursing care, in the home; by licensed practical nurse, per hour ☑

S9125 Respite care, in the home, per diem ☑

S9126 Hospice care, in the home, per diem ☑

CMS: 100-04,11,10

S9127 Social work visit, in the home, per diem ☑

S9128 Speech therapy, in the home, per diem ☑

S9129 Occupational therapy, in the home, per diem ☑

S9131 Physical therapy; in the home, per diem ☑

S9140 Diabetic management program, follow-up visit to non-MD provider ☑

S9141 Diabetic management program, follow-up visit to MD provider ☑

S9145 Insulin pump initiation, instruction in initial use of pump (pump not included)

S9150 Evaluation by ocularist

S9152 Speech therapy, re-evaluation

S9208 Home management of preterm labor, including administrative services, professional pharmacy services, care coordination, and all necessary supplies or equipment (drugs and nursing visits coded separately), per diem (do not use this code with any home infusion per diem code) M☑

S9209 Home management of preterm premature rupture of membranes (PPROM), including administrative services, professional pharmacy services, care coordination, and all necessary supplies or equipment (drugs and nursing visits coded separately), per diem (do not use this code with any home infusion per diem code) M☑

S9211 Home management of gestational hypertension, includes administrative services, professional pharmacy services, care coordination and all necessary supplies and equipment (drugs and nursing visits coded separately); per diem (do not use this code with any home infusion per diem code) M☑

Temporary National Codes (Non-Medicare) S8450 — S9211

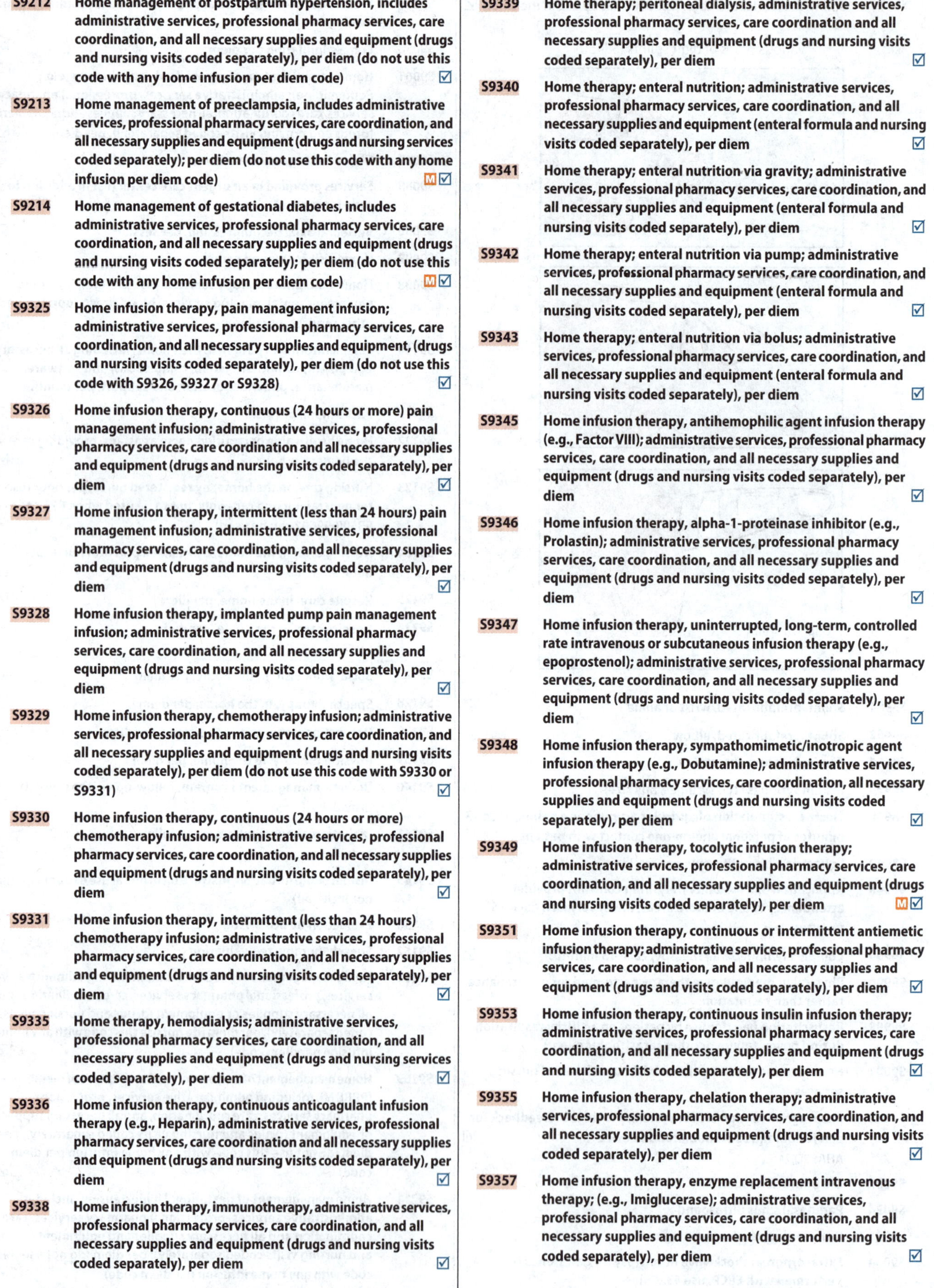

S9212 Home management of postpartum hypertension, includes administrative services, professional pharmacy services, care coordination, and all necessary supplies and equipment (drugs and nursing visits coded separately), per diem (do not use this code with any home infusion per diem code) ☑

S9213 Home management of preeclampsia, includes administrative services, professional pharmacy services, care coordination, and all necessary supplies and equipment (drugs and nursing services coded separately); per diem (do not use this code with any home infusion per diem code) M ☑

S9214 Home management of gestational diabetes, includes administrative services, professional pharmacy services, care coordination, and all necessary supplies and equipment (drugs and nursing visits coded separately); per diem (do not use this code with any home infusion per diem code) M ☑

S9325 Home infusion therapy, pain management infusion; administrative services, professional pharmacy services, care coordination, and all necessary supplies and equipment, (drugs and nursing visits coded separately), per diem (do not use this code with S9326, S9327 or S9328) ☑

S9326 Home infusion therapy, continuous (24 hours or more) pain management infusion; administrative services, professional pharmacy services, care coordination and all necessary supplies and equipment (drugs and nursing visits coded separately), per diem ☑

S9327 Home infusion therapy, intermittent (less than 24 hours) pain management infusion; administrative services, professional pharmacy services, care coordination, and all necessary supplies and equipment (drugs and nursing visits coded separately), per diem ☑

S9328 Home infusion therapy, implanted pump pain management infusion; administrative services, professional pharmacy services, care coordination, and all necessary supplies and equipment (drugs and nursing visits coded separately), per diem ☑

S9329 Home infusion therapy, chemotherapy infusion; administrative services, professional pharmacy services, care coordination, and all necessary supplies and equipment (drugs and nursing visits coded separately), per diem (do not use this code with S9330 or S9331) ☑

S9330 Home infusion therapy, continuous (24 hours or more) chemotherapy infusion; administrative services, professional pharmacy services, care coordination, and all necessary supplies and equipment (drugs and nursing visits coded separately), per diem ☑

S9331 Home infusion therapy, intermittent (less than 24 hours) chemotherapy infusion; administrative services, professional pharmacy services, care coordination, and all necessary supplies and equipment (drugs and nursing visits coded separately), per diem ☑

S9335 Home therapy, hemodialysis; administrative services, professional pharmacy services, care coordination, and all necessary supplies and equipment (drugs and nursing services coded separately), per diem ☑

S9336 Home infusion therapy, continuous anticoagulant infusion therapy (e.g., Heparin), administrative services, professional pharmacy services, care coordination and all necessary supplies and equipment (drugs and nursing visits coded separately), per diem ☑

S9338 Home infusion therapy, immunotherapy, administrative services, professional pharmacy services, care coordination, and all necessary supplies and equipment (drugs and nursing visits coded separately), per diem ☑

S9339 Home therapy; peritoneal dialysis, administrative services, professional pharmacy services, care coordination and all necessary supplies and equipment (drugs and nursing visits coded separately), per diem ☑

S9340 Home therapy; enteral nutrition; administrative services, professional pharmacy services, care coordination, and all necessary supplies and equipment (enteral formula and nursing visits coded separately), per diem ☑

S9341 Home therapy; enteral nutrition via gravity; administrative services, professional pharmacy services, care coordination, and all necessary supplies and equipment (enteral formula and nursing visits coded separately), per diem ☑

S9342 Home therapy; enteral nutrition via pump; administrative services, professional pharmacy services, care coordination, and all necessary supplies and equipment (enteral formula and nursing visits coded separately), per diem ☑

S9343 Home therapy; enteral nutrition via bolus; administrative services, professional pharmacy services, care coordination, and all necessary supplies and equipment (enteral formula and nursing visits coded separately), per diem ☑

S9345 Home infusion therapy, antihemophilic agent infusion therapy (e.g., Factor VIII); administrative services, professional pharmacy services, care coordination, and all necessary supplies and equipment (drugs and nursing visits coded separately), per diem ☑

S9346 Home infusion therapy, alpha-1-proteinase inhibitor (e.g., Prolastin); administrative services, professional pharmacy services, care coordination, and all necessary supplies and equipment (drugs and nursing visits coded separately), per diem ☑

S9347 Home infusion therapy, uninterrupted, long-term, controlled rate intravenous or subcutaneous infusion therapy (e.g., epoprostenol); administrative services, professional pharmacy services, care coordination, and all necessary supplies and equipment (drugs and nursing visits coded separately), per diem ☑

S9348 Home infusion therapy, sympathomimetic/inotropic agent infusion therapy (e.g., Dobutamine); administrative services, professional pharmacy services, care coordination, all necessary supplies and equipment (drugs and nursing visits coded separately), per diem ☑

S9349 Home infusion therapy, tocolytic infusion therapy; administrative services, professional pharmacy services, care coordination, and all necessary supplies and equipment (drugs and nursing visits coded separately), per diem M ☑

S9351 Home infusion therapy, continuous or intermittent antiemetic infusion therapy; administrative services, professional pharmacy services, care coordination, and all necessary supplies and equipment (drugs and visits coded separately), per diem ☑

S9353 Home infusion therapy, continuous insulin infusion therapy; administrative services, professional pharmacy services, care coordination, and all necessary supplies and equipment (drugs and nursing visits coded separately), per diem ☑

S9355 Home infusion therapy, chelation therapy; administrative services, professional pharmacy services, care coordination, and all necessary supplies and equipment (drugs and nursing visits coded separately), per diem ☑

S9357 Home infusion therapy, enzyme replacement intravenous therapy; (e.g., Imiglucerase); administrative services, professional pharmacy services, care coordination, and all necessary supplies and equipment (drugs and nursing visits coded separately), per diem ☑

S9359 Home infusion therapy, antitumor necrosis factor intravenous therapy; (e.g., Infliximab); administrative services, professional pharmacy services, care coordination, and all necessary supplies and equipment (drugs and nursing visits coded separately), per diem ☑

S9361 Home infusion therapy, diuretic intravenous therapy; administrative services, professional pharmacy services, care coordination, and all necessary supplies and equipment (drugs and nursing visits coded separately), per diem ☑

S9363 Home infusion therapy, antispasmotic therapy; administrative services, professional pharmacy services, care coordination, and all necessary supplies and equipment (drugs and nursing visits coded separately), per diem ☑

S9364 Home infusion therapy, total parenteral nutrition (TPN); administrative services, professional pharmacy services, care coordination, and all necessary supplies and equipment including standard TPN formula (lipids, specialty amino acid formulas, drugs other than in standard formula and nursing visits coded separately), per diem (do not use with home infusion codes S9365-S9368 using daily volume scales) ☑

S9365 Home infusion therapy, total parenteral nutrition (TPN); one liter per day, administrative services, professional pharmacy services, care coordination, and all necessary supplies and equipment including standard TPN formula (lipids, specialty amino acid formulas, drugs other than in standard formula and nursing visits coded separately), per diem ☑

S9366 Home infusion therapy, total parenteral nutrition (TPN); more than one liter but no more than two liters per day, administrative services, professional pharmacy services, care coordination, and all necessary supplies and equipment including standard TPN formula (lipids, specialty amino acid formulas, drugs other than in standard formula and nursing visits coded separately), per diem ☑

S9367 Home infusion therapy, total parenteral nutrition (TPN); more than two liters but no more than three liters per day, administrative services, professional pharmacy services, care coordination, and all necessary supplies and equipment including standard TPN formula (lipids, specialty amino acid formulas, drugs other than in standard formula and nursing visits coded separately), per diem ☑

S9368 Home infusion therapy, total parenteral nutrition (TPN); more than three liters per day, administrative services, professional pharmacy services, care coordination, and all necessary supplies and equipment including standard TPN formula (lipids, specialty amino acid formulas, drugs other than in standard formula and nursing visits coded separately), per diem ☑

S9370 Home therapy, intermittent antiemetic injection therapy; administrative services, professional pharmacy services, care coordination, and all necessary supplies and equipment (drugs and nursing visits coded separately), per diem ☑

S9372 Home therapy; intermittent anticoagulant injection therapy (e.g., Heparin); administrative services, professional pharmacy services, care coordination, and all necessary supplies and equipment (drugs and nursing visits coded separately), per diem (do not use this code for flushing of infusion devices with Heparin to maintain patency) ☑

S9373 Home infusion therapy, hydration therapy; administrative services, professional pharmacy services, care coordination, and all necessary supplies and equipment (drugs and nursing visits coded separately), per diem (do not use with hydration therapy codes S9374-S9377 using daily volume scales) ☑

S9374 Home infusion therapy, hydration therapy; 1 liter per day, administrative services, professional pharmacy services, care coordination, and all necessary supplies and equipment (drugs and nursing visits coded separately), per diem ☑

S9375 Home infusion therapy, hydration therapy; more than 1 liter but no more than 2 liters per day, administrative services, professional pharmacy services, care coordination, and all necessary supplies and equipment (drugs and nursing visits coded separately), per diem ☑

S9376 Home infusion therapy, hydration therapy; more than 2 liters but no more than 3 liters per day, administrative services, professional pharmacy services, care coordination, and all necessary supplies and equipment (drugs and nursing visits coded separately), per diem ☑

S9377 Home infusion therapy, hydration therapy; more than 3 liters per day, administrative services, professional pharmacy services, care coordination, and all necessary supplies (drugs and nursing visits coded separately), per diem ☑

S9379 Home infusion therapy, infusion therapy, not otherwise classified; administrative services, professional pharmacy services, care coordination, and all necessary supplies and equipment (drugs and nursing visits coded separately), per diem ☑

S9381 Delivery or service to high risk areas requiring escort or extra protection, per visit

S9401 Anticoagulation clinic, inclusive of all services except laboratory tests, per session

S9430 Pharmacy compounding and dispensing services

S9432 Medical foods for noninborn errors of metabolism

S9433 Medical food nutritionally complete, administered orally, providing 100% of nutritional intake

S9434 Modified solid food supplements for inborn errors of metabolism

S9435 Medical foods for inborn errors of metabolism

S9436 Childbirth preparation/Lamaze classes, nonphysician provider, per session M ☑

S9437 Childbirth refresher classes, nonphysician provider, per session M

S9438 Cesarean birth classes, nonphysician provider, per session M ☑

S9439 VBAC (vaginal birth after cesarean) classes, nonphysician provider, per session M ☑

S9441 Asthma education, nonphysician provider, per session ☑

S9442 Birthing classes, nonphysician provider, per session M ☑

S9443 Lactation classes, nonphysician provider, per session M ☑

S9444 Parenting classes, nonphysician provider, per session ☑

S9445 Patient education, not otherwise classified, nonphysician provider, individual, per session ☑

S9446 Patient education, not otherwise classified, nonphysician provider, group, per session ☑

S9447 Infant safety (including CPR) classes, nonphysician provider, per session ☑

S9449 Weight management classes, nonphysician provider, per session ☑

S9451 Exercise classes, nonphysician provider, per session

S9452 Nutrition classes, nonphysician provider, per session

S9453 Smoking cessation classes, nonphysician provider, per session

S9454 Stress management classes, nonphysician provider, per session

S9455 Diabetic management program, group session

S9460 Diabetic management program, nurse visit

S9465 Diabetic management program, dietitian visit

S9470 Nutritional counseling, dietitian visit

S9472 Cardiac rehabilitation program, nonphysician provider, per diem

S9473 Pulmonary rehabilitation program, nonphysician provider, per diem

S9474 Enterostomal therapy by a registered nurse certified in enterostomal therapy, per diem

S9475 Ambulatory setting substance abuse treatment or detoxification services, per diem

S9476 Vestibular rehabilitation program, nonphysician provider, per diem

S9480 Intensive outpatient psychiatric services, per diem

S9482 Family stabilization services, per 15 minutes ☑

S9484 Crisis intervention mental health services, per hour ☑

S9485 Crisis intervention mental health services, per diem

S9490 Home infusion therapy, corticosteroid infusion; administrative services, professional pharmacy services, care coordination, and all necessary supplies and equipment (drugs and nursing visits coded separately), per diem ☑

S9494 Home infusion therapy, antibiotic, antiviral, or antifungal therapy; administrative services, professional pharmacy services, care coordination, and all necessary supplies and equipment (drugs and nursing visits coded separately), per diem (do not use this code with home infusion codes for hourly dosing schedules S9497-S9504) ☑

S9497 Home infusion therapy, antibiotic, antiviral, or antifungal therapy; once every 3 hours; administrative services, professional pharmacy services, care coordination, and all necessary supplies and equipment (drugs and nursing visits coded separately), per diem ☑

S9500 Home infusion therapy, antibiotic, antiviral, or antifungal therapy; once every 24 hours; administrative services, professional pharmacy services, care coordination, and all necessary supplies and equipment (drugs and nursing visits coded separately), per diem ☑

S9501 Home infusion therapy, antibiotic, antiviral, or antifungal therapy; once every 12 hours; administrative services, professional pharmacy services, care coordination, and all necessary supplies and equipment (drugs and nursing visits coded separately), per diem ☑

S9502 Home infusion therapy, antibiotic, antiviral, or antifungal therapy; once every 8 hours, administrative services, professional pharmacy services, care coordination, and all necessary supplies and equipment (drugs and nursing visits coded separately), per diem ☑

S9503 Home infusion therapy, antibiotic, antiviral, or antifungal; once every 6 hours; administrative services, professional pharmacy services, care coordination, and all necessary supplies and equipment (drugs and nursing visits coded separately), per diem ☑

S9504 Home infusion therapy, antibiotic, antiviral, or antifungal; once every 4 hours; administrative services, professional pharmacy services, care coordination, and all necessary supplies and equipment (drugs and nursing visits coded separately), per diem ☑

S9529 Routine venipuncture for collection of specimen(s), single homebound, nursing home, or skilled nursing facility patient ☑

S9537 Home therapy; hematopoietic hormone injection therapy (e.g., erythropoietin, G-CSF, GM-CSF); administrative services, professional pharmacy services, care coordination, and all necessary supplies and equipment (drugs and nursing visits coded separately), per diem ☑

S9538 Home transfusion of blood product(s); administrative services, professional pharmacy services, care coordination and all necessary supplies and equipment (blood products, drugs, and nursing visits coded separately), per diem ☑

S9542 Home injectable therapy, not otherwise classified, including administrative services, professional pharmacy services, care coordination, and all necessary supplies and equipment (drugs and nursing visits coded separately), per diem ☑

S9558 Home injectable therapy; growth hormone, including administrative services, professional pharmacy services, care coordination, and all necessary supplies and equipment (drugs and nursing visits coded separately), per diem ☑

S9559 Home injectable therapy, interferon, including administrative services, professional pharmacy services, care coordination, and all necessary supplies and equipment (drugs and nursing visits coded separately), per diem ☑

S9560 Home injectable therapy; hormonal therapy (e.g., leuprolide, goserelin), including administrative services, professional pharmacy services, care coordination, and all necessary supplies and equipment (drugs and nursing visits coded separately), per diem ☑

S9562 Home injectable therapy, palivizumab or other monoclonal antibody for RSV, including administrative services, professional pharmacy services, care coordination, and all necessary supplies and equipment (drugs and nursing visits coded separately), per diem ☑

AHA: 2Q,23

S9563 Home injectable therapy, immunotherapy, including administrative services, professional pharmacy services, care coordination, and all necessary supplies and equipment (drugs and nursing visits coded separately), per diem

AHA: 2Q,23

S9590 Home therapy, irrigation therapy (e.g., sterile irrigation of an organ or anatomical cavity); including administrative services, professional pharmacy services, care coordination, and all necessary supplies and equipment (drugs and nursing visits coded separately), per diem ☑

S9810 Home therapy; professional pharmacy services for provision of infusion, specialty drug administration, and/or disease state management, not otherwise classified, per hour (do not use this code with any per diem code) ☑

S9900 Services by a Journal-listed Christian Science practitioner for the purpose of healing, per diem

S9901 Services by a Journal-listed Christian Science nurse, per hour

S9960 Ambulance service, conventional air services, nonemergency transport, one way (fixed wing)

S9961 Ambulance service, conventional air service, nonemergency transport, one way (rotary wing)

S9970 Health club membership, annual

S9975 Transplant related lodging, meals and transportation, per diem

S9976 Lodging, per diem, not otherwise classified

S9977 Meals, per diem, not otherwise specified

S9981 Medical records copying fee, administrative

S9982 Medical records copying fee, per page ☑

S9986 Not medically necessary service (patient is aware that service not medically necessary)

S9988 Services provided as part of a Phase I clinical trial

S9989 Services provided outside of the United States of America (list in addition to code(s) for services(s))

S9990 Services provided as part of a Phase II clinical trial

S9991 Services provided as part of a Phase III clinical trial

S9992 Transportation costs to and from trial location and local transportation costs (e.g., fares for taxicab or bus) for clinical trial participant and one caregiver/companion

S9994 Lodging costs (e.g., hotel charges) for clinical trial participant and one caregiver/companion

S9996 Meals for clinical trial participant and one caregiver/companion

S9999 Sales tax

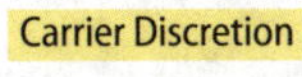
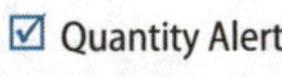
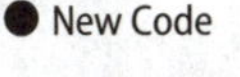
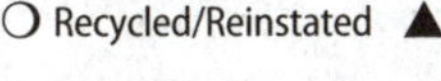

National T Codes Established for State Medicaid Agencies T1000-T5999

The T codes are designed for use by Medicaid state agencies to establish codes for items for which there are no permanent national codes but for which codes are necessary to administer the Medicaid program (T codes are not accepted by Medicare but can be used by private insurers). This range of codes describes nursing and home health-related services, substance abuse treatment, and certain training-related procedures.

T1000 Private duty/independent nursing service(s), licensed, up to 15 minutes ☑

T1001 Nursing assessment/evaluation

T1002 RN services, up to 15 minutes ☑

T1003 LPN/LVN services, up to 15 minutes ☑

T1004 Services of a qualified nursing aide, up to 15 minutes ☑

T1005 Respite care services, up to 15 minutes ☑

T1006 Alcohol and/or substance abuse services, family/couple counseling

T1007 Alcohol and/or substance abuse services, treatment plan development and/or modification

T1009 Child sitting services for children of the individual receiving alcohol and/or substance abuse services

T1010 Meals for individuals receiving alcohol and/or substance abuse services (when meals not included in the program)

T1012 Alcohol and/or substance abuse services, skills development

T1013 Sign language or oral interpretive services, per 15 minutes ☑

T1014 Telehealth transmission, per minute, professional services bill separately

T1015 Clinic visit/encounter, all-inclusive

T1016 Case management, each 15 minutes ☑

T1017 Targeted case management, each 15 minutes ☑

T1018 School-based individualized education program (IEP) services, bundled

T1019 Personal care services, per 15 minutes, not for an inpatient or resident of a hospital, nursing facility, ICF/MR or IMD, part of the individualized plan of treatment (code may not be used to identify services provided by home health aide or certified nurse assistant) ☑

T1020 Personal care services, per diem, not for an inpatient or resident of a hospital, nursing facility, ICF/MR or IMD, part of the individualized plan of treatment (code may not be used to identify services provided by home health aide or certified nurse assistant)

T1021 Home health aide or certified nurse assistant, per visit

T1022 Contracted home health agency services, all services provided under contract, per day

T1023 Screening to determine the appropriateness of consideration of an individual for participation in a specified program, project or treatment protocol, per encounter

T1024 Evaluation and treatment by an integrated, specialty team contracted to provide coordinated care to multiple or severely handicapped children, per encounter A

T1025 Intensive, extended multidisciplinary services provided in a clinic setting to children with complex medical, physical, mental and psychosocial impairments, per diem A

T1026 Intensive, extended multidisciplinary services provided in a clinic setting to children with complex medical, physical, mental, and psychosocial impairments, per hour A

T1027 Family training and counseling for child development, per 15 minutes ☑

T1028 Assessment of home, physical and family environment, to determine suitability to meet patient's medical needs

T1029 Comprehensive environmental lead investigation, not including laboratory analysis, per dwelling

T1030 Nursing care, in the home, by registered nurse, per diem ☑

T1031 Nursing care, in the home, by licensed practical nurse, per diem ☑

T1032 Services performed by a doula birth worker, per 15 minutes
AHA: 4Q,22

T1033 Services performed by a doula birth worker, per diem
AHA: 4Q,22

T1040 Medicaid certified community behavioral health clinic services, per diem

T1041 Medicaid certified community behavioral health clinic services, per month

T1502 Administration of oral, intramuscular and/or subcutaneous medication by health care agency/professional, per visit ☑

T1503 Administration of medication, other than oral and/or injectable, by a health care agency/professional, per visit ☑

T1505 Electronic medication compliance management device, includes all components and accessories, not otherwise classified

T1999 Miscellaneous therapeutic items and supplies, retail purchases, not otherwise classified; identify product in "remarks"

T2001 Nonemergency transportation; patient attendant/escort

T2002 Nonemergency transportation; per diem ☑

T2003 Nonemergency transportation; encounter/trip

T2004 Nonemergency transport; commercial carrier, multipass

T2005 Nonemergency transportation; stretcher van

T2007 Transportation waiting time, air ambulance and nonemergency vehicle, one-half (1/2) hour increments ☑

T2010 Preadmission screening and resident review (PASRR) Level I identification screening, per screen ☑

T2011 Preadmission screening and resident review (PASRR) Level II evaluation, per evaluation

T2012 Habilitation, educational; waiver, per diem ☑

T2013 Habilitation, educational, waiver; per hour ☑

T2014 Habilitation, prevocational, waiver; per diem ☑

T2015 Habilitation, prevocational, waiver; per hour ☑

T2016 Habilitation, residential, waiver; per diem ☑

T2017 Habilitation, residential, waiver; 15 minutes ☑

T2018 Habilitation, supported employment, waiver; per diem ☑

T2019 Habilitation, supported employment, waiver; per 15 minutes ☑

T2020 Day habilitation, waiver; per diem ☑

T2021 Day habilitation, waiver; per 15 minutes ☑

T2022 Case management, per month ☑

T2023 Targeted case management; per month ☑

T2024 Service assessment/plan of care development, waiver

T2025 Waiver services; not otherwise specified (NOS)

T2026 Specialized childcare, waiver; per diem ☑

T2027 Specialized childcare, waiver; per 15 minutes ☑

National T Codes

T1000 — T2027

T2028 Specialized supply, not otherwise specified, waiver

T2029 Specialized medical equipment, not otherwise specified, waiver

T2030 Assisted living, waiver; per month ☑

T2031 Assisted living; waiver, per diem ☑

T2032 Residential care, not otherwise specified (NOS), waiver; per month ☑

T2033 Residential care, not otherwise specified (NOS), waiver; per diem ☑

T2034 Crisis intervention, waiver; per diem ☑

T2035 Utility services to support medical equipment and assistive technology/devices, waiver

T2036 Therapeutic camping, overnight, waiver; each session ☑

T2037 Therapeutic camping, day, waiver; each session ☑

T2038 Community transition, waiver; per service ☑

T2039 Vehicle modifications, waiver; per service ☑

T2040 Financial management, self-directed, waiver; per 15 minutes ☑

T2041 Supports brokerage, self-directed, waiver; per 15 minutes ☑

T2042 Hospice routine home care; per diem ☑
CMS: 100-04,11,10

T2043 Hospice continuous home care; per hour ☑
CMS: 100-04,11,10

T2044 Hospice inpatient respite care; per diem ☑
CMS: 100-04,11,10

T2045 Hospice general inpatient care; per diem ☑
CMS: 100-04,11,10

T2046 Hospice long-term care, room and board only; per diem ☑
CMS: 100-04,11,10

T2047 Habilitation, prevocational, waiver; per 15 minutes

T2048 Behavioral health; long-term care residential (nonacute care in a residential treatment program where stay is typically longer than 30 days), with room and board, per diem ☑

T2049 Nonemergency transportation; stretcher van, mileage; per mile ☑

T2050 Financial management, self-directed, waiver; per diem

T2051 Supports brokerage, self-directed, waiver; per diem

T2101 Human breast milk processing, storage and distribution only

T4521 Adult sized disposable incontinence product, brief/diaper, small, each ☑

T4522 Adult sized disposable incontinence product, brief/diaper, medium, each ☑

T4523 Adult sized disposable incontinence product, brief/diaper, large, each ☑

T4524 Adult sized disposable incontinence product, brief/diaper, extra large, each ☑

T4525 Adult sized disposable incontinence product, protective underwear/pull-on, small size, each ☑

T4526 Adult sized disposable incontinence product, protective underwear/pull-on, medium size, each ☑

T4527 Adult sized disposable incontinence product, protective underwear/pull-on, large size, each ☑

T4528 Adult sized disposable incontinence product, protective underwear/pull-on, extra large size, each ☑

T4529 Pediatric sized disposable incontinence product, brief/diaper, small/medium size, each ☑

T4530 Pediatric sized disposable incontinence product, brief/diaper, large size, each ☑

T4531 Pediatric sized disposable incontinence product, protective underwear/pull-on, small/medium size, each ☑

T4532 Pediatric sized disposable incontinence product, protective underwear/pull-on, large size, each ☑

T4533 Youth sized disposable incontinence product, brief/diaper, each ☑

T4534 Youth sized disposable incontinence product, protective underwear/pull-on, each ☑

T4535 Disposable liner/shield/guard/pad/undergarment, for incontinence, each ☑

T4536 Incontinence product, protective underwear/pull-on, reusable, any size, each ☑

T4537 Incontinence product, protective underpad, reusable, bed size, each ☑

T4538 Diaper service, reusable diaper, each diaper ☑

T4539 Incontinence product, diaper/brief, reusable, any size, each ☑

T4540 Incontinence product, protective underpad, reusable, chair size, each ☑

T4541 Incontinence product, disposable underpad, large, each ☑

T4542 Incontinence product, disposable underpad, small size, each ☑

T4543 Adult sized disposable incontinence product, protective brief/diaper, above extra large, each ☑

T4544 Adult sized disposable incontinence product, protective underwear/pull-on, above extra large, each

T4545 Incontinence product, disposable, penile wrap, each

T5001 Positioning seat for persons with special orthopedic needs

T5999 Supply, not otherwise specified

Coronavirus Services U0001-U0002

U0001 **CDC 2019 Novel Coronavirus (2019-nCoV) Real-Time RT-PCR Diagnostic Panel** A

Use this code for CDC created tests.

AHA: 2Q,20

U0002 **2019-nCoV coronavirus, SARS-CoV-2/2019-nCoV (COVID-19), any technique, multiple types or subtypes (includes all targets), non-CDC** A

Use this code for non-CDC created tests.

AHA: 2Q,20

Vision Services V2020-V2799

These V codes include vision-related supplies, including spectacles, lenses, contact lenses, prostheses, intraocular lenses, and miscellaneous lenses.

Frames

V2020 Frames, purchases

V2025 Deluxe frame
CMS: 100-04,1,30.3.5

Single Vision, Glass, or Plastic

V2100 Sphere, single vision, plano to plus or minus 4.00, per lens

Monofocal spectacles (V2100–V2114)

Trifocal spectacles (V2300–V2314)

Low vision aids mounted to spectacles (V2610)

Telescopic or other compound lens fitted on spectacles as a low vision aid (V2615)

V2101 Sphere, single vision, plus or minus 4.12 to plus or minus 7.00d, per lens

V2102 Sphere, single vision, plus or minus 7.12 to plus or minus 20.00d, per lens

V2103 Spherocylinder, single vision, plano to plus or minus 4.00d sphere, 0.12 to 2.00d cylinder, per lens

V2104 Spherocylinder, single vision, plano to plus or minus 4.00d sphere, 2.12 to 4.00d cylinder, per lens

V2105 Spherocylinder, single vision, plano to plus or minus 4.00d sphere, 4.25 to 6.00d cylinder, per lens

V2106 Spherocylinder, single vision, plano to plus or minus 4.00d sphere, over 6.00d cylinder, per lens

V2107 Spherocylinder, single vision, plus or minus 4.25 to plus or minus 7.00 sphere, 0.12 to 2.00d cylinder, per lens

V2108 Spherocylinder, single vision, plus or minus 4.25d to plus or minus 7.00d sphere, 2.12 to 4.00d cylinder, per lens

V2109 Spherocylinder, single vision, plus or minus 4.25 to plus or minus 7.00d sphere, 4.25 to 6.00d cylinder, per lens

V2110 Spherocylinder, single vision, plus or minus 4.25 to 7.00d sphere, over 6.00d cylinder, per lens

V2111 Spherocylinder, single vision, plus or minus 7.25 to plus or minus 12.00d sphere, 0.25 to 2.25d cylinder, per lens

V2112 Spherocylinder, single vision, plus or minus 7.25 to plus or minus 12.00d sphere, 2.25d to 4.00d cylinder, per lens

V2113 Spherocylinder, single vision, plus or minus 7.25 to plus or minus 12.00d sphere, 4.25 to 6.00d cylinder, per lens

V2114 Spherocylinder, single vision, sphere over plus or minus 12.00d, per lens

V2115 Lenticular (myodisc), per lens, single vision

V2118 Aniseikonic lens, single vision

V2121 Lenticular lens, per lens, single

V2199 Not otherwise classified, single vision lens

Bifocal, Glass, or Plastic

V2200 Sphere, bifocal, plano to plus or minus 4.00d, per lens

V2201 Sphere, bifocal, plus or minus 4.12 to plus or minus 7.00d, per lens

V2202 Sphere, bifocal, plus or minus 7.12 to plus or minus 20.00d, per lens

V2203 Spherocylinder, bifocal, plano to plus or minus 4.00d sphere, 0.12 to 2.00d cylinder, per lens

V2204 Spherocylinder, bifocal, plano to plus or minus 4.00d sphere, 2.12 to 4.00d cylinder, per lens

V2205 Spherocylinder, bifocal, plano to plus or minus 4.00d sphere, 4.25 to 6.00d cylinder, per lens

V2206 Spherocylinder, bifocal, plano to plus or minus 4.00d sphere, over 6.00d cylinder, per lens

V2207 Spherocylinder, bifocal, plus or minus 4.25 to plus or minus 7.00d sphere, 0.12 to 2.00d cylinder, per lens

V2208 Spherocylinder, bifocal, plus or minus 4.25 to plus or minus 7.00d sphere, 2.12 to 4.00d cylinder, per lens

V2209 Spherocylinder, bifocal, plus or minus 4.25 to plus or minus 7.00d sphere, 4.25 to 6.00d cylinder, per lens

V2210 Spherocylinder, bifocal, plus or minus 4.25 to plus or minus 7.00d sphere, over 6.00d cylinder, per lens

V2211 Spherocylinder, bifocal, plus or minus 7.25 to plus or minus 12.00d sphere, 0.25 to 2.25d cylinder, per lens

V2212 Spherocylinder, bifocal, plus or minus 7.25 to plus or minus 12.00d sphere, 2.25 to 4.00d cylinder, per lens

V2213 Spherocylinder, bifocal, plus or minus 7.25 to plus or minus 12.00d sphere, 4.25 to 6.00d cylinder, per lens

V2214 Spherocylinder, bifocal, sphere over plus or minus 12.00d, per lens

V2215 Lenticular (myodisc), per lens, bifocal

V2218 Aniseikonic, per lens, bifocal

V2219 Bifocal seg width over 28mm

V2220 Bifocal add over 3.25d

V2221 Lenticular lens, per lens, bifocal

V2299 Specialty bifocal (by report)
Pertinent documentation to evaluate medical appropriateness should be included when this code is reported.

Trifocal, Glass, or Plastic

V2300 Sphere, trifocal, plano to plus or minus 4.00d, per lens

V2301 Sphere, trifocal, plus or minus 4.12 to plus or minus 7.00d per lens

V2302 Sphere, trifocal, plus or minus 7.12 to plus or minus 20.00, per lens

V2303 Spherocylinder, trifocal, plano to plus or minus 4.00d sphere, 0.12 to 2.00d cylinder, per lens

V2304 Spherocylinder, trifocal, plano to plus or minus 4.00d sphere, 2.25 to 4.00d cylinder, per lens

V2305 Spherocylinder, trifocal, plano to plus or minus 4.00d sphere, 4.25 to 6.00 cylinder, per lens

V2306 Spherocylinder, trifocal, plano to plus or minus 4.00d sphere, over 6.00d cylinder, per lens A ☑ ♿

V2307 Spherocylinder, trifocal, plus or minus 4.25 to plus or minus 7.00d sphere, 0.12 to 2.00d cylinder, per lens A ☑ ♿

V2308 Spherocylinder, trifocal, plus or minus 4.25 to plus or minus 7.00d sphere, 2.12 to 4.00d cylinder, per lens A ☑ ♿

V2309 Spherocylinder, trifocal, plus or minus 4.25 to plus or minus 7.00d sphere, 4.25 to 6.00d cylinder, per lens A ☑ ♿

V2310 Spherocylinder, trifocal, plus or minus 4.25 to plus or minus 7.00d sphere, over 6.00d cylinder, per lens A ☑ ♿

V2311 Spherocylinder, trifocal, plus or minus 7.25 to plus or minus 12.00d sphere, 0.25 to 2.25d cylinder, per lens A ☑ ♿

V2312 Spherocylinder, trifocal, plus or minus 7.25 to plus or minus 12.00d sphere, 2.25 to 4.00d cylinder, per lens A ☑ ♿

V2313 Spherocylinder, trifocal, plus or minus 7.25 to plus or minus 12.00d sphere, 4.25 to 6.00d cylinder, per lens A ☑ ♿

V2314 Spherocylinder, trifocal, sphere over plus or minus 12.00d, per lens A ☑ ♿

V2315 Lenticular, (myodisc), per lens, trifocal A ☑ ♿

V2318 Aniseikonic lens, trifocal A ♿

V2319 Trifocal seg width over 28 mm A ☑ ♿

V2320 Trifocal add over 3.25d A ☑ ♿

V2321 Lenticular lens, per lens, trifocal A ♿

V2399 Specialty trifocal (by report) A

Pertinent documentation to evaluate medical appropriateness should be included when this code is reported.

Variable Asphericity Lens, Glass, or Plastic

V2410 Variable asphericity lens, single vision, full field, glass or plastic, per lens A ☑ ♿

V2430 Variable asphericity lens, bifocal, full field, glass or plastic, per lens A ☑ ♿

V2499 Variable sphericity lens, other type A

Contact Lens

V2500 Contact lens, PMMA, spherical, per lens A ☑ ♿

V2501 Contact lens, PMMA, toric or prism ballast, per lens A ☑ ♿

V2502 Contact lens PMMA, bifocal, per lens A ☑ ♿

V2503 Contact lens, PMMA, color vision deficiency, per lens A ☑ ♿

V2510 Contact lens, gas permeable, spherical, per lens A ☑ ♿

V2511 Contact lens, gas permeable, toric, prism ballast, per lens A ☑ ♿

V2512 Contact lens, gas permeable, bifocal, per lens A ☑ ♿

V2513 Contact lens, gas permeable, extended wear, per lens A ☑ ♿

V2520 Contact lens, hydrophilic, spherical, per lens A ☑ ♿

Hydrophilic contact lenses are covered by Medicare only for aphakic patients. Local contractor if incident to physician services.

V2521 Contact lens, hydrophilic, toric, or prism ballast, per lens A ☑ ♿

Hydrophilic contact lenses are covered by Medicare only for aphakic patients. Local contractor if incident to physician services.

V2522 Contact lens, hydrophilic, bifocal, per lens A ☑ ♿

Hydrophilic contact lenses are covered by Medicare only for aphakic patients. Local contractor if incident to physician services.

V2523 Contact lens, hydrophilic, extended wear, per lens A ☑ ♿

Hydrophilic contact lenses are covered by Medicare only for aphakic patients.

V2524 Contact lens, hydrophilic, spherical, photochromic additive, per lens A

V2525 Contact lens, hydrophilic, dual focus, per lens E1

V2526 Contact lens, hydrophilic, with blue-violet filter, per lens E1

AHA: 4Q,23

V2530 Contact lens, scleral, gas impermeable, per lens (for contact lens modification, see 92325) A ☑ ♿

V2531 Contact lens, scleral, gas permeable, per lens (for contact lens modification, see 92325) A ☑ ♿

V2599 Contact lens, other type A

Local contractor if incident to physician services.

Vision Aids

V2600 Hand held low vision aids and other nonspectacle mounted aids A

V2610 Single lens spectacle mounted low vision aids A

V2615 Telescopic and other compound lens system, including distance vision telescopic, near vision telescopes and compound microscopic lens system A

Prosthetic Eye

V2623 Prosthetic eye, plastic, custom A ♿

Implant

Peg

One type of eye implant

Reverse angle

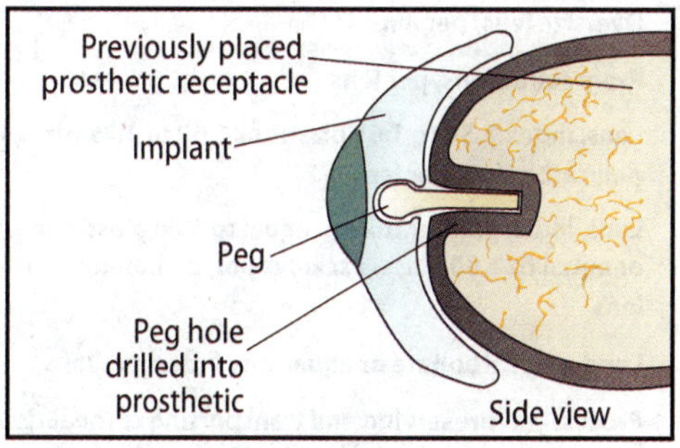

Previously placed prosthetic receptacle

Implant

Peg

Peg hole drilled into prosthetic

Side view

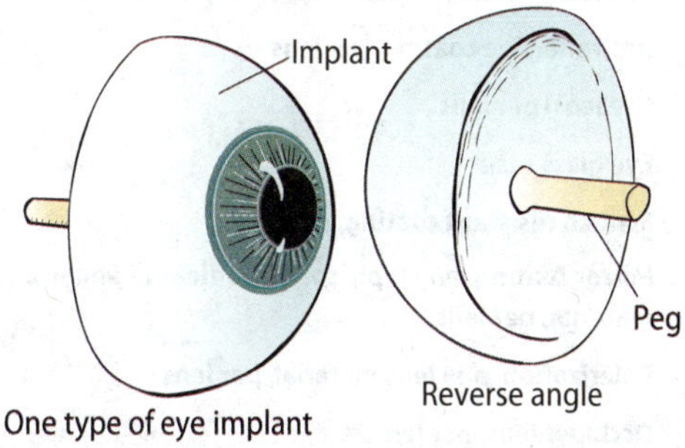

V2624 Polishing/resurfacing of ocular prosthesis A ♿

V2625 Enlargement of ocular prosthesis A ♿

V2626 Reduction of ocular prosthesis A ♿

V2627 Scleral cover shell A ♿

A scleral shell covers the cornea and the anterior sclera. Medicare covers a scleral shell when it is prescribed as an artificial support to a shrunken and sightless eye or as a barrier in the treatment of severe dry eye.

V2628 Fabrication and fitting of ocular conformer A ♿

V2629 Prosthetic eye, other type A

Intraocular Lenses

V2630 **Anterior chamber intraocular lens** N N1 DMEPOS

The IOL must be FDA-approved for reimbursement. Medicare payment for an IOL is included in the payment for ASC facility services. Medicare jurisdiction: local contractor.

V2631 **Iris supported intraocular lens** N N1 DMEPOS

The IOL must be FDA-approved for reimbursement. Medicare payment for an IOL is included in the payment for ASC facility services. Medicare jurisdiction: local contractor.

V2632 **Posterior chamber intraocular lens** N N1 DMEPOS

The IOL must be FDA-approved for reimbursement. Medicare payment for an IOL is included in the payment for ASC facility services. Medicare jurisdiction: local contractor.

CMS: 100-04,32,120.2

Miscellaneous

V2700 **Balance lens, per lens** A ☑ DMEPOS

V2702 **Deluxe lens feature** E

V2710 **Slab off prism, glass or plastic, per lens** A ☑ DMEPOS

V2715 **Prism, per lens** A ☑ DMEPOS

V2718 **Press-on lens, Fresnel prism, per lens** A ☑ DMEPOS

V2730 **Special base curve, glass or plastic, per lens** A ☑ DMEPOS

V2744 **Tint, photochromatic, per lens** A ☑ DMEPOS

V2745 **Addition to lens; tint, any color, solid, gradient or equal, excludes photochromatic, any lens material, per lens** A ☑ DMEPOS

V2750 **Antireflective coating, per lens** A ☑ DMEPOS

V2755 **U-V lens, per lens** A ☑ DMEPOS

V2756 **Eye glass case** E

V2760 **Scratch resistant coating, per lens** E ☑ DMEPOS

V2761 **Mirror coating, any type, solid, gradient or equal, any lens material, per lens** B ☑

V2762 **Polarization, any lens material, per lens** E ☑ DMEPOS

V2770 **Occluder lens, per lens** A ☑ DMEPOS

V2780 **Oversize lens, per lens** A ☑ DMEPOS

V2781 **Progressive lens, per lens** B ☑

V2782 **Lens, index 1.54 to 1.65 plastic or 1.60 to 1.79 glass, excludes polycarbonate, per lens** A ☑ DMEPOS

V2783 **Lens, index greater than or equal to 1.66 plastic or greater than or equal to 1.80 glass, excludes polycarbonate, per lens** A ☑ DMEPOS

V2784 **Lens, polycarbonate or equal, any index, per lens** A ☑ DMEPOS

V2785 **Processing, preserving and transporting corneal tissue** F F4

Medicare jurisdiction: local contractor.

CMS: 100-04,4,200.1

V2786 **Specialty occupational multifocal lens, per lens** E ☑ DMEPOS

V2787 **Astigmatism correcting function of intraocular lens** E

CMS: 100-04,32,120.1; 100-04,32,120.2

V2788 **Presbyopia correcting function of intraocular lens** E

CMS: 100-04,32,120.1; 100-04,32,120.2

V2790 **Amniotic membrane for surgical reconstruction, per procedure** N

Medicare jurisdiction: local contractor.

CMS: 100-04,4,200.4

V2797 **Vision supply, accessory and/or service component of another HCPCS vision code** E

V2799 **Vision item or service, miscellaneous** A

Determine if an alternative HCPCS Level II or a CPT code better describes the service being reported. This code should be used only if a more specific code is unavailable.

Hearing Services V5008-V5364

This range of codes describes hearing tests and related supplies and equipment, speech-language pathology screenings, and repair of augmentative communicative system.

Hearing Services

V5008 **Hearing screening** E

V5010 **Assessment for hearing aid** E

V5011 **Fitting/orientation/checking of hearing aid** E

V5014 **Repair/modification of a hearing aid** E

V5020 **Conformity evaluation** E

Monaural Hearing Aid

V5030 **Hearing aid, monaural, body worn, air conduction** E

V5040 **Hearing aid, monaural, body worn, bone conduction** E

V5050 **Hearing aid, monaural, in the ear** E

V5060 **Hearing aid, monaural, behind the ear** E

Other Hearing Services

V5070 **Glasses, air conduction** E

V5080 **Glasses, bone conduction** E

V5090 **Dispensing fee, unspecified hearing aid** E

V5095 **Semi-implantable middle ear hearing prosthesis** E

V5100 **Hearing aid, bilateral, body worn** E

V5110 **Dispensing fee, bilateral** E

Hearing Aids, Services, and Accessories

V5120 **Binaural, body** E

V5130 **Binaural, in the ear** E

V5140 **Binaural, behind the ear** E

V5150 **Binaural, glasses** E

V5160 **Dispensing fee, binaural** E

V5171 **Hearing aid, contralateral routing device, monaural, in the ear (ITE)** E

V5172 **Hearing aid, contralateral routing device, monaural, in the canal (ITC)** E

V5181 **Hearing aid, contralateral routing device, monaural, behind the ear (BTE)** E

V5190 **Hearing aid, contralateral routing, monaural, glasses** E

V5200 **Dispensing fee, contralateral, monaural** E

V5211 **Hearing aid, contralateral routing system, binaural, ITE/ITE** E

V5212 **Hearing aid, contralateral routing system, binaural, ITE/ITC** E

V5213 **Hearing aid, contralateral routing system, binaural, ITE/BTE** E

V5214 **Hearing aid, contralateral routing system, binaural, ITC/ITC** E

V5215 **Hearing aid, contralateral routing system, binaural, ITC/BTE** E

V5221 **Hearing aid, contralateral routing system, binaural, BTE/BTE** E

V5230 **Hearing aid, contralateral routing system, binaural, glasses** E

V5240 **Dispensing fee, contralateral routing system, binaural** E

V5241 Dispensing fee, monaural hearing aid, any type E1

V5242 Hearing aid, analog, monaural, CIC (completely in the ear canal) E1

V5243 Hearing aid, analog, monaural, ITC (in the canal) E1

V5244 Hearing aid, digitally programmable analog, monaural, CIC E1

V5245 Hearing aid, digitally programmable, analog, monaural, ITC E1

V5246 Hearing aid, digitally programmable analog, monaural, ITE (in the ear) E1

V5247 Hearing aid, digitally programmable analog, monaural, BTE (behind the ear) E1

V5248 Hearing aid, analog, binaural, CIC E1

V5249 Hearing aid, analog, binaural, ITC E1

V5250 Hearing aid, digitally programmable analog, binaural, CIC E1

V5251 Hearing aid, digitally programmable analog, binaural, ITC E1

V5252 Hearing aid, digitally programmable, binaural, ITE E1

V5253 Hearing aid, digitally programmable, binaural, BTE E1

V5254 Hearing aid, digital, monaural, CIC E1

V5255 Hearing aid, digital, monaural, ITC E1

V5256 Hearing aid, digital, monaural, ITE E1

V5257 Hearing aid, digital, monaural, BTE E1

V5258 Hearing aid, digital, binaural, CIC E1

V5259 Hearing aid, digital, binaural, ITC E1

V5260 Hearing aid, digital, binaural, ITE E1

V5261 Hearing aid, digital, binaural, BTE E1

V5262 Hearing aid, disposable, any type, monaural E1

V5263 Hearing aid, disposable, any type, binaural E1

V5264 Ear mold/insert, not disposable, any type E1

V5265 Ear mold/insert, disposable, any type E1

V5266 Battery for use in hearing device E1

V5267 Hearing aid or assistive listening device/supplies/accessories, not otherwise specified E1

Assistive Listening Device

V5268 Assistive listening device, telephone amplifier, any type E1

V5269 Assistive listening device, alerting, any type E1

V5270 Assistive listening device, television amplifier, any type E1

V5271 Assistive listening device, television caption decoder E1

V5272 Assistive listening device, TDD E1

V5273 Assistive listening device, for use with cochlear implant E1

V5274 Assistive listening device, not otherwise specified E1

Miscellaneous Hearing Services

V5275 Ear impression, each E1 ☑

V5281 Assistive listening device, personal FM/DM system, monaural (1 receiver, transmitter, microphone), any type E1

V5282 Assistive listening device, personal FM/DM system, binaural (2 receivers, transmitter, microphone), any type E1

V5283 Assistive listening device, personal FM/DM neck, loop induction receiver E1

V5284 Assistive listening device, personal FM/DM, ear level receiver E1

V5285 Assistive listening device, personal FM/DM, direct audio input receiver E1

V5286 Assistive listening device, personal blue tooth FM/DM receiver E1

V5287 Assistive listening device, personal FM/DM receiver, not otherwise specified E1

V5288 Assistive listening device, personal FM/DM transmitter assistive listening device E1

V5289 Assistive listening device, personal FM/DM adapter/boot coupling device for receiver, any type E1

V5290 Assistive listening device, transmitter microphone, any type E1

V5298 Hearing aid, not otherwise classified E1

V5299 Hearing service, miscellaneous B ⃠

Determine if an alternative HCPCS Level II or a CPT code better describes the service being reported. This code should be used only if a more specific code is unavailable.

Speech-Language Pathology Services

V5336 Repair/modification of augmentative communicative system or device (excludes adaptive hearing aid) E1

Medicare jurisdiction: DME regional contractor.

V5362 Speech screening E1

V5363 Language screening E1

V5364 Dysphagia screening E1

Appendix 1 — Table of Drugs and Biologicals

INTRODUCTION AND DIRECTIONS

The HCPCS 2025 Table of Drugs and Biologicals is designed to quickly and easily direct the user to drug names and their corresponding codes. Both generic and brand or trade names are alphabetically listed in the "Drug Name" column of the table. The associated A, C, J, K, Q, or S code is given only for the generic name of the drug. While every effort is made to make the table comprehensive, it is not all-inclusive.

The "Unit Per" column lists the stated amount for the referenced generic drug as provided by CMS. "Up to" listings are inclusive of all quantities up to and including the listed amount. All other listings are for the amount of the drug as listed. The editors recognize that the availability of some drugs in the quantities listed is dependent on many variables beyond the control of the clinical ordering clerk. The availability in your area of regularly used drugs in the most cost-effective quantities should be relayed to your third-party payers.

The "Route of Administration" column addresses the most common methods of delivering the referenced generic drug as described in current pharmaceutical literature. The official definitions for Level II drug codes generally describe administration other than by oral method. Therefore, with a handful of exceptions, oral-delivered options for most drugs are omitted from the Route of Administration column.

Intravenous administration includes all methods, such as gravity infusion, injections, and timed pushes. When several routes of administration are listed, the first listing is simply the first, or most common, method as described in current reference literature. The "VAR" posting denotes various routes of administration and is used for drugs that are commonly administered into joints, cavities, tissues, or topical applications, in addition to other parenteral administrations. Listings posted with "OTH" alert the user to other administration methods, such as suppositories or catheter injections.

Please be reminded that the Table of Drugs and Biologicals, as well as all HCPCS Level II national definitions and listings, constitutes a post-treatment medical reference for billing purposes only. Although the editors have exercised all normal precautions to ensure the accuracy of the table and related material, the use of any of this information to select medical treatment is entirely inappropriate. Do not code directly from the table. Refer to the tabular section for complete information.

See Appendix 3 for abbreviations.

Drug Name	Units Per	Route	Code
10% LMD	500 ML	IV	J7100
5% DEXTROSE AND .45% NORMAL SALINE	1000 ML	IV	S5010
5% DEXTROSE IN LACTATED RINGERS	1000 CC	IV	J7121
5% DEXTROSE WITH POTASSIUM CHLORIDE	1000 ML	IV	S5012
5% DEXTROSE/.45% NS WITH KCL AND MAG SULFATE	1000ML	IV	S5013
5% DEXTROSE/.45% NS WITH KCL AND MAG SULFATE	1500 ML	IV	S5014
5% DEXTROSE/NORMAL SALINE	5%	VAR	J7042
5% DEXTROSE/WATER	500 ML	IV	J7060
A-HYDROCORT	100 MG	IV, IM, SC	J1720
~~A-METHAPRED~~	~~125 MG~~	~~IM, IV~~	~~J2930~~
~~A-METHAPRED~~	~~40 MG~~	~~IM, IV~~	~~J2920~~
ABATACEPT	10 MG	IV	J0129
ABCIXIMAB	10 MG	IV	J0130
ABECMA	UP TO 510 MILLION CELLS	IV	Q2055
ABELCET	10 MG	IV	J0287
ABILIFY	0.25 MG	IM	J0400
ABILIFY ASIMTUFII	1 MG	IM	J0402
ABILIFY MAINTENA KIT	1 MG	IM	J0401
ABLAVAR	1 ML	IV	A9583
ABOBOTULINUMTOXINA	5 UNITS	IM	J0586
ABRAXANE	1 MG	IV	J9264
~~ABRILADA~~	~~10 MG~~	~~SC~~	~~Q5132~~
ABRILADA	1 MG	SC	Q5145
AC5 ADVANCED WOUND SYSTEM (AC5)	SQ CM	OTH	A2020
ACAPATCH	SQ CM	OTH	Q4325
ACCELULAR PERICARDIAL TISSUE MATRIX NONHUMAN	SQ CM	OTH	C9354
ACCUNEB NONCOMPOUNDED, CONCENTRATED	1 MG	INH	J7611
ACCUNEB NONCOMPOUNDED, UNIT DOSE	1 MG	INH	J7613
ACESSO	SQ CM	OTH	Q4311
ACESSO AC	SQ CM	OTH	Q4312
ACESSO DL	SQ CM	OTH	Q4293
ACESSO TL	SQ CM	OTH	Q4300
ACETADOTE	1 G	INH	J7608
ACETADOTE	100 MG	IV	J0132
ACETAMINOPHEN (B. BRAUN), NOT THERAPEUTICALLY EQUIVALENT TO J0131	10 MG	IV	J0136
ACETAMINOPHEN (FRESENIUS KABI), NOT THERAPEUTICALLY EQUIVALENT TO J0131	10 MG	IV	J0134
ACETAMINOPHEN (HIKMA) NOT THERAPEUTICALLY EQUIVALENT TO J0131	10 MG	IV	J0137
ACETAMINOPHEN/IBUPROFEN	10 MG/3 MG	ORAL	J0138
ACETAZOLAMIDE SODIUM	500 MG	IM, IV	J1120
ACETYLCYSTEINE COMPOUNDED	PER G	INH	J7604
ACETYLCYSTEINE NONCOMPOUNDED	1 G	INH	J7608
ACTEMRA	1 MG	IV	J3262
ACTEMRA	1 MG	IV	Q0249
ACTHAR GEL	UP TO 40 UNITS	IM/SC	J0801
ACTHAR GEL (ANI)	UP TO 40 UNITS	IM/SC	J0802
ACTHREL	1 MCG	IV	J0795
ACTIMMUNE	3 MU	SC	J9216
ACTIVASE	1 MG	IV	J2997
ACTIVATE MATRIX	SQ CM	OTH	Q4301
ACUTECT	STUDY DOSE UP TO 20 MCI	IV	A9504
ACYCLOVIR	5 MG	IV	J0133
ADAGEN	25 IU	IM	J2504
ADAKVEO	5 MG	IV	J0791
~~ADALIMUMAB~~	~~20 MG~~	~~SC~~	~~J0135~~
ADALIMUMAB	1 MG	SC	J0139
ADALIMUMAB-AACF	1 MG	SC	Q5144
~~ADALIMUMAB-AACF, BIOSIMILAR~~	~~20 MG~~	~~SC~~	~~Q5131~~
ADALIMUMAB-AATY	1 MG	SC	Q5141
ADALIMUMAB-ADBM	1 MG	SC	Q5143
~~ADALIMUMAB-AFZB~~	~~10 MG~~	~~SC~~	~~Q5132~~
ADALIMUMAB-AFZB	1 MG	SC	Q5145
ADALIMUMAB-FKJP	1 MG	SC	Q5140
ADALIMUMAB-RYVK	1 MG	SC	Q5142
~~ADAMTS13, RECOMBINANT-KRHN~~	~~10 IU~~	~~IV~~	~~C9167~~
ADAMTS13, RECOMBINANT-KRHN	10 IU	IV	J7171
ADASUVE	1 MG	INH	J2062
ADCETRIS	1 MG	IV	J9042
ADENOCARD	1 MG	IV	J0153

Drug Name	Units Per	Route	Code
ADENOSINE	1 MG	IV	J0153
ADENSOSCAN	1 MG	IV	J0153
ADO-TRASTUZUMAB EMTANSINE	1 MG	IV	J9354
ADRENALIN	0.1 MG	IM, IV, SC	J0171
ADRENOCORT	1 MG	IM, IV, OTH	J1100
ADRIAMYCIN	10 MG	IV	J9000
ADRUCIL	500 MG	IV	J9190
ADSTILADRIN	THERAPEUTIC DOSE	OTH	J9029
ADUCANUMAB-AVWA	2 MG	IV	J0172
ADUHELM	2 MG	IV	J0172
ADYNOVATE	1 IU	IV	J7207
~~ADZYNMA~~	~~10 IU~~	~~IV~~	~~C9167~~
ADZYNMA	10 IU	IV	J7171
AEROBID	1 MG	INH	J7641
AFAMELANOTIDE IMPLANT	1 MG	OTH	J7352
AFFINITY	SQ CM	OTH	Q4159
AFINITOR	0.25 MG	ORAL	J7527
AFLIBERCEPT	1 MG	OTH	J0178
~~AFLIBERCEPT HD~~	~~1 MG~~	~~INJ~~	~~C9161~~
AFLIBERCEPT HD	1 MG	INJ	J0177
AFLURIA	EA	IM	Q2035
AFSTYLA	1 IU	IV	J7210
AGALSIDASE BETA	1 MG	IV	J0180
AGGRASTAT	12.5 MG	IM, IV	J3246
AGRIFLU	UNKNOWN	IM	Q2034
AJOVY	1 MG	SC	J3031
AKYNZEO	300 MG/0.5 MG	ORAL	J8655
AKYNZEO	235 MG/0.25 MG	IV	J1454
ALATROFLOXACIN MESYLATE	100 MG	IV	J0200
ALBUTEROL AND IPRATROPIUM BROMIDE NONCOMPOUNDED	2.5MG/0.5 MG	INH	J7620
ALBUTEROL COMPOUNDED, CONCENTRATED	1 MG	INH	J7610
ALBUTEROL COMPOUNDED, UNIT DOSE	1 MG	INH	J7609
ALBUTEROL NONCOMPOUNDED, UNIT DOSE	1 MG	INH	J7613
ALBUTEROL, NONCOMPOUNDED, CONCENTRATED FORM	1 MG	INH	J7611
ALDESLEUKIN	1 VIAL	IV	J9015
ALDURAZYME	0.1 MG	IV	J1931
ALEFACEPT	0.5 MG	IV, IM	J0215
ALEMTUZUMAB	1 MG	IV	J0202
ALFENTANIL HCL	500 MCG	IV	J0216
ALFERON N	250,000 IU	IM	J9215
ALGLUCERASE	10 U	IV	J0205
ALGLUCOSIDASE ALFA (LUMIZYME)	10 MG	IV	J0221
ALIQOPA	1 MG	IV	J9057
ALKERAN	2 MG	ORAL	J8600
ALLODERM	SQ CM	OTH	Q4116
ALLOGEN	1 CC	OTH	Q4212
ALLOGRAFT, CYMETRA	1 CC	INJ	Q4112
ALLOGRAFT, GRAFTJACKET EXPRESS	1 CC	INJ	Q4113
ALLOPATCHHD	SQ CM	OTH	Q4128
ALLOPLY	SQ CM	OTH	Q4323
ALLOPURINOL SODIUM	1 MG	IV	J0206
ALLOSKIN	SQ CM	OTH	Q4115
ALLOSKIN AC	SQ CM	OTH	Q4141
ALLOSKIN RT	SQ CM	OTH	Q4123
ALLOWRAP DS OR DRY	SQ CM	OTH	Q4150
ALOXI	25 MCG	IV	J2469
ALPHA 1-PROTENIASE INHIBITOR (HUMAN) (GLASSIA)	10 MG	IV	J0257
ALPHANATE	FACTOR VIII IU	IV	J7186
ALPHANINE SD	1 IU	IV	J7193
ALPROLIX	IU	IV	J7201
ALPROSTADIL	1.25 MCG	IV	J0270
ALPROSTADIL	EA	OTH	J0275
ALTEPLASE RECOMBINANT	1 MG	IV	J2997
ALTIPLY	SQ CM	OTH	Q4235
ALTUVIIIO	IU	IV	J7214
ALUPENT, NONCOMPOUNDED, CONCENTRATED	10 MG	INH	J7668
ALUPENT, NONCOMPOUNDED, UNIT DOSE	10 MG	INH	J7669
ALYGLO	500 MG	IV	J1552
ALYMSYS	10 MG	IV	Q5126
AMANTADINE HCL (DEMONSTRATION PROJECT)	100 MG	ORAL	G9017
AMANTADINE HYDROCHLORIDE (BRAND NAME) (DEMONSTRTION PROJECT)	100 MG	ORAL	G9033
AMANTADINE HYDROCHLORIDE (GENERIC)	100 MG	ORAL	G9017
AMBISOME	10 MG	IV	J0289
AMCHOPLAST	SQ CM	OTH	Q4316
AMCORT	5 MG	IM	J3302
AMELUZ	10 MG	OTH	J7345
AMERGAN	12.5 MG	ORAL	Q0169
AMERICAN AMNION	SQ CM	OTH	Q4307
AMERICAN AMNION AC	SQ CM	OTH	Q4306
AMERICAN AMNION AC TRI-LAYER	SQ CM	OTH	Q4305
AMEVIVE	0.5 MG	IV, IM	J0215
AMICAR	5 G	IV	S0017
AMIFOSTINE	500 MG	IV	J0207
AMIKACIN SULFATE	100 MG	IM, IV	J0278
AMINOCAPRIOC ACID	5 G	IV	S0017
AMINOLEVULINIC ACID HCL	354 MG	OTH	J7308
AMINOLEVULINIC ACID HCL	10 MG	OTH	J7345
AMINOPHYLLINE	250 MG	IV	J0280
AMIODARONE HCL	30 MG	IV	J0282
AMIODARONE HCL	30 MG	IV	J0283
AMISULPRIDE	1 MG	IV	J0184
AMITRIPTYLINE HCL	20 MG	IM	J1320
AMIVANTAMAB-VMJW	2 MG	IV	J9061
AMMONIA N-13	STUDY DOSE UP TO 40 MCI	IV	A9526
AMNICORE PRO	SQ CM	OTH	Q4298
AMNICORE PRO+	SQ CM	OTH	Q4299
AMNIO QUAD-CORE	SQ CM	OTH	Q4294
AMNIO TRI-CORE AMNIOTIC	SQ CM	OTH	Q4295
AMNIO-MAXX	SQ CM	OTH	Q4239
AMNIO-MAXX LITE	SQ CM	OTH	Q4239
AMNIOAMP-MP	SQ CM	OTH	Q4250
AMNIOARMOR	SQ CM	OTH	Q4188
AMNIOBAND	SQ CM	OTH	Q4151
AMNIOBAND	1 MG	OTH	Q4168
AMNIOBIND	SQ CM	OTH	Q4225
AMNIOCORE	SQ CM	OTH	Q4227
AMNIOCYTE PLUS	0.5 CC	OTH	Q4242

Drug Name	Units Per	Route	Code
AMNIOEXCEL	SQ CM	OTH	**Q4137**
AMNIOEXCEL PLUS	SQ CM	OTH	**Q4137**
AMNIOMATRIX	1 CC	OTH	**Q4139**
AMNION BIO	SQ CM	OTH	**Q4211**
AMNIOPLAST 1	SQ CM	OTH	**Q4334**
AMNIOPLAST 2	SQ CM	OTH	**Q4335**
AMNIOREPAIR	SQ CM	OTH	**Q4235**
AMNIOTEXT	1 CC	OTH	**Q4245**
AMNIOTEXT PATCH	SQ CM	OTH	**Q4247**
AMNIOTX	SQ CM	OTH	**Q4324**
AMNIOWOUND	SQ CM	OTH	**Q4181**
AMNIOWRAP2	SQ CM	OTH	**Q4221**
AMNIPLY	SQ CM	OTH	**Q4249**
AMOBARBITAL	125 MG	IM, IV	**J0300**
AMONDYS 45	10 MG	IV	**J1426**
AMPHOCIN	50 MG	IV	**J0285**
AMPHOTEC	10 MG	IV	**J0287**
AMPHOTERICIN B	50 MG	IV	**J0285**
AMPHOTERICIN B CHOLESTERYL SULFATE COMPLEX	10 MG	IV	**J0288**
AMPHOTERICIN B LIPID COMPLEX	10 MG	IV	**J0287**
AMPHOTERICIN B LIPOSOME	10 MG	IV	**J0289**
AMPICILLIN SODIUM	500 MG	IM, IV	**J0290**
AMPICILLIN SODIUM/SULBACTAM SODIUM	1.5 G	IM, IV	**J0295**
AMVUTTRA	1 MG	SC	**J0225**
AMYGDALIN	VAR	INJ	**J3570**
AMYTAL	125 MG	IM, IV	**J0300**
AMYVID	UP TO 10 MILLICUIRES	IV	**A9586**
AN-DTPA DIAGNOSTIC	STUDY DOSE UP TO 25 MCI	IV	**A9539**
AN-DTPA THERAPEUTIC	STUDY DOSE UP TO 25 MCI	INH	**A9567**
ANACAULASE-BCDB, 8.8% GEL	1 G	OTH	**J7353**
ANASCORP	UP TO 120 MG	IV	**J0716**
ANASTROZOLE	1 MG	ORAL	**S0170**
ANAVIP	120 MG	IV	**J0841**
ANCEF	500 MG	IM, IV	**J0690**
ANDEXXA	10 MG	IV	**J7169**
ANECTINE	20 MG	IM, IV	**J0330**
ANGIOMAX	1 MG	IV	**J0583**
ANIDULAFUNGIN	1 MG	IV	**J0348**
ANIFROLUMAB-FNIA	1 MG	IV	**J0491**
ANISTREPLASE	30 U	IV	**J0350**
ANJESO	1 MG	IV	**J1738**
~~ANKTIVA~~	~~1 MCG~~	~~IVES~~	~~**C9169**~~
ANKTIVA	1 MCG	OTH	**J9028**
ANNOVERA VAGINAL RING	0.15 MG/0.013 MG	OTH	**J7294**
ANTAGON	250 MCG	SC	**S0132**
ANTI-INHIBITOR	1 IU	IV	**J7198**
ANTI-THYMOCYTE GLOBULIN,EQUINE	250 MG	OTH	**J7504**
ANTIEMETIC DRUG NOS	VAR	ORAL	**J8597**
ANTIHEMOPHILIC FACTOR (RECOMBINANT), FC-VWF-XTEN FUSION PROTEIN-EHTL	IU	IV	**J7214**
ANTIHEMOPHILIC FACTOR PORCINE	1 IU	IV	**J7191**
ANTIHEMOPHILIC FACTOR VIII, XYNTHA, RECOMBINANT	1 IU	IV	**J7185**
ANTIHEMOPHILIC FACTOR VIII/VON WILLEBRAND FACTOR COMPLEX, HUMAN	FACTOR VIII IU	IV	**J7186**
ANTITHROMBIN RECOMBINANT	50 IU	IV	**J7196**
ANTIZOL	15 MG	IV	**J1451**
ANZEMET	10 MG	IV	**J1260**
ANZEMET	50 MG	ORAL	**S0174**
ANZEMET	100 MG	ORAL	**Q0180**
APHEXDA	0.25 MG	SC	**J2277**
APIS	SQ CM	OTH	**A2010**
APLIGRAF	SQ CM	OTH	**Q4101**
APOKYN	1 MG	SC	**J0364**
APOMORPHINE HYDROCHLORIDE	1 MG	SC	**J0364**
APONVIE	1 MG	IV	**C9145**
APREPITANT	1 MG	IV	**J0185**
APREPITANT	1 MG	IV	**C9145**
APREPITANT	5 MG	ORAL	**J8501**
APRETUDE	1 MG	IM	**J0739**
APROTININ	10,000 KIU	IV	**J0365**
AQUAMEPHYTON	1 MG	IM, SC, IV	**J3430**
ARA-C	100 MG	SC, IV	**J9100**
ARALEN	UP TO 250 MG	IM, IV	**J0390**
ARAMINE	10 MG	IV, IM, SC	**J0380**
ARANESP, ESRD USE	1 MCG	SC, IV	**J0882**
ARANESP, NON-ESRD USE	1 MCG	SC, IV	**J0881**
ARBUTAMINE HCL	1 MG	IV	**J0395**
ARCALYST	1 MG	SC	**J2793**
ARCHITECT EXTRACELLULAR MATRIX	SQ CM	OTH	**Q4147**
ARDEOGRAFT	SQ CM	OTH	**Q4333**
AREDIA	30 MG	IV	**J2430**
ARFORMOTEROL	15 MCG	INH	**J7605**
ARGATROBAN	1 MG	IV	**J0883**
ARGATROBAN	1 MG	IV	**J0884**
ARGATROBAN (ACCORD), NOT THERAPEUTICALLY EQUIVALENT TO J0883 (FOR NON-ESRD USE)	1 MG	IV	**J0891**
ARGATROBAN (ACCORD), NOT THERAPEUTICALLY EQUIVALENT TO J0884 (FOR ESRD ON DIALYSIS)	1 MG	IV	**J0892**
ARGATROBAN (AUROMEDICS), NOT THERAPEUTICALLY EQUIVALENT TO J0883 (FOR ESRD ON DIALYSIS)	1 MG	IV	**J0899**
ARGATROBAN (AUROMEDICS), NOT THERAPEUTICALLY EQUIVALENT TO J0883 (FOR NON-ESRD USE)	1 MG	IV	**J0898**
ARIDOL	5 MG	INH	**J7665**
ARIMIDEX	1 MG	ORAL	**S0170**
ARIPIPRAZOLE	0.25 MG	IM	**J0400**
ARIPIPRAZOLE	1 MG	IM	**J0402**
ARIPIPRAZOLE LAUROXIL	1 MG	IM	**J1943**
ARIPIPRAZOLE LAUROXIL	1 MG	IM	**J1944**
ARIPIPRAZOLE, EXTENDED RELEASE	1 MG	IM	**J0401**
ARISTADA	1 MG	IM	**J1944**
ARISTADA INITIO	1 MG	IM	**J1943**
ARISTOCORT	5 MG	IM	**J3302**
ARISTOCORTE FORTE	5 MG	IM	**J3302**
ARISTOCORTE INTRALESIONAL	5 MG	OTH	**J3302**
ARISTOSPAN	5 MG	VAR	**J3303**
ARIXTRA	0.5 MG	SC	**J1652**
AROMASIN	25 MG	ORAL	**S0156**
ARRANON	50 MG	IV	**J9261**

Drug Name	Units Per	Route	Code
ARRESTIN	200 MG	IM	J3250
ARSENIC TRIOXIDE	1 MG	IV	J9017
ARTACENT AC	1 MG	OTH	Q4189
ARTACENT AC	SQ CM	OTH	Q4190
ARTACENT C	SQ CM	OTH	Q4336
ARTACENT CORD	SQ CM	OTH	Q4216
ARTACENT TRIDENT	SQ CM	OTH	Q4337
ARTACENT VELOS	SQ CM	OTH	Q4338
ARTACENT VERICLEN	SQ CM	OTH	Q4339
ARTACENT WOUND	SQ CM	OTH	Q4169
ARTESUNATE	1 MG	IV	J0391
ARTHROFLEX	SQ CM	OTH	Q4125
ARTISS FIBRIN SEALANT	2 ML	OTH	C9250
ARZERRA	10 MG	IV	J9302
ASCENIV	500 MG	IV	J1554
ASCENT	0.5 MG	OTH	Q4213
ASPARAGINASE	1,000 IU	IM,IV,SC	J9019
ASPARAGINASE, RECOMBINANT	0.1 MG	IM	J9021
ASPARLAS	10 UNITS	IV	J9118
ASTAGRAF XL	0.1 MG	ORAL	J7508
ASTRAMORPH PF	10 MG	OTH	J2274
ATEZOLIZUMAB	10 MG	INF	J9022
ATGAM	250 MG	OTH	J7504
ATIVAN	2 MG	IM, IV	J2060
ATOPICLAIR	ANY SIZE	OTH	A6250
ATROPEN	0.01 MG	IM	J0461
ATROPINE SULFATE	0.01 MG	IM, IV, SC	J0461
ATROPINE, COMPOUNDED, CONCENTRATED	I MG	INH	J7635
ATROPINE, COMPOUNDED, UNIT DOSE	1 MG	INH	J7636
ATROVENT, NONCOMPOUNDED, UNIT DOSE	1 MG	INH	J7644
ATRYN	50 IU	IV	J7196
AUROTHIOGLUCOSE	50 MG	IM	J2910
AURYXIA, FOR ESRD ON DIALYSIS	3 MG	ORAL	J0609
AUTOPLEX T	1 IU	IV	J7198
~~AVACINCAPTAD PEGOL~~	~~0.1 MG~~	~~INJ~~	~~C9162~~
AVACINCAPTAD PEGOL	0.1 MG	INJ	J2782
AVALGLUCOSIDASE ALFA-NGPT	4 MG	IV	J0219
AVASTIN	0.25 MG	IV	C9257
AVASTIN	10 MG	IV	J9035
AVEED	1 MG	IM	J3145
AVELOX	100 MG	IV	J2280
AVELUMAB	10 MG	INF	J9023
AVONEX	30 MCG	IM	J1826
AVONEX	1 MCG	IM	Q3027
AVSOLA	10 MG	IV	Q5121
AVYCAZ	0.5 G/0.125 G	IV	J0714
AXICABTAGENE CILOLEUCEL	UP TO 200 MILLION CELLS	IV	Q2041
AXOBIOMEMBRANE	SQ CM	OTH	Q4211
AXOLOTL AMBIENT, AXOLOTL CRYO	0.1 MG	OTH	Q4215
AXOLOTL DUALGRAFT	SQ CM	OTH	Q4332
AXOLOTL GRAFT	SQ CM	OTH	Q4331
~~AXOLOTL GRAFT, AXOLOTL DUALGRAFT~~	~~SQ CM~~	~~OTH~~	~~Q4210~~
AXUMIN	1 MCI	IV	A9588
AZACITIDINE	1 MG	SC	J9025
AZACTAM	100 MG	IM/IV	J0457
AZASAN	50 MG	ORAL	J7500
AZATHIOPRINE	50 MG	ORAL	J7500
AZATHIOPRINE	100 MG	OTH	J7501
AZEDRA	1 MCI	IV	A9590
AZITHROMYCIN	1 G	ORAL	Q0144
AZITHROMYCIN	500 MG	IV	J0456
AZMACORT	1 MG	INH	J7684
AZMACORT CONCENTRATED	1 MG	INH	J7683
AZTREONAM	100 MG	IM/IV	J0457
BACLOFEN	50 MCG	IT	J0476
BACLOFEN	10 MG	IT	J0475
BACTOCILL	250 MG	IM, IV	J2700
BACTRIM IV	10 ML	IV	S0039
BAL	100 MG	IM	J0470
~~BALFAXAR~~	~~IU~~	~~IV~~	~~C9159~~
BALFAXAR	IU	IV	J7165
BAMLANIVIMAB AND ETESEVIMAB	2100 MG	IV	Q0245
BARHEMSYS	1 MG	IV	J0184
BARRERA SL OR BARRERA DL	SQ CM	OTH	Q4281
BASILIXIMAB	20 MG	IV	J0480
BAVENCIO	10 MG	INF	J9023
BAXDELA	1 MG	ORAL, IV	C9462
BCG LIVE INTRAVESICAL	1 MG	OTH	J9030
BEBTELOVIMAB	175 MG	IV	Q0222
BEBULIN VH	1 IU	IV	J7194
BECAPLERMIN GEL 0.01%	0.5 G	OTH	S0157
BECLOMETHASONE COMPOUNDED	1 MG	INH	J7622
BECLOVENT COMPOUNDED	1 MG	INH	J7622
BECONASE COMPOUNDED	1 MG	INH	J7622
BELANTAMAB MAFODOTIN-BLMF	0.5 MG	IV	J9037
BELATACEPT	1 MG	IV	J0485
BELEODAQ	10 MG	IV	J9032
BELIMUMAB	10 MG	IV	J0490
BELINOSTAT	10 MG	IV	J9032
BELLACELL HD	SQ CM	OTH	Q4220
BELRAPZO	1 MG	IV	J9036
BENA-D 10	50 MG	IV, IM	J1200
BENA-D 50	50 MG	IV, IM	J1200
BENADRYL	50 MG	IV, IM	J1200
BENAHIST 10	50 MG	IV, IM	J1200
BENAHIST 50	50 MG	IV, IM	J1200
BENDAMUSTINE HCL	1 MG	IV	J9033
BENDAMUSTINE HCL	1 MG	IV	J9056
BENDAMUSTINE HCL	1 MG	IV	J9034
~~BENDAMUSTINE HCL (APOTEX)~~	~~1 MG~~	~~IV~~	~~J9058~~
~~BENDAMUSTINE HCL (BAXTER)~~	~~1 MG~~	~~IV~~	~~J9059~~
BENDAMUSTINE HYDROCHLORIDE	1 MG	IV	J9036
BENDEKA	1 MG	IV	J9034
BENLYSTA	10 MG	IV	J0490
BENOJECT-10	50 MG	IV, IM	J1200
BENOJECT-50	50 MG	IV, IM	J1200
BENRALIZUMAB	1 MG	SC	J0517
BENTYL	20 MG	IM	J0500
BENZTROPINE MESYLATE	1 MG	IM, IV	J0515
BEOVU	1 MG	INJ	J0179
~~BEQVEZ~~	~~THERAPEUTIC DOSE~~	~~IV~~	~~C9172~~
BEQVEZ	THERAPEUTIC DOSE	IV	J1414
BEREMAGENE GEPERPAVEC-SVDT	0.1 ML	OTH	J3401

Drug Name	Units Per	Route	Code
BERINERT	10 U	IV	J0597
BERUBIGEN	1,000 MCG	SC, IM	J3420
BESPONSA	0.1 MG	IV	J9229
BETA-2	1 MG	INH	J7648
BETALIN 12	1,000 MCG	SC, IM	J3420
BETAMETHASONE ACETATE AND BETAMETHASONE SODIUM PHOSPHATE	3 MG/3 MG	IM	J0702
BETAMETHASONE COMPOUNDED, UNIT DOSE	1 MG	INH	J7624
BETASERON	0.25 MG	SC	J1830
BETHANECHOL CHLORIDE, MYOTONACHOL OR URECHOLINE	5 MG	SC	J0520
BETIBEGLOGENE AUTOTEMCEL	PER TREATMENT	IV	J3393
BEVACIZUMAB	10 MG	IV	J9035
BEVACIZUMAB	0.25 MG	IV	C9257
BEVACIZUMAB-ADCD	10 MG	IV	Q5129
BEVACIZUMAB-AWWB, BIOSIMILAR	10 MG	IV	Q5107
BEVACIZUMAB-BVZR, BIOSIMILAR	10 MG	IV	Q5118
BEVACIZUMAB-MALY, BIOSIMILAR, (ALYMSYS)	10 MG	IV	Q5126
BEZLOTOXUMAB	10 MG	INF	J0565
BICILLIN CR	100,000 UNITS	IM	J0558
BICILLIN CR 900/300	100,000 UNITS	IM	J0558
BICILLIN CR TUBEX	100,000 UNITS	IM	J0558
BICILLIN LA	100,000 U	IM	J0561
BICNU	100 MG	IV	J9050
BIMATOPROST, INTRACAMERAL IMPLANT	1 MCG	OTH	J7351
BIO-CONNEKT	SQ CM	OTH	Q4161
BIO-CONNEKT WOUND MATRIX	SQ CM	OTH	A2003
BIODEXCEL	SQ CM	OTH	Q4137
BIODFENCE	SQ CM	OTH	Q4140
BIODFENCE DRYFLEX	SQ CM	OTH	Q4138
BIODMATRIX	1 CC	OTH	Q4139
BIOSKIN	SQ CM	OTH	Q4163
BIOSKIN FLOW	SQ CM	OTH	Q4162
BIOTROPIN	1 MG	SC	J2941
BIOVANCE	SQ CM	OTH	Q4154
BIOVANCE TRI-LAYER OR BIOVANCE 3L	SQ CM	OTH	Q4283
BIOWOUND, BIOWOUND PLUS, BIOWOUND XPLUS	SQ CM	OTH	Q4217
BIPERIDEN LACTATE	5 MG	IM, IV	J0190
BITOLTEROL MESYLATE, COMPOUNDED CONCENTRATED	1 MG	INH	J7628
BITOLTEROL MESYLATE, COMPOUNDED UNIT DOSE	MG	INH	J7629
BIVALIRUDIN	1 MG	IV	J0583
BIVIGAM	500 MG	IV	J1556
BKEMV	10 MG	IV	Q5139
BLENOXANE	15 U	IM, IV, SC	J9040
BLENREP	0.5 MG	IV	J9037
BLEOMYCIN LYOPHILLIZED	15 U	IM, IV, SC	J9040
BLEOMYCIN SULFATE	15 U	IM, IV, SC	J9040
BLINATUMOMAB	1 MCG	IV	J9039
BLINCYTO	1 MCG	IV	J9039
BONIVA	1 MG	IV	J1740
BORTEZOMIB	0.1 MG	IV, SC	J9041
BORTEZOMIB (DR. REDDY'S), NOT THERAPEUTICALLY EQUIVALENT TO J9041	0.1 MG	IV, SC	J9046
BORTEZOMIB (FRESENIUS KABI), NOT THERAPEUTICALLY EQUIVALENT TO J9041	0.1 MG	IV	J9048
BORTEZOMIB (HOSPIRA), NOT THERAPEUTICALLY EQUIVALENT TO J9041	0.1 MG	IV	J9049
BORTEZOMIB (MAIA), NOT THERAPEUTICALLY EQUIVALENT TO J9041	0.1 MG	IV	J9051
BOTOX	1 UNIT	IM, OTH	J0585
BOTOX COSMETIC	1 UNIT	IM, OTH	J0585
BOTULINUM TOXIN TYPE A	1 UNIT	IM, OTH	J0585
BOTULINUM TOXIN TYPE B	100 U	OTH	J0587
BRACHYTHERAPY LINEAR SOURCE, NONSTRANDED, PALLADIUM-103	1 MM	OTH	C2636
BRACHYTHERAPY PLANAR SOURCE, PALLADIUM-103	SQ MM	OTH	C2645
BRACHYTHERAPY SOURCE, CESIUM-131 CHLORIDE SOLUTION	MCI	OTH	C2644
BRACHYTHERAPY SOURCE, NONSTRANDED, CESIUM-131	SOURCE	OTH	C2643
BRACHYTHERAPY SOURCE, NONSTRANDED, GOLD-198	SOURCE	OTH	C1716
BRACHYTHERAPY SOURCE, NONSTRANDED, HIGH ACTIVITY, IODINE-125, GREATER THAN 1.01 MCI (NIST)	SOURCE	OTH	C2634
BRACHYTHERAPY SOURCE, NONSTRANDED, HIGH ACTIVITY, PALLADIUM-103, GREATER THAN 2.2 MCI (NIST)	SOURCE	OTH	C2635
BRACHYTHERAPY SOURCE, NONSTRANDED, HIGH DOSE RATE IRIDIUM-192	SOURCE	OTH	C1717
BRACHYTHERAPY SOURCE, NONSTRANDED, IODINE-125	SOURCE	OTH	C2639
BRACHYTHERAPY SOURCE, NONSTRANDED, NONHIGH DOSE RATE IRIDIUM-192	SOURCE	OTH	C1719
BRACHYTHERAPY SOURCE, NONSTRANDED, PALLADIUM-103	SOURCE	OTH	C2641
BRACHYTHERAPY SOURCE, NONSTRANDED, YTTERBIUM-169	SOURCE	OTH	C2637
BRACHYTHERAPY SOURCE, NONSTRANDED, YTTRIUM-90	SOURCE	OTH	C2616
BRACHYTHERAPY SOURCE, STRANDED, CESIUM-131	SOURCE	OTH	C2642
BRACHYTHERAPY SOURCE, STRANDED, IODINE-125	SOURCE	OTH	C2638
BRACHYTHERAPY SOURCE, STRANDED, PALLADIUM-103	SOURCE	OTH	C2640
BRAVELLE	75 IU	SC, IM	J3355
BRENTUXIMAB VENDOTIN	1 MG	IV	J9042
BRETHINE	1 MG	INH	J7681
BRETHINE CONCENTRATED	1 MG	INH	J7680
BREXANOLONE	1 MG	IV	J1632
BREXUCABTAGENE AUTOLEUCEL	UP TO 200 MILLION CELLS	IV	Q2053
BREYANZI	UP TO 110 MILLION CELLS	IV	Q2054
BRICANYL	1 MG	INH	J7681
BRICANYL CONCENTRATED	1 MG	INH	J7680
BRINEURA	1 MG	OTH	J0567
BRIUMVI	1 MG	IV	J2329
~~BRIXADI~~	~~1 MG~~	~~SC~~	~~J0576~~

Drug Name	Units Per	Route	Code
BRIXADI, 8 TO 28 DAYS OF THERAPY	64 MG OR GREATER	SC	J0578
BRIXADI, ≤ 7 DAYS OF THERAPY	≤ 32 MG	SC	J0577
BROLUCIZUMAB-DBLL	1 MG	INJ	J0179
BROM-A-COT	10 MG	IM, SC, IV	J0945
BROMPHENIRAMINE MALEATE	10 MG	IM, SC, IV	J0945
BUDESONIDE COMPOUNDED, CONCETRATED	0.25 MG	INH	J7634
BUDESONIDE, COMPOUNDED, UNIT DOSE	0.5 MG	INH	J7627
BUDESONIDE, NONCOMPOUNDED, CONCENTRATED	0.25 MG	INH	J7633
BUDESONIDE, NONCOMPOUNDED, UNIT DOSE	0.5 MG	INH	J7626
BUMETANIDE	0.5 MG	IM, IV	J1939
BUMEX	0.5 MG	IM, IV	J1939
BUNAVAIL	2.1 MG	ORAL	J0572
BUNAVAIL	6.3 MG	ORAL	J0574
BUNAVAIL	4.2 MG	ORAL	J0573
BUPIVACAINE	1 MG	INJ	C9144
BUPIVACAINE AND MELOXICAM	1 MG/0.03 MG	OTH	C9088
~~BUPIVACAINE LIPOSOME~~	~~1 MG~~	~~VAR~~	~~C9290~~
BUPIVACAINE LIPOSOME	1 MG	INJ	J0666
BUPIVACAINE, COLLAGEN-MATRIX IMPLANT	1 MG	OTH	C9089
BUPRENEX	0.1 MG	IM, IV	J0592
BUPRENORPHIN/NALOXONE	UP TO 3 MG	ORAL	J0572
BUPRENORPHIN/NALOXONE	> 10 MG	ORAL	J0575
BUPRENORPHINE EXTENDED-RELEASE	> 100 MG	SC	Q9992
~~BUPRENORPHINE EXTENDED-RELEASE~~	~~1 MG~~	~~SC~~	~~J0576~~
BUPRENORPHINE EXTENDED-RELEASE	≤ 100 MG	SC	Q9991
BUPRENORPHINE EXTENDED-RELEASE, 8 TO 28 DAYS OF THERAPY	64 MG OR GREATER	SC	J0578
BUPRENORPHINE EXTENDED-RELEASE, ≤ 7 DAYS OF THERAPY	≤ 32 MG	SC	J0577
BUPRENORPHINE HCL	0.1 MG	IM, IV	J0592
~~BUPRENORPHINE IMPLANT~~	~~74.2 MG~~	~~OTH~~	~~J0570~~
BUPRENORPHINE ORAL	1 MG	ORAL	J0571
BUPRENORPHINE/NALOXONE	3.1 TO 6 MG	ORAL	J0573
BUPRENORPHINE/NALOXONE	6.1 TO 10 MG	ORAL	J0574
BUPROPION HCL	150 MG	ORAL	S0106
BUROSUMAB-TWZA	1 MG	SC	J0584
BUSULFAN	1 MG	IV	J0594
BUSULFAN	2 MG	ORAL	J8510
BUSULFEX	2 MG	ORAL	J8510
BUTORPHANOL TARTRATE	2 MG	IM, IV	J0595
BUTORPHANOL TARTRATE	25 MG	OTH	S0012
BYFAVO	1 MG	IV	J2249
BYOOVIZ	0.1 MG	INJ	Q5124
C-1 ESTERASE INHIBITOR (HUMAN)	10 UNITS	SC	J0599
C1 ESTERASE INHIBITOR (HUMAN) (BERINERT)	10 UNITS	IV	J0597
C1 ESTERASE INHIBITOR (HUMAN) (CINRYZE)	10 UNITS	IV	J0598
C1 ESTERASE INHIBITOR (RECOMBINANT)	10 UNITS	IV	J0596
CABAZITAXEL	1 MG	IV	J9043
CABAZITAXEL	1 MG	IV	J9064
CABENUVA	2 MG/3 MG	IM	J0741
CABERGOLINE	0.25 MG	ORAL	J8515
CABLIVI	1 MG	IV, SC	C9047
CABOTEGRAVIR	1 MG	IM	J0739
CABOTEGRAVIR AND RILPIVIRINE	2 MG/3 MG	IM	J0741
CAFCIT	5 MG	IV	J0706
CAFFEINE CITRATE	5 MG	IV	J0706
CALASPARGASE PEGOL-MKNL	10 UNITS	IV	J9118
CALCIJEX	0.25 MCG	INJ	S0169
CALCIJEX	0.1 MCG	IM	J0636
CALCIMAR	UP TO 400 U	SC, IM	J0630
CALCITONIN SALMON	400 U	SC, IM	J0630
CALCITRIOL	0.1 MCG	IM	J0636
CALCITRIOL	0.25 MCG	IM	S0169
CALCIUM ACETATE, FOR ESRD ON DIALYSIS	23 MG	ORAL	J0615
CALCIUM DISODIUM VERSENATE	1,000 MG	IV, SC, IM	J0600
CALCIUM GLUCONATE (WG CRITICAL CARE), NOT THERAPEUTICALLY EQUIVALENT TO J0612	10 MG	IV	J0613
CALCIUM GLYCEROPHOSPHATE AND CALCIUM LACTATE	10 ML	IM, SC	J0620
CALDOLOR	100 MG	IV	J1741
CAMCEVI	1 MG	SC	J1952
CAMPTOSAR	20 MG	IV	J9206
CANAKINUMAB	1 MG	SC	J0638
CANCIDAS	5 MG	IV	J0637
~~CANTHARIDIN FOR TOPICAL ADMINISTRATION~~	~~3.2 MG~~	~~OTH~~	~~C9164~~
CANTHARIDIN FOR TOPICAL ADMINISTRATION	3.2 MG	OTH	J7354
~~CAPECITABINE~~	~~150 MG~~	~~ORAL~~	~~J8520~~
CAPECITABINE	50 MG	ORAL	J8522
CAPLACIZUMAB-YHDP	1 MG	IV, SC	C9047
CAPSAICIN 8% PATCH	1 SQ CM	OTH	J7336
CARBIDOPA/LEVODOPA	5 MG/20 MG	ORAL	J7340
CARBOCAINE	10 ML	VAR	J0670
CARBOPLATIN	50 MG	IV	J9045
CARBOXYDEXTRAN-COATED SUPERPARAMAGNETIC IRON OXIDE	STUDY DOSE	SC	A9697
CARDENE IV	0.1 MG	IV	J2404
CARDIOGEN 82	STUDY DOSE UP TO 60 MCI	IV	A9555
CARDIOLITE	STUDY DOSE	IV	A9500
CAREGRAFT	SQ CM	OTH	Q4322
CAREPATCH	SQ CM	OTH	Q4236
CARFILZOMIB	1 MG	IV	J9047
CARMUSTINE	100 MG	IV	J9050
CARMUSTINE (ACCORD), NOT THERAPEUTICALLY EQUIVALENT TO J9050	100 MG	IV	J9052
CARNITOR	1 G	IV	J1955
CARTICEL		OTH	J7330
CARVYKTI	UP TO 100 MILLION CELLS	IV	Q2056
CASGEVY	TREATMENT DOSE	IV	J3392
CASIMERSEN	10 MG	IV	J1426
CASIRIVIMAB AND IMDEVIMAB	2400 MG	IV	Q0243
CASIRIVIMAB AND IMDEVIMAB	600 MG	IV	Q0240
CASIRIVIMAB AND IMDEVIMAB	1200 MG	IV	Q0244
CASPOFUNGIN ACETATE	5 MG	IV	J0637

Drug Name	Units Per	Route	Code
CATAPRES	1 MG	OTH	J0735
CATHFLO	1 MG	IV	J2997
CAVERJECT	1.25 MCG	VAR	J0270
CEA SCAN	STUDY DOSE UP TO 45 MCI	IV	A9568
CEENU	10 MG	ORAL	S0178
CEFAZOLIN SODIUM	500 MG	IM, IV	J0690
CEFAZOLIN SODIUM (BAXTER), NOT THERAPEUTICALLY EQUIVALENT TO J0690	500 MG	IV	J0689
CEFAZOLIN SODIUM (HIKMA), NOT THERAPEUTICALLY EQUIVALENT TO J0690	500 MG	IV	J0688
CEFAZOLIN SODIUM (WG CRITICAL CARE)	500 MG	IV	J0687
CEFEPIME HCL	500 MG	IV	J0692
CEFEPIME HCL (B. BRAUN), NOT THERAPEUTICALLY EQUIVALENT TO MAXIPIME	500 MG	IV	J0703
CEFEPIME HCL (BAXTER), NOT THERAPEUTICALLY EQUIVALENT TO MAXIPIME	500 MG	IV	J0701
CEFIDEROCOL	10 MG	IV	J0699
CEFIZOX	500 MG	IV, IM	J0715
CEFOBID	1 G	IV	S0021
CEFOPERAZONE SODIUM	1 G	IV	S0021
CEFOTAN	500 MG	IM, IV	S0074
CEFOTAXIME SODIUM	1 GM	IV, IM	J0698
CEFOTETAN DISODIUM	500 MG	IM, IV	S0074
CEFOXITIN SODIUM	1 GM	IV, IM	J0694
CEFTAROLINE FOSAMIL	10 MG	IV	J0712
CEFTAZIDIME	500 MG	IM, IV	J0713
CEFTAZIDIME AND AVIBACTAM	0.5 G/0.125 G	IV	J0714
CEFTIZOXIME SODIUM	500 MG	IV, IM	J0715
CEFTOLOZANE AND TAZOBACTAM	50 MG/25 MG	IV	J0695
CEFTRIAXONE SODIUM	250 MG	IV, IM	J0696
CEFUROXIME	750 MG	IM, IV	J0697
CEFUROXIME SODIUM STERILE	750 MG	IM, IV	J0697
CELERA DUAL LAYER/MEMBRANE	SQ CM	OTH	Q4259
CELESTONE SOLUSPAN	3 MG/3 MG	IM	J0702
CELLCEPT	250 MG	ORAL	J7517
CELLCEPT	10 MG	IV	J7519
CELLESTA CORD	SQ CM	OTH	Q4214
CELLESTA FLOWABLE AMNION	0.5 CC	OTH	Q4185
CELLESTA OR CELLESTA DUO	SQ CM	OTH	Q4184
CEMIPLIMAB-RWLC	1 MG	IV	J9119
CENACORT FORTE	5 MG	IM	J3302
CENTRUROIDES (SCORPION) IMMUNE F(AB)2 (EQUINE)	UP TO 120 MG	IV	J0716
CEPHALOTHIN SODIUM	UP TO 1 G	INJ	J1890
CEPHAPIRIN SODIUM	1 G	IV	J0710
CEPTAZ	500 MG	IM, IV	J0713
CEREBRYX	50 MG	IM, IV	Q2009
CEREBRYX	750 MG	IM, IV	S0078
CEREDASE	10 U	IV	J0205
CERETEC	STUDY DOSE UP TO 25 MCI	IV	A9521
CEREZYME	10 U	IV	J1786
CERIANNA	1 MCI	IV	A9591
CERLIPONASE ALFA	1 MG	OTH	J0567
CERTOLIZUMAB PEGOL	1 MG	SC	J0717
CERUBIDINE	10 MG	IV	J9150
CESAMET	1 MG	ORAL	J8650
CETIRIZINE HCL	0.5 MG	IV	J1201
CETUXIMAB	10 MG	IV	J9055
CHEALAMIDE	150 MG	IV	J3520
CHLORAMBUCIL	2 MG	ORAL	S0172
CHLORAMPHENICOL SODIUM SUCCINATE	1 G	IV	J0720
CHLORDIAZEPOXIDE HCL	100 MG	IM, IV	J1990
CHLOROMYCETIN	1 G	IV	J0720
CHLOROPROCAINE HCL	1 MG	INJ	J2401
CHLOROPROCAINE HCL (CLOROTEKAL)	1 MG	INJ	J2402
CHLOROPROCAINE HCL OPHTHALMIC, 3% GEL	1 MG	OTH	J2403
CHLOROQUINE HCL	UP TO 250 MG	IM, IV	J0390
CHLOROTHIAZIDE SODIUM	500 MG	IV	J1205
CHLORPROMAZINE HCL	5 MG	ORAL	Q0161
CHLORPROMAZINE HCL	50 MG	IM, IV	J3230
CHOLETEC	STUDY DOSE UP TO 15 MCI	IV	A9537
CHOLINE C 11, DIAGNOSTIC, PER STUDY DOSE	UP TO 20 MCI	IV	A9515
CHOREX	1000 USP	IM	J0725
CHORIONIC GONADOTROPIN	1,000 USP U	IM	J0725
CHROMIC PHOSPHATE P32 (THERAPEUTIC)	1 MCI	IV	A9564
CHROMITOPE SODIUM	STUDY DOSE UP TO 250 UCI	IV	A9553
CHROMIUM CR-51 SODIUM IOTHALAMATE, DIAGNOSTIC	STUDY DOSE UP TO 250 UCI	IV	A9553
CIDOFOVIR	375 MG	IV	J0740
CILASTATIN SODIUM	250 MG	IV, IM	J0743
CILTACABTAGENE AUTOLEUCEL	UP TO 100 MILLION CELLS	IV	Q2056
CIMERLI	0.1 MG	INJ	Q5128
CIMETIDINE HCL	300 MG	IM, IV	S0023
CIMZIA	1 MG	SC	J0717
CINACALCET	1 MG	ORAL	J0604
CINQUAIR	1 MG	IV	J2786
CINRZYE	10 UNITS	IV	J0598
CINVANTI	1 MG	IV	J0185
CIPAGLUCOSIDASE ALFA-ATGA	5 MG	IV	J1203
CIPLA	1 MG	SC, INJ	J1932
CIPLA	7.5 MG	IM	J1954
CIPRO	200 MG	IV	J0744
CIPROFLOXACIN FOR INTRAVENOUS INFUSION	200 MG	IV	J0744
CIPROFLOXACIN OTIC SUSPENSION	6 MG	OTIC	J7342
CIS-MDP	STUDY DOSE UP TO 30 MCI	IV	A9503
CIS-PYRO	STUDY DOSE UP TO 25 MCI	IV	A9538
CISPLATIN	10 MG	IV	J9060
CLADRIBINE	1 MG	IV	J9065
CLAFORAN	1 GM	IV, IM	J0698
CLARIX 100	SQ MC	OTH	Q4156
CLARIX CORD 1K	SQ CM	OTH	Q4148
CLARIXFLO	1 MG	OTH	Q4155
CLEVIDIPINE BUTYRATE	1 MG	IV	C9248
CLEVIPREX	1 MG	IV	C9248
CLINDAMYCIN PHOSPHATE	300 MG	IV	J0736

Drug Name	Units Per	Route	Code
CLINDAMYCIN PHOSPHATE (BAXTER) NOT THERAPEUTICALLY EQUIVALENT TO J0736	300 MG	IV	J0737
CLOFARABINE	1 MG	IV	J9027
CLOLAR	1 MG	IV	J9027
CLONIDINE HCL	1 MG	OTH	J0735
CLOZAPINE	25 MG	ORAL	S0136
CLOZARIL	25 MG	ORAL	S0136
COAGADEX	1 IU	IV	J7175
COAGULATION FACTOR IX (RECOMBINANT)	1 IU	IV	J7213
COAGULATION FACTOR XA (RECOMBINANT), INACTIVATED-ZHZO	10 MG	IV	J7169
COBAL	1,000 MCG	IM, SC	J3420
COBALT CO-57 CYNOCOBALAMIN, DIAGNOSTIC	STUDY DOSE UP TO 1 UCI	ORAL	A9559
COBATOPE 57	STUDY DOSE UP TO 1 UCI	ORAL	A9559
COBEX	1,000 MCG	SC, IM	J3420
COCAINE HYDROCHLORIDE NASAL SOLUTION	1 MG	OTH	C9046
COCAINE HYDROCHLORIDE NASAL SOLUTION (NUMBRINO)	1 MG	OTH	C9143
COCOON MEMBRANE	SQ CM	OTH	Q4264
CODEINE PHOSPHATE	30 MG	IM, IV, SC	J0745
COGENEX AMNIOTIC MEMBRANE	SQ CM	OTH	Q4229
COGENEX FLOWABLE AMNION	0.5 CC	OTH	Q4230
COGENTIN	1 MG	IM, IV	J0515
COGNEX	10 MG	ORAL	S0014
COLCHICINE	1 MG	IV	J0760
COLHIST	10 MG	IM, SC, IV	J0945
COLISTIMETHATE SODIUM	1 MG	INH	S0142
COLISTIMETHATE SODIUM	150 MG	IM, IV	J0770
COLL-E-DERM	SQ CM	OTH	Q4193
COLLAGEN BASED WOUND FILLER DRY FOAM	1 GM	OTH	A6010
COLLAGEN BASED WOUND FILLER, GEL/PASTE	1 GM	OTH	A6011
COLLAGEN MATRIX NERVE WRAP	0.5 CM	OTH	C9361
COLLAGEN NERVE CUFF	0.5 CM LENGTH	OTH	C9355
COLLAGEN WOUND DRESSING	SQ CM	OTH	Q4164
COLLAGENASE, CLOSTRIDIUM HISTOLYTICUM	0.01 MG	OTH	J0775
COLUMVI	2.5 MG	IV	J9286
COLY-MYCIN M	150 MG	IM, IV	J0770
COMBOGESIC	10 MG/3 MG	ORAL	J0138
COMPAZINE	10 MG	IM, IV	J0780
COMPAZINE	5 MG	ORAL	S0183
COMPAZINE	5 MG	ORAL	Q0164
COMPLETE AA	SQ CM	OTH	Q4303
COMPLETE ACA	SQ CM	OTH	Q4302
COMPLETE FT	SQ CM	OTH	Q4271
COMPLETE SL	SQ CM	OTH	Q4270
CONIVAPTAN HYDROCHLORIDE	1 MG	INJ	C9488
CONTRACEPTIVE INTRAUTERINE DEVICE	EA	OTH	S4989
CONTRACEPTIVE SUPPLY, HORMONE CONTAINING PATCH	EACH	OTH	J7304
CONTRACEPTIVE SUPPLY, SPERMICIDE	EA	OTH	A4269
CONTRAST FOR ECHOCARDIOGRAM	STUDY	IV	A9700
COPANLISIB	1 MG	IV	J9057
COPAXONE	20 MG	SC	J1595
COPPER CU-64, DOTATATE, DIAGNOSTIC	1 MCI	IV	A9592
COPPER T MODEL TCU380A IUD COPPER WIRE/COPPER COLLAR	EA	OTH	J7300
CORDARONE	30 MG	IV	J0282
CORECYTE	0.5 CC	OTH	Q4240
CORETEXT	1 CC	OTH	Q4246
CORIFACT	1 IU	IV	J7180
CORPLEX	SQ CM	OTH	Q4232
CORPLEX P	1 CC	OTH	Q4231
CORTASTAT	1 MG	IM, IV, OTH	J1100
CORTASTAT LA	1 MG	IM	J1094
CORTICORELIN OVINE TRIFLUTATE	1 MCG	IV	J0795
~~CORTIMED~~	~~80 MG~~	~~IM~~	~~J1040~~
CORTROSYN	0.25 MG	IM, IV	J0834
CORVERT	1 MG	IV	J1742
COSELA	1 MG	IV	J1448
~~COSENTYX~~	~~1 MG~~	~~IV~~	~~C9166~~
COSENTYX	1 MG	IV	J3247
COSMEGEN	0.5 MG	IV	J9120
COSYNTROPIN	0.25 MG	IM, IV	J0834
COTOLONE	5 MG	ORAL	J7510
CRESEMBA	1 MG	IV	J1833
CRIZANLIZUMAB-TMCA	5 MG	IV	J0791
CROFAB	UP TO 1 GM	IV	J0840
CROMOLYN SODIUM COMPOUNDED	PER 10 MG	INH	J7632
CROMOLYN SODIUM NONCOMPOUNDED	10 MG	INH	J7631
CROTALIDAE IMMUNE F(AB')2 (EQUINE)	120 MG	IV	J0841
CROTALIDAE POLYVALENT IMMUNE FAB (OVINE)	UP TO 1 GM	IV	J0840
CROVALIMAB-AKKZ	10 MG	IV, SC	J1307
CRYO-CORD	SQ CM	OTH	Q4237
CRYSTAL B12	1,000 MCG	IM, SC	J3420
CRYSTICILLIN 300 A.S.	600,000 UNITS	IM, IV	J2510
CRYSTICILLIN 600 A.S.	600,000 UNITS	IM, IV	J2510
CRYSVITA	1 MG	SC	J0584
CUBICIN	1 MG	IV	J0878
CUTAQUIG	100 MG	IV	J1551
CUVITRU	100 MG	SC	J1555
CYANO	1,000 MCG	IM, SC	J3420
CYANOCOBALAMIN	1,000 MCG	IM, SC	J3420
CYANOCOBALAMIN COBALT 57/58	STUDY DOSE UP TO 1 UCI	IV	A9546
CYANOCOBALAMIN COBALT CO-57	STUDY DOSE UP TO 1 UCI	ORAL	A9559
CYANOKIT	25 MG	IV	J3424
CYCLOPHOSPHAMIDE	25 MG	ORAL	J8530
~~CYCLOPHOSPHAMIDE~~	~~100 MG~~	~~IV~~	~~J9070~~
CYCLOPHOSPHAMIDE (AUROMEDICS)	5 MG	IV	J9071
CYCLOPHOSPHAMIDE (AVYXA)	5 MG	IV	J9072
CYCLOPHOSPHAMIDE (BAXTER)	5 MG	IV	J9076
~~CYCLOPHOSPHAMIDE (DR. REDDY'S)~~	~~5 MG~~	~~IV~~	~~J9072~~
CYCLOPHOSPHAMIDE (INGENUS)	5 MG	IV	J9073
CYCLOPHOSPHAMIDE (SANDOZ)	5 MG	IV	J9074
CYCLOSPORINE	25 MG	ORAL	J7515

Drug Name	Units Per	Route	Code
CYCLOSPORINE	100 MG	ORAL	J7502
CYCLOSPORINE	250 MG	IV	J7516
CYGNUS	SQ CM	OTH	Q4170
CYGNUS DUAL	SQ CM	OTH	Q4282
CYGNUS MATRIX	SQ CM	OTH	Q4199
CYLTEZO	1 MG	SC	Q5143
CYMETRA	1 CC	INJ	Q4112
CYRAMZA	5 MG	IV	J9308
CYSVIEW	STUDY DOSE	OTH	A9589
CYTAL	SQ CM	OTH	Q4166
CYTALUX	0.1 MG	IV	A9603
CYTARABINE	100 MG	SC, IV	J9100
CYTARABINE LIPOSOME	10 MG	IT	J9098
CYTOGAM	VIAL	IV	J0850
CYTOMEGALOVIRUS IMMUNE GLOB	VIAL	IV	J0850
CYTOSAR-U	100 MG	SC, IV	J9100
CYTOTEC	200 MCG	ORAL	S0191
CYTOVENE	500 MG	IV	J1570
CYTOXAN	25 MG	ORAL	J8530
~~CYTOXAN~~	~~100 MG~~	~~IV~~	~~J9070~~
D.H.E. 45	1 MG	IM, IV	J1110
DACARBAZINE	100 MG	IV	J9130
DACLIZUMAB	25 MG	OTH	J7513
DACOGEN	1 MG	IV	J0894
DACTINOMYCIN	0.5 MG	IV	J9120
DALALONE	1 MG	IM, IV, OTH	J1100
DALALONE LA	1 MG	IM	J1094
DALBAVANCIN	5 MG	IV	J0875
DALTEPARIN SODIUM	2,500 IU	SC	J1645
DALVANCE	5 MG	IV	J0875
DANYELZA	1 MG	IV	J9348
DAPRODUSTAT	1 MG	ORAL	J0889
DAPTOMYCIN	1 MG	IV	J0878
DAPTOMYCIN (HOSPIRA), NOT THERAPEUTICALLY EQUIVALENT TO J0878	1 MG	IV	J0877
DAPTOMYCIN (XELLIA), NOT THERAPEUTICALLY EQUIVALENT TO J0878 OR J0872	1 MG	IV	J0873
DAPTOMYCIN (XELLIA), UNREFRIGERATED, NOT THERAPEUTICALLY EQUIVALENT TO J0878 OR J0873	1 MG	IV	J0872
DAPTOMYCIN IN SODIUM CHLORIDE INJECTION	1 MG	IV	J0874
DARATUMUMAB	10 MG	IV	J9145
DARATUMUMAB AND HYALURONIDASE-FIHJ	10 MG	SC	J9144
DARBEPOETIN ALFA, ESRD USE	1 MCG	SC, IV	J0882
DARBEPOETIN ALFA, NON-ESRD USE	1 MCG	SC, IV	J0881
DARZALEX	10 MG	IV	J9145
DARZALEX FASPRO	10 MG	SC	J9144
DATSCAN	STUDY DOSE	IV	A9584
DAUNORUBICIN	10 MG	IV	J9150
DAUNORUBICIN CITRATE, LIPOOSOMAL FORMULATION	10 MG	IV	J9151
DAUNOXOME	10 MG	IV	J9151
~~DAXIBOTULINUMTOXINA-LANM~~	~~1 UNIT~~	~~IM~~	~~C9160~~
DAXIBOTULINUMTOXINA-LANM	PER UNIT	IM	J0589
~~DAXXIFY~~	~~1 UNIT~~	~~IM~~	~~C9160~~
DAXXIFY	PER UNIT	IM	J0589

Drug Name	Units Per	Route	Code
DDAVP	1 MCG	IV, SC	J2597
DECADRON	0.25 MG	ORAL	J8540
DECAJECT	1 MG	IM, IV, OTH	J1100
DECITABINE	1 MG	IV	J0894
DECITABINE (SUN PHARMA), NOT THERAPEUTICALLY EQUIVALENT TO J0894	1 MG	IV	J0893
DECOLONE-50	50 MG	IM	J2320
DEFENCATH	1.35 MG/100 UNITS	OTH	J0911
DEFEROXAMINE MESYLATE	500 MG	IM, SC, IV	J0895
DEGARELIX	1 MG	SC	J9155
DELAFLOXACIN	1 MG	ORAL, IV	C9462
DELANDISTROGENE MOXEPARVOVEC-ROKL	THERAPEUTIC DOSE	IV	J1413
DELATESTRYL	1 MG	IM	J3121
DELESTROGEN	10 MG	IM	J1380
DELTA-CORTEF	5 MG	ORAL	J7510
DEMADEX	10 MG	IV	J3265
DEMEROL	100 MG	IM, IV, SC	J2175
DENOSUMAB	1 MG	SC	J0897
DENOSUMAB-BBDZ (JUBBONTI/ WYOST), BIOSIMILAR	1 MG	SC	Q5136
DEOXYCHOLIC ACID	1 MG	SC	J0591
DEPGYNOGEN	UP TO 5 MG	IM	J1000
DEPHENACEN-50	50 MG	IM, IV	J1200
~~DEPMEDALONE~~	~~40 MG~~	~~IM~~	~~J1030~~
~~DEPMEDALONE~~	~~80 MG~~	~~IM~~	~~J1040~~
DEPO-ESTRADIOL CYPIONATE	UP TO 5 MG	IM	J1000
~~DEPO-MEDROL~~	~~20 MG~~	~~IM, OTH~~	~~J1020~~
DEPO-MEDROL	1 MG	IM	J1010
~~DEPO-MEDROL~~	~~80 MG~~	~~IM, OTH~~	~~J1040~~
~~DEPO-MEDROL~~	~~40 MG~~	~~IM, OTH~~	~~J1030~~
DEPO-TESTOSTERONE	1 MG	IM	J1071
DEPOCYT	10 MG	IT	J9098
DEPOGEN	UP TO 5 MG	IM	J1000
DERM-MAXX	SQ CM	OTH	Q4238
DERMA-GIDE	SQ CM	OTH	Q4203
DERMABIND CH	SQ CM	OTH	Q4288
DERMABIND DL	SQ CM	OTH	Q4287
DERMABIND FM	SQ CM	OTH	Q4313
DERMABIND SL	SQ CM	OTH	Q4284
DERMABIND TL	SQ CM	OTH	Q4225
DERMACELL, DERMACELL AWM OR DERMACELL AWM POROUS	SQ CM	OTH	Q4122
DERMACYTE AC MATRIX AMNIOTIC MEMBRANE ALLOGRAFT	SQ CM	OTH	Q4343
DERMACYTE AMNIOTIC MEMBRANE ALLOGRAFT	SQ CM	OTH	Q4248
DERMAGRAFT	SQ CM	OTH	Q4106
DERMAL SUBSTITUTE, NATIVE, NONDENATURED COLLAGEN, FETAL	0.5 SQ CM	OTH	C9358
DERMAL SUBSTITUTE, NATIVE, NONDENATURED COLLAGEN, NEONATAL	0.5 SQ CM	OTH	C9360
DERMAPURE	SQ CM	OTH	Q4152
DERMAVEST AND PLURIVEST	SQ CM	OTH	Q4153
DESCOVY	200 MG/25 MG	ORAL	J0751
DESFERAL	500 MG	IM, SC, IV	J0895
DESMOPRESSIN ACETATE	1 MCG	IV, SC	J2597
DETECTNET	1 MCI	IV	A9592
DEXAMETHASONE	0.25 MG	ORAL	J8540

Drug Name	Units Per	Route	Code
DEXAMETHASONE	0.25 MG	ORAL	J8541
DEXAMETHASONE 9%	1 MCG	OTH	J1095
DEXAMETHASONE ACETATE	1 MG	IM	J1094
DEXAMETHASONE ACETATE ANHYDROUS	1 MG	IM	J1094
DEXAMETHASONE INTRAVITREAL IMPLANT	0.1 MG	OTH	J7312
DEXAMETHASONE SODIUM PHOSPHATE	1 MG	IM, IV, OTH	J1100
DEXAMETHASONE, COMPOUNDED, CONCENTRATED	1 MG	INH	J7637
DEXAMETHASONE, COMPOUNDED, UNIT DOSE	1 MG	INH	J7638
DEXAMETHASONE, LACRIMAL OPHTHALMIC INSERT	0.1 MG	OTH	J1096
DEXASONE	1 MG	IM, IV, OTH	J1100
DEXEDRINE	5 MG	ORAL	S0160
DEXIM	1 MG	IM, IV, OTH	J1100
DEXMEDETOMIDINE	1 MCG	ORAL	J1105
DEXONE	0.25 MG	ORAL	J8540
DEXONE	1 MG	IM, IV, OTH	J1100
DEXONE LA	1 MG	IM	J1094
DEXRAZOXANE HCL	250 MG	IV	J1190
DEXTENZA	0.1 MG	OTH	J1096
DEXTRAN 40	500 ML	IV	J7100
DEXTROAMPHETAMINE SULFATE	5 MG	ORAL	S0160
DEXTROSE	500 ML	IV	J7060
DEXTROSE, STERILE WATER, AND/OR DEXTROSE DILUENT/FLUSH	10 ML	VAR	A4216
DEXTROSE/SODIUM CHLORIDE	5%	VAR	J7042
DEXTROSE/THEOPHYLLINE	40 MG	IV	J2810
DEXTROSTAT	5 MG	ORAL	S0160
DEXYCU	1 MCG	OTH	J1095
DI-SPAZ	UP TO 20 MG	IM	J0500
DIALYSIS/STRESS VITAMINS	100 CAPS	ORAL	S0194
DIAMOX	500 MG	IM, IV	J1120
DIASTAT	5 MG	IV, IM	J3360
DIAZEPAM	5 MG	IV, IM	J3360
DIAZOXIDE	300 MG	IV	J1730
DIBENT	UP TO 20 MG	IM	J0500
DICLOFENAC SODIUM	0.5 MG	OTH	J1130
DICYCLOMINE HCL	20 MG	IM	J0500
DIDANOSINE (DDI)	25 MG	ORAL	S0137
DIDRONEL	300 MG	IV	J1436
DIETHYLSTILBESTROL DIPHOSPHATE	250 MG	INJ	J9165
DIFELIKEFALIN	0.1 MCG	IV	J0879
DIFLUCAN	200 MG	IV	J1450
DIGIBIND	VIAL	IV	J1162
DIGIFAB	VIAL	IV	J1162
DIGOXIN	0.5 MG	IM, IV	J1160
DIGOXIN IMMUNE FAB	VIAL	IV	J1162
DIHYDROERGOTAMINE MESYLATE	1 MG	IM, IV	J1110
DILANTIN	50 MG	IM, IV	J1165
DILAUDID	250 MG	OTH	S0092
DILAUDID	0.1 MG	IM, IV, SC	J1171
~~DILAUDID~~	~~4 MG~~	~~SC, IM, IV~~	~~J1170~~
DILAUDID-HP	0.1 MG	IM, IV, SC	J1171
DIMENHYDRINATE	50 MG	IM, IV	J1240
DIMERCAPROL	100 MG	IM	J0470
DIMINE	50 MG	IV, IM	J1200
DINATE	50 MG	IM, IV	J1240
DIOVAL	10 MG	IM	J1380
DIOVAL 40	10 MG	IM	J1380
DIOVAL XX	10 MG	IM	J1380
DIPHENHYDRAMINE HCL	50 MG	ORAL	Q0163
DIPHENHYDRAMINE HCL	50 MG	IV, IM	J1200
DIPRIVAN	10 MG	IV	J2704
DIPYRIDAMOLE	10 MG	IV	J1245
DISOTATE	150 MG	IV	J3520
DIURIL	500 MG	IV	J1205
DIURIL SODIUM	500 MG	IV	J1205
DIZAC	5 MG	IV, IM	J3360
DMSO, DIMETHYL SULFOXIDE	50%, 50 ML	OTH	J1212
DOBUTAMINE HCL	250 MG	IV	J1250
DOBUTREX	250 MG	IV	J1250
DOCETAXEL	1 MG	IV	J9171
DOCETAXEL	1 MG	IV	J9172
DOCIVYX	1 MG	IV	J9172
DOLASETRON MESYLATE	100 MG	ORAL	Q0180
DOLASETRON MESYLATE	10 MG	IV	J1260
DOLASETRON MESYLATE	50 MG	ORAL	S0174
DOLOPHINE	5 MG	ORAL	S0109
DOLOPHINE HCL	10 MG	IM, SC	J1230
DOMMANATE	50 MG	IM, IV	J1240
DONANEMAB-AZBT	2 MG	IV	J0175
DOPAMINE HCL	40 MG	IV	J1265
DORIBAX	10 MG	IV	J1267
DORIPENEM	10 MG	IV	J1267
DORNASE ALPHA, NONCOMPOUNDED, UNIT DOSE	1 MG	INH	J7639
DOSTARLIMAB-GXLY	10 MG	IV	J9272
DOSTINEX	0.25 MG	ORAL	J8515
DOTAREM	0.1 ML	IV	A9575
DOXERCALCIFEROL	1 MG	IV	J1270
DOXORUBICIN HCL	10 MG	IV	J9000
DOXORUBICIN HYDROCHLORIDE, LIPOSOMAL, IMPORTED LIPODOX	10 MG	IV	Q2049
DRAMAMINE	50 MG	IM, IV	J1240
DRAMANATE	50 MG	IM, IV	J1240
DRAMILIN	50 MG	IM, IV	J1240
DRAMOCEN	50 MG	IM, IV	J1240
DRAMOJECT	50 MG	IM, IV	J1240
DRAXIMAGE MDP-10	STUDY DOSE UP TO 30 MCI	IV	A9503
DRAXIMAGE MDP-25	STUDY DOSE UP TO 30 MCI	IV	A9503
DRONABINAL	2.5 MG	ORAL	Q0167
DRONABINOL	0.1 MG	ORAL	Q0155
DROPERIDOL	5 MG	IM, IV	J1790
DROPERIDOL AND FENTANYL CITRATE	2 ML	IM, IV	J1810
DROXIA	500 MG	ORAL	S0176
DTIC-DOME	100 MG	IV	J9130
DTPA	STUDY DOSE UP TO 25 MCI	IV	A9539
DTPA	STUDY DOSE UP TO 25 MCI	INH	A9567
DUAL LAYER IMPAX MEMBRANE	SQ CM	OTH	Q4262
DUOAMNION	SQ CM	OTH	Q4327
DUOPA	5 MG/20 MG	ORAL	J7340
DURACILLIN A.S.	600,000 UNITS	IM, IV	J2510

Drug Name	Units Per	Route	Code
DURACLON	1 MG	OTH	J0735
DURAGEN-10	10 MG	IM	J1380
DURAGEN-20	10 MG	IM	J1380
DURAGEN-40	10 MG	IM	J1380
DURAMORPH	500 MG	OTH	S0093
DURAMORPH PF	10 MG	OTH	J2274
~~DURO CORT~~	~~80 MG~~	~~IM~~	~~J1040~~
DUROLANE	1 MG	INJ	J7318
DURVALUMAB	10 MG	IV	J9173
DURYSTA	1 MCG	OTH	J7351
DYLOJECT	0.5 MG	OTH	J1130
DYMENATE	50 MG	IM, IV	J1240
DYPHYLLINE	500 MG	IM	J1180
DYSPORT	5 UNITS	IM	J0586
E-GRAFT	SQ CM	OTH	Q4318
E.D.T.A.	150 MG	IV	J3520
ECALLANTIDE	1 MG	SC	J1290
ECHOCARDIOGRAM IMAGE ENHANCER OCTAFLUOROPROPANE	1 ML	IV	Q9956
ECHOCARDIOGRAM IMAGE ENHANCER PERFLEXANE	1 ML	IV	Q9955
ECULIZUMAB	10 MG	IV	J1300
ECULIZUMAB-AEEB	10 MG	IV	Q5139
EDARAVONE	1 MG	IV	J1301
EDETATE CALCIUM DISODIUM	1,000 MG	IV, SC, IM	J0600
EDETATE DISODIUM	150 MG	IV	J3520
EDEX	1.25 MCG	VAR	J0270
EFBEMALENOGRASTIM ALFA-VUXW	0.5 MG	SC	J9361
EFGARTIGIMOD ALFA-FCAB	2 MG	IV	J9332
EFGARTIGIMOD ALFA/ HYALURONIDASE-QVFC	2 MG	IV	J9334
ELAHERE	1 MG	IV	J9063
ELAPRASE	1 MG	IV	J1743
ELAVIL	20 MG	IM	J1320
ELELYSO	10 U	IV	J3060
ELEVIDYS	THERAPEUTIC DOSE	IV	J1413
ELFABRIO	1 MG	IV	J2508
ELFLAPEGRASTIM-XNST	0.1 MG	SC	J1449
ELIGARD	7.5 MG	SC	J9217
ELITEK	0.5 MG	IM	J2783
ELLENCE	2 MG	IV	J9178
ELLIOTTS B SOLUTION	1 ML	IV, IT	J9175
ELOCTATE	IU	IV	J7205
ELOSULFASE ALFA	1 MG	IV	J1322
ELOTUZUMAB	1 MG	IV	J9176
ELOXATIN	0.5 MG	IV	J9263
~~ELRANATAMAB-BCMM~~	~~1 MG~~	~~SC~~	~~C9165~~
ELRANATAMAB-BCMM	1 MG	SC	J1323
~~ELREXFIO~~	~~1 MG~~	~~SC~~	~~C9165~~
ELREXFIO	1 MG	SC	J1323
ELSPAR	1,000 IU	IM,IV, SC	J9019
ELUCIREM	1 ML	IV	A9573
ELZONRIS	10 MCG	IV	J9269
EMAPALUMAB-LZSG	1 MG	IV	J9210
EMEND	5 MG	ORAL	J8501
EMEND	1 MG	IV	J1453
EMERGE MATRIX	SQ CM	OTH	Q4297
EMICIZUMAB-KXWH	0.5 MG	SC	J7170
EMINASE	30 U	IV	J0350
EMPLICITI	1 MG	IV	J9176
EMTRICITABINE/TENOFOVIR ALAFENAMIDE	200 MG/25 MG	ORAL	J0751
EMTRICITABINE/TENOFOVIR DISOPROXIL FUMARATE	200 MG/300 MG	ORAL	J0750
ENBREL	25 MG	IM, IV	J1438
ENCLOSE TL MATRIX	SQ CM	OTH	Q4351
~~ENDOXAN-ASTA~~	~~100 MG~~	~~IV~~	~~J9070~~
ENDRATE	150 MG	IV	J3520
ENFORTUMAB VEDOTIN-EJFV	0.25 MG	IV	J9177
ENFUVIRTIDE	1 MG	SC	J1324
ENHERTU	1 MG	IV	J9358
ENJAYMO	10 MG	IV	J1302
ENOXAPARIN SODIUM	10 MG	SC	J1650
ENSIFENTRINE, INHALATION SUSPENSION	3 MG	INH	J7601
ENTYVIO	1 MG	IV	J3380
ENVARSUS XR	0.25 MG	ORAL	J7503
ENVERSE	SQ CM	OTH	Q4258
EOVIST	1 ML	IV	A9581
EPCORITAMAB-BYSP	0.16 MG	SC	J9321
EPICORD	SQ CM	OTH	Q4187
EPIEFFECT	SQ CM	OTH	Q4278
EPIFIX	SQ CM	OTH	Q4186
EPIFIX, INJECTABLE	1 MG	OTH	Q4145
EPINEPHRINE	0.1 MG	IM, IV, SC	J0171
EPINEPHRINE (BELCHER), NOT THERAPEUTICALLY EQUIVALENT TO J0171	0.1 MG	IV	J0173
EPIRUBICIN HCL	2 MG	IV	J9178
EPKINLY	0.16 MG	SC	J9321
EPOETIN ALFA FOR ESRD DIALYSIS	100 U	INJ	Q4081
EPOETIN ALFA, BIOSIMILAR	100 UNITS	INJ, IV	Q5105
EPOETIN ALFA, BIOSIMILAR	1000 UNITS	INJ, IV	Q5106
EPOETIN ALFA, NON-ESRD USE	1,000 U	SC, IV	J0885
EPOETIN BETA FOR ESRD ON DIALYSIS	1 MCG	IV	J0887
EPOETIN BETA FOR NON-ESRD	1 MCG	IV, SC	J0888
EPOGEN/NON-ESRD	1,000 U	SC, IV	J0885
EPOPROSTENOL	0.5 MG	IV	J1325
EPOPROSTENOL STERILE DILUTANT	50 ML	IV	S0155
EPTIFIBATIDE	5 MG	IM, IV	J1327
EPTINEZUMAB-JJMR	1 MG	IV	J3032
ERAVACYCLINE	1 MG	IV	J0122
ERAXIS	1 MG	IV	J0348
ERBITUX	10 MG	IV	J9055
ERGAMISOL	50 MG	ORAL	S0177
ERGONOVINE MALEATE	0.2 MG	IM, IV	J1330
ERIBULIN MESYLATE	0.1 MG	IV	J9179
ERTAPENEM SODIUM	500 MG	IM, IV	J1335
ERYTHROCIN LACTOBIONATE	500 MG	IV	J1364
ESANO A	SQ CM	OTH	Q4272
ESANO AAA	SQ CM	OTH	Q4273
ESANO AC	SQ CM	OTH	Q4274
ESANO ACA	SQ CM	OTH	Q4275
ESKETAMINE, NASAL SPRAY	1 MG	OTH	S0013
ESMOLOL HCL	10 MG	IV	J1805
ESMOLOL HCL (WG CRITICAL CARE) NOT THERAPEUTICALLY EQUIVALENT TO J1805	10 MG	IV	J1806
ESPEROCT	1 IU	IV	J7204

Drug Name	Units Per	Route	Code
ESTONE AQUEOUS	1 MG	IM, IV	J1435
ESTRA-L 20	10 MG	IM	J1380
ESTRA-L 40	10 MG	IM	J1380
ESTRADIOL CYPIONATE	UP TO 5 MG	IM	J1000
ESTRADIOL L.A.	10 MG	IM	J1380
ESTRADIOL L.A. 20	10 MG	IM	J1380
ESTRADIOL L.A. 40	10 MG	IM	J1380
ESTRADIOL VALERATE	10 MG	IM	J1380
ESTRAGYN	1 MG	IV, IM	J1435
ESTRO-A	1 MG	IV, IM	J1435
ESTROGEN CONJUGATED	25 MG	IV, IM	J1410
ESTRONE	1 MG	IV, IM	J1435
ESTRONOL	1 MG	IM, IV	J1435
ETANERCEPT	25 MG	IM, IV	J1438
ETELCALCETIDE	0.1 MG	IV	J0606
ETEPLIRSEN	10 MG	INF	J1428
ETHAMOLIN	100 MG	IV	J1430
ETHANOLAMINE OLEATE	100 MG	IV	J1430
ETHINYL ESTRADIOL AND ETONOGESTREL VAGINAL RING	0.015 MG/0.12 MG	OTH	J7295
ETHYOL	500 MG	IV	J0207
ETIDRONATE DISODIUM	300 MG	IV	J1436
ETONOGESTREL	IMPLANT	OTH	J7307
ETOPOSIDE	50 MG	ORAL	J8560
ETOPOSIDE	10 MG	IV	J9181
ETRANACOGEN DEXAPARVOVEC-DRLB	THERAPEUTIC DOSE	IV	J1411
EUFLEXXA	DOSE	INJ	J7323
EULEXIN	125 MG	ORAL	S0175
EVENITY	1 MG	SC	J3111
EVEROLIMUS	0.25 MG	ORAL	J7527
EVINACUMAB-DGNB	5 MG	IV	J1305
EVKEEZA	5 MG	IV	J1305
EVOMELA	1 MG	IV	J9246
EVUSHELD	300 MG	IM	Q0220
EVUSHELD	600 MG	IM	Q0221
EXAGAMGLOGENE AUTOTEMCEL	TREATMENT DOSE	IV	J3392
EXAMETAZIME LABELED AUTOLOGOUS WHITE BLOOD CELLS, TECHNETIUM TC-99M	STUDY DOSE	IV	A9569
EXCELLAGEN	0.1 CC	OTH	Q4149
EXMESTANE	25 MG	ORAL	S0156
EXONDYS 51	10 MG	INF	J1428
~~EXPAREL~~	~~1 MG~~	~~VAR~~	~~C9290~~
EXPAREL	1 MG	INJ	J0666
~~EYLEA HD~~	~~1 MG~~	~~INJ~~	~~C9161~~
EYLEA HD	1 MG	INJ	J0177
EZ-DERM	SQ CM	OTH	Q4136
FABRAZYME	1 MG	IV	J0180
FACTOR IX (ANTIHEMOPHILIC FACTOR, RECOMBINANT), RIXIBUS, PER I.U.	IU	IV	J7200
FACTOR IX NON-RECOMBINANT	1 IU	IV	J7193
FACTOR IX+ COMPLEX	1 IU	IV	J7194
FACTOR IX, (ANTIHEMOPHILIC FACTOR, RECOMBINANT), GLYCOPEGYLATED	1 IU	IV	J7203
FACTOR IX, ALBUMIN FUSION PROTEIN, (RECOMBINANT)	1 IU	IV	J7202
FACTOR IX, FC FUSION PROTEIN (ANTIHEMOPHILIC FACTOR, RECOMBINANT), ALPROLIX	IU	IV	J7201
FACTOR VIIA (ANTIHEMOPHILIC FACTOR, RECOMBINANT)-JNCW	1 MCG	IV	J7212
FACTOR VIIA RECOMBINANT	1 MCG	IV	J7189
FACTOR VIII (ANTIHEMOPHILIC FACTOR, RECOMBINANT)	1 IU	IV	J7209
FACTOR VIII (ANTIHEMOPHILIC FACTOR, RECOMBINANT)	IU	IV	J7188
FACTOR VIII (ANTIHEMOPHILIC FACTOR, RECOMBINANT) (NOVOEIGHT), PER IU	IU	IV	J7182
FACTOR VIII (ANTIHEMOPHILIC FACTOR, RECOMBINANT) PEGYLATED	1 IU	IV	J7207
FACTOR VIII FC FUSION (RECOMBINANT)	IU	IV	J7205
FACTOR VIII PORCINE	1 IU	IV	J7191
FACTOR VIII, (ANTIHEMOPHILIC FACTOR, RECOMBINANT) (AFSTYLA)	1 IU	IV	J7210
FACTOR VIII, (ANTIHEMOPHILIC FACTOR, RECOMBINANT) (KOVALTRY)	1 IU	IV	J7211
FACTOR VIII, (ANTIHEMOPHILIC FACTOR, RECOMBINANT), PEGYLATED-AUCL	1 IU	IV	J7208
FACTOR VIII, ANTIHEMOPHILIC FACTOR (RECOMBINANT), GLYCOPEGYLATED-EXEI	1 IU	IV	J7204
FACTOR VIII, HUMAN	1 IU	IV	J7190
FACTOR X (HUMAN)	1 IU	IV	J7175
FACTOR XIII (ANTIHEMOPHILIC FACTOR, HUMAN)	1 IU	IV	J7180
FACTOR XIII A-SUBUNIT (RECOMBINANT)	10 IU	IV	J7181
FACTREL	100 MCG	SC, IV	J1620
FAM-TRASTUZUMAB DERUXTECAN-NXKI	1 MG	IV	J9358
FAMOTIDINE	20 MG	IV	S0028
FARICIMAB-SVOA	0.1 MG	INJ	J2777
FASENRA	1 MG	SC	J0517
FASLODEX	25 MG	IM	J9395
FDG	STUDY DOSE UP TO 45 MCI	IV	A9552
FECAL MICROBIOTA, LIVE-JSLM	1 ML	OTH	J1440
FEIBA-VH AICC	1 IU	IV	J7198
FENSOLVI	0.25 MG	SC	J1951
FENTANYL CITRATE	0.1 MG	IM, IV	J3010
FERAHEME (FOR ESRD)	1 MG	IV	Q0139
FERAHEME (NON-ESRD)	1 MG	IV	Q0138
FERIDEX IV	1 ML	IV	Q9953
FERRIC CARBOXYMALTOSE	1 MG	IV	J1439
FERRIC CITRATE, FOR ESRD ON DIALYSIS	3 MG	ORAL	J0609
FERRIC DERISOMALTOSE	10 MG	IV	J1437
FERRIC PYROPHOSPHATE CITRATE POWDER	0.1 MG	IV	J1444
FERRIC PYROPHOSPHATE CITRATE SOLUTION	0.1 MG	IV	J1443
FERRIC PYROPHOSPHATE CITRATE SOLUTION	0.1 MG	IV	J1445
FERRLECIT	12.5 MG	IV	J2916
FERTINEX	75 IU	SC	J3355
FERUMOXYTOL (FOR ESRD)	1 MG	IV	Q0139

Drug Name	Units Per	Route	Code
FERUMOXYTOL (NON-ESRD)	1 MG	IV	**Q0138**
FETROJA	10 MG	IV	**J0699**
FIASP	5 U	SC, IV	**J1812**
FIASP	50 U	SC, IV	**J1811**
FIBRIN SEALANT (HUMAN)	2 ML	OTH	**C9250**
FIBRYGA	1 MG	IV	**J7177**
~~**FIDANACOGENE ELAPARVOVEC-DZKT**~~	~~THERAPEUTIC DOSE~~	~~IV~~	~~**C9172**~~
FIDANACOGENE ELAPARVOVEC-DZKT	THERAPEUTIC DOSE	IV	**J1414**
FILGRASTIM	1 MCG	SC, IV	**J1442**
FILGRASTIM-AAFI, BIOSIMILAR	1 MCG	INJ	**Q5110**
FILGRASTIM-AYOW, BIOSIMILAR	1 MCG	SC, IV	**Q5125**
FILGRASTIM-SNDZ, BIOSIMILAR	1 MCG	IV, SC	**Q5101**
FILGRASTIM-TXID	1 MCG	IV, SC	**C9173**
FINASTERIDE	5 MG	ORAL	**S0138**
FIRAZYR	1 MG	SC	**J1744**
FIRMAGON	1 MG	SC	**J9155**
FISH OIL TRIGLYCERIDES	10 G	IV	**B4187**
FLEBOGAMMA	500 MG	IV	**J1572**
FLEXHD	SQ CM	OTH	**Q4128**
FLEXON	60 MG	IV, IM	**J2360**
FLOLAN	0.5 MG	IV	**J1325**
FLORBETABEN F18, DIAGNOSTIC	STUDY DOSE UP TO 8.1 MCI	IV	**Q9983**
FLORTAUCIPIR F-18, DIAGNOSTIC	1 MCI	IV	**A9601**
FLOTUFOLASTAT F18, DIAGNOSTIC	1 MCI	IV	**A9608**
FLOWERAMNIOFLO	SQ CM	OTH	**Q4177**
FLOWERAMNIOPATCH	SQ CM	OTH	**Q4178**
FLOWERDERM	SQ CM	OTH	**Q4179**
FLOXIN IV	400 MG	IV	**S0034**
FLOXURIDINE	500 MG	IV	**J9200**
FLUCICLOVINE F-18, DIAGNOSTIC	1 MCI	IV	**A9588**
FLUCONAZOLE	200 MG	IV	**J1450**
FLUDARA	50 MG	IV	**J9185**
FLUDARABINE PHOSPHATE	10 MG	ORAL	**J8562**
FLUDARABINE PHOSPHATE	50 MG	IV	**J9185**
FLUDEOXYGLUCOSE F18	STUDY DOSE UP TO 45 MCI	IV	**A9552**
FLUDEOXYGLUCOSE F18	UP TO 15 MCI	IV	**A9609**
FLUID FLOW, FLUID GF	1 CC	OTH	**Q4206**
FLULAVAL	EA	IM	**Q2036**
FLUMADINE (DEMONSTATION PROJECT)	100 MG	ORAL	**G9036**
FLUNISOLIDE, COMPOUNDED, UNIT DOSE	1 MG	INH	**J7641**
FLUOCINOLONE ACETONIDE INTRAVITREAL IMPLANT	IMPLANT	OTH	**J7311**
FLUOCINOLONE ACETONIDE, INTRAVITREAL IMPLANT	0.01 MG	OTH	**J7313**
FLUOCINOLONE ACETONIDE, INTRAVITREAL IMPLANT	0.01 MG	OTH	**J7314**
FLUORODEOXYGLUCOSE F-18 FDG, DIAGNOSTIC	STUDY DOSE UP TO 45 MCI	IV	**A9552**
FLUORODOPA F-18, DIAGNOSTIC	1 MCI	IV	**A9602**
FLUOROESTRADIOL F 18, DIAGNOSTIC	1 MCI	IV	**A9591**
FLUOROURACIL	500 MG	IV	**J9190**
FLUPHENAZINE DECANOATE	25 MG	SC, IM	**J2680**
FLUPHENAZINE HCL	1.25 MG	IM	**J2679**
FLUTAMIDE	125 MG	ORAL	**S0175**
FLUTEMETAMOL F18, DIAGNOSTIC	STUDY DOSE UP TO 5 MCI	IV	**Q9982**
FLUVIRIN	EA	IM	**Q2037**
FLUZONE	EA	IM	**Q2038**
FOCINVEZ	1 MG	IV	**J1434**
FOLEX	50 MG	IV, IM, IT, IA	**J9260**
~~**FOLEX**~~	~~5 MG~~	~~IV, IM, IT, IA~~	~~**J9250**~~
FOLEX PFS	50 MG	IV, IM, IT, IA	**J9260**
~~**FOLEX PFS**~~	~~5 MG~~	~~IV, IM, IT, IA~~	~~**J9250**~~
FOLLISTIM	75 IU	SC, IM	**S0128**
FOLLITROPIN ALFA	75 IU	SC	**S0126**
FOLLITROPIN BETA	75 IU	SC, IM	**S0128**
FOLOTYN	1 MG	IV	**J9307**
FOMEPIZOLE	15 MG	IV	**J1451**
FOMIVIRSEN SODIUM	1.65 MG	OTH	**J1452**
FONDAPARINUX SODIUM	0.5 MG	SC	**J1652**
FORMOTEROL FUMERATE NONCOMPOUNDED UNIT DOSE FORM	20 MCG	INH	**J7606**
FORMOTEROL, COMPOUNDED, UNIT DOSE	12 MCG	INH	**J7640**
FORTAZ	500 MG	IM, IV	**J0713**
FORTEO	10 MCG	SC	**J3110**
FORTOVASE	200 MG	ORAL	**S0140**
FOSAPREPITANT	1 MG	IV	**J1453**
FOSAPREPITANT	1 MG	IV	**J1434**
FOSAPREPITANT (TEVA), NOT THERAPEUTICALLY EQUIVALENT TO J1453	1 MG	IV	**J1456**
FOSCARNET SODIUM	1,000 MG	IV	**J1455**
FOSCAVIR	1,000 MG	IV	**J1455**
FOSNETUPITANT AND PALONOSETRON	235 MG/0.25 MG	IV	**J1454**
FOSPHENYTOIN	50 MG	IM, IV	**Q2009**
FOSPHENYTOIN SODIUM	750 MG	IM, IV	**S0078**
FOSRENOL, FOR ESRD ON DIALYSIS	5 MG	ORAL	**J0607**
FOSRENOL, POWDER, FOR ESRD ON DIALYSIS, NOT THERAPEUTICALLY EQUIVALENT TO J0607	5 MG	ORAL	**J0608**
FRAGMIN	2,500 IU	SC	**J1645**
FREMANEZUMAB-VFRM	1 MG	SC	**J3031**
FUDR	500 MG	IV	**J9200**
FULPHILA	0.5 MG	SC	**Q5108**
FULVESTRANT	25 MG	IM	**J9395**
FULVESTRANT (FRESENIUS KABI) NOT THERAPEUTICALLY EQUIVALENT TO J9395	25 MG	IM	**J9394**
FULVESTRANT (TEVA), NOT THERAPEUTICALLY EQUIVALENT TO J9395	25 MG	IM	**J9393**
FUNGIZONE	50 MG	IV	**J0285**
FUROSCIX	20 MG	SC	**J1941**
FUROSEMIDE	20 MG	IM, IV	**J1940**
FUROSEMIDE	20 MG	SC	**J1941**
FUZEON	1 MG	SC	**J1324**
FYARRO	1 MG	IV	**J9331**
FYLNETRA	0.5 MG	SC	**Q5130**
GABLOFEN	10 MG	IT	**J0475**
GABLOFEN	50 MCG	IT	**J0476**
GADAVIST	0.1 ML	IV	**A9585**
GADOBENATE DIMEGLUMINE (MULTIHANCE MULTIPACK)	1 ML	IV	**A9577**

Drug Name	Units Per	Route	Code
GADOBUTROL	0.1 ML	IV	A9585
GADOFOSVESET TRISODIUM	1 ML	IV	A9583
GADOPICLENOL	1 ML	IV	A9573
GADOTERATE MEGLUMINE	0.1 ML	IV	A9575
GADOTERIDOL (PROHANCE MULTIPACK)	1 ML	IV	A9576
GADOXETATE DISODIUM	1 ML	IV	A9581
GALLIUM GA-67	1 MCI	IV	A9556
GALLIUM GA-68 GOZETOTIDE, DIAGNOSTIC	1 MCI	IV	A9596
GALLIUM GA-68 GOZETOTIDE, DIAGNOSTIC	1 MCI	IV	A9800
GALLIUM GA-68 PSMA-11, DIAGNOSTIC, (UCLA)	1 MCI	IV	A9594
GALLIUM GA-68 PSMA-11, DIAGNOSTIC, (UCSF)	1 MCI	IV	A9593
GALLIUM GA-68, DOTATATE, DIAGNOSTIC	0.1 MCI	IV	A9587
GALLIUM GA-68, DOTATOC, DIAGNOSTIC	0.01 MCI	IV	C9067
GALLIUM NITRATE	1 MG	IV	J1457
GALSULFASE	1 MG	IV	J1458
GAMASTAN	1 CC	IM	J1460
GAMASTAN	OVER 10 CC	IM	J1560
GAMASTAN SD	1 CC	IM	J1460
GAMASTAN SD	OVER 10 CC	IM	J1560
GAMIFANT	1 MG	IV	J9210
GAMMA GLOBULIN	1 CC	IM	J1460
GAMMA GLOBULIN	OVER 10 CC	IM	J1560
GAMMAGARD	500 MG	IV	J1569
GAMMAGRAFT	SQ CM	OTH	Q4111
GAMMAKED	500 MG	IV, SC	J1561
GAMMAPLEX	500 MG	IV	J1557
GAMUNEX	500 MG	IV, SQ	J1561
GAMUNEX-C	500 MG	IV, SC	J1561
GANCICLOVIR	4.5 MG	OTH	J7310
GANCICLOVIR SODIUM	500 MG	IV	J1570
GANCICLOVIR SODIUM (EXELA) NOT THERAPEUTICALLY EQUIVALENT TO J1570	1 MG	IV	J1574
GANIRELIX ACETATE	250 MCG	SC	S0132
GANITE	1 MG	IV	J1457
GARAMYCIN	80 MG	IM, IV	J1580
GASTROCROM	10 MG	INH	J7631
GASTROMARK	1 ML	ORAL	Q9954
GATIFLOXACIN	10 MG	IV	J1590
GAZYVA	10 MG	IV	J9301
GEFITINIB	250 MG	ORAL	J8565
GEL-ONE	DOSE	INJ	J7326
GELSYN-3	0.1 MG	INJ	J7328
GEMCITABINE HCL (ACCORD), NOT THERAPEUTICALLY EQUIVALENT TO J9201	200 MG	IV	J9196
GEMCITABINE HYDROCHLORIDE	100 MG	IV	J9198
GEMTUZUMAB OZOGAMICIN	0.1 MG	INF	J9203
GENESIS AMNIOTIC MEMBRANE	SQ CM	OTH	Q4198
GENGRAF	25 MG	ORAL	J7515
GENGRAF	100 MG	ORAL	J7502
GENOTROPIN	1 MG	SC	J2941
GENOTROPIN MINIQUICK	1 MG	SC	J2941
GENOTROPIN NUTROPIN	1 MG	SC	J2941
GENTAMICIN	80 MG	IM, IV	J1580
GENTRAN	500 ML	IV	J7100
GENTRAN 75	500 ML	IV	J7110
GENVISC 850	1 MG	INJ	J7320
GEODON	10 MG	IM	J3486
GEREF	1MCG	SC	Q0515
GIVLAARI	0.5 MG	SC	J0223
GIVOSIRAN	0.5 MG	SC	J0223
GLASSIA	10 MG	IV	J0257
GLATIRAMER ACETATE	20 MG	SC	J1595
GLEEVEC	100 MG	ORAL	S0088
GLOFIL-125	STUDY DOSE UP TO 10 UCI	IV	A9554
GLOFITAMAB-GXBM	2.5 MG	IV	J9286
GLUCAGEN	1 MG	SC, IM, IV	J1610
GLUCAGON	1 MG	SC, IM, IV	J1610
GLUCAGON HCL (FRESENIUS KABI), NOT THERAPEUTICALLY EQUIVALENT TO J1610	1 MG	INJ	J1611
GLUCOTOPE	STUDY DOSE UP TO 45 MCI	IV	A9552
GLYCOPYRROLATE	0.1 MG	IM, IV	J1596
GLYCOPYRROLATE	0.1 MG	IM,IV	J1597
GLYCOPYRROLATE (FRESENIUS KABI)	0.1 MG	IM,IV	J1598
GLYCOPYRROLATE, COMPOUNDED CONCENTRATED	1 MG	INH	J7642
GLYCOPYRROLATE, COMPOUNDED, UNIT DOSE	1 MG	INH	J7643
GLYRX-PF	0.1 MG	IM,IV	J1597
GOLD SODIUM THIOMALATE	50 MG	IM	J1600
GOLIMUMAB	1 MG	IV	J1602
GOLODIRSEN	10 MG	IV	J1429
GONADORELIN HCL	100 MCG	SC, IV	J1620
GONAL-F	75 IU	SC	S0126
GOPRELTO	1 MG	OTH	C9046
GOSERELIN ACETATE	3.6 MG	SC	J9202
GRAFIX CORE	SQ CM	OTH	Q4132
GRAFIX PLUS	SQ CM	OTH	Q4304
GRAFIX PRIME	SQ CM	OTH	Q4133
GRAFIXPL CORE	SQ CM	OTH	Q4132
GRAFIXPL PRIME	SQ CM	OTH	Q4133
GRAFTJACKET	SQ CM	OTH	Q4107
GRAFTJACKET EXPRESS	1 CC	INJ	Q4113
GRANISETRON HCL	1 MG	ORAL	Q0166
GRANISETRON HCL	100 MCG	IV	J1626
GRANISETRON HCL	1 MG	IV	S0091
GRANISETRON, EXTENDED-RELEASE	0.1 MG	SC	J1627
GRANIX	1 MCG	IV	J1447
GUARDIAN	SQ CM	OTH	Q4151
GUSELKUMAB	1 MG	SC	J1628
GYNOGEN L.A. 10	10 MG	IM	J1380
GYNOGEN L.A. 20	10 MG	IM	J1380
GYNOGEN L.A. 40	10 MG	IM	J1380
HAEGARDA	10 UNITS	SC	J0599
HALAVEN	0.1 MG	IV	J9179
HALDOL	5 MG	IM, IV	J1630
HALDOL DECANOATE	50 MG	IM	J1631
HALOPERIDOL	5 MG	IM, IV	J1630
HECTOROL	1 MG	IV	J1270
HELICOLL	SQ CM	OTH	Q4164
HEMADY	0.25 MG	ORAL	J8541

Drug Name	Units Per	Route	Code
HEMGENIX	THERAPEUTIC DOSE	IV	**J1411**
HEMIN	1 MG	IV	**J1640**
HEMLIBRA	0.5 MG	SC	**J7170**
HEMOFIL-M	1 IU	IV	**J7190**
HEMOSPRAY	UNKNOWN	OTH	**C1052**
HEMOSTATIC AGENT, GASTROINTESTINAL	UNKNOWN	OTH	**C1052**
HEP LOCK	10 U	IV	**J1642**
HEP-PAK	10 UNITS	IV	**J1642**
HEPAGAM B	0.5 ML	IM	**J1571**
HEPAGAM B	0.5 ML	IV	**J1573**
HEPARIN SODIUM	10 U	IV	**J1642**
HEPARIN SODIUM	1,000 U	IV, SC	**J1644**
HEPARIN SODIUM (PFIZER), NOT THERAPEUTICALLY EQUIVALENT TO J1644	1000 UNITS	INJ, IV, SC, OTH	**J1643**
HEPATITIS B IMMUNE GLOBULIN	0.5 ML	IV	**J1573**
HEPATOLITE	STUDY DOSE UP TO 15 MCI	IV	**A9510**
HEPZATO	1 MG	IA	**J9248**
HERCEPTIN HYLECTA	10 MG	SC	**J9356**
HERCEPTIN, EXCLUDES BIOSIMILAR	10 MG	IV	**J9355**
HERCESSI	10 MG	IV	**Q5146**
HERZUMA	10 MG	IV	**Q5113**
HEXADROL	0.25 MG	ORAL	**J8540**
HEXAMINOLEVULINATE HYDROCHLORIDE	STUDY DOSE	OTH	**A9589**
HIGH OSMOLAR CONTRAST MATERIAL, UP TO 149 MG/ML IODINE CONCENTRATION	1 ML	IV	**Q9958**
HIGH OSMOLAR CONTRAST MATERIAL, UP TO 150-199 MG/ML IODINE CONCENTRATION	1 ML	IV	**Q9959**
HIGH OSMOLAR CONTRAST MATERIAL, UP TO 200-249 MG/ML IODINE CONCENTRATION	1 ML	IV	**Q9960**
HIGH OSMOLAR CONTRAST MATERIAL, UP TO 250-299 MG/ML IODINE CONCENTRATION	1 ML	IV	**Q9961**
HIGH OSMOLAR CONTRAST MATERIAL, UP TO 300-349 MG/ML IODINE CONCENTRATION	1 ML	IV	**Q9962**
HIGH OSMOLAR CONTRAST MATERIAL, UP TO 350-399 MG/ML IODINE CONCENTRATION	1 ML	IV	**Q9963**
HIGH OSMOLAR CONTRAST MATERIAL, UP TO 400 OR GREATER MG/ML IODINE CONCENTRATION	1 ML	IV	**Q9964**
HISTERLIN IMPLANT (VANTAS)	50 MG	OTH	**J9225**
HISTRELIN ACETATE	10 MG	INJ	**J1675**
HISTRELIN IMPLANT (SUPPRELIN LA)	50 MG	OTH	**J9226**
HIZENTRA	100 MG	SC	**J1559**
HMATRIX	SQ CM	OTH	**Q4134**
HULIO	1 MG	SC	**Q5140**
HUMALOG	5 U	SC	**J1815**
HUMALOG	50 U	SC	**J1817**
HUMAN FIBRINOGEN CONCENTRATE	1 MG	IV	**J7177**
HUMAN HEALTH FACTOR 10 AMNIOTIC PATCH (HHF10-P)	SQ CM	OTH	**Q4224**
HUMATE-P	1 IU	IV	**J7187**
HUMATROPE	1 MG	SC	**J2941**

Drug Name	Units Per	Route	Code
~~**HUMIRA**~~	~~20 MG~~	~~SC~~	~~**J0135**~~
HUMIRA	1 MG	SC	**J0139**
HUMULIN	5 U	SC	**J1815**
HUMULIN	50 U	SC	**J1817**
HUMULIN R	5 U	SC	**J1815**
HUMULIN R U-500	5 U	SC	**J1815**
HYALGAN	DOSE	INJ	**J7321**
HYALOMATRIX	SQ CM	OTH	**Q4117**
HYALURONAN	0.1 MG	INJ	**J7328**
HYALURONAN	DOSE	INJ	**J7327**
HYALURONAN	DOSE	INJ	**J7326**
HYALURONAN	DOSE	INJ	**J7323**
HYALURONAN	DOSE	INJ	**J7321**
HYALURONAN	DOSE	INJ	**J7324**
HYALURONAN	1 MG	INJ	**J7322**
HYALURONAN	1 MG	INJ	**J7325**
HYALURONAN	1 MG	INJ	**J7320**
HYALURONAN	1 MG	INJ	**J7332**
HYALURONAN	1 MG	INJ	**J7331**
HYALURONAN	1 MG	INJ	**J7329**
HYALURONAN	1 MG	INJ	**J7318**
HYALURONIDASE	150 UNITS	VAR	**J3470**
HYALURONIDASE RECOMBINANT	1 USP UNIT	SC	**J3473**
HYALURONIDASE, OVINE, PRESERVATIVE FREE	1000 USP	OTH	**J3472**
HYALURONIDASE, OVINE, PRESERVATIVE FREE	1 USP	OTH	**J3471**
HYCAMTIN	0.1 MG	IV	**J9351**
HYCAMTIN	0.25 MG	ORAL	**J8705**
HYDRALAZINE HCL	20 MG	IV, IM	**J0360**
HYDRATE	50 MG	IM, IV	**J1240**
HYDREA	500 MG	ORAL	**S0176**
HYDROCORTISONE ACETATE	25 MG	IV, IM, SC	**J1700**
HYDROCORTISONE SODIUM PHOSPHATE	50 MG	IV, IM, SC	**J1710**
HYDROCORTISONE SODIUM SUCCINATE	100 MG	IV, IM, SC	**J1720**
HYDROCORTONE PHOSPHATE	50 MG	SC, IM, IV	**J1710**
HYDROMORPHONE	0.1 MG	IM, IV, SC	**J1171**
HYDROMORPHONE HCL	250 MG	OTH	**S0092**
~~**HYDROMORPHONE HCL**~~	~~4 MG~~	~~SC, IM, IV~~	~~**J1170**~~
HYDROXOCOBALAMIN	1,000 MCG	IM, SC	**J3420**
HYDROXOCOBALAMIN	10 MCG	IM	**J3425**
HYDROXOCOBALAMIN	25 MG	IV	**J3424**
HYDROXYCOBAL	1,000 MCG	IM, SC	**J3420**
HYDROXYPROGESTERONE CAPROATE (MAKENA)	10 MG	IM	**J1726**
HYDROXYUREA	500 MG	ORAL	**S0176**
HYDROXYZINE HCL	25 MG	IM	**J3410**
HYDROXYZINE PAMOATE	25 MG	ORAL	**Q0177**
HYMOVIS	1 MG	INJ	**J7322**
HYOSCYAMINE SULFATE	0.25 MG	SC, IM, IV	**J1980**
HYPERRHO S/D	300 MCG	IV	**J2790**
HYPERTET SD	UP TO 250 MG	IM	**J1670**
HYPERTONIC SALINE SOLUTION	1 ML	VAR	**J7131**
HYQVIA	100 MG	IV	**J1575**
HYREXIN	50 MG	IV, IM	**J1200**
HYZINE	25 MG	IM	**J3410**
HYZINE-50	25 MG	IM	**J3410**
IBALIZUMAB-UIYK	10 MG	IV	**J1746**

Appendix 1 — Table of Drugs and Biologicals

Drug Name	Units Per	Route	Code
IBANDRONATE SODIUM	1 MG	IV	J1740
IBRITUMOMAB TUXETAN, DIAGNOSTIC	STUDY DOSE UP TO 5 MCI	IV	A9542
IBUPROFEN	100 MG	IV	J1741
IBUTILIDE FUMARATE	1 MG	IV	J1742
ICATIBANT	1 MG	SC	J1744
IDACIO	1 MG	SC	Q5144
~~IDACIO, BIOSIMILAR~~	~~20 MG~~	~~SC~~	~~Q5131~~
IDAMYCIN	5 MG	IV	J9211
IDAMYCIN PFS	5 MG	IV	J9211
IDARUBICIN HCL	5 MG	IV	J9211
IDECABTAGENE VICLEUCEL	UP TO 510 MILLION CELLS	IV	Q2055
IDELVION	1 IU	IV	J7202
IDOSE TR	1 MCG	OTH	J7355
IDURSULFASE	1 MG	IV	J1743
IFEX	1 G	IV	J9208
IFOSFAMIDE	1 G	IV	J9208
IGALMI	1 MCG	ORAL	J1105
IHEEZO	1 MG	OTH	J2403
IL-2	1 VIAL	IV	J9015
ILARIS	1 MG	SC	J0638
ILETIN	5 UNITS	SC	J1815
ILETIN II NPH PORK	50 U	SC	J1817
ILETIN II REGULAR PORK	5 U	SC	J1815
ILLUCCIX	1 MCI	IV	A9596
ILOPROST	0.1 MCG	INH	J1749
ILOPROST INHALATION SOLUTION	DOSE UP TO 20 MCG	INH	Q4074
ILUMYA	1 MG	SC	J3245
ILUVIEN	0.01 MG	OTH	J7313
IMAGENT	1 ML	IV	Q9955
IMATINIB	100 MG	ORAL	S0088
~~IMDELLTRA~~	~~1 MG~~	~~IV~~	~~C9170~~
IMDELLTRA	1 MG	IV	J9026
IMETELSTAT	1 MG	IV	J0870
IMFINZI	10 MG	IV	J9173
IMIGLUCERASE	10 U	IV	J1786
IMIPENEM, CILASTATIN, AND RELEBACTAM	4 MG/4 MG/2 MG	IV	J0742
IMITREX	6 MG	SC	J3030
IMJUDO	1 MG	IV	J9347
IMLYGIC	1 MILLION	INTRALESIONAL	J9325
IMMPHENTIV	20 MCG	IV	J2373
IMMUNE GLOBULIN	100 MG	IV	J1551
IMMUNE GLOBULIN (ALYGLO)	500 MG	IV	J1552
IMMUNE GLOBULIN (ASCENIV)	500 MG	IV	J1554
IMMUNE GLOBULIN (BIVIGAM)	500 MG	IV	J1556
IMMUNE GLOBULIN (CIVITRU)	100 MG	SC	J1555
IMMUNE GLOBULIN (FLEBOGAMMA, FLEBOGAMMA DIF)	500 MG	IV	J1572
IMMUNE GLOBULIN (GAMMAGARD LIQUID)	500 MG	IV	J1569
IMMUNE GLOBULIN (GAMMAPLEX)	500 MG	IV	J1557
IMMUNE GLOBULIN (GAMUNEX)	500 MG	IV	J1561
IMMUNE GLOBULIN (HIZENTRA)	100 MG	SC	J1559
IMMUNE GLOBULIN (OCTAGAM)	500 MG	IV	J1568
IMMUNE GLOBULIN (PRIVIGEN) NONLYOPHILIZED	500 MG	IV	J1459
IMMUNE GLOBULIN (RHOPHYLAC)	100 IU	IM, IV	J2791
IMMUNE GLOBULIN (XEMBIFY)	100 MG	SC	J1558
IMMUNE GLOBULIN SUBCUTANEOUS	100 MG	SC	J1562
IMMUNE GLOBULIN, NON-LYOPHILIZED	500 MG	IV	J1576
IMMUNE GLOBULIN/ HYALURONIDASE	100 MG	IV	J1575
IMPLANON	IMPLANT	OTH	J7307
IMURAN	50 MG	ORAL	J7500
INAPSINE	5 MG	IM, IV	J1790
INCLISIRAN	1 MG	SC	J1306
INCOBUTULINUMTOXINA	1 UNIT	IM	J0588
INDERAL	1 MG	IV	J1800
INDIUM IN-111 CAPROMAB PENDETIDE, DIAGNOSTIC	STUDY DOSE UP TO 10 MCI	IV	A9507
INDIUM IN-111 IBRITUMOMAB TIUXETAN, DIAGNOSTIC	STUDY DOSE UP TO 5 MCI	IV	A9542
INDIUM IN-111 LABELED AUTOLOGOUS PLATELETS	STUDY DOSE	IV	A9571
INDIUM IN-111 LABELED AUTOLOGOUS WHITE BLOOD CELLS	STUDY DOSE	IV	A9570
INDIUM IN-111 OXYQUINOLINE, DIAGNOSTIC	0.5 MCI	IV	A9547
INDIUM IN-111 PENTETATE, DIAGNOSTIC	0.5 MCI	INJ	A9548
INDIUM IN-111 PENTETREOTIDE	STUDY DOSE UP TO 6 MCI	IV	A9572
INDIUM IN-111 SATUMOMAB PENDETIDE, DIAGNOSTIC	STUDY DOSE UP TO 6MCI	IV	A4642
INDURSALFASE	1 MG	IV	J1743
INEBILIZUMAB-CDON	1 MG	IV	J1823
INFED	50 MG	IM, IV	J1750
INFERGEN	1 MCG	SC	J9212
INFLECTRA	10 MG	IV	Q5103
INFLIXIMAB	10 MG	IV	J1745
INFLIXIMAB-ABDA, BIOSIMILAR	10 MG	IV	Q5104
INFLIXIMAB-AXXQ, BIOSIMILAR	10 MG	IV	Q5121
INFLIXIMAB-DYYB	10 MG	SC	J1748
INFLIXIMAB-DYYB, BIOSIMILAR	10 MG	IV	Q5103
INFLIXIMAB-QBTX, BIOSIMILAR	10 MG	IV	Q5109
INFLUENZA VACCINE, AGRIFLU	UNKNOWN	IM	Q2034
INFLUENZA VIRUS VACCINE (AFLURIA)	EA	IM	Q2035
INFLUENZA VIRUS VACCINE (FLULAVAL)	EA	IM	Q2036
INFLUENZA VIRUS VACCINE (FLUVIRIN)	EA	IM	Q2037
INFLUENZA VIRUS VACCINE (FLUZONE)	EA	IM	Q2038
INFUGEM	100 MG	IV	J9198
INFUMORPH	10 MG	IM, IV, SC	J2270
INJECTAFER	1 MG	IV	J1439
INNOHEP	1,000 IU	SC	J1655
INNOVABURN OR INNOVAMATRIX XL	SQ CM	OTH	A2022
INNOVAMATRIX AC	SQ CM	OTH	A2001
INNOVAMATRIX FS	SQ CM	OTH	A2013
INNOVAMATRIX PD	SQ CM	OTH	A2023
INOTUZUMAB OZOGAMICIN	0.1 MG	IV	J9229
INSULIN	5 U	SC	J1815
INSULIN	50 U	SC	J1817
INSULIN LISPRO	5 U	SC	S5551
INSULIN LISPRO	5 U	SC	J1815

Drug Name	Units Per	Route	Code
INSULIN PURIFIED REGULAR PORK	5 U	SC	J1815
INTAL	10 MG	INH	J7631
INTEGRA BILAYER MATRIX DRESSING	SQ CM	OTH	Q4104
INTEGRA DERMAL REGENERATION TEMPLATE	SQ CM	OTH	Q4105
INTEGRA FLOWABLE WOUND MATRIX	1 CC	INJ	Q4114
INTEGRA MATRIX	SQ CM	OTH	Q4108
INTEGRA MESHED BILAYER WOUND MATRIX	SQ CM	OTH	C9363
INTEGRA MOZAIK OSTEOCONDUCTIVE SCAFFOLD PUTTY	0.5 CC	OTH	C9359
INTEGRA MOZAIK OSTEOCONDUCTIVE SCAFFOLD STRIP	0.5 CC	OTH	C9362
INTEGRA OMNIGRAFT DERMAL REGENERATION MATRIX	SQ CM	OTH	Q4105
INTEGRA OS OSTEOCONDUCTIVE SCAFFOLD PUTTY	0.5 CC	OTH	C9359
INTEGRILIN	5 MG	IM, IV	J1327
INTERFERON ALFA-2A	3,000,000 U	SC, IM	J9213
INTERFERON ALFA-2B	1,000,000 U	SC, IM	J9214
INTERFERON ALFA-N3	250,000 IU	IM	J9215
INTERFERON ALFACON-1	1 MCG	SC	J9212
INTERFERON BETA-1A	1 MCG	IM	Q3027
INTERFERON BETA-1A	30 MCG	IM, SC	J1826
INTERFERON BETA-1A	1 MCG	SC	Q3028
INTERFERON BETA-1B	0.25 MG	SC	J1830
INTERFERON, ALFA-2A, RECOMBINANT	3,000,000 U	SC, IM	J9213
INTERFERON, ALFA-2B, RECOMBINANT	1,000,000 U	SC, IM	J9214
INTERFERON, ALFA-N3, (HUMAN LEUKOCYTE DERIVED)	250,000 IU	IM	J9215
INTERFERON, GAMMA 1-B	3,000,000 U	SC	J9216
INTERFYL	1 MG	OTH	Q4171
INTERLUEKIN	1 VIAL	IV	J9015
INTRON A	1,000,000 U	SC, IM	J9214
INVANZ	500 MG	IM, IV	J1335
INVEGA HAFYERA	1 MG	IM	J2427
INVEGA SUSTENNA	1 MG	IM	J2426
INVEGA TRINZA	1 MG	IM	J2427
INVIRASE	200 MG	ORAL	S0140
IOBENGUANE SULFATE I-131	0.5 MCI	IV	A9508
IOBENGUANE, I-123, DIAGNOSTIC	STUDY DOSE UP TO 15 MCI	IV	A9582
IODINE I-123 IOBENGUANE, DIAGNOSTIC	STUDY DOSE UP TO 15 MCI	IV	A9582
IODINE I-123 IOFLUPANE	STUDY DOSE UP TO 5 MCI	IV	A9584
IODINE I-123 SODIUM IODIDE CAPSULE(S), DIAGNOSTIC	100-9999 UCI	ORAL	A9516
IODINE I-123 SODIUM IODIDE, DIAGNOSTIC	1 MCI	IV	A9509
IODINE I-125 SERUM ALBUMIN, DIAGNOSTIC	5 UCI	IV	A9532
IODINE I-125 SODIUM IOTHALAMATE, DIAGNOSTIC	STUDY DOSE UP TO 10 UCI	IV	A9554
IODINE I-125, SODIUM IODIDE SOLUTION, THERAPEUTIC	1 MCI	OTH	A9527
IODINE I-131 IOBENGUANE SULFATE, DIAGNOSTIC	0.5 MCI	IV	A9508
IODINE I-131 IODINATED SERUM ALBUMIN, DIAGNOSTIC	PER 5 UCI	IV	A9524
IODINE I-131 SODIUM IODIDE CAPSULE(S), DIAGNOSTIC	1 MCI	ORAL	A9528
IODINE I-131 SODIUM IODIDE CAPSULE(S), THERAPEUTIC	1 MCI	ORAL	A9517
IODINE I-131 SODIUM IODIDE SOLUTION, DIAGNOSTIC	1 MCI	ORAL	A9529
IODINE I-131 SODIUM IODIDE SOLUTION, THERAPEUTIC	1 MCI	ORAL	A9530
IODINE I-131 SODIUM IODIDE, DIAGNOSTIC	UCI UP TO 100 UCI	IV	A9531
IODINE I-131, IOBENGUANE	1 MCI	IV	A9590
IODOTOPE THERAPEUTIC CAPSULE(S)	1 MCI	ORAL	A9517
IODOTOPE THERAPEUTIC SOLUTION	1 MCI	ORAL	A9530
IOFLUPANE	STUDY DOSE UP TO 5 MCI	IV	A9584
ION-BASED MAGNETIC RESONANCE CONTRAST AGENT	1 ML	IV	Q9953
IOTHALAMATE SODIUM I-125	STUDY DOSE UP TO 10 UCI	IV	A9554
IPILIMUMAB	1 MG	IV	J9228
IPLEX	1 MG	SC	J2170
IPRATROPIUM BROMIDE, NONCOMPOUNDED, UNIT DOSE	1 MG	INH	J7644
IPTRATROPIUM BROMIDE COMPOUNDED, UNIT DOSE	1 MG	INH	J7645
IRESSA	250 MG	ORAL	J8565
IRINOTECAN	20 MG	IV	J9206
IRINOTECAN LIPOSOME	1 MG	IV	J9205
IRON DEXTRAN, 50 MG	50 MG	IM, IV	J1750
IRON SUCROSE	1 MG	IV	J1756
ISATUXIMAB-IRFC	10 MG	IV	J9227
ISAVUCONAZONIUM	1 MG	IV	J1833
ISOCAINE	10 ML	VAR	J0670
ISOETHARINE HCL COMPOUNDED, CONCENTRATED	1 MG	INH	J7647
ISOETHARINE HCL COMPOUNDED, UNIT DOSE	1 MG	INH	J7650
ISOETHARINE HCL, NONCOMPOUNDED CONCENTRATED	1 MG	INH	J7648
ISOETHARINE HCL, NONCOMPOUNDED, UNIT DOSE	1 MG	INH	J7649
ISOJEX	5 UCI	IV	A9532
ISOPROTERENOL HCL COMPOUNDED, CONCENTRATED	1 MG	INH	J7657
ISOPROTERENOL HCL COMPOUNDED, UNIT DOSE	1 MG	INH	J7660
ISOPROTERENOL HCL, NONCOMPOUNDED CONCENTRATED	1 MG	INH	J7658
ISOPROTERNOL HCL, NONCOMPOUNDED, UNIT DOSE	1MG	INH	J7659
ISOSULFAN BLUE	1 MG	SC	Q9968
ISTODAX	0.1 MG	IV	J9319
ISUPREL	1 MG	INH	J7658
ISUPREL	1 MG	INH	J7659
ITRACONAZOLE	50 MG	IV	J1835
IXABEPILONE	1 MG	IV	J9207
IXEMPRA	1 MG	IV	J9207
IXIFI	10 MG	IV	Q5109
IXINITY	1 IU	IV	J7213

Drug Name	Units Per	Route	Code
~~IZERVAY~~	~~0.1 MG~~	~~INJ~~	~~C9162~~
IZERVAY	0.1 MG	INJ	J2782
JELMYTO	1 MG	OTH	J9281
JEMPERLI	10 MG	IV	J9272
JESDUVROQ	1 MG	ORAL	J0889
JETREA	0.125 MG	OTH	J7316
JEVTANA	1 MG	IV	J9043
JIVI	1 IU	IV	J7208
JUBBONTI	1 MG	SC	Q5136
JYLAMVO	2.5 MG	ORAL	J8611
KADCYLA	1 MG	IV	J9354
KALBITOR	1 MG	SC	J1290
~~KANAMYCIN~~	~~500 MG~~	~~IM, IV~~	~~J1840~~
~~KANAMYCIN~~	~~75 MG~~	~~IM, IV~~	~~J1850~~
KANJINTI	10 MG	IV	Q5117
~~KANTREX~~	~~500 MG~~	~~IM, IV~~	~~J1840~~
~~KANTREX~~	~~75 MG~~	~~IM, IV~~	~~J1850~~
KANUMA	1 MG	IV	J2840
KCENTRA	1 IU	IV	J7168
KEFZOL	500 MG	IM, IV	J0690
KEPIVANCE	50 MCG	IV	J2425
KEPPRA	10 MG	IV	J1953
KERAMATRIX OR KERASORB	SQ CM	OTH	Q4165
KERECIS OMEGA3	SQ CM	OTH	Q4158
KERECIS OMEGA3 MARIGEN SHIELD	SQ CM	OTH	A2019
KEROXX	1 CC	OTH	Q4202
KESTRONE	1 MG	IV, IM	J1435
KETOROLAC TROMETHAMINE	15 MG	IM, IV	J1885
KEYTRUDA	1 MG	IV	J9271
KHAPZORY	0.5 MG	IV	J0642
KIMMTRAK	1 MCG	IV	J9274
KIMYRSA	10 MG	IV	J2406
KINEVAC	5 MCG	IV	J2805
KISUNLA	2 MG	IV	J0175
KOATE-DVI	1 IU	IV	J7190
KONAKION	1 MG	SC, IM, IV	J3430
KONYNE 80	1 IU	IV	J7194
KORSUVA	0.1 MCG	IV	J0879
KOVALTRY	1 IU	IV	J7211
KRYSTEXXA	1 MG	IV	J2507
KYBELLA	1 MG	SC	J0591
KYLEENA	19.5 MG	OTH	J7296
KYMRIAH	UP TO 600 MILLION CELLS	IV	Q2042
KYPROLIS	1 MG	IV	J9047
KYTRIL	1 MG	IV	S0091
KYTRIL	1 MG	ORAL	Q0166
KYTRIL	100 MCG	IV	J1626
L.A.E. 20	10 MG	IM	J1380
LABETALOL HCL	5 MG	IV	J1920
LABETALOL HCL (HIKEMA)	5 MG	IV	J1921
LACOSAMIDE	1 MG	IV	C9254
LAETRILE	VAR	INJ	J3570
LAMELLAS	SQ CM	OTH	Q4292
LAMELLAS XT	SQ CM	OTH	Q4291
LAMZEDE	1 MG	IV	J0217
LANADELUMAB-FLYO	1 MG	SC	J0593
LANOXIN	0.5 MG	IM, IV	J1160
LANREOTIDE	1 MG	SC	J1930
LANREOTIDE	1 MG	SC, INJ	J1932
LANTHANUM CARBONATE, FOR ESRD ON DIALYSIS	5 MG	ORAL	J0607
LANTHANUM CARBONATE, POWDER, FOR ESRD ON DIALYSIS, NOT THERAPEUTICALLY EQUIVALENT TO J0607	5 MG	ORAL	J0608
LANTUS	5 U	SC	J1815
LARONIDASE	0.1 MG	IV	J1931
LARTRUVO	10 MG	INF	J9285
LASIX	20 MG	IM, IV	J1940
LECANEMAB-IRMB	1 MG	IV	J0174
LEFAMULIN	1 MG	IV	J0691
LEMTRADA	1 MG	IV	J0202
LENACAPAVIR	1 MG	SC	J1961
LENTE ILETIN I	5 U	SC	J1815
LEPIRUDIN	50 MG	IV	J1945
LEQEMBI	1 MG	IV	J0174
LEQVIO	1 MG	SC	J1306
LEUCOVORIN CALCIUM	50 MG	IM, IV	J0640
LEUKERAN	2 MG	ORAL	S0172
LEUKINE	50 MCG	IV	J2820
LEUPROLIDE	1 MG	SC	J1952
LEUPROLIDE ACETATE	7.5 MG	SC	J9217
LEUPROLIDE ACETATE	1 MG	IM	J9218
LEUPROLIDE ACETATE (FOR DEPOT SUSPENSION)	3.75 MG	IM	J1950
LEUPROLIDE ACETATE DEPOT	7.5 MG	SC	J9217
LEUPROLIDE ACETATE FOR DEPOT SUSPENSION	0.25 MG	SC	J1951
LEUPROLIDE ACETATE FOR DEPOT SUSPENSION	7.5 MG	IM	J1954
LEUPROLIDE ACETATE IMPLANT	65 MG	OTH	J9219
LEUSTATIN	1 MG	IV	J9065
LEVABUTEROL COMPOUNDED, UNIT DOSE	1 MG	INH	J7615
LEVABUTEROL, COMPOUNDED, CONCENTRATED	0.5 MG	INH	J7607
LEVALBUTEROL NONCOMPOUNDED, CONCENTRATED FORM	0.5 MG	INH	J7612
LEVALBUTEROL, NONCOMPOUNDED, UNIT DOSE	0.5 MG	INH	J7614
LEVAMISOLE HCL	50 MG	ORAL	S0177
LEVAQUIN	250 MG	IV	J1956
LEVEMIR	5 U	SC	J1815
LEVETIRACETAM	10 MG	IV	J1953
LEVO-DROMORAN	UP TO 2 MG	IV, IM	J1960
LEVOCARNITINE	1 G	IV	J1955
LEVOFLOXACIN	250 MG	IV	J1956
LEVOLEUCOVORIN	0.5 MG	IV	J0642
LEVONORGESTREL IMPLANT	IMPLANT	OTH	J7306
LEVONORGESTREL-RELEASING INTRAUTERINE CONTRACEPTIVE (MIRENA)	52 MG	OTH	J7298
LEVONORGESTREL-RELEASING INTRAUTERINE CONTRACEPTIVE (LILETTA)	52 MG	OTH	J7297
LEVONORGESTREL-RELEASING INTRAUTERINE CONTRACEPTIVE SYSTEM (KYLEENA)	19.5 MG	OTH	J7296

Drug Name	Units Per	Route	Code
LEVONORGESTREL-RELEASING INTRAUTERINE CONTRACEPTIVE SYSTEM (SKYLA)	13.5 MG	OTH	J7301
LEVONORGESTREL-RELEASING INTRAUTERINE SYSTEM	EA	OTH	S4981
LEVORPHANOL TARTRATE	2 MG	SC, IV, IM	J1960
LEVOTHYROXINE SODIUM (FRESENIUS KABI) NOT THERAPEUTICALLY EQUIVALENT TO J0650	10 MCG	IV	J0651
LEVOTHYROXINE SODIUM (HIKMA) NOT THERAPEUTICALLY EQUIVALENT TO J0650	10 MCG	IV	J0652
LEVSIN	0.25 MG	SC, IM, IV	J1980
LEVULAN KERASTICK	354 MG	OTH	J7308
LEXISCAN	0.1 MG	IV	J2785
LIBRIUM	100 MG	IM, IV	J1990
LIBTAYO	1 MG	IV	J9119
LIDOCAINE 70 MG/TETRACAINE 70 MG	PATCH	OTH	C9285
~~LIDOCAINE HCL~~	~~10 MG~~	~~IV~~	~~J2001~~
LIDOCAINE HCL	1 MG	IM, IV	J2003
LIDOCAINE HCL IN 5% DEXTROSE	1 MG	IV	J2002
LIDOCAINE HCL WITH EPINEPHRINE	1 MG	INJ	J2004
LILETTA	52 MG	OTH	J7297
LINCOCIN HCL	300 MG	IV	J2010
LINCOMYCIN HCL	300 MG	IM, IV	J2010
LINEZOLID	200 MG	IV	J2020
LINEZOLID (HOSPIRA) NOT THERAPEUTICALLY EQUIVALENT TO J2020	200 MG	IV	J2021
LIORESAL	10 MG	IT	J0475
LIORESAL INTRATHECAL REFILL	50 MCG	IT	J0476
LIPODOX	10 MG	IV	Q2049
LIPOSOMAL, DAUNORUBICIN AND CYTARABINE	1 MG/2.27 MG	IV	J9153
LIQUAEMIN SODIUM	1,000 UNITS	SC, IV	J1644
LISOCABTAGENE MARALEUCEL	UP TO 110 MILLION CELLS	IV	Q2054
LISPRO-PFC	50 U	SC	J1817
LOCAMETZ	1 MCI	IV	A9800
LOK-PAK	10 UNITS	IV	J1642
LOMUSTINE	10 MG	ORAL	S0178
LONCASTUXIMAB TESIRINE-LPYL	1 MG	IV	J9359
LOQTORZI	1 MG	IV	J3263
LORAZEPAM	2 MG	IM, IV	J2060
LOVENOX	10 MG	SC	J1650
LOVOTIBEGLOGENE AUTOTEMCEL	PER TREATMENT	IV	J3394
LOW OSMOLAR CONTRAST MATERIAL, 100-199 MG/ML IODINE CONCENTRATIONS	1 ML	IV	Q9965
LOW OSMOLAR CONTRAST MATERIAL, 200-299 MG/ML IODINE CONCENTRATION	1 ML	IV	Q9966
LOW OSMOLAR CONTRAST MATERIAL, 300-399 MG/ML IODINE CONCENTRATION	1 ML	IV	Q9967
LOW OSMOLAR CONTRAST MATERIAL, 400 OR GREATER MG/ML IODINE CONCENTRATION	1 ML	IV	Q9951
LOXAPINE	1 MG	INH	J2062
LUCENTIS	0.1 MG	IV	J2778
LUMASIRAN	0.5 MG	SC	J0224
LUMASON	1 ML	IV	Q9950

Drug Name	Units Per	Route	Code
~~LUMISIGHT~~	~~1 MG~~	~~IV~~	~~C9171~~
LUMISIGHT	1 MG	IV	A9615
LUMIZYME	10 MG	IV	J0221
LUMOXITI	0.01 MG	IV	J9313
LUNSUMIO	1 MG	IV	J9350
LUPRON	1 MG	SC	J9218
LUPRON DEPOT	7.5 MG	SC	J9217
LUPRON DEPOT	3.75 MG	IM	J1950
LUPRON IMPLANT	65 MG	OTH	J9219
LURBINECTEDIN	0.1 MG	IV	J9223
LUSPATERCEPT-AAMT	0.25 MG	SC	J0896
LUTATHERA	1 MCI	IM	A9513
LUTETIUM LU 177 VIPIVOTIDE TETRAXETAN, THERAPEUTIC	1 MCI	IV	A9607
LUTETIUM LU 177, DOTATATE, THERAPEUTIC	1 MCI	IM	A9513
LUTREPULSE	100 MCG	SC, IV	J1620
LUXTURNA	1 BILLION VECTOR GENOMES	OTH	J3398
LYFGENIA	PER TREATMENT	IV	J3394
LYMPHAZURIN	1 MG	SC	Q9968
LYMPHOCYTE IMMUNE GLOBULIN, ANTITHYMOCYTE GLOBULIN, EQUINE	250 MG	OTH	J7504
LYMPHOCYTE IMMUNE GLOBULIN, ANTITHYMOCYTE GLOBULIN, RABBIT	25 MG	OTH	J7511
LYMPHOSEEK	0.5 MCI	SC, OTH	A9520
LYMUJEV	5 U	SC, IV	J1814
LYMUJEV	50 U	SC, IV	J1813
MACUGEN	0.3 MG	OTH	J2503
MAGNESIUM SULFATE	500 MG	IV	J3475
MAGNETIC RESONANCE CONTRAST AGENT	1 ML	ORAL	Q9954
MAGROTEC	STUDY DOSE UP TO 10 MCI	IV	A9540
MAGTRACE	STUDY DOSE	SC	A9697
MAKENA	10 MG	IM	J1726
MANNITOL	25% IN 50 ML	IV	J2150
MANNITOL	5 MG	INH	J7665
MANTLE DL MATRIX	SQ CM	OTH	Q4349
MARGENZA	5 MG	IV	J9353
MARGETUXIMAB-CMKB	5 MG	IV	J9353
MARINOL	2.5 MG	ORAL	Q0167
MARMINE	50 MG	IM, IV	J1240
~~MARQIBO KIT~~	~~5 MG~~	~~IV~~	~~J9371~~
MATRIDERM	SQ CM	OTH	A2027
MATRION	SQ CM	OTH	Q4201
MATRISTEM MICROMATRIX	1 MG	OTH	Q4118
MATRIX HD ALLOGRAFT DERMIS	SQ CM	OTH	Q4345
MATULANE	50 MG	ORAL	S0182
MAXIPIME	500 MG	IV	J0692
MDP-BRACCO	STUDY DOSE UP TO 30 MCI	IV	A9503
MECASERMIN	1 MG	SC	J2170
MECHLORETHAMINE HCL (NITROGEN MUSTARD)	10 MG	IV	J9230
MEDIDEX	1 MG	IM, IV, OTH	J1100
MEDISKIN	SQ CM	OTH	Q4135
MEDROL	4 MG	ORAL	J7509
MEDROXYPROGESTERONE ACETATE	1 MG	IM	J1050

Appendix 1 — Table of Drugs and Biologicals

Drug Name	Units Per	Route	Code
MEFOXIN	1 G	IV	J0694
MEGACE	20 MG	ORAL	S0179
MEGESTROL ACETATE	20 MG	ORAL	S0179
MELOXICAM	1 MG	IV	J1738
MELPHALAN	1 MG	IV	J9246
MELPHALAN	1 MG	IV	J9249
MELPHALAN	1 MG	IA	J9248
MELPHALAN	2 MG	ORAL	J8600
MELPHALAN FLUFENAMIDE	1 MG	IV	J9247
MEMBRANE GRAFT OR MEMBRANE WRAP	SQ CM	OTH	Q4205
MEMBRANE WRAP-HYDRO	SQ CM	OTH	Q4290
MEMODERM	SQ CM	OTH	Q4126
MENADIONE	1 MG	IM, SC, IV	J3430
MENOTROPINS	75 IU	SC, IM, IV	S0122
MEPERGAN	50 MG	IM, IV	J2180
MEPERIDINE AND PROMETHAZINE HCL	50 MG	IM, IV	J2180
MEPERIDINE HCL	100 MG	IM, IV, SC	J2175
MEPIVACAINE HCL	10 ML	VAR	J0670
MEPOLIZUMAB	1 MG	SQ	J2182
MEPSEVII	1 MG	IV	J3397
MERCAPTOPURINE	50 MG	ORAL	S0108
MERITATE	150 MG	IV	J3520
MEROPENEM	100 MG	IV	J2185
MEROPENEM (B. BRAUN) NOT THERAPEUTICALLY EQUIVALENT TO J2185	100 MG	IV	J2184
MEROPENEM (WG CRITICAL CARE)	100 MG	IV	J2183
MEROPENEM, VABORBACTAM	10 MG/10 MG	IV	J2186
MERREM	100 MG	IV	J2185
MESNA	200 MG	IV	J9209
MESNEX	200 MG	IV	J9209
METAPROTERENOL SULFATE COMPOUNDED, UNIT DOSE	10 MG	INH	J7670
METAPROTERENOL SULFATE, NONCOMPOUNDED, CONCENTRATED	10 MG	INH	J7668
METAPROTERENOL SULFATE, NONCOMPOUNDED, UNIT DOSE	10 MG	INH	J7669
METARAMINOL BITARTRATE	10 MG	IV, IM, SC	J0380
METASTRON STRONTIUM 89 CHLORIDE	1 MCI	IV	A9600
METATRACE	STUDY DOSE UP TO 45 MCI	IV	A9552
METHACHOLINE CHLORIDE	1 MG	INH	J7674
METHADONE	5 MG	ORAL	S0109
METHADONE HCL	10 MG	IM, SC	J1230
METHAPREL, COMPOUNDED, UNIT DOSE	10 MG	INH	J7670
METHAPREL, NONCOMPOUNDED, CONCENTRATED	10 MG	INH	J7668
METHAPREL, NONCOMPOUNDED, UNIT DOSE	10 MG	INH	J7669
METHERGINE	0.2 MG	IM, IV	J2210
METHOTREXATE	2.5 MG	ORAL	J8610
METHOTREXATE	2.5 MG	ORAL	J8612
METHOTREXATE	2.5 MG	ORAL	J8611
~~METHOTREXATE~~	~~5 MG~~	~~IV, IM, IT, IA~~	~~J9250~~
METHOTREXATE	50 MG	IV, IM, IT, IA	J9260

Drug Name	Units Per	Route	Code
METHOTREXATE (ACCORD), NOT THERAPEUTICALLY EQUIVALENT TO J9260	50 MG	INJ	J9255
METHOTREXATE LPF	50 MG	IV, IM, IT, IA	J9260
~~METHOTREXATE LPF~~	~~5 MG~~	~~IV, IM, IT, IA~~	~~J9250~~
METHYL AMINOLEVULINATE 16.8%	1 G	OTH	J7309
~~METHYLCOTOLONE~~	~~80 MG~~	~~IM~~	~~J1040~~
METHYLDOPA HCL	UP TO 250 MG	IV	J0210
METHYLDOPATE HCL	UP TO 250 MG	IV	J0210
METHYLENE BLUE	1 MG	SC	Q9968
METHYLERGONOVINE MALEATE	0.2 MG	IM, IV	J2210
METHYLNALTREXONE	0.1 MG	SC	J2212
METHYLPRED	4 MG	ORAL	J7509
METHYLPREDNISOLONE	4 MG	ORAL	J7509
~~METHYLPREDNISOLONE~~	~~UP TO 40 MG~~	~~IM, IV~~	~~J2920~~
~~METHYLPREDNISOLONE~~	~~125 MG~~	~~IM, IV~~	~~J2930~~
~~METHYLPREDNISOLONE ACETATE~~	~~20 MG~~	~~IM~~	~~J1020~~
METHYLPREDNISOLONE ACETATE	1 MG	IM	J1010
~~METHYLPREDNISOLONE ACETATE~~	~~80 MG~~	~~IM~~	~~J1040~~
~~METHYLPREDNISOLONE ACETATE~~	~~40 MG~~	~~IM~~	~~J1030~~
METHYLPREDNISOLONE SODIUM SUCCINATE	5 MG	IM, IV	J2919
METOCLOPRAMIDE	10 MG	IV	J2765
METRONIDAZOLE	10 MG	IV	J1836
METVIXIA 16.8%	1 G	OTH	J7309
MIACALCIN	400 U	SC, IM	J0630
MIBG	0.5 MCI	IV	A9508
MICAFUNGIN IN SODIUM (BAXTER)	1 MG	IV	J2246
MICAFUNGIN SODIUM	1 MG	IV	J2248
MICAFUNGIN SODIUM (PAR PHARM) NOT THERAPEUTICALLY EQUIVALENT TO J2248	1 MG	IV	J2247
MICRHOGAM	50 MCG	IV	J2788
MICROLYTE MATRIX	SQ CM	OTH	A2005
MICROMATRIX FLEX	1 MG	OTH	A2028
MICROPOROUS COLLAGEN IMPLANTABLE SLIT TUBE	1 CM LENGTH	OTH	C9353
MICROPOROUS COLLAGEN IMPLANTABLE TUBE	1 CM LENGTH	OTH	C9352
MIDAZOLAM (SEIZALAM)	1 MG	IM	J2253
MIDAZOLAM HCI	1 MG	IM, IV	J2250
MIDAZOLAM IN 0.8% SODIUM CHLORIDE, NOT THERAPEUTICALLY EQUIVALENT TO J2250	1 MG	IV	J2252
MIDAZOLAM IN 0.9% SODIUM CHLORIDE	1 MG	IV	J2251
MIFEPRISTONE	200 MG	ORAL	S0190
MIGLUSTAT	65 MG	ORAL	J1202
MILRINONE LACTATE	5 MG	IV	J2260
MINOCIN	1 MG	IV	J2265
MINOCYCLINE HCL	1 MG	IV	J2265
MINOXIDIL	10 MG	ORAL	S0139
MIRCERA	1 MCG	IV	J0887
MIRCERA	1 MCG	SC	J0888
MIRENA	52 MG	OTH	J7298
~~MIRIKIZUMAB-MRKZ~~	~~1 MG~~	~~IV, SC~~	~~C9168~~
MIRIKIZUMAB-MRKZ	1 MG	IV, SC	J2267
MIRO3D	CU CM	OTH	A2025
MIRODERM	SQ CM	OTH	Q4175
MIROTRACT WOUND MATRIX SHEET	1 CC	OTH	A2029
MIRRAGEN ADVANCED WOUND MATRIX	SQ CM	OTH	A2002

Drug Name	Units Per	Route	Code
MIRVETUXIMAB SORAVTANSINE-GYNX	1 MG	IV	J9063
MISOPROSTOL	200 MG	ORAL	S0191
MITHRACIN	2.5 MG	IV	J9270
MITOMYCIN	5 MG	IV	J9280
MITOMYCIN	0.2 MG	OTH	J7315
MITOMYCIN PYELOCALYCEAL INSTILLATION	1 MG	OTH	J9281
MITOSOL	0.2 MG	OTH	J7315
MITOXANA	1 G	IV	J9208
MITOXANTRONE HCL	5 MG	IV	J9293
MLG-COMPLETE	SQ CM	OTH	Q4256
MOGAMULIZUMAB-KPKC	1 MG	IV	J9204
MOMETASONE FUROATE SINUS IMPLANT	10 MCG	OTH	J7402
MONARC-M	1 IU	IV	J7190
MONJUVI	2 MG	IV	J9349
MONOCLATE-P	1 IU	IV	J7190
MONOFERRIC	10 MG	IV	J1437
MONONINE	1 IU	IV	J7193
MONOPUR	75 IU	SC, IM	S0122
MONOVISC	DOSE	INJ	J7327
MORPHINE SULFATE	10 MG	IM, IV, SC	J2270
MORPHINE SULFATE	500 MG	OTH	S0093
MORPHINE SULFATE (FRESENIUS KABI) NOT THERAPEUTICALLY EQUIVALENT TO J2270	10 MG	INJ, IV, SC	J2272
MORPHINE SULFATE, PRESERVATIVE-FREE FOR EPIDURAL OR INTRATHECAL USE	10 MG	OTH	J2274
MOST	SQ CM	OTH	Q4328
MOSUNETUZUMAB-AXGB	1 MG	IV	J9350
MOTIXAFORTIDE	0.25 MG	SC	J2277
MOXETUMOMAB PASUDOTOX-TDFK	0.01 MG	IV	J9313
MOXIFLOXACIN	100 MG	IV	J2280
MOXIFLOXACIN (FRESENIUS KABI) NOT THERAPEUTICALLY EQUIVALENT TO J2280	100 MG	IV	J2281
MOZOBIL	1 MG	SC	J2562
MPI INDIUM DTPA	0.5 MCI	INJ	A9548
MS CONTIN	500 MG	OTH	S0093
MUCOMYST	1 G	INH	J7608
MUCOSIL	1 G	INH	J7608
MUGARD	1 ML	OTH	A9156
MULTIHANCE	1 ML	IV	A9577
MULTIHANCE MULTIPACK	1 ML	IV	A9578
MUROMONAB-CD3	5 MG	OTH	J7505
MUSE	EA	OTH	J0275
MUSTARGEN	10 MG	IV	J9230
MUTAMYCIN	5 MG	IV	J9280
MVASI	10 MG	IV	Q5107
MYCAMINE	1 MG	IV	J2248
MYCOPHENOLATE	10 MG	IV	J7519
MYCOPHENOLATE MOFETIL	250 MG	ORAL	J7517
MYCOPHENOLATE MOFETIL	100 MG	ORAL	J7514
MYCOPHENOLIC ACID	180 MG	ORAL	J7518
MYFORTIC DELAYED RELEASE	180 MG	ORAL	J7518
MYHIBBIN	100 MG	ORAL	J7514
MYLERAN	2 MG	ORAL	J8510
MYLOCEL	500 MG	ORAL	S0176
MYLOTARG	0.1 MG	INF	J9203
MYOBLOC	100 U	IM	J0587
MYOCHRYSINE	50 MG	IM	J1600
MYOWN SKIN	SQ CM	OTH	Q4226
MYOZYME	10 MG	IV	J0220
NABILONE	1 MG	ORAL	J8650
NADOFARAGENE FIRADENOVEC-VNCG	THERAPEUTIC DOSE	OTH	J9029
NAFCILLIN SODIUM	2 GM	IM, IV	S0032
NAFCILLIN SODIUM	20 MG	IV	J2290
NAGLAZYME	1 MG	IV	J1458
NALBUPHINE HCL	10 MG	IM, IV, SC	J2300
NALLPEN	2 GM	IM, IV	S0032
NALOXONE HCL	1 MG	IM, IV, SC	J2310
NALOXONE HCL (ZIMHI)	1 MG	SC	J2311
NALTREXONE, DEPOT FORM	1 MG	IM	J2315
NANDROLONE DECANOATE	50 MG	IM	J2320
NARCAN	1 MG	IM, IV, SC	J2310
NAROPIN	1 MG	VAR	J2795
NASALCROM	10 MG	INH	J7631
NATALIZUMAB	1 MG	IV	J2323
NATALIZUMAB-SZTN	1 MG	IV	Q5134
NATRECOR	0.1 MG	IV	J2325
NATURAL ESTROGENIC SUBSTANCE	1 MG	IM, IV	J1410
NAVELBINE	10 MG	IV	J9390
NAXITAMAB-GQGK	1 MG	IV	J9348
ND-STAT	10 MG	IM, SC, IV	J0945
NEBCIN	80 MG	IM, IV	J3260
NEBUPENT	300 MG	IM, IV	S0080
NEBUPENT	300 MG	INH	J2545
NECITUMUMAB	1 MG	IV	J9295
NELARABINE	50 MG	IV	J9261
NEMBUTAL SODIUM	50 MG	IM, IV, OTH	J2515
NEOMATRIX	SQ CM	OTH	A2021
NEOPATCH	SQ CM	OTH	Q4176
NEORAL	25 MG	ORAL	J7515
NEORAL	250 MG	ORAL	J7516
~~NEOSAR~~	~~100 MG~~	~~IV~~	~~J9070~~
NEOSCAN	1 MCI	IV	A9556
NEOSTIGMINE METHYLSULFATE	0.5 MG	IM, IV	J2710
NEOSTIM DL	SQ CM	OTH	Q4267
NEOSTIM MEMBRANE	SQ CM	OTH	Q4266
NEOSTIM TL	SQ CM	OTH	Q4265
NEOTECT	STUDY DOSE UP TO 35 MCI	IV	A9536
NEOX 100	SQ CM	OTH	Q4156
NEOX CORD 1K	SQ CM	OTH	Q4148
NEOX CORD RT	SQ EM	OTH	Q4148
NEOXFLO	1 MG	OTH	Q4155
NESIRITIDE	0.1 MG	IV	J2325
NETSPOT	0.1 MCI	IV	A9587
NETUPITANT AND PALONOSETRON	300 MG/0.5 MG	ORAL	J8655
NEULASTA	0.5 MG	SC	J2506
NEUMEGA	5 MG	SC	J2355
NEUPOGEN	1 MCG	SC, IV	J1442
NEURAGEN NERVE GUIDE	1 CM LENGTH	OTH	C9352
NEUROLITE	STUDY DOSE UP TO 25 MCI	IV	A9557
NEUROMATRIX	0.5 CM LENGTH	OTH	C9355
NEUROMEND NERVE WRAP	0.5 CM	OTH	C9361
NEUROWRAP NERVE PROTECTOR	1 CM LENGTH	OTH	C9353

Appendix 1 — Table of Drugs and Biologicals

Drug Name	Units Per	Route	Code
NEUTREXIN	25 MG	IV	J3305
NEUTROSPEC	STUDY DOSE UP TO 25 MCI	IV	A9566
NEXOBRID	1 G	OTH	J7353
NEXPLANON	IMPLANT	OTH	J7307
NEXTERONE	30 MG	IV	J0283
NEXVIAZYME	4 MG	IV	J0219
NICARDIPINE	0.1 MG	IV	J2404
NIPENT	10 MG	IV	J9268
NITHIODOTE	3 MG/125 MG	IV	J0211
NITROGEN MUSTARD	10 MG	IV	J9230
NITROGEN N-13 AMMONIA, DIAGNOSTIC	STUDY DOSE UP TO 40 MCI	INJ	A9526
NITROGLYCERIN	5 MG	IV	J2305
NIVESTYM	1 MCG	INJ	Q5110
NIVOLUMAB	1 MG	IV	J9299
NIVOLUMAB AND RELATLIMAB-RMBW	3 MG/1 MG	IV	J9298
~~NOGAPENDEKIN ALFA INBAKICEPT-PMLN~~	~~1 MCG~~	~~IVES~~	~~C9169~~
NOGAPENDEKIN ALFA INBAKICEPT-PMLN	1 MCG	OTH	J9028
NOLVADEX	10 MG	ORAL	S0187
NORDITROPIN	1 MG	SC	J2941
NORDYL	50 MG	IV, IM	J1200
NORFLEX	60 MG	IV, IM	J2360
NORMAL SALINE SOLUTION	1000 CC	IV	J7030
NORMAL SALINE SOLUTION	250 CC	IV	J7050
NORMAL SALINE SOLUTION	500 ML	IV	J7040
NOVACHOR	SQ CM	OTH	Q4194
NOVAFIX	SQ CM	OTH	Q4208
NOVAFIX DL	SQ CM	OTH	Q4254
NOVANTRONE	5 MG	IV	J9293
NOVAREL	1,000 USP U	IM	J0725
NOVOEIGHT	IU	IV	J7182
NOVOLIN	50 U	SC	J1817
NOVOLIN R	5 U	SC	J1815
NOVOLOG	50 U	SC	J1817
NOVOSEVEN	1 MCG	IV	J7189
NOVOSORB SYNPATH DERMAL MATRIX	SQ CM	OTH	A2006
NPH	5 UNITS	SC	J1815
~~NPLATE~~	~~10 MCG~~	~~SC~~	~~J2796~~
NPLATE	1 MCG	SC	J2802
NUBAIN	10 MG	IM, IV, SC	J2300
NUCALA	1 MG	SQ	J2182
NUDYN	0.5 CC	OTH	Q4233
NUDYN DL, DL MESH	SQ CM	OTH	Q4285
NUDYN SL, SLW	SQ CM	OTH	Q4286
NULOJIX	1 MG	IV	J0485
NUMBRINO	1 MG	OTH	C9143
NUMORPHAN	1 MG	IV, SC, IM	J2410
NUSHIELD	SQ CM	OTH	Q4160
NUSINERSEN	0.1 MG	INJ	J2326
NUTRI-TWELVE	1,000 MCG	IM, SC	J3420
NUTROPIN	1 MG	SC	J2941
NUTROPIN A.Q.	1 MG	SC	J2941
NUVARING VAGINAL RING	0.015 MG/0.12 MG	OTH	J7295
NUWIQ	1 IU	IV	J7209
NUZYRA	1 MG	IV	J0121
NYPOZI	1 MCG	IV, SC	C9173
NYVEPRIA	0.5 MG	SC	Q5122
OASIS BURN MATRIX	SQ CM	OTH	Q4103
OASIS ULTRA TRI-LAYER WOUND MATRIX	SQ CM	OTH	Q4124
OASIS WOUND MATRIX	SQ CM	OTH	Q4102
OBINUTUZUMAB	10 MG	IV	J9301
OBIZUR	IU	IV	J7188
OCRELIZUMAB	1 MG	INJ	J2350
OCREVUS	1 MG	INJ	J2350
OCRIPLASMIN	0.125 MG	OTH	J7316
OCTAFLUOROPROPANE UCISPHERES	1 ML	IV	Q9956
OCTAGAM	500 MG	IV	J1568
OCTREOSCAN	STUDY DOSE UP TO 6 MCI	IV	A9572
OCTREOTIDE ACETATE DEPOT	1 MG	IM	J2353
OCTREOTIDE, NON-DEPOT FORM	25 MCG	SC, IV	J2354
OFATUMUMAB	10 MG	IV	J9302
OFLOXACIN	400 MG	IV	S0034
OFORTA	10 MG	ORAL	J8562
OGIVRI	10 MG	IV	Q5114
OHTUVAYRE	3 MG	INH	J7601
OLANZAPINE	0.5 MG	IM	J2359
OLANZAPINE LONG ACTING	1 MG	IM	J2358
OLARATUMAB	10 MG	INF	J9285
OLICERIDINE	0.1 MG	IV	C9101
OLINVYK	0.1 MG	IV	C9101
OLIPUDASE ALFA-RPCP	1 MG	IV	J0218
OMACETAXINE MEPESUCCINATE	0.01 MG	SC	J9262
OMADACYCLINE	1 MG	IV	J0121
OMALIZUMAB	5 MG	SC	J2357
OMEGAVEN	10 G	IV	B4187
OMEZA COLLAGEN MATRIX	100 MG	OTH	A2014
OMIDRIA	1 ML	OTH	J1097
OMNIPAQUE 140	1 ML	IV	Q9965
OMNIPAQUE 180	1 ML	IV	Q9965
OMNIPAQUE 240	1 ML	IV	Q9966
OMNIPAQUE 300	1 ML	IV	Q9967
OMNIPAQUE 350	1 ML	IV	Q9967
OMONTYS (FOR ESRD ON DIALYSIS)	0.1 MG	SC, IV	J0890
~~OMVOH~~	~~1 MG~~	~~IV, SC~~	~~C9168~~
OMVOH	1 MG	IV, SC	J2267
ONABOTULINUMTOXINA	1 UNIT	IM, OTH	J0585
ONASEMNOGENE ABEPARVOVEC-XIOI	UP TO $5X10^{15}$ VECTOR GENOMES	IV	J3399
ONCASPAR	VIAL	IM, IV	J9266
ONCOSCINT CR/OV	STUDY DOSE UP TO 6 MCI	IV	A4642
ONDANSETRON	1 MG	ORAL	Q0162
ONDANSETRON	4 MG	ORAL	S0119
ONDANSETRON HYDROCHLORIDE	1 MG	IV	J2405
ONIVYDE	1 MG	IV	J9205
ONPATTRO	0.1 MG	IV	J0222
ONTRUZANT	10 MG	IV	Q5112
OPDIVO	1 MG	IV	J9299
OPDUALAG	3 MG/1 MG	IV	J9298
OPFOLDA	65 MG	ORAL	J1202
OPRELVEKIN	5 MG	SC	J2355

Drug Name	Units Per	Route	Code
OPTIRAY	1 ML	IV	Q9967
OPTIRAY 160	1 ML	IV	Q9965
OPTIRAY 240	1 ML	IV	Q9966
OPTIRAY 300	1 ML	IV	Q9967
OPTIRAY 320	1 ML	IV	Q9967
OPTISON	1 ML	IV	Q9956
ORAL MAGNETIC RESONANCE CONTRAST AGENT, PER 100 ML	100 ML	ORAL	Q9954
ORAL MUCOADHESIVE, ANY TYPE	1 ML	OTH	A9156
ORBACTIV	10 MG	IV	J2407
ORENCIA	10 MG	IV	J0129
ORION	SQ CM	OTH	Q4276
ORITAVANCIN	10 MG	IV	J2407
ORITAVANCIN	10 MG	IV	J2406
ORPHENADRINE CITRATE	60 MG	IV, IM	J2360
ORTHADAPT BIOIMPLANT	SQ CM	OTH	C1781
ORTHOCLONE OKT3	5 MG	OTH	J7505
ORTHOVISC	DOSE	INJ	J7324
OSELTAMIVIR PHOSPHATE (BRAND NAME) (DEMONSTRATION PROJECT)	75 MG	ORAL	G9035
OSELTAMIVIR PHOSPHATE (GENERIC) (DEMONSTRATION PROJECT)	75 MG	ORAL	G9019
OSMITROL	25% IN 50 ML	IV	J2150
OTIPRIO	6 MG	OTIC	J7342
OVERLAY SL MATRIX	SQ CM	OTH	Q4352
OXACILLIN SODIUM	250 MG	IM, IV	J2700
OXALIPLATIN	0.5 MG	IV	J9263
OXILAN 300	1 ML	IV	Q9967
OXILAN 350	1 ML	IV	Q9967
OXLUMO	0.5 MG	SC	J0224
OXYMORPHONE HCL	1 MG	IV, SC, IM	J2410
OXYTETRACYCLINE HCL	50 MG	IM	J2460
OXYTOCIN	10 U	IV, IM	J2590
OZURDEX	0.1 MG	OTH	J7312
PACIS BCG	1 MG	OTH	J9030
PACLITAXEL	1 MG	IV	J9267
PACLITAXEL PROTEIN-BOUND PARTICLES	1 MG	IV	J9264
~~PACLITAXEL PROTEIN-BOUND PARTICLES (AMERICAN REGENT)~~	~~1 MG~~	~~IV~~	~~J9259~~
~~PACLITAXEL PROTEIN-BOUND PARTICLES (TEVA), NOT THERAPEUTICALLY EQUIVALENT TO J9264~~	~~1 MG~~	~~IV~~	~~J9258~~
PADCEV	0.25 MG	IV	J9177
PAFOLACIANINE	0.1 MG	IV	A9603
PALIFERMIN	50 MCG	IV	J2425
PALINGEN OR PALINGEN XPLU	SQ CM	OTH	Q4173
PALINGEN OR PROMATRX	0.36 MG/0.25 CC	OTH	Q4174
PALIPERIDONE PALMITATE EXTENDED RELEASE	1 MG	IM	J2427
PALIPERIDONE PALMITATE EXTENDED RELEASE (INVEGA SUSTENNA)	1 MG	IM	J2426
PALISADE DM MATRIX	SQ CM	OTH	Q4350
PALONOSETRON HCL	25 MCG	IV	J2469
PALONOSETRON HCL	25 MCG	IV	J2468
PAMIDRONATE DISODIUM	30 MG	IV	J2430
PANHEMATIN	1 MG	IV	J1640
PANITUMUMAB	10 MG	IV	J9303
PANTOPRAZOLE (HIKMA)	40 MG	IV	J2471
~~PANTOPRAZOLE SODIUM~~	~~40 MG~~	~~IV~~	~~S0164~~
PANTOPRAZOLE SODIUM	40 MG	IV	J2470
~~PANTOPRAZOLE SODIUM~~	~~VIAL~~	~~IV~~	~~C9113~~
PANTOPRAZOLE SODIUM (BAXTER)	40 MG	IV	J2472
PANZYGA	500 MG	IV	J1576
PAPAVERINE HCL	60 MG	IV, IM	J2440
PARAGARD T380A	EA	OTH	J7300
PARAPLANTIN	50 MG	IV	J9045
PARICALCITOL	1 MCG	IV, IM	J2501
PARSABIV	0.1 MG	IV	J0606
PASIREOTIDE LONG ACTING	1 MG	IV	J2502
PATISIRAN	0.1 MG	IV	J0222
PEDIAPRED	5 MG	ORAL	J7510
PEDMARK	100 MG	IV	J0208
PEG-INTRON	180 MCG	SC	S0145
PEGADEMASE BOVINE	25 IU	IM	J2504
PEGAPTANIB SODIUM	0.3 MG	OTH	J2503
PEGASPARGASE	VIAL	IM, IV	J9266
PEGCETACOPLAN	1 MG	INJ	J2781
PEGFILGRASTIM, EXCLUDES BIOSIMILAR	0.5 MG	SC	J2506
PEGFILGRASTIM-APGF, BIOSIMILAR	0.5 MG	SC	Q5122
PEGFILGRASTIM-BMEZ, BIOSIMILAR	0.5 MG	SC	Q5120
PEGFILGRASTIM-CBQV, BIOSIMILAR	0.5 MG	SC	Q5111
PEGFILGRASTIM-FPGK, BIOSIMILAR	0.5 MG	SC	Q5127
PEGFILGRASTIM-JMDB, BIOSIMILAR	0.5 MG	SC	Q5108
PEGFILGRASTIM-PBBK	0.5 MG	SC	Q5130
PEGINESATIDE (FOR ESRD ON DIALYSIS)	0.1 MG	SC, IV	J0890
PEGINTERFERON ALFA-2A	180 MCG	SC	S0145
PEGLOTICASE	1 MG	IV	J2507
~~PEGULICIANINE~~	~~1 MG~~	~~IV~~	~~C9171~~
PEGULICIANINE	1 MG	IV	A9615
PEGUNIGALSIDASE ALFA-IWXJ	1 MG	IV	J2508
PEGYLATED INTERFERON ALFA-2A	180 MCG	SC	S0145
PEGYLATED INTERFERON ALFA-2B	10 MCG	SC	S0148
PELLOGRAFT	SQ CM	OTH	Q4320
PEMBROLIZUMAB	1 MG	IV	J9271
PEMETREXED	10 MG	IV	J9304
PEMETREXED	10 MG	IV	J9324
PEMETREXED (ACCORD), NOT THERAPEUTICALLY EQUIVALENT TO J9305	10 MG	IV	J9296
PEMETREXED (AVYXA), NOT THERAPEUTICALLY EQUIVALENT TO J9305	10 MG	IV	J9292
PEMETREXED (BLUEPOINT), NOT THERAPEUTICALLY EQUIVALENT TO J9305	10 MG	IV	J9322
PEMETREXED (HOSPIRA), NOT THERAPEUTICALLY EQUIVALENT TO J9305	10 MG	IV	J9294
PEMETREXED (SANDOZ), NOT THERAPEUTICALLY EQUIVALENT TO J9305	10 MG	IV	J9297
PEMETREXED (TEVA), NOT THERAPEUTICALLY EQUIVALENT TO J9305	10 MG	IV	J9314
PEMETREXED DITROMETHAMINE	10 MG	IV	J9323
PEMFEXY	10 MG	IV	J9304
PEMGARDA	4500 MG	IV	Q0224

Appendix 1 — Table of Drugs and Biologicals

Drug Name	Units Per	Route	Code
PEMIVIBART, PRE-EXPOSURE PROPHYLAXIS	4500 MG	IV	Q0224
PEMRYDI RTU	10 MG	IV	J9324
PENICILLIN G BENZATHINE	100,000 U	IM	J0561
PENICILLIN G BENZATHINE AND PENICILLIN G PROCAINE	100,000 UNITS	IM	J0558
PENICILLIN G POTASSIUM	600,000 U	IM, IV	J2540
PENICILLIN G PROCAINE	600,000 U	IM, IV	J2510
PENTACARINAT	300 MG	INH	S0080
PENTAM	300 MG	IM, IV	J2545
PENTAM 300	300 MG	IM, IV	S0080
PENTAMIDINE ISETHIONATE	300 MG	IM, IV	S0080
PENTAMIDINE ISETHIONATE COMPOUNDED	300 MG	INH	J7676
PENTAMIDINE ISETHIONATE NONCOMPOUNDED	300 MG	INH	J2545
PENTASPAN	100 ML	IV	J2513
PENTASTARCH 10% SOLUTION	100 ML	IV	J2513
PENTATE CALCIUM TRISODIUM	STUDY DOSE UP TO 75 MCI	INH	A9567
PENTATE CALCIUM TRISODIUM	STUDY DOSE UP TO 25 MCI	IV	A9539
PENTATE ZINC TRISODIUM	STUDY DOSE UP TO 25 MCI	IV	A9539
PENTATE ZINC TRISODIUM	STUDY DOSE UP TO 75 MCI	INH	A9567
PENTAZOCINE	30 MG	IM, SC, IV	J3070
PENTOBARBITAL SODIUM	50 MG	IM, IV, OTH	J2515
PENTOSTATIN	10 MG	IV	J9268
PEPAXTO	1 MG	IV	J9247
PEPCID	20 MG	IV	S0028
PERAMIVIR	1 MG	IV	J2547
PERFLEXANE LIPID MICROSPHERE	1 ML	IV	Q9955
PERFLUTREN LIPID MICROSPHERE	1 ML	IV	Q9957
PERFOROMIST	20 MCG	INH	J7606
PERJETA	1 MG	IV	J9306
PERMACOL	SQ CM	OTH	C9364
PERMEADERM B	SQ CM	OTH	A2016
PERMEADERM C	SQ CM	OTH	A2018
PERMEADERM GLOVE	EA	OTH	A2017
PERPHENAZINE	5 MG	IM, IV	J3310
PERPHENAZINE	4 MG	ORAL	Q0175
PERSANTINE	10 MG	IV	J1245
PERSERIS	0.5 MG	SC	J2798
PERTUZUMAB	1 MG	IV	J9306
PERTUZUMAB, TRASTUZUMAB, AND HYALURONIDASE-ZZXF	10 MG	SC	J9316
PFIZERPEN A.S.	600,000 U	IM, IV	J2510
PHENERGAN	50 MG	IM, IV	J2550
PHENERGAN	12.5 MG	ORAL	Q0169
PHENOBARBITAL SODIUM	120 MG	IM, IV	J2560
PHENOBARBITAL SODIUM	1 MG	IV	J2561
PHENTOLAMINE MESYLATE	5 MG	IM, IV	J2760
PHENYLEPHRINE 10.16 MG/ML AND KETOROLAC 2.88 MG/ML OPHTHALMIC IRRIGATION SOLUTION	1 ML	OTH	J1097
PHENYLEPHRINE HCL	20 MCG	IV	J2371
PHENYLEPHRINE HCL (BIORPHEN)	20 MCG	IV	J2372
PHENYLEPHRINE HYDROCHLORIDE	20 MCG	IV	J2373
PHENYTOIN SODIUM	50 MG	IM, IV	J1165
PHESGO	10 MG	SC	J9316
PHOENIX WOUND MATRIX	SQ CM	OTH	A2015
PHOSLO, FOR ESRD ON DIALYSIS	23 MG	ORAL	J0615
PHOSPHOCOL	1 MCI	IV	A9563
PHOSPHOTEC	STUDY DOSE UP TO 25 MCI	IV	A9538
PHOTOFRIN	75 MG	IV	J9600
PHOTREXA VISCOUS	UP TO 3 ML	OTH	J2787
PHYTONADIONE	1 MG	IM, SC, IV	J3430
PIASKY	10 MG	IV, SC	J1307
PIFLUFOLASTAT F-18, DIAGNOSTIC	1 MCI	IV	A9595
PIPERACILLIN SODIUM	500 MG	IM, IV	S0081
PIPERACILLIN SODIUM/ TAZOBACTAM SODIUM	1 G/1.125 GM	IV	J2543
PITOCIN	10 U	IV, IM	J2590
PLASMINOGEN, HUMAN-TVMH	1 MG	IV	J2998
PLATINOL AQ	10 MG	IV	J9060
PLAZOMICIN	5 MG	IV	J0291
PLERIXAFOR	1 MG	SC	J2562
PLICAMYCIN	2.5 MG	IV	J9270
PLUVICTO	1 MCI	IV	A9607
PNEUMOCOCCAL CONJUGATE	EA	IM	S0195
PNEUMOVAX II	EA	IM	S0195
POLATUZUMAB VEDOTIN-PIIQ	1 MG	IV	J9309
POLIVY	1 MG	IV	J9309
POLOCAINE	10 ML	VAR	J0670
POLYCYTE	0.5 CC	OTH	Q4241
POMBILITI	5 MG	IV	J1203
PORCINE IMPLANT, PERMACOL	SQ CM	OTH	C9364
PORFIMER SODIUM	75 MG	IV	J9600
PORK INSULIN	5 U	SC	J1815
POROUS PURIFIED COLLAGEN MATRIX BONE VOID FILLER	0.5 CC	OTH	C9362
POROUS PURIFIED COLLAGEN MATRIX BONE VOID FILLER, PUTTY	0.5 CC	OTH	C9359
PORTRAZZA	1 MG	IV	J9295
POSFREA	25 MCG	IV	J2468
POSIMIR	1 MG	INJ	C9144
POSLUMA	1 MCI	IV	A9608
POTASSIUM CHLORIDE	2 MEQ	IV	J3480
POTELIGEO	1 MG	IV	J9204
POZELIMAB-BBFG	1 MG	IV, SC	J9376
PRALATREXATE	1 MG	IV	J9307
PRALIDOXIME CHLORIDE	1 MG	IV, IM, SC	J2730
PREDNISOLONE	5 MG	ORAL	J7510
PREDNISOLONE ACETATE	1 ML	IM	J2650
PREDNISONE, IMMEDIATE RELEASE OR DELAYED RELEASE	1 MG	ORAL	J7512
PREDNORAL	5 MG	ORAL	J7510
PREGNYL	1,000 USP U	IM	J0725
PRELONE	5 MG	ORAL	J7510
PREMARIN	25 MG	IV, IM	J1410
PRENATAL VITAMINS	30 TABS	ORAL	S0197
~~PRI-METHYLATE~~	~~80 MG~~	~~IM~~	~~J1040~~
PRIALT	1 MCG	OTH	J2278
PRIMACOR	5 MG	IV	J2260
PRIMATRIX	SQ CM	OTH	Q4110
PRIMAXIN	250 MG	IV, IM	J0743
PRIMESTRIN AQUEOUS	1 MG	IM, IV	J1410
PRIMETHASONE	1 MG	IM, IV, OTH	J1100
PRIVIGEN	500 MG	IV	J1459

Drug Name	Units Per	Route	Code
~~PROBUPHINE IMPLANT~~	~~74.2 MG~~	~~OTH~~	~~J0570~~
PROCAINAMIDE HCL	1 G	IM, IV	J2690
PROCARBAZINE HCL	50 MG	ORAL	S0182
~~PROCENTA~~	~~200 MG~~	~~OTH~~	~~Q4244~~
PROCENTA	100 MG	OTH	Q4310
PROCHLOPERAZINE MALEATE	5 MG	ORAL	S0183
PROCHLORPERAZINE	10 MG	IM, IV	J0780
PROCHLORPERAZINE MALEATE	5 MG	ORAL	Q0164
PROCRIT, NON-ESRD USE	1,000 U	SC, IV	J0885
PROFILNINE HEAT-TREATED	1 IU	IV	J7194
PROFILNINE SD	1 IU	IV	J7194
~~PROFONIX~~	~~VIAL~~	~~INJ~~	~~C9113~~
PROGENAMATRIX	SQ CM	OTH	Q4222
PROGESTASERT IUD	EA	OTH	S4989
PROGESTERONE	50 MG	IM	J2675
PROGRAF	5 MG	OTH	J7525
PROGRAF	1 MG	ORAL	J7507
PROLEUKIN	1 VIAL	VAR	J9015
PROLIA	1 MG	SC	J0897
PROLIXIN DECANOATE	25 MG	SC, IM	J2680
PROMAZINE HCL	25 MG	IM	J2950
PROMETHAZINE HCL	12.5 MG	ORAL	Q0169
PROMETHAZINE HCL	50 MG	IM, IV	J2550
PRONESTYL	1 G	IM, IV	J2690
PROPECIA	5 MG	ORAL	S0138
PROPLEX SX-T	1 IU	IV	J7194
PROPLEX T	1 IU	IV	J7194
PROPOFOL	10 MG	IV	J2704
PROPRANOLOL HCL	1 MG	IV	J1800
PROREX	50 MG	IM, IV	J2550
PROSCAR	5 MG	ORAL	S0138
PROSTASCINT	STUDY DOSE UP TO 10 MCI	IV	A9507
PROSTIGMIN	0.5 MG	IM, IV	J2710
PROSTIN VR	1.25 MCG	INJ	J0270
PROTAMINE SULFATE	10 MG	IV	J2720
PROTEIN C CONCENTRATE	10 IU	IV	J2724
PROTEXT	1 CC	OTH	Q4246
PROTHROMBIN COMPLEX CONCENTRATE (HUMAN)	1 IU	IV	J7168
~~PROTHROMBIN COMPLEX CONCENTRATE (HUMAN)~~	~~IU~~	~~IV~~	~~C9159~~
PROTHROMBIN COMPLEX CONCENTRATE, HUMAN-LANS	IU	IV	J7165
PROTIRELIN	250 MCG	IV	J2725
~~PROTONIX IV~~	~~40 MG~~	~~IV~~	~~S0164~~
~~PROTONIX IV~~	~~VIAL~~	~~IV~~	~~C9113~~
PROTOPAM CHLORIDE	1 G	SC, IM, IV	J2730
PROTROPIN	1 MG	SC, IM	J2940
PROVENGE	INFUSION	IV	Q2043
PROVENTIL NONCOMPOUNDED, CONCENTRATED	1 MG	INH	J7611
PROVENTIL NONCOMPOUNDED, UNIT DOSE	1 MG	INH	J7613
PROVOCHOLINE POWDER	1 MG	INH	J7674
PROZINE-50	25 MG	IM	J2950
PULMICORT	0.25 MG	INH	J7633
PULMICORT RESPULES	0.5 MG	INH	J7627
PULMICORT RESPULES NONCOMPOUNDED, CONCETRATED	0.25 MG	INH	J7626
PULMOZYME	1 MG	INH	J7639

Drug Name	Units Per	Route	Code
PURAPLY	SQ CM	OTH	Q4195
PURAPLY AM	SQ CM	OTH	Q4196
PURAPLY XT	SQ CM	OTH	Q4197
PURINETHOL	50 MG	ORAL	S0108
PYLARIFY	1 MCI	IV	A9595
PYRIDOXINE HCL	100 MG	IM, IV	J3415
PYZCHIVA	1 MG	IV	Q9997
PYZCHIVA	1 MG	SC	Q9996
QALSODY	1 MG	INJ	J1304
QUADRAMET	DOSE UP TO 150 MCI	IV	A9604
QUELICIN	20 MG	IM, IV	J0330
QUINUPRISTIN/DALFOPRISTIN	500 MG	IV	J2770
QUTENZA	1 SQ CM	OTH	J7336
QUZYTIIR	0.5 MG	IV	J1201
RADICAVA	1 MG	IV	J1301
RADIESSE	0.1 ML	OTH	Q2026
RADIOELEMENTS FOR BRACHYTHERAPY, ANY TYPE	EA	OTH	Q3001
RADIUM (RA) 223 DICHLORIDE THERAPEUTIC	MICROCURIE	IV	A9606
RAMPART DL MATRIX	SQ CM	OTH	Q4347
RAMUCIRUMAB	5 MG	IV	J9308
RANIBIZUMAB	0.1 MG	OTH	J2778
RANIBIZUMAB	0.1 MG	OTH	J2779
RANIBIZUMAB-EQRN	0.1 MG	INJ	Q5128
RANIBIZUMAB-NUNA	0.1 MG	INJ	Q5124
~~RANITIDINE HCL~~	~~25 MG~~	~~INJ~~	~~J2780~~
RAPAMUNE	1 MG	ORAL	J7520
RAPIVAB	1 MG	IV	J2547
RASBURICASE	0.5 MG	IM	J2783
RAVULIZUMAB-CWVZ	10 MG	IV	J1303
REBETRON KIT	1,000,000 U	SC, IM	J9214
REBIF	30 MCG	SC	J1826
REBIF	1 MCG	SC	Q3028
REBINYN	1 IU	IV	J7203
REBLOZYL	0.25 MG	SC	J0896
REBOUND MATRIX	SQ CM	OTH	Q4296
REBYOTA	1 ML	OTH	J1440
RECARBRIO	4 MG/4 MG/2 MG	IV	J0742
RECLAST	1 MG	IV	J3489
REDISOL	1,000 MCG	SC, IM	J3420
REEVA FT	SQ CM	OTH	Q4314
REFLUDAN	50 MG	IM, IV	J1945
REGADENOSON	0.1 MG	IV	J2785
REGEN-COV	1200 MG	IV	Q0244
REGENELINK AMNIOTIC MEMBRANE ALLOGRAFT	SQ CM	OTH	Q4315
REGITINE	5 MG	IM, IV	J2760
REGLAN	10 MG	IV	J2765
REGRANEX GEL	0.5 G	OTH	S0157
REGUARD	SQ CM	OTH	Q4255
REGULAR INSULIN	5 UNITS	SC	J1815
RELAXIN	10 ML	IV, IM	J2800
RELENZA (DEMONSTRATION PROJECT)	10 MG	INH	G9034
RELESE	SQ CM	OTH	Q4257
RELEUKO	1 MCG	SC, IV	Q5125
RELION	5 U	SC	J1815
RELION NOVOLIN	50 U	SC	J1817

Drug Name	Units Per	Route	Code
RELISTOR	0.1 MG	SC	J2212
REMDESIVIR	1 MG	IV	J0248
REMICADE	10 MG	IV	J1745
REMIMAZOLAM	1 MG	IV	J2249
REMODULIN	1 MG	SC	J3285
RENAGEL OR THERAPEUTICALLY EQUIVALENT, FOR ESRD ON DIALYSIS	20 MG	ORAL	J0603
RENFLEXIS	10 MG	IV	Q5104
RENOGRAFT	SQ CM	OTH	Q4321
RENVELA OR THERAPEUTICALLY EQUIVALENT, FOR ESRD ON DIALYSIS	20 MG	ORAL	J0601
RENVELA OR THERAPEUTICALLY EQUIVALENT, POWDER, FOR ESRD ON DIALYSIS	20 MG	ORAL	J0602
REODULIN	1 MG	SC	J3285
REOPRO	10 MG	IV	J0130
REPRIZA	SQ CM	OTH	Q4143
REPRONEX	75 IU	SC, IM, IV	S0122
RESLIZUMAB	1 MG	IV	J2786
RESOLVE MATRIX	SQ CM	OTH	A2024
RESPIROL NONCOMPOUNDED, CONCENTRATED	1 MG	INH	J7611
RESPIROL NONCOMPOUNDED, UNIT DOSE	1 MG	INH	J7613
RESTORIGIN	1 CC	INJ	Q4192
RESTORIGIN	SQ CM	OTH	Q4191
RESTRATA	SQ CM	OTH	A2007
RESTRATA MINIMATRIX	5 MG	OTH	A2026
RETACRIT	100 UNITS	INJ, IV	Q5105
RETACRIT	1000 UNITS	INJ, IV	Q5106
RETAVASE	18.1 MG	IV	J2993
RETEPLASE	18.1 MG	IV	J2993
RETIFANLIMAB-DLWR	1 MG	IV	J9345
RETISERT	IMPLANT	OTH	J7311
RETROVIR	10 MG	IV	J3485
RETROVIR	100 MG	ORAL	S0104
REVEFENACIN INHALATION	1 MCG	INH	J7677
REVITA	SQ CM	OTH	Q4180
REVITALON	SQ CM	OTH	Q4157
REVOSHIELD+ AMNIOTIC BARRIER	SQ CM	OTH	Q4289
REZAFUNGIN	0.1 MG	IV	J0349
REZZAYO	0.1 MG	IV	J0349
RHEOMACRODEX	500 ML	IV	J7100
RHEUMATREX	2.5 MG	ORAL	J8610
RHEUMATREX DOSE PACK	2.5 MG	ORAL	J8610
RHO D IMMUNE GLOBULIN	300 MCG	IV	J2790
RHO D IMMUNE GLOBULIN (RHOPHYLAC)	100 IU	IM, IV	J2791
RHO D IMMUNE GLOBULIN MINIDOSE	50 MCG	IM	J2788
RHO D IMMUNE GLOBULIN SOLVENT DETERGENT	100 IU	IV	J2792
RHOGAM	50 MCG	IM	J2788
RHOGAM	300 MCG	IM	J2790
RHOPHYLAC	100 IU	IM, IV	J2791
RIABNI	10 MG	IV	Q5123
RIBOFLAVIN 5'-PHOSPHATE, OPHTHALMIC SOLUTION	UP TO 3 ML	OTH	J2787
RILONACEPT	1 MG	SC	J2793

Drug Name	Units Per	Route	Code
RIMANTADINE HCL (DEMONSTRATION PROJECT)	100 MG	ORAL	G9020
RIMANTADINE HCL (DEMONSTRATION PROJECT)	100 MG	ORAL	G9036
RIMSO 50	50 ML	IV	J1212
RINGERS LACTATE INFUSION	UP TO 1000 CC	IV	J7120
RISANKIZUMAB-RZAA	1 MG	IV	J2327
RISPERDAL CONSTA	0.5 MG	IM	J2794
RISPERIDONE	0.5 MG	SC	J2798
RISPERIDONE	0.5 MG	IM	J2801
RISPERIDONE	1 MG	SC	J2799
RISPERIDONE	0.5 MG	IM	J2794
RITUXAN	10 MG	IV	J9312
RITUXAN HYCELA	10 MG	SC	J9311
RITUXIMAB	10 MG	IV	J9312
RITUXIMAB 10 MG AND HYALURONIDASE	10 MG	SC	J9311
RITUXIMAB-ABBS, BIOSIMILAR	10 MG	IV	Q5115
RITUXIMAB-ARRX, BIOSIMILAR	10 MG	IV	Q5123
RITUXIMAB-PVVR, BIOSIMILAR	10 MG	IV	Q5119
RIXUBIS	IU	IV	J7200
ROBAXIN	10 ML	IV, IM	J2800
ROCEPHIN	250 MG	IV, IM	J0696
ROCTAVIAN	1 ML	IV	J1412
ROFERON-A	3,000,000 U	SC, IM	J9213
ROLAPITANT	1 MG	ORAL	J8670
ROLAPITANT	0.5 MG	ORAL, IV	J2797
ROLVEDON	0.1 MG	SC	J1449
ROMIDEPSIN, LYOPHILIZED	0.1 MG	IV	J9319
ROMIDEPSIN, NONLYOPHILIZED	0.1 MG	IV	J9318
~~ROMIPLOSTIM~~	~~10 MCG~~	~~SC~~	~~J2796~~
ROMIPLOSTIM	1 MCG	SC	J2802
ROMOSOZUMAB-AQQG	1 MG	SC	J3111
ROPIVACAINE HYDROCHLORIDE	1 MG	VAR	J2795
ROZANOLIXIZUMAB-NOLI	1 MG	SC	J9333
RUBEX	10 MG	IV	J9000
RUBIDIUM RB-82	STUDY DOSE UP TO 60 MCI	IV	A9555
RUBRAMIN PC	1,000 MCG	SC, IM	J3420
RUBRATOPE 57	STUDY DOSE UP TO 1 UCI	ORAL	A9559
RUCONEST	10 UNITS	IV	J0596
RUXIENCE	10 MG	IV	Q5119
RYBREVANT	2 MG	IV	J9061
RYKINDO	0.5 MG	IM	J2801
RYLAZE	0.1 MG	IM	J9021
RYPLAZIM	1 MG	IV	J2998
RYSTIGGO	1 MG	SC	J9333
RYTELO	1 MG	IV	J0870
RYZNEUTA	0.5 MG	SC	J9361
SACITUZUMAB GOVITECAN-HZIY	2.5 MG	IV	J9317
SAIZEN	1 MG	SC	J2941
SAIZEN SOMATROPIN RDNA ORIGIN	1 MG	SC	J2941
SALINE OR STERILE WATER, METERED DOSE DISPENSER	10 ML	INH	A4218
SALINE, STERILE WATER, AND/OR DEXTROSE DILUENT/FLUSH	10 ML	VAR	A4216
SALINE/STERILE WATER	500 ML	VAR	A4217
SAMARIUM LEXIDRONAM	DOSE UP TO 150 MCI	IV	A9604
SANDIMMUNE	100 MG	ORAL	J7502

Drug Name	Units Per	Route	Code
SANDIMMUNE	250 MG	IV	J7516
SANDIMMUNE	25 MG	ORAL	J7515
SANDOSTATIN	25 MCG	SC, IV	J2354
SANDOSTATIN LAR	1 MG	IM	J2353
SANGCYA	100 MG	ORAL	J7502
~~SANO-DROL~~	~~40 MG~~	~~IM~~	~~J1030~~
~~SANO-DROL~~	~~80 MG~~	~~IM~~	~~J1040~~
SANOGRAFT	SQ CM	OTH	Q4319
SANOPELLIS	SQ CM	OTH	Q4308
SAPHNELLO	1 MG	IV	J0491
SAQUINAVIR	200 MG	ORAL	S0140
SARCLISA	10 MG	IV	J9227
SARGRAMOSTIM (GM-CSF)	50 MCG	IV	J2820
SCANDONEST	10 ML	IV	J0670
SCENESSE	1 MG	OTH	J7352
SCULPTRA	0.5 ML	OTH	Q2028
SEBELIPASE ALFA	1 MG	IV	J2840
SECREFLO	1 MCG	IV	J2850
SECRETIN, SYNTHETIC, HUMAN	1 MCG	IV	J2850
~~SECUKINUMAB~~	~~1 MG~~	~~IV~~	~~C9166~~
SECUKINUMAB	1 MG	IV	J3247
SEGESTERONE ACETATE AND ETHINYL ESTRADIOL VAGINAL RING	0.15 MG/0.013 MG	OTH	J7294
SEIZALAM	1 MG	IM	J2253
SELARSDI	1 MG	SC	Q9998
SENSIPAR	1 MG	ORAL	J0604
SENTIMAG	STUDY DOSE	SC	A9697
SENTRY SL MATRIX	SQ CM	OTH	Q4348
SEPTRA IV	10 ML	IV	S0039
SERMORELIN ACETATE	1 MCG	IV	Q0515
SEROSTIM	1 MG	SC	J2941
SEROSTIM RDNA ORIGIN	1 MG	SC	J2941
SEVELAMER CARBONATE, FOR ESRD ON DIALYSIS	20 MG	ORAL	J0601
SEVELAMER CARBONATE, POWDER, FOR ESRD ON DIALYSIS	20 MG	ORAL	J0602
SEVELAMER HCL, FOR ESRD ON DIALYSIS	20 MG	ORAL	J0603
SEVENFACT	1 MCG	IV	J7212
SEZABY	1 MG	IV	J2561
SHELTER DM MATRIX	SQ CM	OTH	Q4346
SIGNATURE APATCH	SQ CM	OTH	Q4260
SIGNIFOR LAR	1 MG	IV	J2502
SILDENAFIL CITRATE	25 MG	ORAL	S0090
SILTUXIMAB	10 MG	IV	J2860
SIMLANDI	1 MG	SC	Q5142
SIMPLIGRAFT	SQ CM	OTH	Q4340
SIMPLIMAX	SQ CM	OTH	Q4341
SIMPONI	1 MG	IV	J1602
SIMULECT	20 MG	IV	J0480
SINCALIDE	5 MCG	IV	J2805
~~SINCALIDE (MAIA)~~	~~5 MCG~~	~~IV~~	~~J2806~~
SINGLAY	SQ CM	OTH	Q4329
SINUVA	10 MCG	OTH	J7402
SIPULEUCEL-T	INFUSION	IV	Q2043
SIROLIMUS	1 MG	ORAL	J7520
SIROLIMUS PROTEIN-BOUND PARTICLES	1 MG	IV	J9331
SIVEXTRO	1 MG	IV	J3090
SKINTE	SQ CM	OTH	Q4200
SKYLA	13.5 MG	OTH	J7301
SKYRIZI	1 MG	IV	J2327
SMZ-TMP	10 ML	IV	S0039
SODIUM FERRIC GLUCONATE COMPLEX IN SUCROSE	12.5 MG	IV	J2916
SODIUM FLUORIDE F-18, DIAGNOSTIC	STUDY DOSE UP TO 30 MCI	IV	A9580
SODIUM IODIDE I-131 CAPSULE DIAGNOSTIC	1 MCI	ORAL	A9528
SODIUM IODIDE I-131 CAPSULE THERAPEUTIC	1 MCI	ORAL	A9517
SODIUM IODIDE I-131 SOLUTION THERAPEUTIC	1 MCI	ORAL	A9530
SODIUM NITRITE/SODIUM THIOSULFATE	3 MG/125 MG	IV	J0211
SODIUM PHOSPHATE P32	1 MCI	IV	A9563
SODIUM THIOSULFATE	100 MG	IV	J0208
SODIUM THIOSULFATE (HOPE)	100 MG	IV	J0209
SOLGANAL	50 MG	IM	J2910
SOLIRIS	10 MG	IV	J1300
SOLTAMOX	10 MG	ORAL	S0187
SOLU-CORTEF	100 MG	IV, IM, SC	J1720
~~SOLU-MEDROL~~	~~125 MG~~	~~IM, IV~~	~~J2930~~
SOLU-MEDROL	5 MG	IM, IV	J2919
~~SOLU-MEDROL~~	~~40 MG~~	~~IM, IV~~	~~J2920~~
SOLUREX	1 MG	IM, IV, OTH	J1100
SOMATREM	1 MG	SC, IM	J2940
SOMATROPIN	1 MG	SC	J2941
SOMATULINE	1 MG	SC	J1930
SOTALOL HYDROCHLORIDE	1 MG	IV	C9482
SOTROVIMAB	500 MG	IV	Q0247
SPECTINOMYCIN DIHYDROCHLORIDE	2 G	IM	J3320
SPECTRO-DEX	1 MG	IM, IV, OTH	J1100
SPESOLIMAB-SBZO	1 MG	IV	J1747
SPEVIGO	1 MG	IV	J1747
SPINRAZA	0.1 MG	INJ	J2326
SPORANOX	50 MG	IV	J1835
SPRAVATO	1 MG	OTH	S0013
STADOL	1 MG	IM, IV	J0595
STADOL NS	25 MG	OTH	S0012
STELARA	1 MG	SC	J3357
STELARA	1 MG	SC, IV	J3358
STERILE WATER OR SALINE, METERED DOSE DISPENSER	10 ML	INH	A4218
STERILE WATER, SALINE, AND/OR DEXTROSE DILUENT/FLUSH	10 ML	VAR	A4216
STERILE WATER/SALINE	500 ML	VAR	A4217
STIMUFEND	0.5 MG	SC	Q5127
STRATTICE TM	SQ CM	OTH	Q4130
STRAVIX	SQ CM	OTH	Q4133
STRAVIXPL	SQ CM	OTH	Q4133
STREPTASE	250,000 IU	IV	J2995
STREPTOKINASE	250,000 IU	IV	J2995
STREPTOMYCIN	1 G	IM	J3000
STREPTOZOCIN	1 G	IV	J9320
STRONTIUM 89 CHLORIDE	1 MCI	IV	A9600
SUBLIMAZE	0.1 MG	IM, IV	J3010
SUBLOCADE	> 100 MG	SC	Q9992
SUBLOCADE	<=100 MG	SC	Q9991
SUBOXONE	4 MG	ORAL	J0573

Drug Name	Units Per	Route	Code
SUBOXONE	2 MG	ORAL	J0572
SUBOXONE	12 MG	ORAL	J0575
SUBOXONE	8 MG	ORAL	J0574
SUBUTEX	1 MG	ORAL	J0571
SUCCINYLCHOLINE CHLORIDE	20 MG	IM, IV	J0330
SUCROFERRIC OXYHYDROXIDE, FOR ESRD ON DIALYSIS	5 MG	ORAL	J0605
SULFAMETHOXAZOLE AND TRIMETHOPRIM	10 ML	IV	S0039
SULFUR HEXAFLUORIDE LIPID MICROSPHERES	1 ML	IV	Q9950
SULFUTRIM	10 ML	IV	S0039
SUMATRIPTAN SUCCINATE	6 MG	SC	J3030
SUNLENCA	1 MG	SC	J1961
SUPARTZ	DOSE	INJ	J7321
SUPPRELIN LA	10 MCG	OTH	J1675
SUPRA SDRM	SQ CM	OTH	A2011
SUPRATHEL	SQ CM	OTH	A2012
SUREDERM	SQ CM	OTH	Q4220
SURFACTOR	0.5 CC	OTH	Q4233
SURGICORD	SQ CM	OTH	Q4218
SURGIGRAFT	SQ CM	OTH	Q4183
SURGIGRAFT-DUAL	SQ CM	OTH	Q4219
SURGIMEND COLLAGEN MATRIX, FETAL	0.5 SQ CM	OTH	C9358
SURGIMEND COLLAGEN MATRIX, NEONATAL	0.5 SQ CM	OTH	C9360
SURGRAFT	SQ CM	OTH	Q4209
SURGRAFT FT	SQ CM	OTH	Q4268
SURGRAFT TL	SQ CM	OTH	Q4263
SURGRAFT XT	SQ CM	OTH	Q4269
SUSTOL	0.1 MG	SC	J1627
SUSVIMO	0.1 MG	OTH	J2779
SUTIMLIMAB-JOME	10 MG	IV	J1302
SYFOVRE	1 MG	INJ	J2781
SYLVANT	10 MG	IV	J2860
SYMMETREL (DEMONSTRATION PROJECT)	100 MG	ORAL	G9033
SYMPHONY	SQ CM	OTH	A2009
SYNDROS	0.1 MG	ORAL	Q0155
SYNERA	70 MG/70 MG	OTH	C9285
SYNERCID	500 MG	IV	J2770
SYNOJOYNT	1 MG	INJ	J7331
SYNRIBO	0.01 MG	SC	J9262
SYNTOCINON	10 UNITS	IV	J2590
SYNVISC/SYNVISC-ONE	1 MG	INJ	J7325
SYTOBEX	1,000 MCG	SC, IM	J3420
T-GEN	250 MG	ORAL	Q0173
TACRINE HCL	10 MG	ORAL	S0014
TACROLIMUS	1 MG	ORAL	J7507
TACROLIMUS	5 MG	OTH	J7525
TACROLIMUS, EXTENDED RELEASE	0.25 MG	ORAL	J7503
TACROLIMUS, EXTENDED RELEASE	0.1 MG	ORAL	J7508
TAFASITAMAB-CXIX	2 MG	IV	J9349
TAG	SQ CM	OTH	Q4261
TAGAMET HCL	300 MG	IM, IV	S0023
TAGRAXOFUSP-ERZS	10 MCG	IV	J9269
TAKHZYRO	1 MG	SC	J0593
TALIGLUCERASE ALFA	10 U	IV	J3060
TALIMOGENE LAHERPAREPVEC	1 MILLION	INTRALESIONAL	J9325
~~TALQUETAMAB-TGVS~~	~~0.25 MG~~	~~SC~~	~~C9163~~
TALQUETAMAB-TGVS	0.25 MG	SC	J3055
~~TALVEY~~	~~0.25 MG~~	~~SC~~	~~C9163~~
TALVEY	0.25 MG	SC	J3055
TALWIN	30 MG	IM, SC, IV	J3070
TALYMED	SQ CM	OTH	Q4127
TAMIFLU (DEMONSTRATION PROJECT)	75 MG	ORAL	G9019
TAMIFLU (DEMONSTRATION PROJECT)	75 MG	ORAL	G9035
TAMOXIFEN CITRATE	10 MG	ORAL	S0187
~~TARLATAMAB-DLLE~~	~~1 MG~~	~~IV~~	~~C9170~~
TARLATAMAB-DLLE	1 MG	IV	J9026
TAUROLIDINE AND HEPARIN SODIUM	1.35 MG/100 UNITS	OTH	J0911
TAUVID	1 MCI	IV	A9601
TAXOL	1 MG	IV	J9267
TAXOTERE	1 MG	IV	J9171
TAZICEF	500 MG	IM, IV	J0713
TBO-FILGRASTIM	1 MCG	IV	J1447
TC 99M TILOMANOCEPT	0.5 MCI	SC, OTH	A9520
TEBAMIDE	250 MG	ORAL	Q0173
TEBENTAFUSP-TEBN	1 MCG	IV	J9274
TEBOROXIME TECHNETIUM TC 99M	STUDY DOSE	IV	A9501
TEBOROXIME, TECHNETIUM	STUDY DOSE	IV	A9501
TECARTUS	UP TO 200 MILLION CELLS	IV	Q2053
TECENTRIQ	10 MG	INF	J9022
TECHNEPLEX	STUDY DOSE UP TO 25 MCI	IV	A9539
TECHNESCAN	STUDY DOSE UP TO 30 MCI	IV	A9561
TECHNESCAN FANOLESOMAB	STUDY DOSE UP TO 25 MCI	IV	A9566
TECHNESCAN MAA	STUDY DOSE UP TO 10 MCI	IV	A9540
TECHNESCAN MAG3	STUDY DOSE UP TO 15 MCI	IV	A9562
TECHNESCAN PYP	STUDY DOSE UP TO 25 MCI	IV	A9538
TECHNESCAN PYP KIT	STUDY DOSE UP TO 25 MCI	IV	A9538
TECHNETIUM SESTAMBI	STUDY DOSE	IV	A9500
TECHNETIUM TC 99M APCITIDE	STUDY DOSE UP TO 20 MCI	IV	A9504
TECHNETIUM TC 99M ARCITUMOMAB, DIAGNOSTIC	STUDY DOSE UP TO 45 MCI	IV	A9568
TECHNETIUM TC 99M BICISATE	STUDY DOSE UP TO 25 MCI	IV	A9557
TECHNETIUM TC 99M DEPREOTIDE	STUDY DOSE UP TO 35 MCI	IV	A9536
TECHNETIUM TC 99M EXAMETAZIME	STUDY DOSE UP TO 25 MCI	IV	A9521
TECHNETIUM TC 99M FANOLESOMAB	STUDY DOSE UP TO 25 MCI	IV	A9566
TECHNETIUM TC 99M LABELED RED BLOOD CELLS	STUDY DOSE UP TO 30 MCI	IV	A9560
TECHNETIUM TC 99M MACROAGGREGATED ALBUMIN	STUDY DOSE UP TO 10 MCI	IV	A9540
TECHNETIUM TC 99M MDI-MDP	STUDY DOSE UP TO 30 MCI	IV	A9503
TECHNETIUM TC 99M MEBROFENIN	STUDY DOSE UP TO 15 MCI	IV	A9537

Drug Name	Units Per	Route	Code
TECHNETIUM TC 99M MEDRONATE	STUDY DOSE UP TO 30 MCI	IV	A9503
TECHNETIUM TC 99M MERTIATIDE	STUDY DOSE UP TO 15 MCI	IV	A9562
TECHNETIUM TC 99M OXIDRONATE	STUDY DOSE UP TO 30 MCI	IV	A9561
TECHNETIUM TC 99M PENTETATE	STUDY DOSE UP TO 25 MCI	IV	A9539
TECHNETIUM TC 99M PYROPHOSPHATE	STUDY DOSE UP TO 25 MCI	IV	A9538
TECHNETIUM TC 99M SODIUM GLUCEPTATE	STUDY DOSE UP TO 25 MCI	IV	A9550
TECHNETIUM TC 99M SUCCIMER	STUDY DOSE UP TO 10 MCI	IV	A9551
TECHNETIUM TC 99M SULFUR COLLOID	STUDY DOSE UP TO 20 MCI	IV	A9541
TECHNETIUM TC 99M TETROFOSMIN, DIAGNOSTIC	STUDY DOSE	IV	A9502
TECHNETIUM TC-99M EXAMETAZIME LABELED AUTOLOGOUS WHITE BLOOD CELLS	STUDY DOSE	IV	A9569
TECHNETIUM TC-99M PERTECHNETATE, DIAGNOSTIC	1 MCI	IV	A9512
TECHNETIUM TC-99M TEBOROXIME	STUDY DOSE	IV	A9501
TECHNILITE	1 MCI	IV	A9512
TECLISTAMAB-CQYV	0.5 MG	SC	J9380
TECVAYLI	0.5 MG	SC	J9380
TEDIZOLID PHOSPHATE	1 MG	IV	J3090
TEFLARO	10 MG	IV	J0712
TELAVANCIN	10 MG	IV	J3095
TEMODAR	5 MG	ORAL	J8700
TEMODAR	1 MG	IV	J9328
TEMOZOLOMIDE	5 MG	ORAL	J8700
TEMOZOLOMIDE	1 MG	IV	J9328
TEMSIROLIMUS	1 MG	IV	J9330
TENDON, POROUS MATRIX	SQ CM	OTH	C9356
TENDON, POROUS MATRIX CROSS-LINKED AND GLYCOSAMINOGLYCAN MATRIX	SQ CM	OTH	C9356
TENECTEPLASE	1 MG	IV	J3101
TENIPOSIDE	50 MG	IV	Q2017
TENOGLIDE TENDON PROTECTOR	SQ CM	OTH	C9356
TENOGLIDE TENDON PROTECTOR SHEET	SQ CM	OTH	C9356
TENSIX	SQ CM	OTH	Q4146
TEPEZZA	10 MG	IV	J3241
TEPLIZUMAB-MZWV	5 MCG	IV	J9381
TEPROTUMUMAB-TRBW	10 MG	IV	J3241
TEQUIN	10 MG	IV	J1590
TERBUTALINE SULFATE	1 MG	SC, IV	J3105
TERBUTALINE SULFATE, COMPOUNDED, CONCENTRATED	1 MG	INH	J7680
TERBUTALINE SULFATE, COMPOUNDED, UNIT DOSE	1 MG	INH	J7681
TERIPARATIDE	10 MCG	SC	J3110
TERRAMYCIN	50 MG	IM	J2460
TESTOSTERONE CYPIONATE	1 MG	IM	J1071
TESTOSTERONE ENANTHATE	1 MG	IM	J3121
TESTOSTERONE PELLET	75 MG	OTH	S0189
TESTOSTERONE UNDECANOATE	1 MG	IM	J3145
TETANUS IMMUNE GLOBULIN	250 U	IM	J1670
TETRACYCLINE HCL	250 MG	IV	J0120
TEVIMBRA	1 MG	IV	J9329
TEZEPELUMAB-EKKO	1 MG	SC	J2356
TEZSPIRE	1 MG	SC	J2356
THALLOUS CHLORIDE	1 MCI	IV	A9505
THALLOUS CHLORIDE TL-201	1 MCI	IV	A9505
THALLOUS CHLORIDE USP	1 MCI	IV	A9505
THEELIN AQUEOUS	1 MG	IM, IV	J1435
THEOPHYLLINE	40 MG	IV	J2810
THERAGENESIS	SQ CM	OTH	A2008
THERAMEND	SQ CM	OTH	Q4342
THERASKIN	SQ CM	OTH	Q4121
THERION	SQ CM	OTH	Q4176
THIAMINE HCL	100 MG	INJ	J3411
THIETHYLPERAZINE MALEATE	10 MG	IM	J3280
THIETHYLPERAZINE MALEATE	10 MG	ORAL	Q0174
THIMAZIDE	250 MG	ORAL	Q0173
THIOTEPA	15 MG	IV	J9340
THORAZINE	50 MG	IM, IV	J3230
THROMBATE III	1 IU	IV	J7197
THYMOGLOBULIN	25 MG	OTH	J7511
THYROGEN	0.9 MG	IM, SC	J3240
THYROTROPIN ALPHA	0.9 MG	IM, SC	J3240
TICARCILLIN DISODIUM AND CLAVULANATE	3.1 G	IV	S0040
TICE BCG	1 MG	OTH	J9030
TICON	250 MG	IM	Q0173
TIGAN	200 MG	IM	J3250
TIGECYCLINE	1 MG	IV	J3243
TIGECYCLINE (ACCORD) NOT THERAPEUTICALLY EQUIVALENT TO J3243	1 MG	IV	J3244
TIJECT-20	200 MG	IM	J3250
TILDRAKIZUMAB	1 MG	SC	J3245
TIMENTIN	3.1 G	IV	S0040
TINZAPARIN	1,000 IU	SC	J1655
TIROFIBAN HCL	0.25 MG	IM, IV	J3246
TISAGENLECLEUCEL	UP TO 600 MILLION CELLS	IV	Q2042
TISLELIZUMAB-JSGR	1 MG	IV	J9329
TISOTUMAB VEDOTIN-TFTV	1 MG	IV	J9273
TIVDAK	1 MG	IV	J9273
TIXAGEVIMAB AND CILGAVIMAB	300 MG	IM	Q0220
TIXAGEVIMAB AND CILGAVIMAB	600 MG	IM	Q0221
TNKASE	1 MG	IV	J3101
TOBI	300 MG	INH	J7682
TOBRAMYCIN COMPOUNDED, UNIT DOSE	300 MG	INH	J7685
TOBRAMYCIN SULFATE	80 MG	IM, IV	J3260
TOBRAMYCIN, NONCOMPOUNDED, UNIT DOSE	300 MG	INH	J7682
TOCILIZUMAB	1 MG	IV	J3262
TOCILIZUMAB	1 MG	IV	Q0249
TOCILIZUMAB-AAZG, BIOSIMILAR	1 MG	IV, SC	Q5135
TOCILIZUMAB-BAVI	1 MG	IV	Q5133
TOFERSEN	1 MG	INJ	J1304
TOFIDENCE	1 MG	IV	Q5133
TOLAZOLINE HCL	25 MG	IV	J2670
TOPOSAR	10 MG	IV	J9181
TOPOTECAN	0.25 MG	ORAL	J8705
TOPOTECAN	0.1 MG	IV	J9351
TORADOL	15 MG	IV	J1885

Drug Name	Units Per	Route	Code
TORIPALIMAB-TPZI	1 MG	IV	J3263
TORISEL	1 MG	IV	J9330
TORNALATE	MG	INH	J7629
TORNALATE CONCENTRATE	1 MG	INH	J7628
TORSEMIDE	10 MG	IV	J3265
TOSITUMOMAB	450 MG	IV	G3001
TOTAL	SQ CM	OTH	Q4330
TOTECT	250 MG	IV	J1190
TRABECTEDIN	0.1 MG	IV	J9352
TRANSCYTE	SQ CM	OTH	Q4182
TRASTUZUMAB AND HYALURONIDASE-OYSK	10 MG	SC	J9356
TRASTUZUMAB, EXCLUDES BIOSIMILAR	10 MG	IV	J9355
TRASTUZUMAB-ANNS, BIOSIMILAR	10 MG	IV	Q5117
TRASTUZUMAB-DKST, BIOSIMILAR	10 MG	IV	Q5114
TRASTUZUMAB-DTTB, BIOSIMILAR	10 MG	IV	Q5112
TRASTUZUMAB-PKRB, BIOSIMILAR	10 MG	IV	Q5113
TRASTUZUMAB-QYYP, BIOSIMILAR	10 MG	IV	Q5116
TRASTUZUMAB-STRF	10 MG	IV	Q5146
TRASYLOL	10,000 KIU	IV	J0365
TRAVOPROST, INTRACAMERAL IMPLANT	1 MCG	OTH	J7355
TRAZIMERA	10 MG	IV	Q5116
TREANDA	1 MG	IV	J9033
TRELSTAR DEPOT	3.75 MG	IM	J3315
TRELSTAR DEPOT PLUS DEBIOCLIP KIT	3.75 MG	IM	J3315
TRELSTAR LA	3.75 MG	IM	J3315
TREMELIMUMAB-ACTL	1 MG	IV	J9347
TREMFYA	1 MG	SC	J1628
TREPROSTINIL	1 MG	SC	J3285
TREPROSTINIL, INHALATION SOLUTION	1.74 MG	INH	J7686
TRETINOIN	5 G	OTH	S0117
TRETTEN	10 IU	IV	J7181
TRI-MEMBRANE WRAP	SQ CM	OTH	Q4344
TRIAMCINOLONE ACETONIDE	1 MG	INJ	J3299
TRIAMCINOLONE ACETONIDE, PRESERVATIVE FREE	1 MG	INJ	J3300
TRIAMCINOLONE ACETONIDE, PRESERVATIVE-FREE, EXTENDED-RELEASE, MICROSPHERE FORMULATION	1 MG	OTH	J3304
TRIAMCINOLONE DIACETATE	5 MG	IM	J3302
TRIAMCINOLONE HEXACETONIDE	5 MG	VAR	J3303
TRIAMCINOLONE, COMPOUNDED, CONCENTRATED	1 MG	INH	J7683
TRIAMCINOLONE, COMPOUNDED, UNIT DOSE	1 MG	INH	J7684
TRIBAN	250 MG	ORAL	Q0173
TRIESENCE	1 MG	OTH	J3300
TRIFERIC AVNU	0.1 MG	IV	J1445
TRIFERIC POWDER	0.1 MG	IV	J1444
TRIFERIC SOLUTION	0.1 MG	IV	J1443
TRIFLUPROMAZINE HCL	UP TO 20 MG	INJ	J3400
TRILACICLIB	1 MG	IV	J1448
TRILIFON	4 MG	ORAL	Q0175
TRILONE	5 MG	IM	J3302
TRILURON	1 MG	INJ	J7332
TRIMETHOBENZAMIDE HCL	200 MG	IM	J3250
TRIMETHOBENZAMIDE HCL	250 MG	ORAL	Q0173

Drug Name	Units Per	Route	Code
TRIMETREXATE GLUCURONATE	25 MG	IV	J3305
TRIPTODUR	3.75 MG	IM	J3316
TRIPTORELIN PAMOATE	3.75 MG	IM	J3315
TRIPTORELIN, EXTENDED-RELEASE	3.75 MG	IM	J3316
TRISENOX	1 MG	IV	J9017
TRIVARIS	1 MG	VAR	J3300
TRIVISC	1 MG	INJ	J7329
TROBICIN	2 G	IM	J3320
TRODELVY	2.5 MG	IV	J9317
TROGARZO	10 MG	IV	J1746
TRUSKIN	SQ CM	OTH	Q4167
TRUVADA	200 MG/300 MG	ORAL	J0750
TRUXADRYL	50 MG	IV, IM	J1200
TRUXIMA	10 MG	IV	Q5115
TYENNE	1 MG	IV, SC	Q5135
TYGACIL	1 MG	IV	J3243
TYPE A BOTOX	1 UNIT	IM, OTH	J0585
TYRUKO	1 MG	IV	Q5134
TYSABRI	1 MG	IV	J2323
TYVASO	1.74 MG	INH	J7686
TZIELD	5 MCG	IV	J9381
UBLITUXIMAB-XIIY	1 MG	IV	J2329
UDENYCA	0.5 MG	SC	Q5111
ULTOMIRIS	10 MG	IV	J1303
ULTRA-TECHNEKOW	1 MCI	IV	A9512
ULTRALENTE	5 U	SC	J1815
ULTRATAG	STUDY DOSE UP TO 30 MCI	IV	A9560
ULTRAVIST 150	1 ML	IV	Q9965
ULTRAVIST 240	1 ML	IV	Q9966
ULTRAVIST 300	1 ML	IV	Q9967
ULTRAVIST 370	1 ML	IV	Q9967
UNASYN	1.5 G	IM, IV	J0295
UPLIZNA	1 MG	IV	J1823
UREA	40 G	IV	J3350
URECHOLINE	UP TO 5 MG	SC	J0520
UROFOLLITROPIN	75 IU	SC, IM	J3355
UROKINASE	5,000 IU	IV	J3364
UROKINASE	250,000 IU	IV	J3365
USTEKINUMAB	1 MG	SC	J3357
USTEKINUMAB	1 MG	SC, IV	J3358
USTEKINUMAB-AEKN	1 MG	SC	Q9998
USTEKINUMAB-AUUB	1 MG	IV	Q5138
USTEKINUMAB-AUUB	1 MG	SC	Q5137
USTEKINUMAB-TTWE	1 MG	IV	Q9997
USTEKINUMAB-TTWE	1 MG	SC	Q9996
UZEDY	1 MG	SC	J2799
VABOMERE	10 MG/10 MG	IV	J2186
VABYSMO	0.1 MG	INJ	J2777
VADADUSTAT, FOR ESRD ON DIALYSIS	1 MG	ORAL	J0901
VAFSEO, FOR ESRD ON DIALYSIS	1 MG	ORAL	J0901
VALERGEN	10 MG	IM	J1380
VALIUM	5 MG	IV, IM	J3360
VALOCTOCOGENE ROXAPARVOVEC-RVOX	1 ML	IV	J1412
VALRUBICIN INTRAVESICAL	200 MG	OTH	J9357
VALSTAR	200 MG	OTH	J9357
VANCOCIN	500 MG	IM, IV	J3370
VANCOMYCIN HCL	500 MG	IV, IM	J3370

Drug Name	Units Per	Route	Code
VANCOMYCIN HCL (MYLAN) NOT THERAPEUTICALLY EQUIVALENT TO J3370	500 MG	IV	J3371
VANCOMYCIN HCL (XELLIA) NOT THERAPEUTICALLY EQUIVALENT TO J3370	500 MG	IV	J3372
VANTAS	50 MG	OTH	J9225
VAPRISOL	1 MG	INJ	C9488
VARUBI	1 MG	ORAL	J8670
VARUBI	0.5 MG	ORAL, IV	J2797
VASOPRESSIN	1 U	IV	J2598
VASOPRESSIN (AMERICAN REGENT)	1 U	IV	J2599
VASOPRESSIN (BAXTER)	1 UNIT	IV	J2601
VECTIBIX	10 MG	IV	J9303
VEDOLIZUMAB	1 MG	IV	J3380
VEGZELMA	10 MG	IV	Q5129
VEKLURY	1 MG	IV	J0248
VELAGLUCERASE ALFA	100 U	IV	J3385
VELBAN	1 MG	IV	J9360
VELETRI	0.5 MG	IV	J1325
VELMANASE ALFA-TYCV	1 MG	IV	J0217
VELOSULIN	5 U	SC	J1815
VELOSULIN BR	5 U	SC	J1815
VELPHORO, FOR ESRD ON DIALYSIS	5 MG	ORAL	J0605
VENDAJE	SQ CM	OTH	Q4252
VENDAJE AC	SQ CM	OTH	Q4279
VENOFER	1 MG	IV	J1756
VENTAVIS	0.1 MCG	INH	J1749
VENTOLIN NONCOMPOUNDED, CONCENTRATED	1 MG	INH	J7611
VENTOLIN NONCOMPOUNDED, UNIT DOSE	1 MG	INH	J7613
VEOPOZ	1 MG	IV, SC	J9376
VEPESID	50 MG	ORAL	J8560
VEPESID	10 MG	IV	J9181
VERITAS	SQ CM	OTH	C9354
VERSED	1 MG	IM, IV	J2250
VERTEPORFIN	0.1 MG	IV	J3396
VESTRONIDASE ALFA-VJBK	1 MG	IV	J3397
VFEND	200 MG	IV	J3465
VIA MATRIX	SQ CM	OTH	Q4309
VIAGRA	25 MG	ORAL	S0090
VIBATIV	10 MG	IV	J3095
VIDAZA	1 MG	SC	J9025
VIDEX	25 MG	ORAL	S0137
VILTEPSO	10 MG	IV	J1427
VILTOLARSEN	10 MG	IV	J1427
VIM	SQ CM	OTH	Q4251
VIMIZIM	1 MG	IV	J1322
VIMPAT	1 MG	IV, ORAL	C9254
VINBLASTINE SULFATE	1 MG	IV	J9360
VINCASCAR	1 MG	IV	J9370
VINCRISTINE SULFATE	1 MG	IV	J9370
~~VINCRISTINE SULFATE LIPOSOME~~	~~5 MG~~	~~IV~~	~~J9371~~
VINORELBINE TARTRATE	10 MG	IV	J9390
VIRILON	1 CC, 200 MG	IM	J1080
VISCO-3	DOSE	INJ	J7321
VISTAJECT-25	25 MG	IM	J3410
VISTARIL	25 MG	IM	J3410
VISTARIL	25 MG	ORAL	Q0177

Drug Name	Units Per	Route	Code
VISTIDE	375 MG	IV	J0740
VISUDYNE	0.1 MG	IV	J3396
VITAMIN B-12 CYANOCOBALAMIN	1,000 MCG	IM, SC	J3420
VITAMIN B-17	VAR	INJ	J3570
VITOGRAFT	SQ CM	OTH	Q4317
VITRASE	1 USP	OTH	J3471
VITRASE	1,000 USP	OTH	J3472
VITRASERT	4.5 MG	OTH	J7310
VITRAVENE	1.65 MG	OTH	J1452
VIVIMUSTA	1 MG	IV	J9056
VIVITROL	1 MG	IM	J2315
VON WILLEBRAND FACTOR (RECOMBINANT)	1 IU	IV	J7179
VON WILLEBRAND FACTOR COMPLEX (HUMAN) (WILATE)	1 IU	IV	J7183
VON WILLEBRAND FACTOR COMPLEX, HUMATE-P	1 IU	IV	J7187
VON WILLEBRAND FACTOR VIII COMPLEX, HUMAN	FACTOR VIII IU	IV	J7186
VONVENDI	1 IU	IV	J7179
VORAXAZE	10 UNITS	IV	C9293
VORETIGENE NEPARVOVEC-RZYL	1 BILLION VECTOR GENOMES	OTH	J3398
VORICONAZOLE	200 MG	IV	J3465
VPRIV	100 U	IV	J3385
VUEWAY	1 ML	IV	A9573
VUMON	50 MG	IV	Q2017
VUTRISIRAN	1 MG	SC	J0225
VYEPTI	1 MG	IV	J3032
VYJUVEK	0.1 ML	OTH	J3401
VYONDYS 53	10 MG	IV	J1429
VYVGART	2 MG	IV	J9332
VYVGART HYTRULO	2 MG	IV	J9334
VYXEOS	1 MG/2.27 MG	IV	J9153
WEHAMINE	50 MG	IM, IV	J1240
WEHDRYL	50 MG	IM, IV	J1200
WELBUTRIN SR	150 MG	ORAL	S0106
WEZLANA	1 MG	IV	Q5138
WEZLANA	1 MG	SC	Q5137
WILATE	1 IU	IV	J7183
WINRHO SDF	100 IU	IV	J2792
WOUNDEX	SQ CM	OTH	Q4163
WOUNDEX FLOW	0.5 CC	OTH	Q4162
WOUNDFIX, WOUNDFIX PLUS, WOUNDFIX XPLUS	SQ CM	OTH	Q4217
WOUNDPLUS	SQ CM	OTH	Q4326
~~WOUNDPLUS MEMBRANE OR E-GRAFT~~	~~SQ CM~~	~~OTH~~	~~Q4277~~
WYCILLIN	600,000 U	IM, IV	J2510
WYOST	1 MG	SC	Q5136
XARACOLL	1 MG	OTH	C9089
XATMEP	2.5 MG	ORAL	J8612
XCEED TL MATRIX	SQ CM	OTH	Q4353
XCELL AMNIO MATRIX	SQ CM	OTH	Q4280
XCELLERATE	SQ CM	OTH	Q4234
XCELLISTEM	1 MG	OTH	A2004
XCM BIOLOGIC TISSUE MATRIX	SQ CM	OTH	Q4142
~~XELODA~~	~~150 MG~~	~~ORAL~~	~~J8520~~
XELODA	50 MG	ORAL	J8522
~~XELODA~~	~~500 MG~~	~~ORAL~~	~~J8521~~

Appendix 1 — Table of Drugs and Biologicals

Drug Name	Units Per	Route	Code
XEMBIFY	100 MG	SC	J1558
XENLETA	1 MG	IV	J0691
~~XENON XE-129 HYPERPOLARIZED GAS, DIAGNOSTIC~~	~~STUDY DOSE~~	~~INH~~	~~C9150~~
XENON XE-129 HYPERPOLARIZED GAS, DIAGNOSTIC	STUDY DOSE	INH	A9610
XENON XE-133	10 MCI	INH	A9558
XENOPATCH	SQ CM	OTH	A2024
~~XENOVIEW~~	~~STUDY DOSE~~	~~INH~~	~~C9150~~
XENOVIEW	STUDY DOSE	INH	A9610
XENPOZYME	1 MG	IV	J0218
XEOMIN	1 UNIT	IM	J0588
XERAVA	1 MG	IV	J0122
XGEVA	1 MG	SC	J0897
XIAFLEX	0.01 MG	OTH	J0775
XIPERE	1 MG	INJ	J3299
XOFIGO	MICROCURIE	IV	A9606
XOLAIR	5 MG	SC	J2357
XWRAP	SQ CM	OTH	Q4204
~~XYLOCAINE~~	~~10 MG~~	~~IV~~	~~J2001~~
XYNTHA	1 IU	IV	J7185
~~YCANTH~~	~~3.2 MG~~	~~OTH~~	~~C9164~~
YCANTH	3.2 MG	OTH	J7354
YERVOY	1 MG	IV	J9228
YESCARTA	UP TO 200 MILLION CELLS	IV	Q2041
YONDELIS	0.1 MG	IV	J9352
YTTRIUM-90 IBRITUMOMAB TIUXETAN, THERAPEUTIC	TX DOSE UP TO 40 MCI	IV	A9543
YUFLYMA	1 MG	SC	Q5141
YUPELRI	1 MCG	INH	J7677
YUTIQ	0.01 MG	OTH	J7314
ZALTRAP	1 MG	IV	J9400
ZANAMIVIR (BRAND) (DEMONSTRATION PROJECT)	10 MG	INH	G9034
ZANAMIVIR (GENERIC) (DEMONSTRATION PROJECT)	10 MG	INH	G9018
ZANOSAR	1 GM	IV	J9320
~~ZANTAC~~	~~25 MG~~	~~INJ~~	~~J2780~~
ZARXIO	1 MCG	IV, SC	Q5101
ZEMDRI	5 MG	IV	J0291
ZEMPLAR	1 MCG	IV, IM	J2501
ZENAPAX	25 MG	OTH	J7513
ZENITH AMNIOTIC MEMBRANE	SQ CM	OTH	Q4253
ZEPZELCA	0.1 MG	IV	J9223
ZERBAXA	50 MG/25 MG	IV	J0695
ZEVALIN, DIAGNOSTIC	STUDY DOSE UP TO 5 MCI	IV	A9542
ZEVALIN, THERAPEUTIC	TX DOSE UP TO 40 MCI	IV	A9543
ZICONOTIDE	1 MCG	IT	J2278
ZIDOVUDINE	100 MG	ORAL	S0104
ZIDOVUDINE	10 MG	IV	J3485
ZIEXTENZO	0.5 MG	SC	Q5120
ZILRETTA	1 MG	OTH	J3304
ZIMHI	1 MG	SC	J2311
ZINACEFT	750 MG	IM, IV	J0697
ZINECARD	250 MG	IV	J1190
ZINPLAVA	10 MG	INF	J0565
ZIPRASIDONE MESYLATE	10 MG	IM	J3486
ZIRABEV	10 MG	IV	Q5118
ZITHROMAX	500 MG	IV	J0456
ZITHROMAX	1 G	ORAL	Q0144
ZIV-AFLIBERCEPT	1 MG	IV	J9400
ZOFRAN	1 MG	IV	J2405
ZOFRAN	4 MG	ORAL	S0119
ZOFRAN	1 MG	ORAL	Q0162
ZOLADEX	3.6 MG	SC	J9202
ZOLEDRONIC ACID	1 MG	IV	J3489
ZOLGENSMA	UP TO $5X10^{15}$ VECTOR GENOMES	IV	J3399
ZOMETA	1 MG	IV	J3489
ZORBTIVE	1 MG	SC	J2941
ZORTRESS	0.25 MG	ORAL	J7527
ZOSYN	1 G/1.125 GM	IV	J2543
ZOVIRAX	5 MG	IV	J0133
ZUBSOLV	1.4 MG	ORAL	J0572
ZUBSOLV	5.7 MG	ORAL	J0573
ZULRESSO	1 MG	IV	J1632
ZUPLENZ	4 MG	ORAL	S0119
ZUPLENZ	1 MG	ORAL	Q0162
ZYLONTA	1 MG	IV	J9359
ZYMFENTRA	10 MG	SC	J1748
ZYNRELEF	1 MG/0.03 MG	OTH	C9088
ZYNTEGLO	PER TREATMENT	IV	J3393
ZYNYZ	1 MG	IV	J9345
ZYPREXA RELPREVV	1 MG	IM	J2358
ZYVOX	200 MG	IV	J2020

NOT OTHERWISE CLASSIFIED DRUGS

Drug Name	Unit Per	Route	Code
ALGLUCOSIDASE ALFA NOS	10 MG	IV	J0220
ALPHA 1 - PROTEINASE INHIBITOR (HUMAN), NOS	10 MG	IV	J0256
ANTIEMETIC NOC	VAR	ORAL	Q0181
ANTIEMETIC DRUG, ORAL, NOS	VAR	ORAL	J8597
ANTIEMETIC DRUG, RECTAL/ SUPPOSITORY, NOS	1 EA	OTH	J8498
ASPARAGINASE, NOS	10,000 U	IM, IV, SC	J9020
BRACHYTHERAPY SOURCE, NONSTRANDED, NOS	SOURCE	OTH	C2699
BRACHYTHERAPY SOURCE, STRANDED, NOS	SOURCE	OTH	C2698
BUPIVICAINE, NOS	0.5 MG	INJ	J0665
CALCIUM GLUCONATE, NOS	10 MG	IV	J0612
COMPOUNDED DRUG, NOC	VAR	VAR	J7999
CYCLOPHOSPHAMIDE, NOS	5 MG	IV	J9075
DOXORUBICIN HCL, LIPOSOMAL, NOS	10 MG	IV	Q2050
DRUG OR BIOLOGICAL, NOC, PART B DRUG COMPETITIVE ACQUISITION PROGRAM (CAP)	VAR	VAR	Q4082
FACTOR IX (ANTIHEMOPHILIC FACTOR, RECOMBINANT), NOS	1 IU	IV	J7195
FACTOR VIII (ANTIHEMOPHILIC FACTOR, RECOMBINANT), NOS	1 IU	IV	J7192
FDA-APPROVED PRESCRIPTION DRUG, ONLY FOR USE AS HIV PRE-EXPOSURE PROPHYLAXIS	VAR	VAR	J0799
GADOLINIUM -BASED CONTRAST, NOS	1 ML	IV	A9579

Drug Name	Unit Per	Route	Code
GEMCITABINE HCL, NOS	200 MG	IV	J9201
HEMOPHILIA CLOTTING FACTOR, NOC	VAR	INJ	J7199
HUMAN FIBRINOGEN CONCENTRATE, NOS	1 MG	IV	J7178
HYDROXYPROGESTERONE CAPROATE, NOS	10 MG	IM	J1729
IMMUNE GLOBULIN LYOPHILIZED, NOS	500 MG	IV	J1566
IMMUNE GLOBULIN, NONLYOPHILIZED (NOS)	500 MG	IV	J1599
IMMUNOSUPPRESSIVE DRUG, NOC	VAR	VAR	J7599
INFLUENZA VIRUS VACCINE, NOS	EA	IM	Q2039
LEVOLEUCOVORIN, NOS	0.5 MG	IV	J0641
LEVOTHYROXINE SODIUM, NOS	10 MCG	IV	J0650
MELPHALAN HCL, NOS	50 MG	IV	J9245
MULTIPLE VITAMINS, WITH OR WITHOUT MINERALS AND TRACE ELEMENTS	VAR	ORAL	A9153
NOC DRUGS, INHALATION SOLUTION ADMINISTERED THROUGH DME	1 EA	OTH	J7699
NOC DRUGS, OTHER THAN INHALATION DRUGS, ADMINISTERED THROUGH DME	1 EA	OTH	J7799
NONRADIOACTIVE CONTRACT IMAGING MATERIAL	STUDY DOSE	IV	A9698
NOT OTHERWISE CLASSIFIED, ANTINEOPLASTIC DRUGS	VAR	VAR	J9999
PEMETREXED, NOS	10 MG	IV	J9305
POSITRON EMISSION TOMOGRAPHY RADIOPHARMACEUTICAL, DIAGNOSTIC, FOR NON-TUMOR IDENTIFICATION	STUDY DOSE	IV	A9598
POSITRON EMISSION TOMOGRAPHY RADIOPHARMACEUTICAL, DIAGNOSTIC, FOR TUMOR IDENTIFICATION	STUDY DOSE	IV	A9597
PRESCRIPTION DRUG, ORAL, CHEMOTHERAPEUTIC, NOS	VAR	ORAL	J8999
PRESCRIPTION DRUG, ORAL, NONCHEMOTHERAPEUTIC, NOS	VAR	ORAL	J8499
RADIOPHARMACEUTICAL, DIAGNOSTIC, NOC	VAR	VAR	A4641
RADIOPHARMACEUTICAL, THERAPEUTIC	STUDY DOSE	IV	A9699
SINGLE VITAMIN/MINERAL/TRACE ELEMENT	VAR	ORAL	A9152
SKIN SUBSTITUTE, FDA-CLEARED AS A DEVICE, NOS	SQ CM	OTH	A4100
SKIN SUBSTITUTE, NOS	VAR	OTH	Q4100
TRIAMCINOLONE ACETONIDE, NOS	10 MG	IM	J3301
UNCLASSIFIED BIOLOGICS	VAR	VAR	J3590
UNCLASSIFIED DRUG OR BIOLOGICAL USED FOR ESRD ON DIALYSIS	VAR	VAR	J3591
UNCLASSIFIED DRUGS	VAR	VAR	J3490
UNCLASSIFIED DRUGS OR BIOLOGICALS	VAR	VAR	C9399
WOUND FILLER, DRY FORM, PER G, NOS	1 G	OTH	A6262
WOUND FILLER, GEL/PASTE, PER FL OZ, NOS	1 OZ	OTH	A6261

Appendix 2 — HCPCS Modifiers and Expanded Guidance

HCPCS Level II code modifiers play an important role in expert coding practices. A modifier is a two-character code that is added to the end of a code to clarify the services being reported. Modifiers provide a means by which a service can be altered without changing the procedure code. They add more information, such as the anatomical site, to the code. In addition, they help eliminate the appearance of duplicate billing and unbundling. Modifiers are appended to increase accuracy in reimbursement, coding consistency, editing, and to capture payment data.

This appendix includes:

- *Introduction to Modifiers*, providing general information about modifiers
- *Ambulance Modifiers*, providing guidance for reporting ambulance services
- A list of HCPCS Level II modifiers. Select modifiers have additional instructional notes from Optum inside gray boxes below the official descriptor to assist with appropriate reporting
- Additional regulatory and coding guidance for appropriate reporting of modifiers

Introduction to Modifiers

Over the years, physicians and hospitals have learned that coding and billing are inextricably entwined processes. Coding provides the common language through which the physician and hospital can communicate – or report – their services to third-party payers, including managed care organizations, the federal Medicare program, and state Medicaid programs.

The use of modifiers is an important part of coding and billing for healthcare services. Modifier use has increased as various commercial payers, who in the past did not incorporate modifiers into their reimbursement protocol, recognize and accept codes appended with these specialized billing flags. Correct modifier use is also an important part of avoiding fraud and abuse or noncompliance issues, especially in coding and billing processes involving the federal and state governments. One of the top 10 billing errors determined by federal, state, and private payers involves the incorrect use of modifiers.

Modifiers give payers additional information needed to process a claim. This includes HCPCS Level I (Physician's Current Procedural Terminology [CPT]) and HCPCS Level II codes.

There are two levels of modifiers within the HCPCS coding system. Level I (CPT) and Level II (HCPCS Level II) modifiers apply nationally for many third-party payers and all Medicare Part B claims. Level I, or CPT, modifiers are developed by the American Medical Association (AMA), and HCPCS Level II modifiers are developed by the Centers for Medicare and Medicaid Services (CMS). However, some coding and modifier information issued by CMS differs from the AMA's coding advice in the CPT book; a clear understanding of each payer's rules is necessary to assign such modifiers correctly. Therefore, it is always a good idea to refer to your Medicare provider manual, contractor newsletters, local coverage determinations (LCDs), and national coverage determinations (NCDs) for regional determinations as well as with commercial carriers for specific guidance.

The reporting physician appends a modifier to indicate special circumstances that affect the service provided without affecting the service or procedure description itself. When applicable, the appropriate two-character modifier code should be appended to the usual procedure code number to identify the modifying circumstance.

Similar to the CPT coding system, HCPCS Level II codes also contain modifiers that further define services and items without changing the basic meaning of the CPT or HCPCS code with which they are reported. However, the HCPCS Level II modifiers differ somewhat from their CPT counterparts in that they are composed of either alpha characters or alphanumeric characters that range from A1 to XU.

It is important to note that HCPCS Level II modifiers may be used in conjunction with CPT codes. Likewise, CPT modifiers can be used when reporting HCPCS Level II codes. For example, per Medicare's National Correct Coding Initiative (NCCI) manual, a provider can append modifier 59 to J3471 Injection, hyaluronidase, ovine, preservative free, per 1 USP unit (up to 999 USP units), when reporting the code on more than one line on a claim when greater than 999 units are administered. In some cases, a report may be required to accompany the claim to support the need for a particular modifier's use, especially when the presence of a modifier caused suspension of the claim for manual review and pricing.

For detailed information for reporting CPT modifiers, see appendix A of Optum's *Current Procedural Coding Expert 2025.*

Ambulance Modifiers

For ambulance services modifiers, single alpha characters with distinct definitions are paired to form a two-character modifier. The first character indicates the origin of the patient (e.g., patient's home, physician office, etc.), and the second character indicates the destination of the patient (e.g., hospital, skilled nursing facility, etc.). When ambulance services are reported, the name of the hospital or facility should be included on the claim. If reporting the scene of an accident or acute event (character S) as the origin of the patient, a written description of the actual location of the scene or event must be included with the claim.

The modifier describing the transportation arrangement, either QM or QN, is listed first. The modifier describing the origin and destination are listed second. Each alpha character, with the exception of X, represents either an origin or a destination. Each pair of alpha characters creates one modifier.

First-Listed Ambulance Modifiers

One of the following modifiers must be listed first when reported by institutional-based ambulance provides with every HCPCS code to describe whether the service was provided under arrangement or directly:

QM Ambulance service provided under arrangement by a provider of services

QN Ambulance service furnished directly by a provider of services

Second-Listed Ambulance Modifiers

D Diagnostic or therapeutic site other than "P" or "H" when these are used as origin codes

E Residential, domiciliary, custodial facility (other than 1819 facility)

G Hospital based ESRD facility

H Hospital

I Site of transfer (e.g., airport or helicopter pad) between modes of ambulance transport

J Freestanding ESRD facility

N Skilled nursing facility

P Physician's office

R Residence

S Scene of accident or acute event

X Intermediate stop at physician's office on way to hospital (destination code only)

Note: Modifier X can only be used as a second position modifier representing a destination code. See S0215. For Medicaid, see T codes and T modifiers.

Additional Ambulance Modifiers

GM Multiple patients on one ambulance trip

GY Item or service is statutorily excluded or does not meet the definitions of any Medicare benefit

Note: Append modifier GY when ambulance service is not medically necessary

QL Patient pronounced dead after ambulance called

TP Medical transport, unloaded vehicle

TQ Basic life support transport by a volunteer ambulance provider

HCPCS Modifiers

A1 Dressing for one wound
A2 Dressing for two wounds
A3 Dressing for three wounds
A4 Dressing for four wounds
A5 Dressing for five wounds
A6 Dressing for six wounds
A7 Dressing for seven wounds
A8 Dressing for eight wounds
A9 Dressing for nine or more wounds

Modifiers A1, A2, A3, A4, A5, A6, A7, A8, and A9 wound dressings:

- Modifiers A1–A9 indicate that a primary or secondary dressing on a surgical or debrided wound is being applied. Primary dressings are defined as therapeutic or protective coverings, and secondary dressings are materials applied for a therapeutic or protective function.
- Documentation must indicate the number of wounds being dressed.
- The modifier number reported must correspond to the number of wound dressings applied, not necessarily the number of wounds treated. For example, a patient with three previously debrided wounds may require a secondary dressing on only two wounds, which would be reported with modifier A2.
- Gradient compression stockings are not considered wound dressing and would not be reported with modifiers A1–A9 although A6531 and A6532 are covered for open venous stasis ulcers.

AA Anesthesia services performed personally by anesthesiologist

- Modifier AA has no effect on payment.

AB Audiology service furnished personally by an audiologist without a physician/NPP order for nonacute hearing assessment unrelated to disequilibrium, or hearing aids, or examinations for the purpose of prescribing, fitting, or changing hearing aids; service may be performed once every 12 months, per beneficiary

- This modifier can be appended to certain audiology service codes to indicate that the service was provided without an order by a physician or nonphysician practitioner. Services without an order are allowed once every 12 months per patient for nonacute hearing conditions.

AD Medical supervision by a physician: more than four concurrent anesthesia procedures

- Modifier AD is appended to physician claims when a physician supervised four or more concurrent procedures.
- Payment is made on a 3 base unit amount.
- Base units are assigned by CMS or payers, and the lowest unit value is 3.

Example:

The anesthesiologist is supervising five CRNAs whose services overlapped. The anesthesiologist reports each of these services with modifier AD appended. Each of these services will be reimbursed at the base rate of 3 units regardless of the actual base units assigned.

AE Registered dietician

- Append modifier AE when reporting nutritional services to indicate that an appropriate provider performed the service.

AF Specialty physician
AG Primary physician

Modifiers AF and AG physician designation:

- These modifiers are appended as a physician designation for outpatient services provided in a critical access hospital (CAH) in a designated physician scarcity area (PSA) or health professional shortage area (HPSA).
- Primary care physicians are defined as general practice, family practice, internal medicine, and obstetrics/gynecology for modifier AG.
- Specialty care physicians are defined as specialties other than dental, optometry, chiropractic, or podiatry for modifier AF.

AH Clinical psychologist

- Modifier AH may be appended for services provided by a clinical psychologist who has met the required level of education (PhD) and hours of practice.

AI Principal physician of record

- CMS policies regarding the use of consultation and inpatient services codes were revised in 2010. Under these guidelines the inpatient and office/outpatient consultation services as described by these codes in the CPT book are not covered services. For Medicare patients, inpatient services will be reported only with the initial and subsequent hospital care codes.
- Medicare requires that the initial hospital care code be reported for each physician's first visit with a patient during a specific hospitalization.
- As only one physician may be the admitting physician, CMS has added HCPCS Level II modifier AI Principal physician of record, to be appended to the initial hospital care code reported by the attending physician. All other physicians and consultants report just the initial hospital or nursing facility care code without appending a modifier.
- Subsequent inpatient encounters by any physician are reported using appropriate CPT codes.

AJ Clinical social worker

- Modifier AJ may be appended for services provided by a clinical psychologist who has met the required level of education (MSW) and hours of practice.

AK Nonparticipating physician

- Modifier AK is appended by physicians who are not participating providers with Medicare and are not "opt-out" physicians.
- Nonparticipating providers may see patients in their offices or when providing on-call coverage.
- This is separate from modifier GJ Opt-out physician or practitioner emergency or urgent service.

AM Physician, team member service

- The physician member of a team is required to perform one out of every three visits made by a team member.
- Modifier AM should be appended to indicate a team member visit was performed by the physician.
- Team member visits are denied if only one person rendering services is billing for team services, as this is inappropriate billing practice.
- Modifier AM has no effect on payment.

AO Alternate payment method declined by provider of service
AP Determination of refractive state was not performed in the course of diagnostic ophthalmological examination
AQ Physician providing a service in an unlisted health professional shortage area (HPSA)

- Physician services furnished in a health professional shortage area (HPSA) qualify for a quarterly incentive payment. Global surgery packages may also qualify for these payments. The following guidelines apply for the HPSA incentive payment:
  - If the entire global surgery package is furnished in an HPSA, the procedure code for the surgery should be reported with the applicable HPSA procedure code modifier.
  - If only a portion of the global surgical package is performed in an HPSA, only the portion that is furnished in the HPSA should be reported with the HPSA modifier.
- Only physician services are eligible for the HPSA incentive payment. Do not report nonphysician services with modifier AQ.
- Modifier AQ has no effect on individual claim payment but generates a quarterly bonus payment.
- The name, address, and ZIP code where the service was provided must be included on the electronic or paper billing to be considered for HPSA bonus payment.

AR Physician provider services in a physician scarcity area

- Modifier AR is appended when a physician provides services in an area designated as a physician scarcity area.
- A health scarcity area may be urban or any other area as designated.

AS Physician assistant, nurse practitioner, or clinical nurse specialist services for assistant at surgery

- Medicare will pay assistant-at-surgery services directly at 85 percent of 16 percent of the amount a physician gets under the physician fee schedule (PFS). This is equal to 13.6 percent of the physician amount under the PFS.
- See the PFS for a list of services where modifier AS can be appended.
- Check with third-party payers for their guideline regarding modifier AS.

AT Acute treatment (this modifier should be used when reporting service 98940, 98941, 98942).
- Append to claims for tetanus or rabies injection(s).
- For treatment of an injury or direct exposure to a disease or condition, append modifier AT to both the vaccine code and administration code.
- Modifier AT has no effect on payment for Medicare and many third-party payer claims.
- Do not submit modifier AT on the same line with modifier GA. Per Medicare, effective November 1, 2015, services that include both modifiers on the same detail line will be rejected.

AU Item furnished in conjunction with a urological, ostomy, or tracheostomy supply

AV Item furnished in conjunction with a prosthetic device, prosthetic or orthotic

AW Item furnished in conjunction with a surgical dressing

Modifiers AU, AV, and AW:
- The CMS Pub. 100-04, identifies modifiers AU, AV, and AW for use with durable medical equipment, prosthetics, orthotics, and supplies (DMEPOS).
- Append AU to codes A4217, A4450, A4452, and A5120.
- Append AV to codes A4450, A4452 and A5120.
- Append AW to codes A4450, A4452, A6531, A6532 and A6545
- Payment for these codes is determined by appending the appropriate modifier.
- Other codes for these modifiers may be identified in the future.

AX Item furnished in conjunction with dialysis services
- Modifier AX is appended to the following codes when service is associated with home dialysis: A4215, A4216, A4217, A4244, A4245, A4246, A4247, A4248, A4450, A4452, A4651, A4652, A4657, A4660, A4663, A4670, A4927, A4928, A4930, A4931, A6216, A6250, A6260, A6402, E0210, E1629, E1632, E1637, E1639, J0604, J0606, J0879, J0889, and J1644.
- Drugs eligible for Transitional Drug Add-on Payment Adjustment (TDAPA) must be reported with modifier AX: J0604, J0606, J0879, and J0889
- Items identified as Transitional Add-on Payment Adjustment for New and Innovative Equipment and Supplies (TPNIES) must be reported with modifier AX

AY Item or service furnished to an ESRD patient that is not for the treatment of ESRD

AZ Physician providing a service in a dental health professional shortage area for the purpose of an electronic health record incentive payment

BA Item furnished in conjunction with parenteral enteral nutrition (PEN) services
- Modifier BA is appended to HCPCS code E0776, for IV pole.
- If the IV pole is rented, modifier RR should be listed first, followed by BA.

BL Special acquisition of blood and blood products
- Modifier BL is appended for the blood and blood products as well as the processing and storage of the blood or blood products in the OPPS setting.
- The same date and number of units for the supply, processing, and storage must be reported.
- The OCE editor will reject claims that do not report the supply of the blood and blood products with the processing and storage for the same dates of service and number of units.
- Applies to blood and blood products purchased from another approved agency or from the facility when a charge is made to the patient.

BO Orally administered nutrition, not by feeding tube

BP The beneficiary has been informed of the purchase and rental options and has elected to purchase the item

BR The beneficiary has been informed of the purchase and rental options and has elected to rent the item

BU The beneficiary has been informed of the purchase and rental options and after 30 days has not informed the supplier of his/her decision

Modifiers BP, BR, and BU:
- A purchase decision for a capped rental item must be received prior to the 13th month.
- Modifier BP, BR, or BU must be appended by the 11th month of rental.
- Modifier BU should be replaced with BP or BR if possible.
- Failure to report modifier BP, BR, or BU will result in Medicare error message D911.

CA Procedure payable only in the inpatient setting when performed emergently on an outpatient who expires prior to admission
- CMS instructions (Transmittal A-02-129) indicate that the patient must be an outpatient and must have an emergent, life-threatening condition.
- The procedure reported must be considered an inpatient service (status indicator C) as identified in OPPS.
- The patient must have died without having been admitted as an inpatient. The surgical service, including medical necessity, must be documented and provided upon request.
- Only one inpatient procedure will be considered.
- CMS applies the packaging concept to all services.

CB Service ordered by a renal dialysis facility (RDF) physician as part of the ESRD beneficiary's dialysis benefit, is not part of the composite rate, and is separately reimbursable
- Beginning July 1, 2019, modifier CB is no longer applicable for ESRD dialysis-related lab services outside of the SNF facility.

CC Procedure code change (use CC when the procedure code submitted was changed either for administrative reasons or because an incorrect code was filed)
- Modifier CC is appended by the contractor when the procedure code submitted had to be changed either for administrative reasons or because an incorrect code was filed.
- Payment rule: Payment determination will be based on the new code used by the contractor.
- Modifier CC has no effect on payment.

CD AMCC test has been ordered by an ESRD facility or MCP physician that is part of the composite rate and is not separately billable

CE AMCC test has been ordered by an ESRD facility or MCP physician that is a composite rate test but is beyond the normal frequency covered under the rate and is separately reimbursable based on medical necessity

CF AMCC test has been ordered by an ESRD facility or MCP physician that is not part of the composite rate and is separately billable

Modifiers CD, CE, and CF:
- Automated multichannel chemistry (AMCC) tests are performed to monitor the patient with end-stage renal disease (ESRD).
- AMCC is permitted when more than 50 percent of the AMCC tests are not part of the composite rate.
- All chemistries ordered for an ESRD patient must be reported individually and not as a panel.
- The physician is responsible for determining the appropriate modifier to be appended.

CG Policy criteria applied
- Rural health clinics (RHC) are required to report a HCPCS code for each service provided. RHCs must report modifier CG along with the HCPCS code that best describes the primary reason for the face-to-face visit.
- When a problem-focused service and preventive service are furnished on the same day, modifier CG should be appended only to the code for the service that represents the primary reason for the medically necessary face-to-face visit.
- Modifier CG may be reported twice on the same date of service when reported once for a qualified medical visit and once for a qualified mental health visit.
- Modifier CG should be appended to claims for hemodialysis treatments in excess of the 13 or 14 monthly allowable treatments. This modifier should be submitted by the ESRD facility on the claim line for the date of service that reflects the excess treatment. In this circumstance, modifier CG indicates that the treatment does not meet medical justification requirements and should not be reimbursed separately.

CH Zero percent impaired, limited or restricted

CI At least 1 percent but less than 20 percent impaired, limited or restricted

CJ At least 20 percent but less than 40 percent impaired, limited or restricted

CK At least 40 percent but less than 60 percent impaired, limited or restricted

CL At least 60 percent but less than 80 percent impaired, limited or restricted

CM At least 80 percent but less than 100 percent impaired, limited or restricted

CN 100 percent impaired, limited or restricted

Modifiers CH, CI, CJ, CK, CL, CM, and CN:

- Modifiers CH, CI, CJ, CK, CL, CM, and CN are informational and no longer required for Medicare therapy functional reporting effective January 1, 2019.

CO Outpatient occupational therapy services furnished in whole or in part by an occupational therapy assistant

CQ Outpatient physical therapy services furnished in whole or in part by a physical therapist assistant

Modifiers CO and CQ:

- For practitioners paid under the physician fee schedule, modifiers CO and CQ apply only to services of physical and occupational therapists in private practice.
- Effective for dates of service on and after January 1, 2020, modifiers CQ and CO are required to be appended, when applicable, for services furnished in whole or in part by physical therapy assistants (PTA) and occupational therapy assistants (OSA) on the claim line of the service alongside the respective GP or GO therapy modifier, to identify those PTA and OTA services furnished under a PT or OT plan of care.
- Modifier CO will be reported with modifier GO and modifier CQ will be reported with modifier GP.

CR Catastrophe/disaster related

- Modifier CR was established for providers to use on disaster-related claims.
- It may be used on claims for disaster-related services, even if not performed in the geographic location of the catastrophe or disaster. This includes those who are directly affected by the disaster and may leave the area, as well as rescue, relief, and volunteers who provide aid in the disaster.
- It may be used by providers and DMERC suppliers.
- Condition code DR, disaster related, may also need to be reported for some services.

CS Cost-sharing waived for specified COVID-19 testing-related services that result in an order for or administration of a COVID-19 test and/or used for cost-sharing waived preventive services furnished via telehealth in rural health clinics and federally qualified health centers during the COVID-19 public health emergency

- Append modifier CS when physician/practitioner services lead to the administration of or order for a new COVID-19 lab test.
- Coinsurance and deductible will not apply.
- Cost sharing does not apply to services related to COVID-19 testing. These include services:
  - provided between March 18, 2020, and the end of the PHE
  - result in an order for administration of a test
  - related to providing a test
  - evaluating an individual for determining the need for a test

CT Computed tomography services furnished using equipment that does not meet each of the attributes of the national electrical manufacturers association (NEMA) XR-29-2013 standard

- Modifier CT is appended by hospitals and suppliers who own and report CT services performed using CT scanners not compliant with the NEMA XR-29-2013 standard.
- Use of this modifier results in a 15 percent reduction of payment.

DA Oral health assessment by a licensed health professional other than a dentist

E1 Upper left, eyelid

E2 Lower left, eyelid

E3 Upper right, eyelid

E4 Lower right, eyelid

Modifiers E1, E2, E3, and E4:

- Modifiers E1, E2, E3, and E4 are appended to identify services performed on separate eyelids.
- Modifiers LT and RT should be appended for procedures on the eye globe or ocular adnexa.
- CMS and some private or third-party payers require these modifiers.

EA Erythropoietic stimulating agent (ESA) administered to treat anemia due to anticancer chemotherapy

EB Erythropoietic stimulating agent (ESA) administered to treat anemia due to anticancer radiotherapy

EC Erythropoietic stimulating agent (ESA) administered to treat anemia not due to anticancer radiotherapy or anticancer chemotherapy

Modifiers EA, EB, and EC:

- Non-ESRD patients often receive erythropoiesis stimulating agents (ESA) as part of treatment for anemia.
- Append modifier EA for patients with anemia due to chemotherapy who receive ESA treatment.
- Append modifier EB for patients with anemia due to radiotherapy who receive ESA treatment.
- Append modifier EC for patients who receive ESA treatment for anemia that is not due to radiotherapy or chemotherapy.
- ESAs include epoetin alfa (Epogen, Procrit) and darbepoetin alfa (Aranesp).

ED Hematocrit level has exceeded 39 percent (or hemoglobin level has exceeded 13.0 G/dl) for three or more consecutive billing cycles immediately prior to and including the current cycle

EE Hematocrit level has not exceeded 39 percent (or hemoglobin level has not exceeded 13.0 G/dl) for three or more consecutive billing cycles immediately prior to and including the current cycle

Modifiers ED and EE:

- ESRD patients often receive erythropoiesis stimulating agents (ESA) as part of treatment for anemia.
- ESAs include epoetin alfa (Epogen, Procrit), darbepoetin alfa (Aranesp).
- See modifiers JA and JB to report route of ESA administration.
- Hematocrit levels are verified using lab values.

EJ Subsequent claims for a defined course of therapy, e.g., EPO, sodium hyaluronate, infliximab

- Modifier EJ is appended to report a single treatment in a defined course of multiple treatments.
- Modifier EJ should not be appended on the initial treatment.
- Examples of treatment courses include medications administered by infusion or injection by a provider and not self-administered by the patient.

EM Emergency reserve supply (for ESRD benefit only)

- Modifier EM is to be appended only for supplies dispensed to patients on home dialysis.
- Modifier EM may be appended for more than one item; however, all supplies must be reported in the same month.
- Nonemergent services for that same billing month are reported without modifier EM.
- An emergency reserve of supplies for one month is allowed by Medicare only once in a patient's lifetime.

EP Service provided as part of Medicaid early periodic screening diagnosis and treatment (EPSDT) program

ER Items and services furnished by a provider-based, off-campus emergency department

ET Emergency services

- Modifier ET should be appended to describe dental procedures (D0120–D9999) performed in emergency situations.
- Append modifier ET for emergency services to a skilled nursing facility or end stage renal disease (ESRD) patient that span more than one day.

EX Expatriate beneficiary

- Append to services provided to expatriate beneficiary.
- Not reported for beneficiary traveling out of country.
- Assigned status code C indicating the carrier will price the code.
- Use to report purchased DMEPOS items provided to US address for beneficiary living outside of the US
  - EX must be appended to all line items of claim
  - Excludes oxygen equipment and supplies, parenteral/enteral nutrition equipment and supplies, and rented DME

EY No physician or other licensed health care provider order for this item or service

- Modifier EY cannot be appended to procedures or services when a home health advance beneficiary notice of non-coverage (HHABN) or standard or ABN is required.
- Modifier EY does not override denial for services requiring an order from a physician or provider.
- Modifier EY may be appended to noncovered services.

F1 Left hand, second digit

F2 Left hand, third digit

F3 Left hand, fourth digit

F4 Left hand, fifth digit

F5 Right hand, thumb

F6 Right hand, second digit

F7 Right hand, third digit

F8 Right hand, fourth digit

F9 Right hand, fifth digit

FA Left hand, thumb

Modifiers F1, F2, F3, F4, F5, F6, F7, F8, F9, and FA:

- Modifiers F1-F9 and FA are appended to procedures performed on the fingers.
- Append modifiers affecting reimbursement first (e.g., 51, 80).
- Procedures should be reported with these modifiers appended to identify the specific finger; it is not sufficient to simply increase the number of services in the unit box.

FB Item provided without cost to provider, supplier or practitioner, or full credit received for replaced device (examples, but not limited to, covered under warranty, replaced due to defect, free samples)

- Modifier FB includes, but is not limited to, items covered under warranty, replaced due to defect, or free samples.
- APC reimbursement to facilities will discount any offset amount for the device or supply furnished to the facility.

FC Partial credit received for replaced device

- Facilities must append modifier FC with the procedure code when the device was furnished without cost to the facility (e.g., when the manufacturer furnishes a replacement device when the original device was recalled or failed.
- Append to procedure code specified by CMS.

FP Service provided as part of family planning program

FQ The service was furnished using audio-only communication technology

- Reported for mental health visits using audio-only technology
- Medicare allows the use of modifier FQ or 93, or both "where appropriate and true, since they are identical in meaning."

FR The supervising practitioner was present through two-way, audio/video communication technology

FS Split (or shared) evaluation and management visit

- Medicare requires this modifier for split (or shared) critical care visits or split (or shared) visits in a facility setting. This means that the service is split between a physician and non-physician practitioner. This modifier does not apply to services performed in an outpatient setting.

FT Unrelated evaluation and management (E/M) visit on the same day as another E/M visit or during a global procedure (preoperative, postoperative period, or on the same day as the procedure, as applicable). (Report when an E/M visit is furnished within the global period but is unrelated, or when one or more additional E/M visits furnished on the same day are unrelated)

- Medicare requires this modifier for unrelated critical care services that are performed during the global surgery period or with an E/M service or procedure on the same day.

FX X-ray taken using film

- Reduces payment amount by 20 percent.

FY X-ray taken using computed radiography technology/cassette-based imaging

- Providers must append modifier FY to the CPT code for x-rays taken using computed radiography.
  - A 7 percent payment reduction applies to the technical component for x-ray services provided using computed radiography for dates of service from January 1, 2018, to December 31, 2022.
  - A 10 percent payment reduction applies to these services for dates of service on and after January 1, 2023

G0 Telehealth services for diagnosis, evaluation, or treatment, of symptoms of an acute stroke

- Valid for the following when submitted to identify acute stroke telehealth services performed on and after January 1, 2019:
  - All telehealth distant site codes with place of-service code 02
  - Critical access hospitals (CAH), CAH method II (revenue codes 096X-098X)
  - Telehealth originating site facility fees reported with code Q3014

G1 Most recent URR reading of less than 60

G2 Most recent URR reading of 60 to 64.9

G3 Most recent URR reading of 65 to 69.9

G4 Most recent URR reading of 70 to 74.9

G5 Most recent URR reading of 75 or greater

G6 ESRD patient for whom less than six dialysis sessions have been provided in a month

Modifiers G1, G2, G3, G4, G5, and G6:

- URR is the urea reduction ratio, a calculation that demonstrates the effectiveness of renal dialysis.
- The Balanced Budget Act (BBA) of 1997 requires CMS to develop and implement a method to measure and report on the quality of dialysis services.
- ESRD facilities must append modifiers on or after January 1, 1998, to reflect the most recent urea reduction ratio (URR), along with the unlisted dialysis code, on all claims filed to Medicare for hemodialysis. Consequently, ESRD facilities must also report a HCPCS code with the dialysis revenue code (820, 821, or 829). ESRD facilities (both hospital-based and free-standing) should report the unlisted dialysis code and one of the G modifiers as appropriate on all claims filed for hemodialysis services on or after January 1, 1998. This information provides data to CMS regarding the adequacy of hemodialysis for quality improvement initiatives. ESRD facilities must monitor hemodialysis adequacy monthly for all facility patients. Home hemodialysis patients may be monitored less frequently, but not less often than quarterly.
- Because CMS profiles facilities based on the URR ranges reported, CMS is recommending that dialysis facilities use a standardized methodology for drawing the pre- and postdialysis blood urea nitrogen (BUN) samples that are used in calculating the URR. Facilities may use either the slow flow/stop pump or blood reinfusing sampling technique.
- Medicare requires the URR reading to determine the adequacy of dialysis.
- If fewer than six dialysis sessions have been provided in a month, report services, with modifier G6 appended, to Medicare.

G7 Pregnancy resulted from rape or incest or pregnancy certified by physician as life threatening

- Modifier G7 is appended to the CPT procedure code(s) for abortion services and indicates that the pregnancy resulted from rape or incest, or that the physician considers the pregnancy to be life-threatening to the mother.
- Appending this modifier on a claim communicates to the contractor the physician certifies the abortion meets Medicare's coverage policy. Medicare will cover an abortion when:
  - the pregnancy is the result of an act of rape or incest
  - the woman suffers from a physical disorder, physical injury, or physical illness, including a life-endangering physical condition caused by or arising from the pregnancy itself that would, as certified by a physician, place the woman in danger of death unless an abortion is performe
- Claims submitted with modifier G7 for abortion services may be subject to post-payment review by the contractor.
- Third-party payers, other than Medicare, may not accept this modifier. Individual payers should be queried for claim submission requirements.

G8 Monitored anesthesia care (MAC) for deep complex, complicated, or markedly invasive surgical procedure

G9 Monitored anesthesia care for patient who has history of severe cardiopulmonary condition

Modifiers G8, G9, and QS:

- Modifier G8 is appended only to anesthesia service codes to identify a circumstance in which MAC is provided and the service is a deeply complex, complicated, or markedly invasive surgical procedure.
- Modifier G9 is appended only to anesthesia service codes to identify those circumstances in which a patient with a history of severe cardio-pulmonary conditions has a surgical procedure with MAC.
- Modifier QS should be appended by the anesthesiologist or CRNA to indicate that the type of anesthesia performed was MAC.
  - Modifier QS has no effect on payment.

Note: MAC services are closely watched to ensure medical necessity is documented. ICD-10-CM codes should accurately describe the condition requiring MAC anesthesia. CMS collects data for MAC, even though it is paid the same as general anesthesia. The anesthesiologist or CRNA monitors the patient's vital signs, furnishes the pre-anesthesia exam, prescribes the necessary anesthesia care, administers medication, and furnishes required postoperative anesthesia care. Documentation must be very clear in the record as to the medical necessity for monitored anesthesia care.

GA Waiver of liability statement issued as required by payer policy, individual case

- Modifier GA indicates the physician's office has a signed advance beneficiary notice (ABN) retained in the patient's chart or has provided the notice to the patient and has documented the patient's refusal to sign the ABN.
- The purpose of the waiver of liability is to ensure that the provider will be paid for the services performed and to protect the beneficiary from receiving unnecessary services. Providers who acquire a waiver of liability for a service should append modifier GA directly following a procedure code to indicate that a beneficiary has signed a waiver of liability form. The provider should keep the form on file. No other statement regarding the waiver of liability is required when modifier GA is used. Modifier GA appended to a procedure code is sufficient evidence that the beneficiary has signed an advance notice and has agreed to pay for the service if it is denied as not medically necessary by Medicare. If the beneficiary subsequently requests a review of the denial, Medicare will request the physician to forward a copy of the notice for its files.
- Fully completing claims is an important preventive measure the physician can use to avoid most claim denials when the services are medically reasonable and necessary. Medical necessity denials are often due to a lack of information on the claim to support the medical necessity of the service.
- An advance notice may be applied to an extended course of treatment, provided the notice identifies each service for which Medicare is likely to deny payment. A separate notice is required, however, if additional services for which Medicare is likely to deny payment are furnished later in the course of treatment.
- The Medicare beneficiary is never liable for payment of services that are unbundled from another service. Examples of unbundled services include two hospital visits on the same day by the same physician, removal of sutures by the same physician who performed the surgical procedure, and administration of an injection on the day of an evaluation and management service.
- Modifier GA has no effect on payment; however, potential liability determinations are based, in part, on the use of this modifier.

GB Claim being resubmitted for payment because it is no longer covered under a global payment demonstration

GC This service has been performed in part by a resident under the direction of a teaching physician

Modifiers GC and QK:

- When a teaching physician's services are reported with modifier GC, the teaching physician is certifying that their presence during the key portions of the service and was immediately available during the other portions of the service.
- When an anesthesiologist appends modifier QK for two to four medically directed procedures, modifier GC would not also be appended to the anesthesia code. Only modifier QK is appended.
- When there is a one-on-one situation with a resident and a teaching anesthesiologist (teaching setting) the anesthesiologist appends modifiers AA and GC.
- Modifiers QK and GC are never appended together.
- Modifier GC has no effect on payment.

GE This service has been performed by a resident without the presence of a teaching physician under the primary care exception

- Modifier GE identifies services being reported under the primary care exception to the guideline for governing presence during the key portions of a service by the teaching physician.
- See MLN006347 for appropriate codes to report.
- Modifier GE has no effect on payment.

GF Nonphysician (e.g., nurse practitioner (NP), certified registered nurse anesthetist (CRNA), certified registered nurse (CRN), clinical nurse specialist (CNS), physician assistant (PA) services in a critical access hospital

- Critical access hospitals may use nonphysician providers (NPPs) to provide patient care.
- The professional services of an NPP in the inpatient setting are reported by appending modifier GF.
- The professional service should be reported with the appropriate revenue code (96x, 97x, or 98x).
- Some Medicare contractors do not cover services of CRNAs with modifier GF.

GG Performance and payment of a screening mammogram and diagnostic mammogram on the same patient, same day

- Append modifier GG when additional films are ordered after a radiologist's interpretation of a screening mammogram results in an additional diagnostic mammogram:
  - Modifier GG must be appended to the claim for the diagnostic mammogram, thus allowing the screening and diagnostic films to be paid.
  - Modifier GH is still required when a screening mammogram is converted to a diagnostic mammogram (screening mammogram will not be reported).

GH Diagnostic mammogram converted from screening mammogram on same day

- If a screening mammography study is converted to a diagnostic mammogram by the ordering of additional views to rule out or to better visualize a suspected abnormality seen on the screening views, report the appropriate CPT codes appended with modifier GH.
- The radiologist is considered the ordering physician in this situation and must furnish his/her national provider identifier (NPI) for Medicare claims. Diagnostic mammography claims submitted to Medicare without the ordering physician's NPI will be denied and returned as unprocessable.

GJ "Opt out" physician or practitioner emergency or urgent service

- Append modifier GJ for claims submitted to Medicare for services rendered by an opt-out provider who has not signed a private contract with the Medicare patient requiring either emergent or urgent medical care.
- The provider may not charge the Medicare beneficiary more than what a nonparticipating provider would be permitted to charge and must submit the claim to Medicare on the beneficiary's behalf.
- If modifier GJ is not reported on the claim for emergency or urgent care rendered to a Medicare beneficiary by the opt-out provider, the claim will be denied and returned as unprocessable.

GK Reasonable and necessary item/service associated with a GA or GZ modifier

- Facilities should not report this modifier. Facility claims with this modifier will be returned to the provider for correction. (Transmittal R1472CP,3/6/08)

GL Medically unnecessary upgrade provided instead of nonupgraded item, no charge, no advance beneficiary notice (ABN)

- Modifier GL is allowable only on HHA claims containing DME and is reportable on type of bill 032X, 033X, or 034X per Transmittal R1472CP,3/6/08).

GM Multiple patients on one ambulance trip

- The total number of patients transported should be listed.
- Some Medicare contractors require that the Medicare number and charges for each patient also be submitted.

GN Services delivered under an outpatient speech language pathology plan of care

GO Services delivered under an outpatient occupational therapy plan of care

GP Services delivered under an outpatient physical therapy plan of care

Modifiers GN, GO, and GP:

- Append modifier GN, GO, or GP to therapy services subject to a financial limitation as defined by CMS.
- Appending these modifiers does change the status of noncovered services.
- These modifiers apply to outpatient services only and should be appended with revenue codes 42x, 43x, and 44x (for facility claims).
- Assign the modifier based upon the type of service rendered: GN for speech-language pathology, GO for occupational therapy, and GP for physical therapy.
- The reimbursement limitations do not apply to audiologists, physicians, and NPPs.

An "always therapy" service is a physical, speech-language pathology, or occupational therapy service that must be performed by a qualified therapist under a certified therapy plan of care. A "sometimes therapy" service may be performed by an individual outside of a certified therapy plan of care.

When physicians or NPPs report "always therapy" codes, they must follow the policies of the type of therapy they are providing (e.g., use a plan of care, bill with the appropriate therapy modifier [GP, GO, GN]). A physician or NPP shall not report an "always therapy" code unless the service is provided under a therapy plan of care. When a "sometimes therapy" code is reported by a physician or NPP as a medical service and not under a therapy plan of care, the therapy modifier should not be appended.

GQ Via asynchronous telecommunications system

Modifiers GQ and GT:

- Modifiers GQ and GT apply to telehealth services provided in an approved remote location as identified in CMS program memorandum AB-01-69.
- Beginning October 1, 2018, modifier GT should only be reported on institutional claims billed by a Critical Access Hospital (CAH) Method II.
- HCPCS code Q3014 Telehealth originating site facility fee, is reported at the patient site.

GQ

- The provider reports the service provided with the appropriate CPT code and modifier GQ appended for service rendered via asynchronous telecommunications or GT for service rendered via interactive audio and video telecommunications.
  - Modifier GQ indicates an asynchronous telecommunications system such as "store and forward" for transmission of medical files.
  - Except for demonstrations in Alaska and Hawaii, all telehealth services must be interactive.

GR This service was performed in whole or in part by a resident in a Department of Veterans Affairs medical center or clinic, supervised in accordance with VA policy

- Modifier GR is appended only for services rendered in a VA medical center or clinic.
- Resident services provided in a non-VA facility are reported with modifiers GC or GE.

GS Dosage of erythropoietin stimulating agent has been reduced and maintained in response to hematocrit or hemoglobin level

- Modifier GS is appended for national claims monitoring for ESA's administered in Medicare dialysis facilities.
- Not applicable to Part B claims.

GT Via interactive audio and video telecommunication systems

See modifier GQ notes.

GU Waiver of liability statement issued as required by payer policy, routine notice

GV Attending physician not employed or paid under arrangement by the patient's hospice provider

GW Service not related to the hospice patient's terminal condition

Modifiers GV and GW:

- Modifier GV must be appended to all services a nurse practitioner provides to hospice patients.
- The patient may choose to receive hospice care from a physician not employed by the hospice provider. These services are not counted towards the hospice financial cap.
- Medically necessary services that are not part of the patient's hospice care should be reported with modifier GW.
- Failure to append modifier GV or GW to the codes for services rendered to beneficiaries enrolled in hospice care will result in denial.

GX Notice of liability issued, voluntary under payer policy

- Modifier GX is appended by providers to identify when a **voluntary** advance beneficiary notice (ABN) was issued for a service.
- Append modifier GA when a **required** ABN was issued for a service.
- Noncovered services submitted with modifier GX will be denied by the contractor as a beneficiary liability so that the claim may be submitted to secondary payers.
- Do not report GX with modifiers EY, GA, GL, GZ, KB, QL, and TQ.

GY Item or service statutorily excluded, does not meet the definition of any Medicare benefit or, for non-Medicare insurers, is not a contract benefit

- Do not append to bundled procedure or add-on codes.
- Append to items or services that are statutorily excluded from Medicare.
- Charges should be shown as noncovered.
- Use will result in claim denial and patient/beneficiary liability.
- An ABN is not necessary for these items/services.
- May be appended in combination with modifier GX.

GZ Item or service expected to be denied as not reasonable and necessary

Charges should be shown as noncovered. Provider is held liable for charges. Append modifier GZ when an ABN has not been issued, but the provider determines after the service has been performed that it was not covered. For example, a laboratory test that has specific diagnosis criteria, but the hospital does not check the diagnosis until after the test has been run.

H9 Court-ordered

HA Child/adolescent program

HB Adult program, nongeriatric

HC Adult program, geriatric

HD Pregnant/parenting women's program

HE Mental health program

HF Substance abuse program

HG Opioid addiction treatment program

HH Integrated mental health/substance abuse program

HI Integrated mental health and intellectual disability/developmental disabilities program

HJ Employee assistance program

HK Specialized mental health programs for high-risk populations

HL Intern

HM Less than bachelor degree level

HN Bachelors degree level

HO Masters degree level

HP Doctoral level

HQ Group setting

HR Family/couple with client present

HS Family/couple without client present

HT Multidisciplinary team

HU Funded by child welfare agency

HV Funded state addictions agency

HW Funded by state mental health agency

HX Funded by county/local agency

HY Funded by juvenile justice agency

HZ Funded by criminal justice agency

Modifiers HA, HB, HC, HD, HE, HF, HG, HH, HI, HJ, HK, HL, HM, HN, HO, HP, HQ, HR, HS, HT, HU, HV, HW, HX, HY, and HZ:

- Modifiers in this section are required for many state Medicaid programs.
- Many of these modifiers are related to behavioral health programs.
- Modifiers HA, HB, HC, and HD may be appended in addition to HE, HF, HG, HH, HI, and HK to further define the type of service rendered.
- Place of service must be coordinated for modifiers HE, HF, HG, HH, HI, and HK.
- Modifier HJ should be appended to report services in conjunction with or by referral from an employee assistance program.
- Modifiers HL, HM, HN, HO, and HP are usually reported in conjunction with behavioral health services.
- Modifier HR and HS may be appended for conjoint therapy/marriage counseling.
- Modifier HU, HV, HW, HX, HY, or HZ should be appended to identify behavioral health or other programs funded by other sources.
- Third-party payers do not recognize many of the modifiers in this section.
- Some state Medicaid programs require NPP providers to report HN, HO, or HP.

J1 Competitive acquisition program no-pay submission for a prescription number

J2 Competitive acquisition program, restocking of emergency drugs after emergency administration

- Modifier J2 is appended only when the participating competitive acquisition program (CAP) physician certifies the following:
  - The drugs were required immediately.
  - The participating CAP physician could not have anticipated the need for the drugs.
  - The approved CAP vendor could not have delivered the drugs in a timely manner.
  - The drugs were administered in an emergency situation.
  - The participating CAP physician is maintaining documentation to validate the information in the four bullets above.
  - The participating CAP physician will provide this documentation to the local contractor upon request.

J3 Competitive acquisition program (CAP), drug not available through CAP as written, reimbursed under average sales price methodology

- Modifier J3 is appended only when the participating CAP physician certifies the following:
  - A specific drug was medically necessary.
  - The selected approved CAP vendor could not provide that specific brand and/or NDC.
  - Documentation to validate the information in the two previous bullets is being maintained by the participating CAP physician and will be provided upon the local contractor's request.

J4 DMEPOS item subject to DMEPOS competitive bidding program that is furnished by a hospital upon discharge

- Modifier J4 is specifically for reporting by hospitals.
- Modifier J4 is appended to identify the dispensing of DMEPOS items that are part of the competitive bidding program.

J5 Off-the-shelf orthotic subject to DMEPOS competitive bidding program that is furnished as part of a physical therapist or occupational therapist professional service

- Modifier J5 should be appended to codes L0450, L0455, L0457, L0467, L0469, L0621, L0623, L0625, L0628, L0641, L0642, L0643, L0648, L0649, L0650, and L0651 for OTS back braces.
- Modifier J5 should be appended to codes L1812, L1830, L1833, L1836, L1850, L1851, and L1852 for OTS knee braces.

JA Administered intravenously

JB Administered subcutaneously

Modifiers JA and JB:

- ESRD patients often receive erythropoiesis stimulating agents (ESA) as part of treatment for anemia.
- ESA is reported with codes Q4081, J0882, and J0887.
- ESAs include epoetin alfa (Epogen, Procrit) and darbepoetin alfa (Aranesp).
- Append modifier JA to report administration of ESA to ESRD patients when administered intravenously.
- Append modifier JB to report administration of ESA to ESRD patients when administered subcutaneously.
- When ESAs are administered both intravenously and subcutaneously, two services must be reported with the appropriate modifiers appended.
- See modifiers ED and EE to report hematocrit and hemoglobin values.
- Report non-ESRD-related ESA treatment with modifier EA, EB, or EC appended.

JC Skin substitute used as a graft

JD Skin substitute not used as a graft

JE Administered via dialysate

- CMS Transmittal 2688 issued April 26, 2013, instruction states that modifier JE is to be appended on all ESRD claims for drugs and biologicals provided to ESRD beneficiaries via the dialysate solution—a solution comprised of purified water, glucose, and electrolytes. The strength of the solution mirrors the electrolytes found naturally in blood and its purpose is to regulate electrolytes and maintain the acid-base balance and eliminate waste products in dialysis patients.
- Modifier JE is the third and newest route of administration (ROA) modifier created to assist CMS in monitoring which specific drugs/biologicals are being provided via dialysate; the other two ROA modifiers are JA and JB.
- It is designed to assist in preventing the inappropriate assignment of modifier AY Item or service furnished to an ESRD patient that is not for the treatment of ESRD.
- Append modifier JE with the following categories of drugs when administered in an ESRD facility by facility staff:
  - Antibiotics
  - Analgesics
  - Anabolics
  - Hematinics
  - Muscle relaxants
  - Sedatives
  - Tranquilizers
  - Thrombolytics (used to declot CVCs)

JG ~~Drug or biological acquired with 340B drug pricing program discount, reported for informational purposes~~

JK One month supply or less of drug or biological

JL Three month supply of drug or biological

JW Drug amount discarded/not administered to any patient

- Modifier JW is appended to CPT and/or HCPCS codes for drugs where the dosage listed is greater than ordered and administered by the provider.
- Modifier JW indicates the overage was discarded and not part of a multidose vial.
- Modifier JW should not be appended to a code describing the highest dose if a code for a lesser dose is available.
- Effective January 2017, CMS requires modifier JW to be appended with Part B claims for unused drugs or biologicals from single-use vials or single-use packages that are properly discarded and that the discarded drug or biological is documented in the patient's medical record.
- Do not append to claims for CAP drugs and biologicals.

JZ Zero drug amount discarded/not administered to any patient

- Effective July 1, 2023, modifier JZ must be appended with Part B claims when there is no drug amount discarded from a single-dose container or single-use package.

K0 Lower extremity prosthesis functional level 0 - does not have the ability or potential to ambulate or transfer safely with or without assistance and a prosthesis does not enhance their quality of life or mobility.

K1 Lower extremity prosthesis functional level 1 - has the ability or potential to use a prosthesis for transfers or ambulation on level surfaces at fixed cadence, typical of the limited and unlimited household ambulator

K2 Lower extremity prosthesis functional level 2 - has the ability or potential for ambulation with the ability to traverse low level environmental barriers such as curbs, stairs or uneven surfaces, typical of the limited community ambulator

K3 Lower extremity prosthesis functional level 3 - has the ability or potential for ambulation with variable cadence, typical of the community ambulator who has the ability to transverse most environmental barriers and may have vocational, therapeutic, or exercise activity that demands prosthetic utilization beyond simple locomotion

K4 Lower extremity prosthesis functional level 4 - has the ability or potential for prosthetic ambulation that exceeds the basic ambulation skills, exhibiting high impact, stress, or energy levels, typical of the prosthetic demands of the child, active adult, or athlete

KA Add on option/accessory for wheelchair

KB Beneficiary requested upgrade for ABN, more than four modifiers identified on claim

KC Replacement of special power wheelchair interface

KD Drug or biological infused through DME

- Modifier KD reportable only by DME suppliers.

KE Bid under round one of the DMEPOS competitive bidding program for use with noncompetitive bid base equipment

KF Item designated by FDA as Class III device

- Reported for elevating/stair climbing power wheelchairs.

KG DMEPOS item subject to DMEPOS competitive bidding program number 1

KH DMEPOS item, initial claim, purchase or first month rental

KI DMEPOS item, second or third month rental

Modifiers KH and KI:

- DMEPOS is the acronym for durable medical equipment, prosthetics, orthotics, and supplies.
- Effective October 1, 2018, modifier KH is no longer required on purchased capped rental DME or parenteral/enteral services.
- Standard hospital beds are reported with HCPCS Level II codes E0250–E0266 or E0290–E0297. Hospital beds with a mattress that is wider than 36 inches and that can support a patient weighing more than 300 pounds must be submitted using code E1399 Durable medical equipment, miscellaneous.
- These beds are considered capped rental and, therefore, payment will be made only on a rental basis. The appropriate modifier (KH, KI) must be appended and the rent/purchase option must be offered in the 10th rental month, as with all capped rental items.
- Append modifier RR for rented DME.

KJ DMEPOS item, parenteral enteral nutrition (PEN) pump or capped rental, months four to fifteen

- Report with modifier RR for rented DME.

KK DMEPOS item subject to DMEPOS competitive bidding program number 2

KL DMEPOS item delivered via mail

KM Replacement of facial prosthesis including new impression/moulage

KN Replacement of facial prosthesis using previous master model

- Report with codes L8040 thru L8047 for replacement of facial prostheses.

KO Single drug unit dose formulation

KP First drug of a multiple drug unit dose formulation

KQ Second or subsequent drug of a multiple drug unit dose formulation

Modifiers KO, KP, and KQ:

- Modifiers KO, KP, and KQ may be appended to report drugs used or supplied by DMERCs.
- Modifier KO may be appended alone.
- Modifiers KP and KQ must both be appended to the same claim; it would be inappropriate to report KP on a line item and not report KQ on one or more subsequent line items.

KR Rental item, billing for partial month

- Report with modifier RR for rented DME.

KS Glucose monitor supply for diabetic beneficiary not treated with insulin

KT Beneficiary resides in a competitive bidding area and travels outside that competitive bidding area and receives a competitive bid item

KU DMEPOS item subject to DMEPOS competitive bidding program number 3

KV DMEPOS item subject to DMEPOS competitive bidding program that is furnished as part of a professional service

KW DMEPOS item subject to DMEPOS competitive bidding program number 4

KX Requirements specified in the medical policy have been met

- Modifier KX is appended to confirm that specific documentation requirements outlined in the Local Coverage Determination (LCD) or other applicable policy have been met.
- Append on claims for speech language pathology, physical therapy, or occupational therapy services.
  - Append to each procedure code when the therapy service has met the monetary limit (cap), is considered reasonable and necessary, and qualifies for the therapy cap exception.
  - Append following the appropriate therapy modifiers (GN, GO, and GP).
- Append on dental codes for dental services that are medically necessary prior to a covered surgical procedure for Medicare claims.
  - Oral infections must be treated prior to some surgeries such as major organ procedures.

KY DMEPOS item subject to DMEPOS competitive bidding program number 5

- Append to report standard power and manual wheelchair accessories
- Append for non-competitive bid wheelchair
  - Append modifier KE for beneficiary who resides in a competitive bid area

KZ New coverage not implemented by managed care

LC Left circumflex coronary artery

LD Left anterior descending coronary artery

LM Left main coronary artery

Modifiers LC, LD, LM, RC, and RI:

- Modifiers LC, LD, LM, RC, and RI are appended when more than one intervention is required on a major vessel and its branches. CPT codes describe codes for coronary angioplasty, atherectomy, and stent procedures in terms of the "initial" vessel and a "subsequent" vessel.
- Note that modifiers LC, LD, and RC are included in the CPT book.
- Modifiers LM and RI are not in the CPT book but should be appended to report these arteries.
- Modifiers LC, LD, LM, RC, and RI may be appended to bypass a CCI edit when correctly applied to an edit that allows a modifier.

  Note: Do not report additional vessel codes without first billing the single vessel code.

  The three procedures (stent, balloon angioplasty, and atherectomy) have two codes each: a single vessel code and an additional vessel code. The single-vessel code is reported only the first time that intervention is used during the interventional session. If the intervention is performed on more than one vessel, the additional vessel code(s) should be reported.

LL Lease/rental (use the LL modifier when DME equipment rental is to be applied against the purchase price)

- Append modifier LL when the DME rental amount is to be applied against the final purchase price of the DME.

LR Laboratory round trip

- Modifier LR should be appended to charges submitted by an independent lab with code P9604.

LS FDA-monitored intraocular lens implant

LT Left side (used to identify procedures performed on the left side of the body)

- Modifier LT indicates the side of the body on which a procedure is performed. It does not indicate a bilateral procedure.
- Many procedure codes require a physician to indicate the side of the body on which a procedure was performed by using modifiers RT and LT.
- When billing for a separately identifiable/unrelated surgical procedure performed during the postoperative period of another surgical procedure, procedure code modifiers RT (right) and LT (left) must be indicated on the claim as appropriate. In addition, modifier 79 Unrelated procedure or service by the same physician or other qualified health care professional during the postoperative period, must be submitted on the subsequent claim.
- Modifiers LT and RT have no effect on payment; however, failure to append when appropriate could result in delay or denial (or partial denial) of the claim.

LU Fractionated payment

M2 Medicare secondary payer (MSP)

MA Ordering professional is not required to consult a Clinical Decision Support Mechanism due to service being rendered to a patient with a suspected or confirmed emergency medical condition

MB Ordering professional is not required to consult a Clinical Decision Support Mechanism due to the significant hardship exception of insufficient internet access

MC Ordering professional is not required to consult a Clinical Decision Support Mechanism due to the significant hardship exception of electronic health record or Clinical Decision Support Mechanism vendor issues

MD Ordering professional is not required to consult a Clinical Decision Support Mechanism due to the significant hardship exception of extreme and uncontrollable circumstances

ME The order for this service adheres to Appropriate Use Criteria in the Clinical Decision Support Mechanism consulted by the ordering professional

MF The order for this service does not adhere to the Appropriate Use Criteria in the Clinical Decision Support Mechanism consulted by the ordering professional

MG The order for this service does not have applicable Appropriate Use Criteria in the qualified Clinical Decision Support Mechanism consulted by the ordering professional

MH Unknown if ordering professional consulted a Clinical Decision Support Mechanism for this service, related information was not provided to the furnishing professional or provider

MS Six month maintenance and servicing fee for reasonable and necessary parts and labor which are not covered under any manufacturer or supplier warranty

N1 Group 1 oxygen coverage criteria met

N2 Group 2 oxygen coverage criteria met

N3 Group 3 oxygen coverage criteria met

NB Nebulizer system, any type, FDA-cleared for use with specific drug

NR New when rented (use the NR modifier when DME which was new at the time of rental is subsequently purchased)

- Append modifier NR when the DME, which was new at the time of its rental, is subsequently purchased.

NU New equipment

P1 A normal healthy patient

P2 A patient with mild systemic disease

P3 A patient with severe systemic disease

P4 A patient with severe systemic disease that is a constant threat to life

P5 A moribund patient who is not expected to survive without the operation

P6 A declared brain-dead patient whose organs are being removed for donor purposes

Modifiers P1-P6:

- Physical status modifiers are reported only with anesthesia procedure codes.
- Report physical status modifiers only on claims being submitted to commercial insurance carriers. Verify specific requirements with the specific payer as some commercial carriers do not recognize physical status modifiers.
- Modifiers P1–P6 should not be appended to anesthesia procedures provided to Medicare patients.

PA Surgical or other invasive procedure on wrong body part

PB Surgical or other invasive procedure on wrong patient

PC Wrong surgery or other invasive procedure on patient

Modifiers PA, PB, and PC:

- Medicare does not reimburse physicians, other healthcare professionals, hospitals, or other facilities for hospitalizations or other services related to a surgical or other invasive procedure performed in error.
- All related services provided during the same hospitalization in which the error occurred are not covered.
- Providers should append modifier PA, PB, or PC to the codes reported to describe the erroneous surgery or invasive procedure performed on the patient. All HCPCS codes containing one of these modifiers will be denied reimbursement.
- Hospitals are required to report a no-pay claim with the noncovered procedures and services related to the erroneous surgery and append the applicable erroneous surgery modifier.

PD Diagnostic or related nondiagnostic item or service provided in a wholly owned or operated entity to a patient who is admitted as an inpatient within three days

- Modifier PD is appended to the entity's preadmission diagnostic- or admission-related nondiagnostic services that are subject to the three-day payment window.
- Addition of modifier PD on a claim will ensure that CMS pays only the professional component of codes with both a professional and technical component if provided in the one- or three-calendar day payment window; additionally, codes that do not have a split between professional and technical components will be processed at the facility rate.

PI Positron emission tomography (PET) or pet/computed tomography (CT) to inform the initial treatment strategy of tumors that are biopsy proven or strongly suspected of being cancerous based on other diagnostic testing

Modifiers PI and PS:

- Providers are required to identify the procedure as either for initial treatment strategy or subsequent treatment strategy by appending the appropriate modifier, PI or PS.
- PI is appended to the code for PET or PET/CT when performed to identify the initial treatment strategy for tumors that are biopsy proven or strongly suspected of being cancerous based on other diagnostic testing.
- PS identifies PET or PET/CT performed to identify the subsequent treatment strategy of cancerous tumors when the treating physician determines that the PET study is needed to inform the payer regarding subsequent anti-tumor strategy.

PL Progressive addition lenses

PM Post mortem

- Modifier PM is appended by hospices for visits by employed nurses, aides, social workers, and therapists, including length of visits (rounded to the nearest 15 minute increment), occurring on the date of death after the patient has expired.
- Report appropriate revenue code with the HCPCS code for the specific discipline in units of 15-minute increments with modifier PM appended.

PN Nonexcepted service provided at an off-campus, outpatient, provider-based department of a hospital

- Modifier PN must be appended to all non-excepted outpatient hospital items and services reported on an institutional claim that is furnished in an off-campus provider-based department of a hospital.
- Modifier PN is not required for dedicated ED services.

PO Excepted service provided at an off-campus, outpatient, provider-based department of a hospital

- Append modifier PO to codes for outpatient hospital services rendered in an off-campus physician-based department of an inpatient facility.
- Modifier PO is not required for ED services.
- Modifier PO is to be appended with **all** outpatient hospital **items and services** furnished in an excepted off-campus provider-based department of a hospital.

PS Positron emission tomography (PET) or pet/computed tomography (CT) to inform the subsequent treatment strategy of cancerous tumors when the beneficiary's treating physician determines that the PET study is needed to inform subsequent antitumor strategy

- See modifier PI.

PT Colorectal cancer screening test; converted to diagnostic test or other procedure

- Append to HCPCS codes G0104, G0105, or G0121.

Q0 Investigational clinical service provided in a clinical research study that is in an approved clinical research study

Q1 Routine clinical service provided in a clinical research study that is in an approved clinical research study

Q2 Demonstration procedure/service

Q3 Live kidney donor surgery and related services

- Append modifier Q3 to identify postoperative live kidney donor services, which are reimbursed at 100 percent of the Medicare fee schedule amount.

Q4 Service for ordering/referring physician qualifies as a service exemption

- Append modifier Q4 when the ordering or referring provider has a financial relationship with the entity performing the service and when the service qualifies as one of the service-related exemptions.

Q5 Service furnished under a reciprocal billing arrangement by a substitute physician or by a substitute physical therapist furnishing outpatient physical therapy services in a health professional shortage area, a medically underserved area, or a rural area

- Modifier Q5 is appended to a procedure code to indicate the service was provided by a substitute physician (locum tenens) in a health professional shortage, medical underserved, or rural area. The regular physician should keep a record on file of each service provided by the substitute physician, associated with the substitute physician's NPI, and make this record available to Medicare upon request.
- Modifier Q5 may also be used to report substitute physical therapy in a health professional shortage, medical underserved, or rural area.
- Modifier Q5 has no effect on payment.

Q6 Service furnished under a fee-for-time compensation arrangement by a substitute physician or by a substitute physical therapist furnishing outpatient physical therapy services in a health professional shortage area, a medically underserved area, or a rural area

- Substitute physicians (locum tenens) generally have no practice of their own; they usually move from area to area as needed. The patient's regular physician typically pays the substitute physician for their services on a per diem or comparable fee-for-time basis.
- The patient's regular physician may submit a claim and receive Medicare Part B payment for a covered and medically necessary visit in a health professional shortage, medical underserved, or rural area of a substitute physician who is not an employee of the regular physician and whose services for patients of the regular physician are not restricted to the regular physician's office.
- The regular physician identifies the visits as substitute physician services by appending modifier Q6 to the services provided by the locum tenens physician.
- The substitute physician should not provide the visit services to Medicare patients for a continuous period of longer than 60 days.
- Modifier Q6 may also be used to report substitute physical therapy in a health professional shortage, medical underserved, or rural area when paid under a time basis.
- Modifier Q6 has no effect on payment.

Q7 One Class A finding

Class A findings:

- Nontraumatic amputation of foot or integral skeletal portions thereof

Q8 Two Class B findings

Class B findings:

- Absent posterior tibial pulse
- Absent dorsalis pedis pulse
- Advance trophic changes such as (three required):
  - Hair growth (decrease or absence)
  - Nail changes (thickening)
  - Pigmentary changes (discoloration)
  - Skin texture (thin, shiny)
  - Skin color (rubor or redness)

Q9 One Class B and two Class C findings

Class C findings:

- Claudication
- Temperature changes (e.g., cold feet)
- Edema
- Paresthesia
- Burning

Modifiers Q7, Q8, and Q9—Foot care:

- Modifiers Q7–Q9 were established to allow the provider to report class findings without needing to write a narrative description on the claim form or submit additional documentation with the claim. This modifier should be appended to foot care procedures to indicate the severity of the patient's systemic condition and justify the medical necessity of a procedure that is usually denied as routine.
- Documentation of the systemic conditions and class findings must be in the patient's record. The record must be maintained in the physician's office and available for medical review by the contractor. Documentation should indicate the course of treatment and length of treatment for infectious conditions. Documentation should include the affected toes, including the clinical evidence of mycosis, the manner in which and to what extent the nails were debrided, and the antifungal agent used in the office note/progress note.
- In addition, a description of the qualifying symptoms should be documented.
- Ambulatory patients must exhibit a marked limitation in ambulation, pain, or secondary infection resulting from thickening and dystrophy.
- Nonambulatory patients must suffer from pain or secondary infection resulting from thickening and dystrophy of the infected nail plate.
- Routine foot care is excluded from Medicare coverage.
- General diagnoses such as arteriosclerotic heart disease (ASHD), circulatory problems, vascular disease, and venous insufficiency are not sufficient to support payment for routine foot care.

QA Prescribed amounts of stationary oxygen for daytime use while at rest and nighttime use differ and the average of the two amounts is less than 1 liter per minute (LPM)

- Modifier QA is appended when the oxygen prescribed is less than 1 liter per minute (LPM) and the prescribed flow rate differs for nighttime and daytime use.
- The monthly allowed amount is reduced by 50 percent.

QB Prescribed amounts of stationary oxygen for daytime use while at rest and nighttime use differ and the average of the two amounts exceeds 4 liters per minute (LPM) and portable oxygen is prescribed

- Modifier QB is appended when stationary oxygen amounts for daytime use and nighttime use differ and the average amount between the two is greater than 4 LPM and portable oxygen is prescribed. This results in an increase to the payment for stationary oxygen. Either an increase of 50 percent to the monthly payment amount or the fee schedule amount for the portable oxygen add-on, whichever is higher is used.
- When different flow rates for the stationary oxygen and portable oxygen are required, use the flow rate for the stationary equipment.

QC Single channel monitoring

QD Recording and storage in solid state memory by a digital recorder

QE Prescribed amount of stationary oxygen while at rest is less than 1 liter per minute (LPM)

QF Prescribed amount of stationary oxygen while at rest exceeds 4 liters per minute (LPM) and portable oxygen is prescribed

QG Prescribed amount of stationary oxygen while at rest is greater than 4 liters per minute (LPM)

QH Oxygen conserving device is being used with an oxygen delivery system

Modifiers QE, QF, QG, and QH:

- CMS Pub. 100-04, Chapter 20, Section 130.6, indicates that modifiers QE, QF, QG, and QH are to be appended when reporting home oxygen.
- Modifier QE is appended when the stationary oxygen prescribed is less than 1 liter per minute (LPM); the allowed amount will be reduced by 50 percent.
- Modifier QF is appended when stationary oxygen at rest is greater than 4 LPM and portable oxygen is also prescribed. This results in an increase to the payment for stationary oxygen. Either an increase of 50 percent to the monthly payment amount or the fee schedule amount for the portable oxygen add-on, whichever is higher is used.
  - When different flow rates for the stationary oxygen and portable oxygen are required, use the flow rate for the stationary equipment.
- Home health agencies and suppliers providing oxygen-conserving devices append modifier QH to the charge for the device.

QJ Services/items provided to a prisoner or patient in state or local custody; however, the state or local government, as applicable, meets the requirements in 42 CFR 411.4 (B)

QK Medical direction of two, three, or four concurrent anesthesia procedures involving qualified individuals

- See modifier GC.

QL Patient pronounced dead after ambulance called

QM Ambulance service provided under arrangement by a provider of services

QN Ambulance service furnished directly by a provider of services

Modifiers QM and QN:

- Modifiers QM and QN should be appended when a patient has an inpatient status at one hospital and is transferred to another hospital or facility for tests or treatment and then is returned to the first hospital.
- These modifiers are valid for Medicare; however, the service would be denied under Medicare Part B since it is considered a Medicare Part A expense.

QP Documentation is on file showing that the laboratory test(s) was ordered individually or ordered as a CPT-recognized panel other than automated profile codes 80002-80019, G0058, G0059, and G0060

- Sufficient documentation includes the requisition form showing that the physician ordered the individual tests either by code or the corresponding code definition.
- The individual tests that constitute an organ- or disease-related CPT panel do not need to be ordered individually for the laboratory to use modifier QP. The laboratory may report using the CPT code for organ- or disease-oriented panel, with modifier QP appended, when the physician orders the components of the panel.
- CMS does not require laboratories to use this modifier, but some contractors strongly advise its use.

QQ Ordering professional consulted a qualified clinical decision support mechanism for this service and the related data was provided to the furnishing professional

QR Prescribed amounts of stationary oxygen for daytime use while at rest and nighttime use differ and the average of the two amounts is greater than 4 liters per minute (LPM)

- Modifier QR is appended when stationary oxygen amounts for daytime use and nighttime use differ and the average amount between the two is greater than 4 LPM.
- The monthly allowed amount is increased by 50 percent.

QS Monitored anesthesiology care service

- See modifiers G8 and G9.

QT Recording and storage on tape by an analog tape recorder

QW CLIA waived test

- Modifier QW is to be appended for all codes that were designated as waived tests after 1996. For codes approved prior to 1996, the existing codes should be reported without the modifier.
- Modifier QW must be appended in the first modifier field.
- For additional information on CLIA-waived tests, refer to the CMS website: https://www.cms.gov/medicare/quality/clinical-laboratory-improvement-amendments.

QX CRNA service: with medical direction by a physician

- Modifier QX is appended on CRNA or anesthetist assistant (AA) claims to inform the payer a CRNA/AA provided the service with direction by an anesthesiologist.
- Reduces payment amount by 50 percent.

QY Medical direction of one certified registered nurse anesthetist (CRNA) by an anesthesiologist

- Modifier QY is appended by the anesthesiologist when directing a CRNA in a single case.

QZ CRNA service: without medical direction by a physician

- Modifier QZ is appended when a CRNA performs the anesthesia without any direction by a physician.
- Payment is usually based on 100 percent of the fee schedule.

RA Replacement of a DME, orthotic or prosthetic item

RB Replacement of a part of a DME, orthotic or prosthetic item furnished as part of a repair

Modifiers RA and RB:

- Modifier RA is specific to replacement of a DME item, not repair of the item.
- Modifier RB is appended to report repair of a DME item by replacing a part of the item.

RC Right coronary artery

- See LC, LD, and LM.

RD Drug provided to beneficiary, but not administered "incident-to"

RE Furnished in full compliance with FDA-mandated risk evaluation and mitigation strategy (REMS)

RI Ramus intermedius coronary artery

- See LC, LD, and LM.

RR Rental (use the RR modifier when DME is to be rented)

- Append modifier RR in conjunction with the appropriate rental modifiers KH, KI, and KJ.
- Modifier RR is listed first on the HCPCS Level II code for the DME followed by the appropriate rental modifier in the above bullet.

RT Right side (used to identify procedures performed on the right side of the body)

- Modifier RT indicates the side of the body on which a procedure is performed. It does not indicate a bilateral procedure.
- Many procedure codes require a physician to indicate the side of the body on which a procedure was performed by using modifiers RT and LT.
- When billing for a separately identifiable/unrelated surgical procedure performed during the postoperative period of another surgical procedure, procedure code modifiers RT (right) and LT (left) must be indicated on the claim as appropriate. In addition, modifier 79 Unrelated procedure or service by the same physician or other qualified health care professional during the postoperative period, must be submitted on the subsequent claim.
- Modifiers LT and RT have no effect on payment; however, failure to append when appropriate could result in delay or denial (or partial denial) of the claim.

SA Nurse practitioner rendering service in collaboration with a physician

SB Nurse midwife

Modifiers SA and SB:

- Modifiers SA and SB are required by some state Medicaid programs and third-party payers to indicate that a nurse practitioner (NP) or certified nurse midwife (CNM) provided the service.
- Modifier SA is appended when the physician reports the NP's services. Some state Medicaid programs do not require modifier SA if the NP bills under his/her own provider number.
- Modifier SB is appended when the service is provided by a CNM. Some states allow a CNM to practice independently if a physician coverage arrangement has been made.

SC Medically necessary service or supply

SD Services provided by registered nurse with specialized, highly technical home infusion training

SE State and/or federally funded programs/services

SF Second opinion ordered by a professional review organization (PRO) per section 9401, p.l. 99-272 (100 percent reimbursement - no Medicare deductible or coinsurance)

- Append modifier SF when the second opinion is ordered or requested by a professional review organization.
- For Medicare beneficiaries, when this modifier is appended the service is eligible for 100 percent reimbursement. The usual deductible and/or coinsurance amounts are not applied.

SG Ambulatory surgical center (ASC) facility service

- ASCs are not required to append modifier SG on ASC facility services they report to Medicare.
- Payment for the ASC facility service for Medicare patients is based on the appropriate APC taken from the ASC payment list upon release of the final rule.

SH Second concurrently administered infusion therapy

SJ Third or more concurrently administered infusion therapy

Modifiers SD, SH, and SJ:

- Modifiers SD, SH, and SJ are required by many state Medicaid programs.
- Modifiers SD, SH, and SJ are appended to codes reported by HHAs.

SK Member of high-risk population (use only with codes for immunization)

SL State supplied vaccine

SM Second surgical opinion

SN Third surgical opinion

SQ Item ordered by home health

SS Home infusion services provided in the infusion suite of the IV therapy provider

ST Related to trauma or injury

SU Procedure performed in physician's office (to denote use of facility and equipment)

SV Pharmaceuticals delivered to patient's home but not utilized

SW Services provided by a certified diabetic educator

SY Persons who are in close contact with member of high-risk population (use only with codes for immunization)

T1 Left foot, second digit

T2 Left foot, third digit

T3 Left foot, fourth digit

T4 Left foot, fifth digit

T5 Right foot, great toe

T6 Right foot, second digit

T7 Right foot, third digit

T8 Right foot, fourth digit

T9 Right foot, fifth digit

TA Left foot, great toe

Modifiers T1, T2, T3, T4, T5, T6, T7, T8, T9, and TA:

- Modifiers T1–T9 and TA are appended to codes for procedures performed on the toes.
- Report modifiers affecting reimbursement first (e.g., 51, 80).
- Procedures should be reported with these modifiers appended to identify the toe; it is not sufficient to just increase the number of services in the unit box.

▲ **TB** Drug or biological acquired with 340B drug pricing program discount, reported for informational purposes

TC Technical component; under certain circumstances, a charge may be made for the technical component alone; under those circumstances the technical component charge is identified by adding modifier TC to the usual procedure number; technical component charges are institutional charges and not reported separately by physicians; however, portable x-ray suppliers only bill for technical component and should utilize modifier TC; the charge data from portable x-ray suppliers will then be used to build customary and prevailing profiles Certain procedures are a combination of a physician component and a technical I component. To report the technical component only, append modifier TC to the procedure code.

- Modifier TC is considered a payment modifier and must be reported first in the modifier field.
- Technical component procedures cannot be reported separately by a provider when the patient is an inpatient, outpatient, or in a covered Part A stay in a skilled nursing facility (SNF) location.
- Modifier TC should be appended to report only the technical component of a global procedure or service code. Remember, typically the technical component is provided by the facility or mobile x-ray unit. This modifier is never reported on E/M service codes.

Example:

PET imaging is performed for initial diagnosis of breast cancer and/or surgical planning for breast cancer. Report code G0252 with modifier TC to identify the facility's services.

TD RN

TE LPN/LVN

Modifiers TD and TE:

- Modifiers TD and TE are required by some state Medicaid and state health departments.
- Community health services provided by RNs and LPN/LVNs are reported with modifiers TD and TE.

TF Intermediate level of care

TG Complex/high tech level of care

TH Obstetrical treatment/services, prenatal or postpartum

TJ Program group, child and/or adolescent

TK Extra patient or passenger, non-ambulance

TL Early intervention/individualized family service plan (IFSP)

TM Individualized education program (IEP)

TN Rural/outside providers' customary service area

TP Medical transport, unloaded vehicle

TQ Basic life support transport by a volunteer ambulance provider

TR School-based individualized education program (IEP) services provided outside the public school district responsible for the student

TS Follow-up service

TT Individualized service provided to more than one patient in same setting

TU Special payment rate, overtime

TV Special payment rates, holidays/weekends

TW Back-up equipment

U1 Medicaid level of care 1, as defined by each state

U2 Medicaid level of care 2, as defined by each state

U3 Medicaid level of care 3, as defined by each state

U4 Medicaid level of care 4, as defined by each state

U5 Medicaid level of care 5, as defined by each state

U6 Medicaid level of care 6, as defined by each state

U7 Medicaid level of care 7, as defined by each state

U8 Medicaid level of care 8, as defined by each state

U9 Medicaid level of care 9, as defined by each state

UA Medicaid level of care 10, as defined by each state

UB Medicaid level of care 11, as defined by each state

UC Medicaid level of care 12, as defined by each state

UD Medicaid level of care 13, as defined by each state

Modifiers U1, U2, U3, U4, U5, U6, U7, U8, U9, UA, UB, UC, and UD:

- Modifiers U1–U9 and UA-UD allow a state Medicaid agency to define specific levels or types of services. Not all state Medicaid agencies have set definitions for all the levels described.
- Providers should obtain manuals/instruction in modifier usage from state Medicaid agencies for specific guidance in using these modifiers.

UE Used durable medical equipment
- Append modifier UE when a beneficiary purchases the used equipment.

UF Services provided in the morning

UG Services provided in the afternoon

UH Services provided in the evening

UJ Services provided at night

UK Services provided on behalf of the client to someone other than the client (collateral relationship)

UN Two patients served

UP Three patients served

UQ Four patients served

UR Five patients served

US Six or more patients served

Modifiers UN, UP, UQ, UR, and US:
- Providers are required to append one of these modifiers to HCPCS code R0075 when billing Medicare carriers for portable x-rays. Modifier selection is based on the number of patients served during a single trip to a particular location.
- Skilled nursing facilities are required to report these modifiers when reporting R0075 to a fiscal intermediary. Modifier selection is based on the number of patients served during a single trip to a facility or specific location.

V1 Demonstration modifier 1

V2 Demonstration modifier 2

V3 Demonstration modifier 3

V4 Demonstration modifier 4

V5 Vascular catheter (alone or with any other vascular access)

V6 Arteriovenous graft (or other vascular access not including a vascular catheter)

V7 Arteriovenous fistula only (in use with two needles)

V8 Infection present

V9 No infection present

VM Medicare Diabetes Prevention Program (MDPP) virtual make-up session

VP Aphakic patient

X1 Continuous/broad services: for reporting services by clinicians, who provide the principal care for a patient, with no planned endpoint of the relationship; services in this category represent comprehensive care, dealing with the entire scope of patient problems, either directly or in a care coordination role; reporting clinician service examples include, but are not limited to, primary care, and clinicians providing comprehensive care to patients in addition to specialty care

X2 Continuous/focused services: for reporting services by clinicians whose expertise is needed for the ongoing management of a chronic disease or a condition that needs to be managed and followed with no planned endpoint to the relationship; reporting clinician service examples include, but are not limited to, a rheumatologist taking care of the patient's rheumatoid arthritis longitudinally but not providing general primary care services

X3 Episodic/broad services: for reporting services by clinicians who have broad responsibility for the comprehensive needs of the patient that is limited to a defined period and circumstance such as a hospitalization; reporting clinician service examples include, but are not limited to, the hospitalist's services rendered providing comprehensive and general care to a patient while admitted to the hospital

X4 Episodic/focused services: for reporting services by clinicians who provide focused care on particular types of treatment limited to a defined period and circumstance; the patient has a problem, acute or chronic, that will be treated with surgery, radiation, or some other type of generally time-limited intervention; reporting clinician service examples include, but are not limited to, the orthopedic surgeon performing a knee replacement and seeing the patient through the postoperative period

X5 Diagnostic services requested by another clinician: for reporting services by a clinician who furnishes care to the patient only as requested by another clinician or subsequent and related services requested by another clinician; this modifier is reported for patient relationships that may not be adequately captured by the above alternative categories; reporting clinician service examples include, but are not limited to, the radiologist's interpretation of an imaging study requested by another clinician

XE Separate encounter, a service that is distinct because it occurred during a separate encounter

XP Separate practitioner, a service that is distinct because it was performed by a different practitioner

XS Separate structure, a service that is distinct because it was performed on a separate organ/structure

XU Unusual nonoverlapping service, the use of a service that is distinct because it does not overlap usual components of the main service

In 2014, CMS established four HCPCS Level II modifiers, collectively referred to as X{EPSU} modifiers, to identify and define specific subsets of modifier 59 Distinct Procedural Service:
- Modifiers 59, XE, XP, XS, and XU indicate a procedure or service was independent from other services performed on the same day.
- If a more descriptive modifier is not available and the use of modifier 59 best explains the circumstance, report the service with this modifier.
- When a procedure or service designated as a separate procedure is conducted independently or considered to be unrelated from the other services provided at the same session, it may be reported by appending modifier 59, XE, XP, XS, or XU to the specific separate procedure code. This indicates the procedure is not considered a component of another procedure but instead is a distinct procedure.
- Medicare and other payers may, in many instances, require one of the four specific subsets of modifier 59 (X{EPSU} modifiers) be reported in lieu of simply reporting the more general modifier 59. In no circumstance should both modifier 59 and an X{EPSU} modifier be reported together.

Regulatory and Coding Guidance

Outpatient Modifier Guidance/Usage

CMS, through hospital Transmittal 726, dated January 1998, initially identified Level I and Level II modifiers for hospital use when reporting outpatient services (effective date July 1, 1998). Modifiers are required to ensure payment accuracy, coding consistency, and accurate editing under the outpatient prospective payment system (OPPS). Modifiers are reported as an attachment to the code as reported in the UB-04 form locator (FL) 44 or for electronic submission field Loop 2400, SV202-3 of the 837i format.

Multiple Modifiers

Sometimes, more than one modifier must be appended for a submitted code. In such a case, the modifier that may affect payment is listed first, followed by additional appropriate modifiers. It may be necessary, for example, to report the nerve repair of a finger was performed on multiple digits. Modifier 51 would be listed first, followed by the HCPCS modifier identifying the specific finger involved.

The CMS claims processing manual lists acceptable combinations of surgery modifiers. The CMS list of possible modifier combinations includes:

- Bilateral surgery (50) and assistant surgeon (80)
- Bilateral surgery (50), two surgeons (62), and surgical care only (54)
- Bilateral surgery (50), team surgery (66), and surgical care only (54)
- Multiple surgery (51) and surgical care only (54)
- Multiple surgery (51) and postoperative care only (55)
- Multiple surgery (51) and two surgeons (62)
- Multiple surgery (51) and surgical team (66)
- Multiple surgery (51) and assistant surgeon (80)
- Multiple surgery (51), two surgeons (62), and surgical care only (54)
- Multiple surgery (51), team surgery (66), and surgical care only (54)
- Two surgeons (62) and surgical care only (54)
- Two surgeons (62) and postoperative care only (55)
- Surgical team (66) and surgical care only (54)
- Surgical team (66) and postoperative care only (55)

If two or more modifiers are appropriate, modifier 99 Multiple modifiers, may be appended immediately after the procedure code to indicate one or more additional modifiers will follow.

Determining Correct Use

Determining correct modifier assignment can be confusing at times. If the medical record documentation does not support the use of a specific modifier, the provider risks denial of the claim based on lack of medical necessity and possible fraud and/or abuse penalties if/when the medical record documentation is reviewed by federal, state, and other third-party payers.

It is important to validate the final modifier determination against the medical record documentation. First, the special circumstance that warrants the use of a modifier must be identified in the medical record. Keep in mind, a modifier provides the way a provider or facility can indicate a service provided to the patient has been changed by some distinctive situation yet the code description itself remains the same. Therefore, the medical record should contain pertinent information and an adequate definition of the service or procedure performed that supports the use of the assigned modifier. If the service is not documented or a special circumstance is not indicated, it is not appropriate to report the modifier.

HCPCS Level II modifiers may be appended to any HCPCS Level I or Level II code. Because the CPT book lists a subset of the Level II modifiers, some incorrectly assume only those modifiers may be appended to CPT codes.

For example, a pediatrician receives free flu vaccine for children under age 3 from the state health department. When the vaccine is administered, the procedure code is reported with modifier SL State supplied vaccine, appended. Although modifier SL is not listed in the CPT book, it would be incorrect to report the service without modifier SL.

Appropriate Use of Professional/Technical Component Modifiers

- Modifier 26 is appended:
  - to the procedure code to report only the professional component.
  - when a physician is providing the interpretation of the diagnostic test/study performed. The interpretation of the diagnostic test/study is a patient-specific service that is separate, distinct, written, and signed.
- Modifier TC is appended:
  - to the procedure code to report only the technical component. Payment includes both the practice and malpractice expenses.
  - to stand-alone procedure codes to describe the technical component only (e.g., staff and equipment costs) of diagnostic tests.
  - to the procedure code by portable x-ray suppliers to report only the technical component.
  - to procedures with a "1" indicator in the PC/TC field of the MPFSDB.
- Modifier TC payment rule: Payment is based solely on the technical value of each individual procedure.
  - Modifier TC is appropriate for use with the following types of services:

    1 = Medical care/injections

    2 = Surgery

    4 = Radiology

    5 = Lab

    6 = Radiation therapy

    8 = Assistant surgeon

    When both the professional and technical components are performed, and the technical component was purchased by an outside entity, report the two components on separate lines on the CMS-1500 claim form.

Inappropriate Use of Professional/Technical Component Modifiers

- Appending modifier 26 for a reread of results of an interpretation initially provided by another provider.
- Appending both modifier 26, indicating that only the professional portion of the service was provided, and modifier 52 for reduced services. It is not necessary to report 52 because the professional component modifier already indicates that only a portion of the complete service was performed.
- Appending modifiers 26 and TC (except for purchased diagnostic tests) when a diagnostic test or radiology service is performed globally (both components are performed by the same provider). When a global service is performed, the code representing the complete service should be reported without modifiers. The payment for the global service reflects the allowances for both components.
- Appending modifier TC to identify procedures that are covered only as diagnostic tests and, therefore, do not have a related professional component. The use of modifier TC on these codes is not appropriate, nor is it correct coding.

Do not append these modifiers to:

- Professional component-only procedure codes, identified in the MPFSDB by an indicator "2" in the PC/TC column.
- Global-only procedures, identified in the MPFSDB with an indicator "4" in the PC/TC column.
- Technical-component-only procedure codes, assigned an indicator "3" in the MPFSDB PC/TC column.

Appropriate Use of Other Modifiers

- Append modifier 59, XE, XP, XS, or XU when reporting a combination of codes that would normally not be reported together. This modifier indicates the ordinarily bundled code represents a service done at a different anatomic site or at a different session on the same date. This may represent a:
  - different session or patient encounter (XE)
  - different practitioner/physician (XP)
  - different site or organ system (e.g., a skin graft and an allograft in different locations) (XS)
  - separate incision/excision (XS)
  - separate lesion (e.g., a biopsy of skin on the neck is performed at the same session as an excision of a 1.0 cm benign lesion of the face) (XS)
  - separate injury (XU)
- Append modifier 59, XE, XP, XS, or XU only on the procedure designated as a separate procedural service. The physician needs to document that the procedure or service was independent of other services rendered on the same day.
- Ensure the medical record documentation is clear as to the separate and distinct procedure before appending modifier 59, XE, XP, XS, or XU to a code. This modifier allows the code to bypass edits; therefore, appropriate documentation must be present in the record.

  Note: Medicare uses the Correct Coding Initiative (CCI) screens when editing claims for possible unbundling. Under CCI screens, specific codes have been identified that should not be reported together, and not all edits allow modifier 59, XE, XP, XS, or XU to override the CCI edit.
- When multiple approaches are taken to obtain a tissue sample (cytological or surgical), report the most invasive procedure performed at the same session/site in order to obtain a specimen. For example, if a fine-needle aspiration is attempted and is unsuccessful and the same physician proceeds to obtain a core biopsy using a cutting needle and ultimately finds it necessary to perform an open biopsy, all occurring at the same session, report only the open biopsy. If different lesions are biopsied using different methodologies, even at the same session, append modifier 59, XE, XP, XS, or XU. If different biopsy procedures are necessary for different reasons (e.g., fine-needle aspiration for diagnosis and needle biopsy for receptors in breast carcinoma), report both procedures.
- When a recurrent hernia requires repair (herniorrhaphy, hernioplasty), report the appropriate recurrent hernia repair code. A code for incisional hernia repair is not to be reported in addition to the recurrent hernia repair unless a medically necessary incisional hernia repair is performed at a different site. In this case, attach modifier 59 or XS to the incisional hernia repair code.
- Modifier 59 is appended only if another modifier such as XE, XS, XP, or XU does not more accurately describe the situation.
- For Medicare reporting purposes, it may be necessary to report one of the more specific X{EPSU} modifiers (XE, XS, XP, or XU) in lieu of appending the general modifier 59.

Inappropriate Use of Other Modifiers

Avoid the following inappropriate use of modifiers:

- Appending modifier 59, XE, XP, XS, or XU to E/M codes.
- Appending modifier 59, XE, XP, XS, or XU as a replacement for modifier 24, 25, 51, 78, or 79.
- Appending modifier 59, XE, XP, XS, or XU when another modifier best describes the distinct service.
- Appending modifier 59, XE, XP, XS, or XU for the sole purpose of bypassing an appropriate CCI edit.
- Appending modifier 59 in conjunction with one of the XE, XP, XS, or XU modifiers on the same line item.

Appropriate Use of Surgical Assistant Modifier AS

Note the following appropriate application of the surgical assistant modifiers:

- Append modifier AS on the appropriate procedure codes. The codes must match those reported by the primary surgeon.
- Append modifier AS on claims with other surgery modifiers, such as 50 and 51.
- Append modifier AS to the code for the procedure the NPP or APP assisted with.
- When reporting modifier AS, the nonphysician practitioner should report the code for the procedure using his or her own provider identification number with the appropriate site-of-service code.

Inappropriate Use of Surgical Assistant Modifier AS

Avoid the following inappropriate application of the surgical assistant modifiers:

- Appending modifier AS when the NPP/APP functions simply as an extra pair of hands for the surgeon and not as a true surgical assistant in place of another surgeon.
- Appending modifier AS to a procedure code when the assistant at surgery is an MD or DO.

Appendix 3 — Abbreviations and Acronyms

HCPCS Abbreviations and Acronyms

The following abbreviations and acronyms are used in the HCPCS descriptions:

/	or
<	less than
<=	less than equal to
>	greater than
>=	greater than equal to
AC	alternating current
ACE/ACEI	angiotensin-converting enzyme inhibitor
AFO	ankle-foot orthosis
AHI	apnea hypopnea index
AICC	anti-inhibitor coagulant complex
AK	above the knee
AKA	above knee amputation
ALS	advanced life support
AMP	ampule
AO	ankle orthosis
ARB	angiotensin receptor blocker
ART	artery
ART	arterial
ASC	ambulatory surgery center
ATT	attached
A-V	arteriovenous
AVF	arteriovenous fistula
BICROS	bilateral routing of signals
BK	below the knee
BLS	basic life support
BMI	body mass index
BP	blood pressure
BTE	behind the ear (hearing aid)
CAPD	continuous ambulatory peritoneal dialysis
Carb	carbohydrate
CBC	complete blood count
cc	cubic centimeter
CCPD	continuous cycling peritoneal analysis
CGM	continuous glucose monitoring
CHF	congestive heart failure
CIC	completely in the canal (hearing aid)
CIM	Coverage Issue Manual
CKD	chronic kidney disease
Clsd	closed
cm	centimeter
CMN	certificate of medical necessity
CMS	Centers for Medicare and Medicaid Services
CMV	cytomegalovirus
Conc	concentrate
Conc	concentrated
Cont	continuous
CP	clinical psychologist
CPAP	continuous positive airway pressure
CPT	Current Procedural Terminology
CRF	chronic renal failure
CRNA	certified registered nurse anesthetist
CROS	contralateral routing of signals
CSW	clinical social worker
CT	computed tomography
CTLSO	cervical-thoracic-lumbar-sacral orthosis
cu	cubic
DC	direct current
DI	diurnal rhythm
Dx	diagnosis
DLI	donor leukocyte infusion
DME	durable medical equipment
DME MAC	durable medical equipment Medicare administrative contractor
DMEPOS	durable medical equipment, prosthetics, orthotics and other supplies
DMERC	durable medical equipment regional carrier
DR	diagnostic radiology
DX	diagnostic
e.g.	for example
Ea	each
ECF	extended care facility
EEG	electroencephalogram
EGFR	estimated glomerular filtration rate
EKG	electrocardiogram
EMG	electromyography
EO	elbow orthosis
EP	electrophysiologic
EPO	epoetin alfa
EPSDT	early periodic screening, diagnosis and treatment
ERCP	endoscopic retrograde cholangiopancreatography
ESRD	end-stage renal disease
EWHO	elbow-wrist-hand orthotic
Ex	extended
Exper	experimental
Ext	external
F	french
FDA	Food and Drug Administration
FDG-PET	positron emission with tomography with 18 fluorodeoxyglucose
Fem	female
FO	finger orthosis
FPD	fixed partial denture
Fr	french
ft	foot
G-CSF	filgrastim (granulocyte colony-stimulating factor)
gm	gram (g)
H2O	water
HCl	hydrochloric acid, hydrochloride
HCPCS	Healthcare Common Procedural Coding System
HCT	hematocrit
HFO	hand-finger orthosis
HHA	home health agency
HI	high
HI-LO	high-low
HIT	home infusion therapy
HKAFO	hip-knee-ankle foot orthosis
HLA	human leukocyte antigen
HMES	heat and moisture exchange system
HNPCC	hereditary non-polyposis colorectal cancer
HO	hip orthosis
HPSA	health professional shortage area
HST	home sleep test
IA	intra-arterial administration
ip	interphalangeal
I-131	Iodine 131
ICF	intermediate care facility
ICU	intensive care unit
IM	intramuscular
in	inch
INF	infusion
INH	inhalation solution
INJ	injection
IOL	intraocular lens
IPD	intermittent peritoneal dialysis
IPPB	intermittent positive pressure breathing
IT	intrathecal administration
ITC	in the canal (hearing aid)
ITE	in the ear (hearing aid)
IU	international units
IV	intravenous
IVF	in vitro fertilization
KAFO	knee-ankle-foot orthosis
KO	knee orthosis
KOH	potassium hydroxide

L	left
LASIK	laser in situ keratomileusis
LAUP	laser assisted uvulopalatoplasty
lbs	pounds
LDL	low density lipoprotein
LDS	lipodystrophy syndrome
Lo	low
LO	lumbar orthosis
LPM	liters per minute
LPN/LVN	Licensed Practical Nurse/Licensed Vocational Nurse
LSO	lumbar-sacral orthosis
lvad	left ventricular assist device
lvef	left ventricular ejection fraction
MAC	Medicare administrative contractor
mp	metacarpophalangeal
mcg	microgram
mCi	millicurie
MCM	Medicare Carriers Manual
MCP	metacarpophalangeal joint
MCP	monthly capitation payment
mEq	milliequivalent
MESA	microsurgical epididymal sperm aspiration
mg	milligram
mgs	milligrams
MHT	megahertz
ml	milliliter
mm	millimeter
mmHg	millimeters of Mercury
MRA	magnetic resonance angiography
MRI	magnetic resonance imaging
NA	sodium
NCI	National Cancer Institute
NEC	not elsewhere classified
NG	nasogastric
NH	nursing home
NMES	neuromuscular electrical stimulation
NOC	not otherwise classified
NOS	not otherwise specified
NRS	numeric rating scale
O2	oxygen
OBRA	Omnibus Budget Reconciliation Act
OMT	osteopathic manipulation therapy
OPPS	outpatient prospective payment system
ORAL	oral administration
OSA	obstructive sleep apnea
Ost	ostomy
OTH	other routes of administration
oz	ounce
PA	physician's assistant
PAR	parenteral
PCA	patient controlled analgesia
PCH	pouch
PEN	parenteral and enteral nutrition
PENS	percutaneous electrical nerve stimulation
PET	positron emission tomography
PHP	pre-paid health plan
PHP	physician hospital plan
PI	paramedic intercept
PICC	peripherally inserted central venous catheter
PKR	photorefractive keratotomy
Pow	powder
PRK	photoreactive keratectomy
PRO	peer review organization
PSA	prostate specific antigen
PTB	patellar tendon bearing
PTK	phototherapeutic keratectomy
PVC	polyvinyl chloride
QPP	Quality Payment Program
R	right
RDI	respiratory disturbance index
REI	respiratory event index
Repl	replace
RN	registered nurse
RP	retrograde pyelogram
Rx	prescription
SACH	solid ankle, cushion heel
SC	subcutaneous
SCT	specialty care transport
SEO	shoulder-elbow orthosis
SEWHO	shoulder-elbow-wrist-hand orthosis
SEXA	single energy x-ray absorptiometry
SGD	speech generating device
SGD	sinus rhythm
SM	samarium
SNCT	sensory nerve conduction test
SNF	skilled nursing facility
SO	sacroiliac orthosis
SO	shoulder orthosis
Sol	solution
SQ	square
SR	screen
ST	standard
ST	sustained release
Syr	syrup
TABS	tablets
Tc	technetium
Tc 99m	technetium isotope
TENS	transcutaneous electrical nerve stimulator
THKAO	thoracic-hip-knee-ankle orthosis
TLSO	thoracic-lumbar-sacral-orthosis
TM	temporomandibular
TMJ	temporomandibular joint
TPN	total parenteral nutrition
U	unit
UACR	urine albumin-creatinine ratio
uCi	microcurie
VAR	various routes of administration
VAS	visual analog scale
VRS	visual rating scale
w	with
w/	with
w/o	without
WAK	wearable artificial kidney
wc	wheelchair
WHFO	wrist-hand-finger orthotic
WHO	wrist-hand orthotic
Wk	week
w/o	without
Xe	xenon (isotope mass of xenon 133)

Appendix 4 — Medicare Internet-only Manuals (IOMs)

The Centers for Medicare and Medicaid Services (CMS) restructured its paper-based manual system as a web-based system on October 1, 2003. Called the online CMS manual system, it combines all of the various program instructions into Internet-only Manuals (IOMs), which are used by all CMS programs and contractors. In many instances, the references from the online manuals in appendix 4 contain a mention of the old paper manuals from which the current information was obtained when the manuals were converted. This information is shown in the header of the text, in the following format, when applicable, as A3-3101, HO-210, and B3-2049.

Effective with implementation of the IOMs, the former method of publishing program memoranda (PMs) to communicate program instructions was replaced by the following four templates:

- One-time notification
- Manual revisions
- Business requirements
- Confidential requirements

The web-based system has been organized by functional area (e.g., eligibility, entitlement, claims processing, benefit policy, program integrity) in an effort to eliminate redundancy within the manuals, simplify updating, and make CMS program instructions available more quickly. The web-based system contains the functional areas included below:

Pub. 100	Introduction
Pub. 100-01	Medicare General Information, Eligibility, and Entitlement Manual
Pub. 100-02	Medicare Benefit Policy Manual
Pub. 100-03	Medicare National Coverage Determinations (NCD) Manual
Pub. 100-04	Medicare Claims Processing Manual
Pub. 100-05	Medicare Secondary Payer Manual
Pub. 100-06	Medicare Financial Management Manual
Pub. 100-07	State Operations Manual
Pub. 100-08	Medicare Program Integrity Manual
Pub. 100-09	Medicare Contractor Beneficiary and Provider Communications Manual
Pub. 100-10	Quality Improvement Organization Manual
Pub. 100-11	Programs of All-Inclusive Care for the Elderly (PACE) Manual
Pub. 100-12	State Medicaid Manual (The new manual is under development. Please continue to use the Paper-Based Manual to make your selection.)
Pub. 100-13	Medicaid State Children's Health Insurance Program (Under Development)
Pub. 100-15	Medicaid Program Integrity Manual
Pub. 100-16	Medicare Managed Care Manual
Pub. 100-17	CMS/Business Partners Systems Security Manual
Pub. 100-18	Medicare Prescription Drug Benefit Manual
Pub. 100-19	Demonstrations
Pub. 100-20	One-Time Notification
Pub. 100-21	Reserved
Pub. 100-22	Medicare Quality Reporting Incentive Programs Manual
Pub. 100-23	Payment Error Rate Measurement (Under Development)
Pub. 100-24	State Payment of Medicare Premiums
Pub. 100-25	Information Security Acceptable Risk Safeguards Manual

A brief description of the Medicare manuals primarily used for *HCPCS Level II* follows:

- The *National Coverage Determinations Manual* (NCD), is organized according to categories such as diagnostic services, supplies, and medical procedures. The table of contents lists each category and subject within that category. Revision transmittals identify any new or background material, recap the changes, and provide an effective date for the change. The manual contains four sections and is organized in accordance with CPT category sequence and contains a list of HCPCS codes related to coverage determinations, where appropriate.
- The *Medicare Benefit Policy Manual* contains Medicare general coverage instructions that are not national coverage determinations. As a general rule, in the past these instructions have been found in chapter II of the *Medicare Carriers Manual*, the *Medicare Intermediary Manual*, other provider manuals, and program memoranda.
- The *Medicare Claims Processing Manual* contains instructions for processing claims for contractors and providers.
- The *Medicare Program Integrity Manual* communicates the priorities and standards for the Medicare integrity programs.

Medicare IOM References

A printed version of the Medicare IOM references will no longer be published in Optum's *HCPCS Level II* product. Complete versions of all the manuals can be found online at https://www.cms.gov/medicare/regulations-guidance/manuals/internet-only-manuals-ioms.

Appendix 5 — New, Revised, and Deleted Codes

NEW CODES

A2026 Restrata MiniMatrix, 5 mg
A2027 MatriDerm, per sq cm
A2028 MicroMatrix Flex, per mg
A2029 MiroTract Wound Matrix sheet, per cc
A4438 Adhesive clip applied to the skin to secure external electrical nerve stimulator controller, each
A4543 Supplies for transcutaneous electrical nerve stimulator, for nerves in the auricular region, per month
A4544 Electrode for external lower extremity nerve stimulator for restless legs syndrome
A4545 Supplies and accessories for external tibial nerve stimulator (e.g., socks, gel pads, electrodes, etc.), needed for one month
A4564 Pessary, disposable, any type
A4593 Neuromodulation stimulator system, adjunct to rehabilitation therapy regime, controller
A4594 Neuromodulation stimulator system, adjunct to rehabilitation therapy regime, mouthpiece, each
A7021 Supplies and accessories for lung expansion airway clearance, continuous high frequency oscillation, and nebulization device (e.g., handset, nebulizer kit, biofilter)
A9293 Fertility cycle (contraception & conception) tracking software application, FDA cleared, per month, includes accessories (e.g., thermometer)
A9506 Graphite crucible for preparation of Technetium Tc 99m-labeled carbon aerosol, each
A9610 Xenon Xe-129 hyperpolarized gas, diagnostic, per study dose
A9615 Injection, pegulicianine, 1 mg
C1605 Pacemaker, leadless, dual chamber (right atrial and right ventricular implantable components), rate-responsive, including all necessary components for implantation
C1606 Adapter, single-use (i.e., disposable), for attaching ultrasound system to upper gastrointestinal endoscope
C1735 Catheter(s), intravascular for renal denervation, radiofrequency, including all single use system components
C1736 Catheter(s), intravascular for renal denervation, ultrasound, including all single use system components
C1737 Joint fusion and fixation device(s), sacroiliac and pelvis, including all system components (implantable)
C1738 Powered, single-use (i.e., disposable) endoscopic ultrasound-guided biopsy device
C1739 Tissue marker, imaging and nonimaging device (implantable)
C7562 Catheter placement in coronary artery(ies) for coronary angiography, including intraprocedural injection(s) for coronary angiography, imaging supervision and interpretation; with right and left heart catheterization including intraprocedural injection(s) for left ventriculography, when performed with intraprocedural coronary fractional flow reserve (FFR) with 3D functional mapping of color-coded FFR values for the coronary tree, derived from coronary angiogram data, for real-time review and interpretation of possible atherosclerotic stenosis(es) intervention
C7563 Transluminal balloon angioplasty (except lower extremity artery(ies) for occlusive disease, intracranial, coronary, pulmonary, or dialysis circuit), open or percutaneous, including all imaging and radiological supervision and interpretation necessary to perform the angioplasty within the same artery, initial artery and all additional arteries
C7564 Percutaneous transluminal mechanical thrombectomy, vein(s), including intraprocedural pharmacological thrombolytic injections and fluoroscopic guidance with intravascular ultrasound (noncoronary vessel(s)) during diagnostic evaluation and/or therapeutic intervention, including radiological supervision and interpretation
C7565 Repair of anterior abdominal hernia(s) (i.e., epigastric, incisional, ventral, umbilical, spigelian), any approach (i.e., open, laparoscopic, robotic), recurrent, including implantation of mesh or other prosthesis when performed, total length of defect(s) less than 3 cm, reducible with removal of total or near total noninfected mesh or other prosthesis at the time of initial or recurrent anterior abdominal hernia repair or parastomal hernia repair
C8000 Support device, extravascular, for arteriovenous fistula (implantable)
C8001 3D anatomical segmentation imaging for preoperative planning, data preparation and transmission, obtained from previous diagnostic computed tomographic or magnetic resonance examination of the same anatomy
C8002 Preparation of skin cell suspension autograft, automated, including all enzymatic processing and device components (do not report with manual suspension preparation)
C8003 Implantation of medial knee extraarticular implantable shock absorber spanning the knee joint from distal femur to proximal tibia, open, includes measurements, positioning and adjustments, with imaging guidance (e.g., fluoroscopy)
C9173 Injection, filgrastim-txid (Nypozi), biosimilar, 1 mcg
C9610 Catheter, transluminal drug delivery with or without angioplasty, coronary, nonlaser (insertable)
C9796 Repair of enterocutaneous fistula small intestine or colon (excluding anorectal fistula) with plug (e.g., porcine small intestine submucosa [SIS])
C9797 Vascular embolization or occlusion procedure with use of a pressure-generating catheter (e.g., one-way valve, intermittently occluding), inclusive of all radiological supervision and interpretation, intraprocedural roadmapping, and imaging guidance necessary to complete the intervention; for tumors, organ ischemia, or infarction
C9804 Elastomeric infusion pump (e.g., On-Q* pump with bolus), including catheter and all disposable system components, nonopioid medical device (must be a qualifying Medicare nonopioid medical device for postsurgical pain relief in accordance with Section 4135 of the CAA, 2023)
C9806 Rotary peristaltic infusion pump (e.g., ambIT pump), including catheter and all disposable system components, nonopioid medical device (must be a qualifying Medicare nonopioid medical device for postsurgical pain relief in accordance with Section 4135 of the CAA, 2023)
C9807 Nerve stimulator, percutaneous, peripheral (e.g., sprint peripheral nerve stimulation system), including electrode and all disposable system components, nonopioid medical device (must be a qualifying Medicare nonopioid medical device for postsurgical pain relief in accordance with Section 4135 of the CAA, 2023)
C9808 Nerve cryoablation probe (e.g., cryoICE, cryoSPHERE, cryoSPHERE MAX, cryo2), including probe and all disposable system components, nonopioid medical device (must be a qualifying Medicare nonopioid medical device for postsurgical pain relief in accordance with Section 4135 of the CAA, 2023)
C9809 Cryoablation needle (e.g., iovera system), including needle/tip and all disposable system components, nonopioid medical device (must be a qualifying Medicare nonopioid medical device for postsurgical pain relief in accordance with Section 4135 of the CAA, 2023)
C9901 Endoscopic defect closure within the entire gastrointestinal tract, including upper endoscopy (including diagnostic, if performed) or colonoscopy (including diagnostic, if performed), with all system and tissue anchoring components
E0152 Walker, battery powered, wheeled, folding, adjustable or fixed height
E0468 Home ventilator, dual-function respiratory device, also performs additional function of cough stimulation, includes all accessories, components and supplies for all functions
E0469 Lung expansion airway clearance, continuous high frequency oscillation, and nebulization device
E0683 Nonpneumatic, nonsequential, peristaltic wave compression pump
E0715 Intravaginal device intended to strengthen pelvic floor muscles during Kegel exercises
E0716 Supplies and accessories for intravaginal device intended to strengthen pelvic floor muscles during Kegel exercises
E0721 Transcutaneous electrical nerve stimulator, stimulates nerves in the auricular region
E0736 Transcutaneous tibial nerve stimulator
E0737 Transcutaneous tibial nerve stimulator, controlled by phone application
E0738 Upper extremity rehabilitation system providing active assistance to facilitate muscle re-education, includes microprocessor, all components and accessories
E0743 External lower extremity nerve stimulator for restless legs syndrome, each

NEW CODES (continued)

E0767 Intrabuccal, systemic delivery of amplitude-modulated, radiofrequency electromagnetic field device, for cancer treatment, includes all accessories

E1803 Dynamic adjustable elbow extension only device, includes soft interface material

E1804 Dynamic adjustable elbow flexion only device, includes soft interface material

E1807 Dynamic adjustable wrist extension only device, includes soft interface material

E1808 Dynamic adjustable wrist flexion only device, includes soft interface material

E1813 Dynamic adjustable knee extension only device, includes soft interface material

E1814 Dynamic adjustable knee flexion only device, includes soft interface material

E1822 Dynamic adjustable ankle extension only device, includes soft interface material

E1823 Dynamic adjustable ankle flexion only device, includes soft interface material

E1826 Dynamic adjustable finger extension only device, includes soft interface material

E1827 Dynamic adjustable finger flexion only device, includes soft interface material

E1828 Dynamic adjustable toe extension only device, includes soft interface material

E1829 Dynamic adjustable toe flexion only device, includes soft interface material

E2104 Home blood glucose monitor for use with integrated lancing/blood sample testing cartridge

E2298 Complex rehabilitative power wheelchair accessory, power seat elevation system, any type

E2513 Accessory for speech generating device, electromyographic sensor

E3200 Gait modulation system, rhythmic auditory stimulation, including restricted therapy software, all components and accessories, prescription only

G0138 IV infusion of cipaglucosidase alfa-atga, including provider/supplier acquisition and clinical supervision of oral administration of miglustat in preparation of receipt of cipaglucosidase alfa-atga

G0519 Management of new patient-caregiver dyad with dementia, low complexity, for use in CMMI model

G0520 Management of new patient-caregiver dyad with dementia, moderate complexity, for use in CMMI model

G0521 Management of new patient-caregiver dyad with dementia, high complexity, for use in CMMI model

G0522 Management of a new patient with dementia, low complexity, for use in CMMI model

G0523 Management of a new patient with dementia, moderate to high complexity, for use in CMMI model

G0524 Management of established patient-caregiver dyad with dementia, low complexity, for use in CMMI model

G0525 Management of established patient-caregiver dyad with dementia, moderate complexity, for use in CMMI model

G0526 Management of established patient-caregiver dyad with dementia, high complexity, for use in CMMI model

G0527 Management of established patient with dementia, low complexity, for use in CMMI model

G0528 Management of established patient with dementia, moderate to high complexity, for use in CMMI model

G0529 In-home respite care, 4-hour unit, for use in CMMI model

G0530 Adult day center, 8-hour unit, for use in CMMI model

G0531 Facility-based respite, 24-hour unit, for use in CMMI model

G0532 Take-home supply of nasal nalmefene HCl; one carton of two, 2.7 mg per 0.1 ml nasal sprays (provision of the services by a Medicare-enrolled opioid treatment program);(list separately in addition to each primary code)

G0533 Medication assisted treatment, buprenorphine (injectable) administered on a weekly basis; weekly bundle including dispensing and/or administration, substance use counseling, individual and group therapy, and toxicology testing if performed (provision of the services by a Medicare-enrolled opioid treatment program)

G0534 Coordinated care and/or referral services, such as to adequate and accessible community resources to address unmet health-related social needs, including harm reduction interventions and recovery support services a patient needs and wishes to pursue, which significantly limit the ability to diagnose or treat an opioid use disorder; each additional 30 minutes of services (provision of the services by a Medicare-enrolled opioid treatment program); (list separately in addition to each primary code)

G0535 Patient navigational services, provided directly or by referral; including helping the patient to navigate health systems and identify care providers and supportive services, to build patient selfadvocacy and communication skills with care providers, and to promote patient-driven action plans and goals; each additional 30 minutes of services (provision of the services by a Medicare-enrolled opioid treatment program); (list separately in addition to each primary code)

G0536 Peer recovery support services, provided directly or by referral; including leveraging knowledge of the condition or lived experience to provide support, mentorship, or inspiration to meet oud treatment and recovery goals; conducting a person-centered interview to understand the patient's life story, strengths, needs, goals, preferences, and desired outcomes; developing and proposing strategies to help meet person-centered treatment goals; assisting the patient in locating or navigating recovery support services; each additional 30 minutes of services (provision of the services by a Medicare-enrolled opioid treatment program); (list separately in addition to each primary code)

G0537 Administration of a standardized, evidence-based atherosclerotic cardiovascular disease (ASCVD) risk assessment, 5-15 minutes, not more often than every 12 months

G0538 Atherosclerotic cardiovascular disease (ASCVD) risk management services; clinical staff time; per calendar month

G0539 Caregiver training in behavior management/modification for caregiver(s) of patients with a mental or physical health diagnosis, administered by physician or other qualified health care professional (without the patient present), face-to-face; initial 30 minutes

G0540 Caregiver training in behavior management/modification for parent(s)/guardian(s)/caregiver(s) of patients with a mental or physical health diagnosis, administered by physician or other qualified health care professional (without the patient present), face-to-face; each additional 15 minutes

G0541 Caregiver training in direct care strategies and techniques to support care for patients with an ongoing condition or illness and to reduce complications (including, but not limited to, techniques to prevent decubitus ulcer formation, wound care, and infection control) (without the patient present), face-to-face; initial 30 minutes

G0542 Caregiver training in direct care strategies and techniques to support care for patients with an ongoing condition or illness and to reduce complications (including, but not limited to, techniques to prevent decubitus ulcer formation, wound care, and infection control) (without the patient present), face-to-face; each additional 15 minutes (list separately in addition to code for primary service) (use G0542 in conjunction with G0541)

G0543 Group caregiver training in direct care strategies and techniques to support care for patients with an ongoing condition or illness and to reduce complications (including, but not limited to, techniques to prevent decubitus ulcer formation, wound care, and infection control) (without the patient present), face-to-face with multiple sets of caregivers

G0544 Post discharge telephonic follow-up contacts performed in conjunction with a discharge from the emergency department for behavioral health or other crisis encounter, 4 calls per calendar month

G0545 Visit complexity inherent to hospital inpatient or observation care associated with a confirmed or suspected infectious disease by an infectious diseases specialist, including disease transmission risk assessment and mitigation, public health investigation, analysis, and testing, and complex antimicrobial therapy counseling and treatment (add-on code, list separately in addition to hospital inpatient or observation evaluation and management visit, initial, same day discharge, subsequent or discharge)

G0546 Interprofessional telephone/internet/electronic health record assessment and management service provided by a practitioner in a specialty whose covered services are limited by statute to services for the diagnosis and treatment of mental illness, including a verbal and written report to the patient's treating/requesting practitioner; 5-10 minutes of medical consultative discussion and review

NEW CODES (continued)

G0547 Interprofessional telephone/internet/electronic health record assessment and management service provided by a practitioner in a specialty whose covered services are limited by statute to services for the diagnosis and treatment of mental illness, including a verbal and written report to the patient's treating/requesting practitioner; 11-20 minutes of medical consultative discussion and review

G0548 Interprofessional telephone/internet/electronic health record assessment and management service provided by a practitioner in a specialty whose covered services are limited by statute to services for the diagnosis and treatment of mental illness, including a verbal and written report to the patient's treating/requesting practitioner; 21-30 minutes of medical consultative discussion and review

G0549 Interprofessional telephone/internet/electronic health record assessment and management service provided by a practitioner in a specialty whose covered services are limited by statute to services for the diagnosis and treatment of mental illness, including a verbal and written report to the patient's treating/requesting practitioner; 31 or more minutes of medical consultative discussion and review

G0550 Interprofessional telephone/internet/electronic health record assessment and management service provided by a practitioner in a specialty whose covered services are limited by statute to services for the diagnosis and treatment of mental illness, including a written report to the patient's treating/requesting practitioner, 5 minutes or more of medical consultative time

G0551 Interprofessional telephone/internet/electronic health record referral service(s) provided by a treating/requesting practitioner in a specialty whose covered services are limited by statute to services for the diagnosis and treatment of mental illness, 30 minutes

G0552 Supply of digital mental health treatment device and initial education and onboarding, per course of treatment that augments a behavioral therapy plan

G0553 First 20 minutes of monthly treatment management services directly related to the patient's therapeutic use of the digital mental health treatment (DMHT) device that augments a behavioral therapy plan, physician/other qualified health care professional time reviewing information related to the use of the DMHT device, including patient observations and patient specific inputs in a calendar month and requiring at least one interactive communication with the patient/caregiver during the calendar month

G0554 Each additional 20 minutes of monthly treatment management services directly related to the patient's therapeutic use of the digital mental health treatment (DMHT) device that augments a behavioral therapy plan, physician/other qualified health care professional time reviewing data generated from the DMHT device from patient observations and patient specific inputs in a calendar month and requiring at least one interactive communication with the patient/caregiver during the calendar month

G0555 Provision of replacement patient electronics system (e.g., system pillow, handheld reader) for home pulmonary artery pressure monitoring

G0556 Advanced primary care management services for a patient with one chronic condition [expected to last at least 12 months, or until the death of the patient, which place the patient at significant risk of death, acute exacerbation/decompensation, or functional decline], or fewer, provided by clinical staff and directed by a physician or other qualified health care professional who is responsible for all primary care and serves as the continuing focal point for all needed health care services; per calendar month, with the following elements, as appropriate:

G0557 Advanced primary care management services for a patient with multiple (two or more) chronic conditions expected to last at least 12 months, or until the death of the patient, which place the patient at significant risk of death, acute exacerbation/decompensation, or functional decline, provided by clinical staff and directed by a physician or other qualified health care professional who is responsible for all primary care and serves as the continuing focal point for all needed health care services, per calendar month, with the following elements, as appropriate:

G0558 Advanced primary care management services for a patient that is a qualified medicare beneficiary with multiple (two or more) chronic conditions expected to last at least 12 months, or until the death of the patient, which place the patient at significant risk of death, acute exacerbation/decompensation, or functional decline, provided by clinical staff and directed by a physician or other qualified health care professional who is responsible for all primary care and serves as the continuing focal point for all needed health care services, per calendar month, with the following elements, as appropriate:

G0559 Postoperative follow-up visit complexity inherent to evaluation and management services addressing surgical procedure(s), provided by a physician or qualified health care professional who is not the practitioner who performed the procedure (or in the same group practice) and is of the same or of a different specialty than the practitioner who performed the procedure, within the 90-day global period of the procedure(s), once per 90-day global period, when there has not been a formal transfer of care and requires the following required elements, when possible and applicable:

G0560 Safety planning interventions, each 20 minutes personally performed by the billing practitioner, including assisting the patient in the identification of the following personalized elements of a safety plan:

G0561 Tympanostomy with local or topical anesthesia and insertion of a ventilating tube when performed with tympanostomy tube delivery device, unilateral (list separately in addition to 69433) (do not use in conjunction with 0583T)

G0562 Therapeutic radiology simulation-aided field setting; complex, including acquisition of PET and CT imaging data required for radiopharmaceutical-directed radiation therapy treatment planning (i.e., modeling)

G0563 Stereotactic body radiation therapy, treatment delivery, per fraction to 1 or more lesions, including image guidance and real-time positron emissions-based delivery adjustments to 1 or more lesions, entire course not to exceed 5 fractions

G0564 Creation of subcutaneous pocket with insertion of 365 day implantable interstitial glucose sensor, including system activation and patient training

G0565 Removal of implantable interstitial glucose sensor with creation of subcutaneous pocket at different anatomic site and insertion of new 365 day implantable sensor, including system activation

G9037 Interprofessional telephone/internet/electronic health record clinical question/request for specialty recommendations by a treating/requesting physician or other qualified health care professional for the care of the patient (i.e., not for professional education or scheduling) and may include subsequent follow up on the specialist's recommendations; 30 minutes

G9038 Co-management services with the following elements: new diagnosis or acute exacerbation and stabilization of existing condition; condition which may benefit from joint care planning; condition for which specialist is taking a co-management role; condition expected to last at least 3 months; comprehensive care plan established, implemented, revised or monitored in partnership with co-managing clinicians; ongoing communication and care coordination between co-managing clinicians furnishing care

G9886 Behavioral counseling for diabetes prevention, in-person, group, 60 minutes

G9887 Behavioral counseling for diabetes prevention, distance learning, 60 minutes

G9888 Maintenance 5% WL from baseline weight in months 7-12

H0051 Traditional healing service

H0052 Missing and murdered indigenous persons (MMIP) mental health and clinical care

H0053 Historical trauma (HT) mental health and clinical care for indigenous persons

J0138 Injection, acetaminophen 10 mg and ibuprofen 3 mg

J0139 Injection, adalimumab, 1 mg

J0175 Injection, donanemab-azbt, 2 mg

J0177 Injection, aflibercept HD, 1 mg

J0209 Injection, sodium thiosulfate (Hope), 100 mg

J0211 Injection, sodium nitrite 3 mg and sodium thiosulfate 125 mg (Nithiodote)

J0577 Injection, buprenorphine extended-release (Brixadi), less than or equal to 7 days of therapy

J0578 Injection, buprenorphine extended-release (Brixadi), greater than 7 days and up to 28 days of therapy

J0589 Injection, daxibotulinumtoxina-lanm, 1 unit

J0601 Sevelamer carbonate (Renvela or therapeutically equivalent), oral, 20 mg (for ESRD on dialysis)

J0602 Sevelamer carbonate (Renvela or therapeutically equivalent), oral, powder, 20 mg (for ESRD on dialysis)

J0603 Sevelamer hydrochloride (Renagel or therapeutically equivalent), oral, 20 mg (for ESRD on dialysis)

NEW CODES (continued)

J0605 Sucroferric oxyhydroxide, oral, 5 mg (for ESRD on dialysis)

J0607 Lanthanum carbonate, oral, 5 mg (for ESRD on dialysis)

J0608 Lanthanum carbonate, oral, powder, 5 mg, not therapeutically equivalent to J0607 (for ESRD on dialysis)

J0609 Ferric citrate, oral, 3 mg ferric iron, (for ESRD on dialysis)

J0615 Calcium acetate, oral, 23 mg (for ESRD on dialysis)

J0650 Injection, levothyroxine sodium, not otherwise specified, 10 mcg

J0666 Injection, bupivacaine liposome, 1 mg

J0687 Injection, cefazolin sodium (WG Critical Care), not therapeutically equivalent to J0690, 500 mg

J0870 Injection, imetelstat, 1 mg

J0872 Injection, daptomycin (Xellia), unrefrigerated, not therapeutically equivalent to J0878 or J0873, 1 mg

J0901 Vadadustat, oral, 1 mg (for ESRD on dialysis)

J0911 Instillation, taurolidine 1.35 mg and heparin sodium 100 units (central venous catheter lock for adult patients receiving chronic hemodialysis)

J1010 Injection, methylprednisolone acetate, 1 mg

J1171 Injection, hydromorphone, 0.1 mg

J1202 Miglustat, oral, 65 mg

J1203 Injection, cipaglucosidase alfa-atga, 5 mg

J1307 Injection, crovalimab-akkz, 10 mg

J1323 Injection, elranatamab-bcmm, 1 mg

J1414 Injection, fidanacogene elaparvovec-dzkt, per therapeutic dose

J1434 Injection, fosaprepitant (Focinvez), 1 mg

J1552 Injection, immune globulin (Alyglo), 500 mg

J1597 Injection, glycopyrrolate (Glyrx-PF), 0.1 mg

J1598 Injection, glycopyrrolate (Fresenius Kabi), not therapeutically equivalent to J1596, 0.1 mg

J1748 Injection, infliximab-dyyb (Zymfentra), 10 mg

J1749 Injection, iloprost, 0.1 mcg

J2002 Injection, lidocaine HCl in 5% dextrose, 1 mg

J2003 Injection, lidocaine HCl , 1 mg

J2004 Injection, lidocaine HCl with epinephrine, 1 mg

J2183 Injection, meropenem (WG Critical Care), not therapeutically equivalent to J2185, 100 mg

J2246 Injection, micafungin in sodium (Baxter), not therapeutically equivalent to J2248, 1 mg

J2252 Injection, midazolam in 0.8% sodium chloride, intravenous, not therapeutically equivalent to J2250, 1 mg

J2253 Injection, midazolam (Seizalam), 1 mg

J2267 Injection, mirikizumab-mrkz, 1 mg

J2277 Injection, motixafortide, 0.25 mg

J2290 Injection, nafcillin sodium, 20 mg

J2373 Injection, phenylephrine hydrochloride (Immphentiv), 20 mcg

J2470 Injection, pantoprazole sodium, 40 mg

J2471 Injection, pantoprazole (Hikma), not therapeutically equivalent to J2470, 40 mg

J2472 Injection, pantoprazole sodium in sodium chloride (Baxter), 40 mg

J2601 Injection, vasopressin (Baxter), 1 unit

J2782 Injection, avacincaptad pegol, 0.1 mg

J2801 Injection, risperidone (Rykindo), 0.5 mg

J2802 Injection, romiplostim, 1 mcg

J2919 Injection, methylprednisolone sodium succinate, 5 mg

J3055 Injection, talquetamab-tgvs, 0.25 mg

J3247 Injection, secukinumab, IV, 1 mg

J3263 Injection, toripalimab-tpzi, 1 mg

J3392 Injection, exagamglogene autotemcel, per treatment

J3393 Injection, betibeglogene autotemcel, per treatment

J3394 Injection, lovotibeglogene autotemcel, per treatment

J3424 Injection, hydroxocobalamin, IV, 25 mg

J7165 Injection, prothrombin complex concentrate, human-lans, per IU of Factor IX activity

J7171 Injection, ADAMTS13, recombinant-krhn, 10 IU

J7354 Cantharidin for topical administration, 0.7%, single unit dose applicator (3.2 mg)

J7355 Injection, travoprost, intracameral implant, 1 mcg

J7514 Mycophenolate mofetil (Myhibbin), oral suspension, 100 mg

J7601 Ensifentrine, inhalation suspension, FDA-approved final product, noncompounded, administered through DME, unit dose form, 3 mg

J8522 Capecitabine, oral, 50 mg

J8541 Dexamethasone (Hemady), oral, 0.25 mg

J8611 Methotrexate (Jylamvo), oral, 2.5 mg

J8612 Methotrexate (Xatmep), oral, 2.5 mg

J9026 Injection, tarlatamab-dlle, 1 mg

J9028 Injection, nogapendekin alfa inbakicept-pmln, for intravesical use, 1 mcg

J9073 Injection, cyclophosphamide (Ingenus), 5 mg

J9074 Injection, cyclophosphamide (Sandoz), 5 mg

J9075 Injection, cyclophosphamide, not otherwise specified, 5 mg

J9076 Injection, cyclophosphamide (Baxter), 5 mg

J9248 Injection, melphalan (Hepzato), 1 mg

J9249 Injection, melphalan (Apotex), 1 mg

J9292 Injection, pemetrexed (Avyxa), not therapeutically equivalent to J9305, 10 mg

J9329 Injection, tislelizumab-jsgr, 1mg

J9361 Injection, efbemalenograstim alfa-vuxw, 0.5 mg

J9376 Injection, pozelimab-bbfg, 1 mg

K1037 Docking station for use with oral device/appliance used to reduce upper airway collapsibility

L1006 Scoliosis orthosis (SO), sagittal-coronal control provided by a rigid lateral frame, extends from axilla to trochanter, includes all accessory pads, straps and interface, prefabricated item that has been trimmed, bent, molded, assembled, or otherwise customized to fit a specific patient by an individual with expertise

L1320 Thoracic, pectus carinatum orthosis, sternal compression, rigid circumferential frame with anterior and posterior rigid pads, custom fabricated

L1653 Hip orthosis (HO), bilateral thigh cuffs with adjustable abductor spreader bar, adult size, prefabricated, off the shelf

L1821 Knee orthosis (KO), elastic with condylar pads and joints, with or without patellar control, prefabricated, off the shelf

L5783 Addition to lower extremity, user adjustable, mechanical, residual limb volume management system

L5841 Addition, endoskeletal knee-shin system, polycentric, pneumatic swing, and stance phase control

L8720 External lower extremity sensory prosthesis, cutaneous stimulation of mechanoreceptors proximal to the ankle, per leg

L8721 Receptor sole for use with L8720, replacement, each

M0224 Intravenous infusion, pemivibart, for the pre-exposure prophylaxis only, for certain adults and adolescents (12 years of age and older weighing at least 40 kg) with no known SARS-CoV-2 exposure, who either have moderate-to-severe immune compromise due to a medical condition or receipt of immunosuppressive medications or treatments, includes infusion and post administration monitoring

M1371 Most recent glycemic status assessment (HbA1c or GMI) level < 7.0%

M1372 Most recent glycemic status assessment (HbA1c or GMI) level >= 7.0% and < 8.0%

M1373 Most recent glycemic status assessment (HbA1c or GMI) level >= 8.0% and <= 9.0%

M1374 An additional encounter with an RA diagnosis during the performance period or prior performance period that is at least 90 days before or after an encounter with an RA diagnosis during the performance period

M1375 An additional encounter with an RA diagnosis during the performance period or prior performance period that is at least 90 days before or after an encounter with an RA diagnosis during the performance period

M1376 An additional encounter with an RA diagnosis during the performance period or prior performance period that is at least 90 days before or after an encounter with an RA diagnosis during the performance period

M1377 Recommended follow-up interval for repeat colonoscopy of 10 years documented in colonoscopy report and communicated with patient

M1378 Documentation of medical reason(s) for not recommending a 10 year follow-up interval (e.g., inadequate prep, familial or personal history of colonic polyps, patient had no adenoma and age is >= 66 years old, or life expectancy < 10 years, other medical reasons)

M1379 A 10 year follow-up interval for colonoscopy not recommended, reason not otherwise specified

NEW CODES (continued)

M1380 Filled at least two prescriptions during the performance period for any combination of the qualifying oral antipsychotic medications listed under "denominator note" or the long-acting injectable antipsychotic medications listed under "denominator note"

M1381 Patients with secondary stroke (e.g., a subsequent stroke that may occur with vasospasm in the setting of subarachnoid hemorrhage) within 5 days of the initial procedure

M1382 Patient encounter during the performance period with Place of Service code 11

M1383 Acute PVD

M1384 Patients who died during the performance period

M1385 Documentation of patient reasons for patients who were not seen for the second PAM survey (e.g., less than 4 months between baseline pam assessment and follow-up)

M1386 Patients with an excisional surgery for melanoma or melanoma in situ in the past 5 years with an initial AJCC staging of 0, I, or II at the start of the performance period

M1387 Patients who died during the performance period

M1388 Patients with documentation of an exam performed for recurrence of melanoma

M1389 Documentation of patient reasons for no examination, i.e., refusal of examination or lost to follow-up (documentation must include information that the clinician was unable to reach the patient by phone, mail or secure electronic mail - at least one method must be documented)

M1390 Patients who do not have a documented exam performed for recurrence of melanoma or no documentation within the performance period

M1391 All patients who were diagnosed with recurrent melanoma during the current performance period

M1392 Documentation of patient reasons for no examination, i.e., refusal of examination or lost to follow-up (documentation must include information that the clinician was unable to reach the patient by phone, mail or secure electronic mail - at least one method must be documented)

M1393 Patients who were not diagnosed with recurrent melanoma during the current performance period

M1394 Stages I-III breast cancer

M1395 Patients receiving an initial chemotherapy regimen with a defined duration with the eligible clinician or group

M1396 Patients on a therapeutic clinical trial

M1397 Patients with recurrence/disease progression

M1398 Patients with baseline and follow-up PROMIS surveys documented in the medical record

M1399 Patients who leave the practice during the follow-up period

M1400 Patients who died during the follow-up period

M1401 Stages I-III breast cancer

M1402 Patients receiving an initial chemotherapy regimen with a defined duration with the eligible clinician or group

M1403 Patients with baseline and follow-up PROMIS surveys documented in the medical record

M1404 Patients on a therapeutic clinical trial

M1405 Patients with recurrence/disease progression

M1406 Patients who leave the practice during the follow-up period

M1407 Patients who died during the follow-up period

M1408 Patients who have germline BRCA testing completed before diagnosis of epithelial ovarian, fallopian tube, or primary peritoneal cancer

M1409 Patients who received germline testing for BRCA1 and BRCA2 or genetic counseling completed within 6 months of diagnosis

M1410 Patients who did not have germline testing for BRCA1 and BRCA2 or genetic counseling completed within 6 months of diagnosis

M1411 Currently on first-line immune checkpoint inhibitors without chemotherapy

M1412 Patients with metastatic NSCLC with epidermal growth factor receptor (EGFR) mutations, ALK genomic tumor aberrations, or other targetable genomic abnormalities with approved first-line targeted therapy, such as NSCLC with ROS1 rearrangement, BRAF V600E mutation, NTRK 1/2/3 gene fusion, METex14 skipping mutation, and RET rearrangement

M1413 Patients who had a positive PD-L1 biomarker expression test result prior to the initiation of first-line immune checkpoint inhibitor therapy

M1414 Documentation of medical reason(s) for not performing the PD-L1 biomarker expression test prior to initiation of first-line immune checkpoint inhibitor therapy (e.g., patient is in an urgent or emergent situation where delay of treatment would jeopardize the patient's health status; other medical reasons/contraindication)

M1415 Patients who did not have a positive PD-L1 biomarker expression test result prior to the initiation of first-line immune checkpoint inhibitor therapy

M1416 Patient received hospice services any time during the performance period

M1417 Patients who are up to date on their Covid-19 vaccinations as defined by CDC recommendations on current vaccination

M1418 Patients who are not up to date on their Covid-19 vaccinations as defined by CDC recommendations on current vaccination because of a medical contraindication documented by clinician

M1419 Patients who are not up to date on their Covid-19 vaccinations as defined by CDC recommendations on current vaccination

M1420 Complete ophthalmologic care MIPS value pathway

M1421 Dermatological care MIPS value pathway

M1422 Gastroenterology care MIPS value pathway

M1423 Optimal care for patients with urologic conditions MIPS value pathway

M1424 Pulmonology care MIPS value pathway

M1425 Surgical care MIPS value pathway

P9027 Red blood cells, leukocytes reduced, oxygen/ carbon dioxide reduced, each unit

Q0155 Dronabinol (Syndros), 0.1 mg, oral, FDA-approved prescription anti-emetic, for use as a complete therapeutic substitute for an IV anti-emetic at the time of chemotherapy treatment, not to exceed a 48 hour dosage regimen

Q0224 Injection, pemivibart, for the pre-exposure prophylaxis only, for certain adults and adolescents (12 years of age and older weighing at least 40 kg) with no known SARS-CoV-2 exposure, and who either have moderate-to-severe immune compromise due to a medical condition or receipt of immunosuppressive medications or treatments, and are unlikely to mount an adequate immune response to COVID-19 vaccination, 4500 mg

Q0521 Pharmacy supplying fee for HIV pre-exposure prophylaxis FDA-approved prescription

Q4305 American Amnion AC Tri-Layer, per sq cm

Q4306 American Amnion AC, per sq cm

Q4307 American Amnion, per sq cm

Q4308 Sanopellis, per sq cm

Q4309 VIA Matrix, per sq cm

Q4310 Procenta, per 100 mg

Q4311 Acesso, per sq cm

Q4312 Acesso AC, per sq cm

Q4313 DermaBind FM, per sq cm

Q4314 Reeva FT, per sq cm

Q4315 RegeneLink Amniotic Membrane Allograft, per sq cm

Q4316 AmchoPlast, per sq cm

Q4317 VitoGraft, per sq cm

Q4318 E-Graft, per sq cm

Q4319 SanoGraft, per sq cm

Q4320 PelloGraft, per sq cm

Q4321 RenoGraft, per sq cm

Q4322 CaregraFT, per sq cm

Q4323 alloPLY, per sq cm

Q4324 AmnioTX, per sq cm

Q4325 ACApatch, per sq cm

Q4326 WoundPlus, per sq cm

Q4327 DuoAmnion, per sq cm

Q4328 MOST, per sq cm

Q4329 Singlay, per sq cm

Q4330 TOTAL, per sq cm

Q4331 Axolotl Graft, per sq cm

Q4332 Axolotl DualGraft, per sq cm

Q4333 ArdeoGraft, per sq cm

Q4334 AmnioPlast 1, per sq cm

NEW CODES (continued)

Q4335 AmnioPlast 2, per sq cm
Q4336 Artacent C, per sq cm
Q4337 Artacent Trident, per sq cm
Q4338 Artacent Velos, per sq cm
Q4339 Artacent Vericlen, per sq cm
Q4340 SimpliGraft, per sq cm
Q4341 SimpliMax, per sq cm
Q4342 TheraMend, per sq cm
Q4343 Dermacyte AC Matrix Amniotic Membrane Allograft, per sq cm
Q4344 Tri-Membrane Wrap, per sq cm
Q4345 Matrix HD Allograft Dermis, per sq cm
Q4346 Shelter DM Matrix, per sq cm
Q4347 Rampart DL Matrix, per sq cm
Q4348 Sentry SL Matrix, per sq cm
Q4349 Mantle DL Matrix, per sq cm
Q4350 Palisade DM Matrix, per sq cm
Q4351 Enclose TL Matrix, per sq cm
Q4352 Overlay SL Matrix, per sq cm
Q4353 Xceed TL Matrix, per sq cm
Q5133 Injection, tocilizumab-bavi (Tofidence), biosimilar, 1 mg
Q5134 Injection, natalizumab-sztn (Tyruko), biosimilar, 1 mg
Q5135 Injection, tocilizumab-aazg (Tyenne), biosimilar, 1 mg
Q5136 Injection, denosumab-bbdz (Jubbonti/Wyost), biosimilar, 1 mg
Q5137 Injection, ustekinumab-auub (Wezlana), biosimilar, SC, 1 mg
Q5138 Injection, ustekinumab-auub (Wezlana), biosimilar, IV, 1 mg
Q5139 Injection, eculizumab-aeeb (bkemv), biosimilar, 10 mg
Q5140 Injection, adalimumab-fkjp, biosimilar, 1 mg
Q5141 Injection, adalimumab-aaty, biosimilar, 1 mg
Q5142 Injection, adalimumab-ryvk biosimilar, 1 mg
Q5143 Injection, adalimumab-adbm, biosimilar, 1 mg
Q5144 Injection, adalimumab-aacf (Idacio), biosimilar, 1 mg
Q5145 Injection, adalimumab-afzb (Abrilada), biosimilar, 1 mg
Q5146 Injection, trastuzumab-strf (Hercessi), biosimilar, 10 mg
Q9996 Injection, ustekinumab-ttwe (Pyzchiva), subcutaneous, 1 mg
Q9997 Injection, ustekinumab-ttwe (Pyzchiva), intravenous, 1 mg
Q9998 Injection, ustekinumab-aekn (Selarsdi), 1 mg
S4988 Penile contracture device, manual, greater than 3 lbs traction force
S9002 Intravaginal motion sensor system, provides biofeedback for pelvic floor muscle rehabilitation device

REVISED CODES

A2024 Resolve Matrix or XenoPatch, per sq cm
A4271 Integrated lancing and blood sample testing cartridges for home blood glucose monitor, per 50 tests
A4561 Pessary, reusable, rubber, any type
A4562 Pessary, reusable, non rubber, any type
C7900 Service for diagnosis, evaluation, or treatment of a mental health or substance use disorder, 15-29 minutes, provided remotely by hospital staff who are licensed to provide mental health services under applicable state law(s), when the patient is in their home, and there is no associated professional service
C7901 Service for diagnosis, evaluation, or treatment of a mental health or substance use disorder, 30-60 minutes, provided remotely by hospital staff who are licensed to provided mental health services under applicable state law(s), when the patient is in their home, and there is no associated professional service
E0739 Rehabilitation system with interactive interface providing active assistance in rehabilitation therapy, includes all components and accessories, motors, microprocessors, sensors
E1800 Dynamic adjustable elbow extension and flexion device, includes soft interface material
E1805 Dynamic adjustable wrist extension and flexion device, includes soft interface material
E1810 Dynamic adjustable knee extension and flexion device, includes soft interface material
E1815 Dynamic adjustable ankle extension and flexion device, includes soft interface material
E1825 Dynamic adjustable finger extension and flexion device, includes soft interface material
E1830 Dynamic adjustable toe extension and flexion device, includes soft interface material
E2001 Suction pump, home model, portable or stationary, electric, any type, for use with external urine and/or fecal management system
G0323 Care management services for behavioral health conditions, at least 20 minutes of clinical psychologist, clinical social worker, mental health counselor, or marriage and family therapist time, per calendar month. (These services include the following required elements: initial assessment or follow-up monitoring, including the use of applicable validated rating scales; behavioral health care planning in relation to behavioral/psychiatric health problems, including revision for patients who are not progressing or whose status changes; facilitating and coordinating treatment such as psychotherapy, coordination with and/or referral to physicians and practitioners who are authorized by medicare to prescribe medications and furnish E/M services, counseling and/or psychiatric consultation; and continuity of care with a designated member of the care team)
G2069 Medication assisted treatment, buprenorphine (injectable) administered on a monthly basis; bundle including dispensing and/or administration, substance use counseling, individual and group therapy, and toxicology testing if performed (provision of the services by a medicare-enrolled opioid treatment program)
G2076 Intake activities, including initial medical examination that is conducted by an appropriately licensed practitioner and preparation of a care plan, which may be informed by administration of a standardized, evidence-based social determinants of health risk assessment to identify unmet health-related social needs, and that includes the patient's goals and mutually agreed-upon actions for the patient to meet those goals, including harm reduction interventions; the patient's needs and goals in the areas of education, vocational training, and employment; and the medical and psychiatric, psychosocial, economic, legal, housing, and other recovery support services that a patient needs and wishes to pursue, conducted by an appropriately licensed/credentialed personnel (provision of the services by a medicare-enrolled opioid treatment program); list separately in addition to each primary code
G2077 Periodic assessment; assessing periodically by an otp practitioner and includes a review of moud dosing, treatment response, other substance use disorder treatment needs, responses and patient-identified goals, and other relevant physical and psychiatric treatment needs and goals; assessment may be informed by administration of a standardized, evidence-based social determinants of health risk assessment to identify unmet health-related social needs, or the need and interest for harm reduction interventions and recovery support services (provision of the services by a medicare-enrolled opioid treatment program); list separately in addition to each primary code
G2091 Patients 66 years of age and older with at least one claim/encounter for frailty during the measurement period and an advanced illness diagnosis during the measurement period or the year prior to the measurement period
G2099 Patients 66 years of age and older with at least one claim/encounter for frailty during the measurement period and an advanced illness diagnosis during the measurement period or the year prior to the measurement period
G2101 Patients 66 years of age and older with at least one claim/encounter for frailty during the measurement period and an advanced illness diagnosis during the measurement period or the year prior to the measurement period
G2107 Patients 66 years of age and older with at least one claim/encounter for frailty during the measurement period and an advanced illness diagnosis during the measurement period or the year prior to the measurement period
G2116 Patients 66 - 80 years of age with at least one claim/encounter for frailty during the measurement period and an advanced illness diagnosis during the measurement period or the year prior to the measurement period
G2126 Patients 66-80 years of age with at least one claim/encounter for frailty during the measurement period and an advanced illness diagnosis during the measurement period or the year prior to the measurement period
G8577 Re-exploration required due to mediastinal bleeding with or without tamponade, unplanned coronary artery intervention (native, vessel, graft, or both), valve dysfunction, aortic reintervention, or other cardiac reason

REVISED CODES (continued)

G8578 Re-exploration not required due to mediastinal bleeding with or without tamponade, unplanned coronary artery intervention (native, vessel, graft, or both), valve dysfunction, aortic reintervention, or other cardiac reason

G8694 Current or prior left ventricular ejection fraction (lvef) < = 40% or documentation of moderate or severe lvsd

G8842 Apnea hypopnea index (ahi), respiratory disturbance index (rdi) or respiratory event index (rei) documented or measured within 2 months after initial evaluation for suspected obstructive sleep apnea

G8843 Documentation of reason(s) for not measuring an apnea hypopnea index (ahi), a respiratory disturbance index (rdi), or a respiratory event index (rei) within 2 months after initial evaluation for suspected obstructive sleep apnea (e.g., medical, neurological, or psychiatric disease that prohibits successful completion of a sleep study, patients for whom a sleep study would present a bigger risk than benefit or would pose an undue burden, dementia, patients previously diagnosed with osa and severity assessed by another provider, patients who decline ahi/rdi/rei measurement, patients who had a financial reason for not completing testing, test was ordered but not completed, patients decline because their insurance (payer) does not cover the expense)

G8844 Apnea hypopnea index (ahi), respiratory disturbance index (rdi), or respiratory event index (rei) not documented or measured within 2 months after initial evaluation for suspected obstructive sleep apnea, reason not given

G8923 Current or prior left ventricular ejection fraction (lvef) <= 40% or documentation of moderately or severely depressed left ventricular systolic function

G8934 Current or prior left ventricular ejection fraction (lvef) <=40% or documentation of moderately or severely depressed left ventricular systolic function

G9246 Patient did not have two eligible encounters at least 90 days apart or one eligible encounter and one hiv viral load test at least 90 days apart

G9247 Patient had two eligible encounters at least 90 days apart or one eligible encounter and one hiv viral load test at least 90 days apart

G9254 Documentation of patient discharged to home later than post-operative day 2 following cea or cas

G9255 Documentation of patient discharged to home no later than post operative day 2 following cea or cas

G9321 Count of previous ct (any type of ct) and cardiac nuclear medicine (myocardial perfusion or infarct avid imaging) studies documented in the 12-month period prior to the current study

G9322 Count of previous ct and cardiac nuclear medicine (myocardial perfusion or infarct avid imaging) studies not documented in the 12-month period prior to the current study, reason not given

G9659 Patients greater than or equal to 86 years of age who underwent a screening colonoscopy and did not have a history of colorectal cancer or other valid medical reason for the colonoscopy, including: iron deficiency anemia, lower gastrointestinal bleeding, familial adenomatous polyposis, lynch syndrome (i.e., hereditary non-polyposis colorectal cancer), inflammatory bowel disease (i.e., crohn's disease or ulcerative colitis), abnormal finding of gastrointestinal tract, weight loss, or changes in bowel habits

G9660 Documentation of medical reason(s) for a colonoscopy performed on a patient greater than or equal to 86 years of age (e.g., iron deficiency anemia, lower gastrointestinal bleeding, familial history of adenomatous polyposis, lynch syndrome (i.e., hereditary non-polyposis colorectal cancer), inflammatory bowel disease (i.e., crohn's disease or ulcerative colitis), abnormal finding of gastrointestinal tract, weight loss, or changes in bowel habits)

G9999 Documentation of system reason(s) for an interval of less than 3 years since the last colonoscopy (e.g., unable to locate previous colonoscopy report, patient cannot provide precise date or details from previous colonoscopy, previous colonoscopy report was incomplete)

J0134 Injection, acetaminophen (Fresenius Kabi), not therapeutically equivalent to J0131, 10 mg

J0136 Injection, acetaminophen (B. Braun), not therapeutically equivalent to J0131, 10 mg

J0137 Injection, acetaminophen (Hikma), not therapeutically equivalent to J0131, 10 mg

J0173 Injection, epinephrine (Belcher), not therapeutically equivalent to J0171, 0.1 mg

J0208 Injection, sodium thiosulfate (Pedmark), 100 mg

J0401 Injection, aripiprazole (Abilify Maintena), 1 mg

J0612 Injection, calcium gluconate, not otherwise specified, 10 mg

J0613 Injection, calcium gluconate (WG Critical Care), not therapeutically equivalent to J0612, 10 mg

J0651 Injection, levothyroxine sodium (Fresenius Kabi), not therapeutically equivalent to J0650, 10 mcg

J0652 Injection, levothyroxine sodium (Hikma), not therapeutically equivalent to J0650, 10 mcg

J0873 Injection, daptomycin (Xellia), not therapeutically equivalent to J0878 or J0872, 1 mg

J0893 Injection, decitabine (Sun Pharma), not therapeutically equivalent to J0894, 1 mg

J1574 Injection, ganciclovir sodium (Exela), not therapeutically equivalent to J1570, 500 mg

J1806 Injection, esmolol hydrochloride (WG Critical Care), not therapeutically equivalent to J1805, 10 mg

J1921 Injection, labetalol hydrochloride (Hikma), not therapeutically equivalent to J1920, 5 mg

J2021 Injection, linezolid (Hospira), not therapeutically equivalent to J2020, 200 mg

J2184 Injection, meropenem (B. Braun), not therapeutically equivalent to J2185, 100 mg

J2251 Injection, midazolam in 0.9% sodium chloride, intravenous, not therapeutically equivalent to J2250, 1 mg

J2272 Injection, morphine sulfate (Fresenius Kabi), not therapeutically equivalent to J2270, up to 10 mg

J2281 Injection, moxifloxacin (Fresenius Kabi), not therapeutically equivalent to J2280, 100 mg

J2468 Injection, palonosetron hydrochloride (posfrea), 25 micrograms

J2599 Injection, vasopressin (American Regent), not therapeutically equivalent to J2598, 1 unit

J3244 Injection, tigecycline (Accord), not therapeutically equivalent to J3243, 1 mg

J3371 Injection, vancomycin HCl (Mylan), not therapeutically equivalent to J3370, 500 mg

J3372 Injection, vancomycin HCl (Xellia), not therapeutically equivalent to J3370, 500 mg

J3380 Injection, vedolizumab, IV, 1 mg

J3425 Injection, hydroxocobalamin, IM, 10 mcg

J7516 Injection, cyclosporine, 250 mg

J9029 Intravesical instillation, nadofaragene firadenovec-vncg, per therapeutic dose

J9033 Injection, bendamustine hydrochloride, 1 mg

J9046 Injection, bortezomib (Dr. Reddy's), not therapeutically equivalent to J9041, 0.1 mg

J9071 Injection, cyclophosphamide (AuroMedics), 5 mg

J9072 Injection, cyclophosphamide (avyxa), 5 mg

J9172 Injection, docetaxel (Docivyx), 1 mg

J9255 Injection, methotrexate (Accord), not therapeutically equivalent to J9260, 50 mg

J9260 Injection, methotrexate sodium, 50 mg

J9294 Injection, pemetrexed (Hospira), not therapeutically equivalent to J9305, 10 mg

J9296 Injection, pemetrexed (Accord), not therapeutically equivalent to J9305, 10 mg

J9314 Injection, pemetrexed (Teva), not therapeutically equivalent to J9305, 10 mg

J9322 Injection, pemetrexed (BluePoint), not therapeutically equivalent to J9305, 10 mg

J9393 Injection, fulvestrant (Teva), not therapeutically equivalent to J9395, 25 mg

L1652 Hip orthosis (HO), bilateral thigh cuffs with adjustable abductor spreader bar, adult size, prefabricated, includes fitting and adjustment, prefabricated item that has been trimmed, bent, molded, assembled, or otherwise customized to fit a specific patient by an individual with expertise

L1820 Knee orthosis (KO), elastic with condylar pads and joints, with or without patellar control, prefabricated item that has been trimmed, bent, molded, assembled, or otherwise customized to fit a specific patient by an individual with expertise

REVISED CODES (continued)

M0004 Quality care for patients with neurological conditions mips value pathway

M1150 Current or prior left ventricular ejection fraction (lvef) less than or equal to 40% or documentation of moderately or severely depressed left ventricular systolic function

M1176 Patient did not receive two doses of the herpes zoster recombinant vaccine (at least 28 days apart) anytime on or after the patient's 50th birthday before or during the measurement period

M1177 Patient received any pneumococcal conjugate or polysaccharide vaccine on or after their 19th birthday and before the end of the measurement period

M1179 Patient did not receive any pneumococcal conjugate or polysaccharide vaccine, on or after their 19th birthday and before or during measurement period

M1211 Most recent glycemic status assessment (hba1c or gmi) level > 9.0%

M1212 Glycemic status assessment (hba1c or gmi) level is missing, or was not performed during the measurement period

M1259 Patient status documented within the first year of initiating dialysis

M1260 Patient status not documented within the first year of initiating dialysis

M1267 Patients not observed in active status on any kidney or kidney-pancreas transplant waitlist as of the last day of each month during the measurement period

M1268 Patients observed in active status on any kidney or kidney-pancreas transplant waitlist as of the last day of each month during the measurement period

M1272 Patients observed on any kidney or kidney-pancreas transplant waitlist as of the last day of each month during the measurement period

M1292 Patients 66 years of age and older with at least one claim/encounter for frailty during the measurement period and an advanced illness diagnosis during the measurement period or the year prior to the measurement period

M1343 Patients who are at pam level 4 at baseline or patients who are flagged with extreme straight line response sets on the pam or with excessive missing responses

M1344 Patients who did not have a baseline pam score and/or a second score within 4 to 12 months of baseline pam score

M1345 Patients who had a baseline pam score and a second score within 4 to 12 month of baseline pam score

M1346 Patients who did not have a net increase in pam score of at least 6 points within a 4 to 12 month period

M1347 Patients who achieved a net increase in pam score of at least 3 points in a 4 to 12 month period (passing)

M1348 Patients who achieved a net increase in pam score of at least 6-points in a 4 to 12 month period (excellent)

M1349 Patients who did not have a net increase in pam score of at least 3 points within a 4 to 12 month period

Q2052 Services, supplies and accessories used in the home for the administration of intravenous immune globulin (IVIG)

Q2055 Idecabtagene vicleucel, up to 510 million autologous B-cell maturation antigen (BCMA) directed CAR-positive T cells, including leukapheresis and dose preparation procedures, per therapeutic dose

DELETED CODES

C7558 C9113 C9150 C9159 C9160 C9161 C9162
C9163 C9164 C9165 C9166 C9167 C9168 C9169
C9170 C9171 C9172 C9290 C9734 C9769 C9786
C9787 C9790 C9794 C9795 E2300 G0106 G0120
G0122 G2012 G2070 G2071 G2072 G8482 G8483
G8484 G8965 G8966 G9402 G9403 G9404 G9405
G9406 G9407 G9458 G9459 G9460 G9707 G9751
G9760 G9892 G9893 G9919 G9920 G9921 G9974
G9975 G9990 G9991 J0135 J0570 J0576 J1020
J1030 J1040 J1170 J1840 J1850 J2001 J2780
J2796 J2806 J2920 J2930 J8520 J8521 J9058
J9059 J9070 J9250 J9258 J9259 J9371 M0003
M1154 M1155 M1219 M1264 Q0516 Q0517 Q0518
Q0519 Q0520 Q4210 Q4244 Q4277 Q5131 Q5132
S0164

Appendix 6 — Place of Service and Type of Service

Place-of-Service Codes for Professional Claims

Listed below are place of service codes and descriptions. These codes should be used on professional claims to specify the entity where service(s) were rendered. Check with individual payers (e.g., Medicare, Medicaid, other private insurance) for reimbursement policies regarding these codes. Comments or questions regarding place-of-service codes or descriptions should be directed to your Medicare administrative contractor (MAC).

Code	Name	Description
01	Pharmacy	A facility or location where drugs and other medically related items and services are sold, dispensed, or otherwise provided directly to patients.
02	Telehealth Provided Other than in Patient's Home	The location where health services and health related services are provided or received, through telecommunication technology. Patient is not located in their home when receiving health services or health related services through telecommunication technology.
03	School	A facility whose primary purpose is education.
04	Homeless Shelter	A facility or location whose primary purpose is to provide temporary housing to homeless individuals (e.g., emergency shelters, individual or family shelters).
05	Indian Health Service Free-standing Facility	A facility or location, owned and operated by the Indian Health Service, which provides diagnostic, therapeutic (surgical and non-surgical), and rehabilitation services to American Indians and Alaska Natives who do not require hospitalization.
06	Indian Health Service Provider-based Facility	A facility or location, owned and operated by the Indian Health Service, which provides diagnostic, therapeutic (surgical and non-surgical), and rehabilitation services rendered by, or under the supervision of, physicians to American Indians and Alaska Natives admitted as inpatients or outpatients.
07	Tribal 638 Free-standing Facility	A facility or location owned and operated by a federally recognized American Indian or Alaska Native tribe or tribal organization under a 638 agreement, which provides diagnostic, therapeutic (surgical and non-surgical), and rehabilitation services to tribal members who do not require hospitalization.
08	Tribal 638 Provider-based Facility	A facility or location owned and operated by a federally recognized American Indian or Alaska Native tribe or tribal organization under a 638 agreement, which provides diagnostic, therapeutic (surgical and non-surgical), and rehabilitation services to tribal members admitted as inpatients or outpatients.
09	Prison/Correctional Facility	A prison, jail, reformatory, work farm, detention center, or any other similar facility maintained by either Federal, State or local authorities for the purpose of confinement or rehabilitation of adult or juvenile criminal offenders.
10	Telehealth Provided in Patient's Home	The location where health services and health related services are provided or received, through telecommunication technology. Patient is located in their home (which is a location other than a hospital or other facility where the patient receives care in a private residence) when receiving health services or health related services through telecommunication technology.
11	Office	Location, other than a hospital, skilled nursing facility (SNF), military treatment facility, community health center, State or local public health clinic, or intermediate care facility (ICF), where the health professional routinely provides health examinations, diagnosis, and treatment of illness or injury on an ambulatory basis.
12	Home	Location, other than a hospital or other facility, where the patient receives care in a private residence.
13	Assisted Living Facility	Congregate residential facility with self-contained living units providing assessment of each resident's needs and on-site support 24 hours a day, 7 days a week, with the capacity to deliver or arrange for services including some health care and other services.
14	Group home	A residence, with shared living areas, where clients receive supervision and other services such as social and/or behavioral services, custodial service, and minimal services (e.g., medication administration).
15	Mobile Unit	A facility/unit that moves from place-to-place equipped to provide preventive, screening, diagnostic, and/or treatment services.
16	Temporary Lodging	A short term accommodation such as a hotel, campground, hostel, cruise ship or resort where the patient receives care, and which is not identified by any other POS code.
17	Walk-in Retail Health Clinic	A walk-in health clinic, other than an office, urgent care facility, pharmacy or independent clinic and not described by any other Place of Service code, that is located within a retail operation and provides, on an ambulatory basis, preventive and primary care services.
18	Place of Employment-Worksite	A location, not described by any other POS code, owned or operated by a public or private entity where the patient is employed, and where a health professional provides on-going or episodic occupational medical, therapeutic or rehabilitative services to the individual.
19	Off Campus-Outpatient Hospital	A portion of an off-campus hospital provider based department which provides diagnostic, therapeutic (both surgical and nonsurgical), and rehabilitation services to sick or injured persons who do not require hospitalization or institutionalization.
20	Urgent Care Facility	Location, distinct from a hospital emergency room, an office, or a clinic, whose purpose is to diagnose and treat illness or injury for unscheduled, ambulatory patients seeking immediate medical attention.
21	Inpatient Hospital	A facility, other than psychiatric, which primarily provides diagnostic, therapeutic (both surgical and nonsurgical), and rehabilitation services by, or under, the supervision of physicians to patients admitted for a variety of medical conditions.
22	On Campus-Outpatient Hospital	A portion of a hospital's main campus which provides diagnostic, therapeutic (both surgical and nonsurgical), and rehabilitation services to sick or injured persons who do not require hospitalization or institutionalization.
23	Emergency Room-Hospital	A portion of a hospital where emergency diagnosis and treatment of illness or injury is provided.
24	Ambulatory Surgical Center	A freestanding facility, other than a physician's office, where surgical and diagnostic services are provided on an ambulatory basis.
25	Birthing center	A facility, other than a hospital's maternity facilities or a physician's office, which provides a setting for labor, delivery, and immediate post-partum care as well as immediate care of new born infants.

26	Military Treatment Facility	A medical facility operated by one or more of the Uniformed services. Military Treatment Facility (MTF) also refers to certain former US Public Health Service (USPHS) facilities now designated as Uniformed Service Treatment Facilities (USTF).
27	Outreach Site/Street	A non-permanent location on the street or found environment, not described by any other POS code, where health professionals provide preventive, screening, diagnostic, and/or treatment services to unsheltered homeless individuals.
28-30	Unassigned	N/A
31	Skilled Nursing Facility	A facility which primarily provides inpatient skilled nursing care and related services to patients who require medical, nursing, or rehabilitative services but does not provide the level of care or treatment available in a hospital.
32	Nursing Facility	A facility which primarily provides to residents skilled nursing care and related services for the rehabilitation of injured, disabled, or sick persons, or, on a regular basis, health-related care services above the level of custodial care to other than individuals with intellectual disabilities.
33	Custodial Care Facility	A facility which provides room, board and other personal assistance services, generally on a long-term basis, and which does not include a medical component.
34	Hospice	A facility, other than a patient's home, in which palliative and supportive care for terminally ill patients and their families are provided.
35-40	Unassigned	N/A
41	Ambulance-Land	A land vehicle specifically designed, equipped and staffed for lifesaving and transporting the sick or injured.
42	Ambulance-Air or Water	An air or water vehicle specifically designed, equipped and staffed for lifesaving and transporting the sick or injured.
43-48	Unassigned	N/A
49	Independent Clinic	A location, not part of a hospital and not described by any other Place-of-Service code, that is organized and operated to provide preventive, diagnostic, therapeutic, rehabilitative, or palliative services to outpatients only.
50	Federally Qualified Health Center	A facility located in a medically underserved area that provides Medicare beneficiaries preventive primary medical care under the general direction of a physician.
51	Inpatient Psychiatric Facility	A facility that provides inpatient psychiatric services for the diagnosis and treatment of mental illness on a 24-hour basis, by or under the supervision of a physician.
52	Psychiatric Facility-Partial Hospitalization	A facility for the diagnosis and treatment of mental illness that provides a planned therapeutic program for patients who do not require full time hospitalization, but who need broader programs than are possible from outpatient visits to a hospital-based or hospital-affiliated facility.
53	Community Mental Health Center	A facility that provides the following services: outpatient services, including specialized outpatient services for children, the elderly, individuals who are chronically ill, and residents of the CMHC's mental health services area who have been discharged from inpatient treatment at a mental health facility; 24 hour a day emergency care services; day treatment, other partial hospitalization services, or psychosocial rehabilitation services; screening for patients being considered for admission to State mental health facilities to determine the appropriateness of such admission; and consultation and education services.
54	Intermediate Care Facility/Individuals with Intellectual Disabilities	A facility which primarily provides health-related care and services above the level of custodial care to individuals but does not provide the level of care or treatment available in a hospital or SNF.
55	Residential Substance Abuse Treatment Facility	A facility which provides treatment for substance (alcohol and drug) abuse to live-in residents who do not require acute medical care. Services include individual and group therapy and counseling, family counseling, laboratory tests, drugs and supplies, psychological testing, and room and board.
56	Psychiatric Residential Treatment Center	A facility or distinct part of a facility for psychiatric care which provides a total 24-hour therapeutically planned and professionally staffed group living and learning environment.
57	Non-residential Substance Abuse Treatment Facility	A location which provides treatment for substance (alcohol and drug) abuse on an ambulatory basis. Services include individual and group therapy and counseling, family counseling, laboratory tests, drugs and supplies, and psychological testing.
58	Non-residential Opioid Treatment Facility	A location that provides treatment for opioid use disorder on an ambulatory basis. Services include methadone and other forms of Medication Assisted Treatment (MAT).
59	Unassigned	N/A
60	Mass Immunization Center	A location where providers administer pneumococcal pneumonia and influenza virus vaccinations and submit these services as electronic media claims, paper claims, or using the roster billing method. This generally takes place in a mass immunization setting, such as, a public health center, pharmacy, or mall but may include a physician office setting.
61	Comprehensive Inpatient Rehabilitation Facility	A facility that provides comprehensive rehabilitation services under the supervision of a physician to inpatients with physical disabilities. Services include physical therapy, occupational therapy, speech pathology, social or psychological services, and orthotics and prosthetics services.
62	Comprehensive Outpatient Rehabilitation Facility	A facility that provides comprehensive rehabilitation services under the supervision of a physician to outpatients with physical disabilities. Services include physical therapy, occupational therapy, and speech pathology services.
63-64	Unassigned	N/A
65	End-Stage Renal Disease Treatment Facility	A facility other than a hospital, which provides dialysis treatment, maintenance, and/or training to patients or caregivers on an ambulatory or home-care basis.

66	Programs of All-Inclusive Care for the Elderly (PACE) Center	A facility or location providing comprehensive medical and social services as part of the Programs of All-Inclusive Care for the Elderly (PACE). This includes, but is not limited to, primary care; social work services; restorative therapies, including physical and occupational therapy; personal care and supportive services; nutritional counseling; recreational therapy; and meals when the individual is enrolled in PACE.
67-70	Unassigned	N/A
71	Public Health Clinic	A facility maintained by either State or local health departments that provides ambulatory primary medical care under the general direction of a physician.
72	Rural Health Clinic	A certified facility which is located in a rural medically underserved area that provides ambulatory primary medical care under the general direction of a physician.
73-80	Unassigned	N/A
81	Independent Laboratory	A laboratory certified to perform diagnostic and/or clinical tests independent of an institution or a physician's office.
82-98	Unassigned	N/A
99	Other Place of Service	Other place of service not identified above.

Type of Service

Common Working File Type of Service (TOS) Indicators

For submitting a claim to the Common Working File (CWF), use the following table to assign the proper TOS. Some procedures may have more than one applicable TOS. CWF will reject codes with incorrect TOS designations. CWF will produce alerts on codes with incorrect TOS designations.

The only exceptions to this annual update are:

- Surgical services billed for dates of service through December 31, 2007, containing the ASC facility service modifier SG must be reported as TOS F. Effective for services on or after January 1, 2008, the SG modifier is no longer applicable for Medicare services. ASC providers should discontinue applying the SG modifier on ASC facility claims. The indicator F does not appear in the TOS table because its use depends upon claims submitted with POS 24 (ASC facility) from an ASC (specialty 49). This became effective for dates of service January 1, 2008, or after.
- Surgical services billed with an assistant-at-surgery modifier (80-82, AS) must be reported with TOS 8. The 8 indicator does not appear on the TOS table because its use is dependent upon the use of the appropriate modifier. (See Pub. 100-04 *Medicare Claims Processing Manual*, chapter 12, "Physician/Nonphysician Practitioner," for instructions on when assistant-at-surgery is allowable.)
- TOS H appears in the list of descriptors. However, it does not appear in the table. In CWF, "H" is used only as an indicator for hospice. The contractor should not submit TOS H to CWF at this time.
- For outpatient services, when a transfusion medicine code appears on a claim that also contains a blood product, the service is paid under reasonable charge at 80 percent; coinsurance and deductible apply. When transfusion medicine codes are paid under the clinical laboratory fee schedule they are paid at 100 percent; coinsurance and deductible do not apply.

Note: For injection codes with more than one possible TOS designation, use the following guidelines when assigning the TOS:

When the choice is L or 1:

- Use TOS L when the drug is used related to ESRD; or
- Use TOS 1 when the drug is not related to ESRD and is administered in the office.

When the choice is G or 1:

- Use TOS G when the drug is an immunosuppressive drug; or
- Use TOS 1 when the drug is used for other than immunosuppression.

When the choice is P or 1:

- Use TOS P if the drug is administered through durable medical equipment (DME); or
- Use TOS 1 if the drug is administered in the office.

The place of service or diagnosis may be considered when determining the appropriate TOS. The descriptors for each of the TOS codes listed in the annual HCPCS update are:

0	Whole blood only
1	Medical care
2	Surgery
3	Consultation
4	Diagnostic radiology
5	Diagnostic laboratory
6	Therapeutic radiology
7	Anesthesia
8	Assistant at surgery
9	Other medical items or services
A	Used durable medical equipment (DME)
D	Ambulance
E	Enteral/parenteral nutrients/supplies
F	Ambulatory surgical center (facility usage for surgical services)
G	Immunosuppressive drugs
J	Diabetic shoes
K	Hearing items and services
L	ESRD supplies
M	Monthly capitation payment for dialysis
N	Kidney donor
P	Lump sum purchase of DME, prosthetics, orthotics
Q	Vision items or services
R	Rental of DME
S	Surgical dressings or other medical supplies
T	Outpatient mental health limitation
U	Occupational therapy
V	Pneumococcal/flu vaccine
W	Physical therapy